Contents

Preface to the second edition ix

Preface to the first edition x

Acknowledgments xii

CHAPTER 1 'Be good women but do not bother with a Code of Ethics' 1

Views on bioethics and nursing practice 3

Issues and recommendations 28

CHAPTER 2 What is ethics? 34

Understanding moral language 35

What is the task of ethics? 57

CHAPTER 3 Western moral philosophy: its modes, theories and conclusions 64

Deontological theories 65

Teleological theories 83

Which theory to choose? 89

Moral principles and moral rules 90

CHAPTER 4 Feminist moral philosophy 103

Feminist moral theory 103

The contributions of women to philosophy 104

The supposed difference between male and female thinking 108

The hypothetical versus the real 115

Issues and recommendations 130

CHAPTER 5 Transcultural ethics   **139**

Culture and its relationship to ethics   **140**

The nature and implications of transcultural ethics   **143**

Issues and recommendations   **153**

CHAPTER 6 Identifying and resolving moral problems   **157**

Types of moral problems   **158**

Dealing with moral problems — a systematic approach   **182**

Dealing with moral problems — an experiential approach   **191**

Should nurses study ethics?   **196**

Issues and recommendations   **199**

CHAPTER 7 Patients' rights   **203**

The issue of patients' rights   **204**

The nursing profession's perspective   **210**

What are patients' rights?   **211**

Issues and recommendations   **261**

CHAPTER 8 The question of nurse–patient advocacy   **270**

The notion of nurse–patient advocacy   **272**

What is advocacy?   **274**

A critical examination of advocacy   **283**

Issues and recommendations   **287**

CHAPTER 9 Matters of life and death: I Abortion   **290**

Abortion — raising the issues   **291**

What is abortion?   **299**

Is abortion morally permissible?   **300**

Fetal and maternal rights   **305**

Issues and recommendations   **312**

Bioethics
a nursing perspective

To my Grandmothers and to Aunty Dora, in fond memory

You should not decide until you have
heard what both have to say.

Aristophanes, *The wasps*

Nobody is infallible; and for that reason many
different points of view are needed.

Mary Midgley, *Can't we make moral judgements?*

Bioethics
a nursing perspective

Megan-Jane Johnstone

RN, BA, PhD, FRCNA, FCN (NSW)
Faculty of Nursing
Royal Melbourne Institute of Technology, Melbourne

W. B. Saunders
Baillière Tindall

Harcourt Brace & Company
Sydney   Philadelphia   London   Toronto

174.2

Acquisitions Editor: Jeremy Fisher
Manager Editorial, Design and
Production: Rema Gnanadickam
Designer: Pamela Horsnell
Senior Production Editor: Fiona Julian

Cover and Page Design: Pamela Horsnell

W. B. Saunders/Baillière Tindall

An imprint of
Harcourt Brace & Company, Australia
30–52 Smidmore Street, Marrickville, NSW 2204

Harcourt Brace & Company
24–28 Oval Road, London NW1 7DX

Harcourt Brace & Company
Orlando, Florida 32887

Copyright © 1994, 1989
by Harcourt Brace & Company, Australia, ACN 000 910 583

National Library of Australia Cataloguing-in-Publication data

Johnstone, Megan-Jane, date.
  Bioethics.

  2nd ed.
  Includes index.
  ISBN 0 7295 1421 8.

  1. Nursing ethics. 2. Bioethics. 3. Strikes and lockouts –
  Nursing – Victoria. 4. Trade-unions – Nurses – Victoria.
  I. Title.

174.2

Edited and proofread by Janet Healey
Typeset in Bookman by Essay Composition, Alexandria, NSW
Printed in Australia by Southwood Press

CHAPTER 10   Matters of life and death: II
Euthanasia   **321**

Euthanasia and its significance for nurses   **323**

The legal status of euthanasia   **324**

What is euthanasia?   **330**

Types of euthanasia   **332**

Is euthanasia morally justified?   **333**

Issues and recommendations   **353**

CHAPTER 11   Matters of life and death: III
Suicide   **359**

Socio-cultural attitudes to suicide: a brief
historical overview   **361**

Defining suicide   **373**

Suicide: some moral considerations   **379**

Suicide prevention: some further considerations   **385**

Issues and recommendations   **385**

CHAPTER 12   Matters of life and death: IV   **391**

Quality of life   **391**

'Not For Resuscitation' (NFR) orders   **397**

Organ harvesting and transplantation   **421**

CHAPTER 13   Taking a stand   **446**

Conscientious objection   **447**

Strike action   **469**

Institutional ethics committees   **480**

CHAPTER 14   Where to from here?   **501**

Education   **502**

Research   **508**

Lobbying   **508**

Policy and law reform   **509**

Conclusion   **510**

APPENDIXES

I   Code for nurses (*International Council of Nurses*)   **515**

II   Consumer health rights   **517**

III   Code of ethics for nurses in Australia (*Australian Nursing Council*)   **520**

IV   Patients' Bill of Rights (*Australian Nursing Federation, Western Australia*)   **525**

V   Patients' Bill of Rights (*Australian Nursing Federation, Victoria*)   **528**

VI   Assuring quality care for those who are dying (*Australian Nursing Federation*)   **532**

VII   Code of ethics (*New Zealand Nurses' Association*)   **535**

VIII   Code of professional conduct (*United Kingdom Central Council for Nursing, Midwifery and Health Visiting*)   **544**

IX   American Nurses' Association Code for nurses   **547**

X   Code of ethics for nursing (*Canadian Nurses Association*)   **550**

INDEX   **561**

Preface

Second edition

THIS NEW EDITION reflects the ongoing and developing debate on bioethical issues in nursing and in health care. Discussion has been expanded on a range of topics, including the involvement of Nazi nurses in Hitler's medicalised killing program during the Second World War; media biases against reporting a nursing perspective on important ethical issues; patients' rights; competency to decide; abortion; euthanasia; 'Not For Resucitation' orders; and conscientious objection.

As well as this, due to popular request, new material has been added. Specifically, attention has been given to: the nature and function of codes of nursing ethics; the importance of transcultural ethics to and in nursing practice; the role of experience in guiding moral decision making in nursing; the ethical aspects of suicide; the problem of homophobia and the moral entitlements of patients who are AIDS/HIV positive; and the nature, development and role of distinct nursing ethics committees. The appendixes have also been expanded to include copies of the United Kingdom Central Council for Nursing, Midwifery and Health Visiting's (1992) *Code of Professional Conduct*; the American Nurses' Association's (1985) *Code for Nurses*; and the Canadian Nurses Association's (1985) *Code of ethics for nursing*.

Both the formal and informal feedback I have received about the first edition has indicated that nurses reading this text have found it useful, informative, realistic, practical and thought provoking. Many have also commented that the text 'put into words what they had been feeling for years, but felt too afraid to speak out about'. I hope that this new edition will succeed doubly in its achievements to date, and will contribute further to nurses finding their own inner strength and courage to 'speak for themselves' and to 'make visible their own experiences', and, in so doing, taking a firm step forward towards challenging the status quo.

First edition

THIS BOOK IS UNIQUE in both its content and its conviction. It raises issues that have not been comprehensively addressed before in nursing texts of this kind, and offers a broad theoretical basis upon which these issues can be examined critically.

Public and professional debates on bioethical issues are flourishing. These debates have prompted major policy and law reforms on issues ranging from reproductive technology, abortion, and the care and treatment of defective newborns through to organ transplantation, the right to refuse orthodox medical treatment, the allocation of scarce health care resources, and many more. The outcomes and implications of these debates and the resulting policy and law reforms have yet to be fully realised, however, and there is room for concern about whether bioethics will bring about the beneficial changes in health care domains that are hoped for.

Regardless of the outcomes of past and current bioethical debates, it is clear that bioethics, as we know it, has serious implications not only for nursing practice (and, of course, its concomitants nursing education, administration and nursing research), but also for nursing theory. In light of this, it is probably true that bioethics is singularly one of the most important issues facing the nursing profession at this time — and one which nurses both individually and collectively cannot afford to ignore.

The nursing profession has a great deal to contribute to the bioethics debate; and the bioethics debate has a great deal to gain by including a nursing perspective. Unfortunately, however, these two obvious points are not always fully appreciated by those advancing bioethics and its associated activities. The media, for example, consistently neglects to include a meaningful nursing perspective on the many bioethical issues it covers. As well, the organisers of so-called interdisciplinary bioethics conferences either do not invite nurses to speak at all, or invite them to perform only a 'token role', such as chairing a session or concluding the conference (neither of which facilitates the input of a substantive nursing view).

There is an important lesson to be learned from this, notably, that the outcome of the bioethics debate will depend very much not only on its content (that is, the issues chosen), but also on who leads it, who contributes to it, and more importantly, how widely it is conducted. Unless this lesson is heeded, there will remain the ever-present danger of bioethics being converted into an unscrupulous power struggle among rival factions of society's elite (including, among others, eminent philosophers, lawyers, doctors and theologians), rather than being a humanistic campaign intent on improving human welfare.

This book does not promise concrete answers to complex problems — no book on bioethics could make such a promise! Neither does it promise to offer a panacea for all the difficulties that nurses are currently facing in this area. What this book does aim to do, however, is first to show that bioethics is an important and legitimate nursing concern. It will also attempt to show that if nurses are to make a worthwhile contribution to the bioethics debate, they need to have at least a working knowledge of what it is about, who is controlling it, who is contributing to it, and what its outcomes are likely to be. It is the contention of this book that, unless nurses have a working knowledge of these issues, and can actively respond to them, they may find themselves in the intolerable position of having to comply with questionable standards of behaviour imposed on them by others, thereby further constraining their attempts to deliver morally responsible and accountable nursing care.

Second, this book aims to show that a nursing perspective has much to contribute to bioethics generally — not only in terms of generating issues for debate, but also in terms of generating a more substantive and cohesive ethical theory, and thus one which can be reliably applied in actual 'flesh and blood' situations. It is hoped that in this way the nursing perspective will become something to be sought after and respected, rather than something to be feared or ignored.

Third, this book aims to provide nurses with a text that will both stimulate their own critical thinking on bioethical issues as these particularly relate to nursing practice, and offer them reliable guidance on how best to decide when dealing with morally troubling situations in nursing practice.

Last, this book represents, for me, the fulfilment of the many pledges I have made (to both patients and colleagues) that one day I would do something about the many injustices personally witnessed during the course of my nursing career. On account of this, *Bioethics: a nursing perspective* is a very personal book. Nevertheless, I hope it accurately reflects the needs of my nursing colleagues and responds to those needs in an honest, meaningful, useful and reliable way. I also hope that this book will contribute in a major way to the community's as well as to allied health professional groups' understanding of the moral nature of nursing and why a nursing perspective on bioethics is both desirable and necessary. More importantly, I hope this book will stimulate reform in the health care arena and will contribute to the realisation of a morally tolerable clinical reality for both patients and health professionals.

Acknowledgments

THE WRITING AND REVISION of this text would not have been possible without the stalwart support of several of my friends and colleagues. My deepest gratitude goes to my colleague and friend, Olga Kanitsaki, of La Trobe University, who read large portions of the original and revised manuscript and made many helpful suggestions. I am particularly indebted to Olga for sharing her views on the fundamental relationship between culture and ethics, and on the important role culture plays in shaping and mediating our ethical thinking and conduct. The final text is, however, entirely my own, as are any weaknesses, omissions or mistakes.

A debt of gratitude is also due to my close friends in New Zealand — both of whom have always taken a keen and supporting interest in my work: Dr Bill McArthur, who tirelessly collected newspaper clippings and kept me informed of the proceedings of the New Zealand Cervical Cancer Inquiry in 1988; and Elaine Henry, who also kept me informed of the proceedings and findings of the inquiry.

I am grateful, too, for the professional support and encouragement of Pam Ryan and June Cochrane (formerly of the Royal College of Nursing, Australia), and of Valda Hext (formerly of the Phillip Institute of Technology); and I am very appreciative of the many helpful 'corridor conversations' with my colleagues in the Faculty of Nursing at the Royal Melbourne Institute of Technology: Carol Jackson, Rhonda Goodwin, Cally Berryman, Chris Poole, Tony Welch, Judy Gillette, and Karen Nightingale.

Special thanks are particularly due to the many people (nurses, counsellors, patients/clients, students, and others) whose generosity in sharing their experiences and views has, in many ways, made writing and revising this text possible. I especially want to thank Naomi Halpern for sharing her insights on the nature of psychogenic suffering and the influential role it plays in shaping our perceptions of 'a life worth living', and what can be done to alleviate this suffering. And I wish to acknowledge Ekura Emery's helpful comments on the case discussed in this text involving a young Maori woman who gave birth prematurely to a 20-week-old fetus.

These acknowledgments would not be complete without thanks being given to the team at Harcourt Brace & Company for their contribution to the successful production of this text: Jeremy Fisher, Janet Healey, Pamela Horsnell and Fiona Julian. Acknowledgment and thanks are also due to Jenny Curtis, Chris Fox and Carol Natsis for their work on the first edition.

Finally, thanks are due to the Executive Director of the International Council of Nurses, Constance Holleran, for her prompt replies to my letters seeking information on the activities of Nazi nurses, and for being instrumental in locating the work of the German nurse historian Hilde Steppe. I also wish to acknowledge the assistance of the staff of the National Archives, Washington DC, the National Library of Australia, the International Red Cross, Geneva, the United Nations Information Centre, and the United Nations in sending me what little information they could concerning the involvement of nurses in Nazi war crimes.

Chapter

1

'Be good women but do not bother with a Code of Ethics'

ONE OF THE EARLIEST ADVOCATES of a code of ethics for nurses in America was advised by a physician: 'Be good women but do not bother with a Code of Ethics' (Dock 1900, p. 37). Fortunately, not only have nurses ignored this advice but, since 1973, they have adopted an international code of ethics that recognises and explicates the nurse's independent responsibility and account-ability for nursing care. Statements that once 'abrogated the nurse's judgment and personal responsibility and showed dependency on physicians' (Kelly 1985, p. 207) were, in 1973, deleted once and for all from nursing codes of conduct around the world, and thus from nursing philosophy. A more significant achievement, however, has been the development of nursing ethics as a distinctive disciplinary area in its own right, as evidenced, among other things, by the proliferation of nursing research and scholarship in this area; by the organisation of conferences, seminars and courses on nursing ethics; and, not least, by the increasing number of nurses who are engaging in the political act of *naming* this new disciplinary area by identifying themselves as *nurse ethicists* (as opposed, for instance, to calling themselves bioethicists or medical ethicists or health care ethicists).

Despite this profound philosophical and intellectual shift in nursing thought, little progress has been made. Even today, in this new era of intensive and supposedly enlightened bioethical debate, morally condescending attitudes towards nurses continue to prevail. Nurses are still expected to be merely 'good women' and, more than ever, it seems, are not expected to have a code of ethics — or, if they do, not to take it too seriously. Nurses are certainly not expected to have a substantive moral position on anything significant, and are most certainly not expected to express a view publicly. Those who do risk being either reprimanded or ridiculed, as examples given later in this text show.

1

Difficult as it may be to believe, there are people in positions of power who trivialise, seek to invalidate, and even actively oppose, the involvement of nurses in the public and professional debate on bioethical issues in health care. Evidence of this is both compelling and thought provoking; at a deeper level it is also shocking and extremely frustrating. For example, some doctors apparently believe that nurses are incapable of sound rational thought or of grasping the essence of sound moral thinking. These doctors are reluctant to accept that nurses have any independent moral responsibility when caring for patients. As these doctors are almost always in positions of power, they are more than able to ensure that a nursing perspective on patient care, and on related moral issues, is effectively constrained.

Doctors are by no means the only ones obstructing a nursing perspective on bioethics. The media (with some notable exceptions involving sympathetic radio commentators and journalists) have also effectively obstructed a credible nursing view on the numerous bioethical issues reported over the past few years. In many respects, the nursing profession today is just as much at the mercy of unscrupulous lay editors as it was in the late 1800s and early 1900s. From the 1890s, the press succeeded in obstructing the professional development of nursing for almost thirty years until, in 1923, the International Council of Nurses (ICN) finally established an international nursing journal, to be controlled by nurses and to reflect nursing opinion and nursing issues (Bridges 1968, p. 10). At the 1923 ICN Executive Committee meeting, at which the proposal to establish an international nursing journal was originally discussed, one of the delegates gave a solemn warning that reports in the lay press were a 'very serious peril to personal and professional liberty' (Bridges 1968, p. 10). Her warning is as pertinent today as it was in 1923, as will be shown shortly.

The courts have also sometimes been unsupportive of the plight of nurses and the considerable difficulties they face in trying to deliver morally responsible and accountable nursing care. Notable legal cases, both in Australia and overseas, have made it abundantly clear that nurses are bound to follow the lawful and reasonable orders of a superior on the one hand, and yet paradoxically are also bound to be independently accountable for their own actions on the other (Johnstone 1994; Sanders 1988). The courts have continued to find in favour of employer hospitals who have dismissed nurses for conscientiously refusing to participate in morally controversial medical procedures. In one notable case, a court even rejected the authority of the local nursing profession's formally adopted code of ethical conduct (Johnstone 1988a). On matters relating to morally responsible nursing practice, evidence suggests that the courts are not only frequently unsympathetic; they have even been a major factor in ensuring that the moral autonomy of nurses and the authority of professional nursing ethics have not achieved either the legal, social or cultural legitimation they deserve (Johnstone 1994).

These claims, of course, warrant some substantiation for at least two reasons. First, substantiation will counteract any accusations that the approach taken here reeks of professional neurosis or hysteria or, more simply, is misguided. Second, substantiation will clarify the social and political context in which nursing is operating and, by virtue of the practical realities and moral implications of this context, will highlight why a special 'nursing perspective' on bioethics is needed. It is to substantiating these comments, and giving concrete examples illustrating the extent to which nurses have been obstructed in contributing to the bioethics debate, that this chapter now turns.

Views on bioethics and nursing practice

A medical perspective

In 1986, a class of registered nurses undertaking a postgraduate diploma course in health administration attended a lecture on ethical issues in professional functioning. The lecturer (a medical doctor) told his audience, some of whom were senior nurse administrators, that 'nurses [were] unable to understand the intellectual concept of ethical models'. His reasoning seemed to be that nurses were 'too simplistic and practical, not generally capable of the objective, abstract thought that is required for this type of [ethical] decision' (*Report of the Study of Professional Issues in Nursing* 1988, p. 165). The lecturer is also alleged to have discouraged those present from attending a session on ethical decision making that was planned for a neurosurgical conference later that year.

The attitude of this lecturer is by no means unique. Anecdotal evidence abounds worldwide on how nurses are continually told by doctors that nursing practice is devoid of any sort of moral complication, and that it is nonsense for nurses to assume that they have any independent moral responsibilities when caring for patients. Examples from the literature also offer compelling evidence. For instance, Yarling and McElmurry (1986) cite the case of an American physician who objected strongly to the suggestion that nurses have a moral duty, even though an attending physician has expressly ordered that no information be given out, to disclose information to terminally ill patients who request it. Medical students present at the time were unanimous in suggesting that 'the nurse had a moral duty to disclose and that the physician's order was unjustifiable' (Yarling and McElmurry 1986, pp. 65–6).

When one of the medical students asked the physician why he disagreed with their view, the physician replied that 'the nurse's relationship with the patient is different than the physician's. It does not require independent moral judgment by the nurse' (Yarling and McElmurry 1986, p. 66). Another example of this kind of attitude can be found among some English physicians who participated in a survey investigating physician opinion on the nurse's duty to tell the truth to questioning patients. Of the nineteen doctors surveyed, most believed that nurses should avoid giving patients precise information in response to queries about their (the patients') health problems (*Nursing Times*, 11 July 1990, p. 9). Significantly, three doctors asserted that 'nurses should lie to patients if they were put on the spot by a direct question' (*Nursing Times*, 11 July 1990, p. 9). Like their American colleagues referred to above, it would seem that these English physicians do not recognise — or at least are reluctant to recognise — the moral nature of the nurse–patient relationship, or to concede that nurses have any independent moral (or professional) responsibilities to their patients (Johnstone 1994).

The perception that nurses are not required to make independent moral judgments is not as uncommon as some would like to believe. Clay (1987), for example, writes:

> Many assume that because it is the doctors who decide when to turn off the ventilator, the lawyers who pronounce on issues such as surrogacy, the scientists who play around with *in vitro* fertilisation, and the managers and politicians who decide where limited health resources are put, then the nurses have no separate responsibilities. And there is a supposedly sympathetic way of thinking that wants to keep nurses out of all this intellectual and moral agonising.
>
> (Clay 1987, pp. 39–40)

Regardless of their popularity among those who choose to hold them, these views — that nursing practice is devoid of moral complication, that it is nonsense for nurses to presume they have any independent moral responsibilities when caring for patients, and that nurses are not required to make independent moral judgments in the nurse–patient relationship — are quite misleading and incorrect. Examples are given in the following chapters to illustrate clearly that nurses are just as much 'responders who encounter the claims of others' (in this instance, patients) as are doctors and other allied health professionals, and are just as stringently bound by moral considerations when responding to these claims (Beauchamp and Childress 1989; Johnstone 1987, pp. 31–2). Arguments are also given to show conclusively that nurses have as much independent moral responsibility for their actions (and omissions) as they have independent legal responsibility, and are just as accountable for their practice morally as they are legally. It is the contention of this book that to regard nurses as 'moral morons' (or even moral automata under the control of doctors and employers and the courts) is naive and possibly subversive. Nurses must be permitted to fulfil their very real moral responsibilities when delivering nursing care. It needs to be recognised that nurses' legal responsibilities when caring for patients are also very real. Nurses cannot be expected to ignore or violate these responsibilities.

A media perspective

Members of the medical profession are not alone in their view that nurses have no independent moral concerns regarding bioethical issues. The media, it seems (with some honourable exceptions), share this view, as revealed by a rough analysis of newspaper articles appearing in a major Melbourne newspaper during a ten-week period in 1988. Between 14 March 1988 and 20 May 1988, *The Age* featured over 38 main articles, 37 'Letters to the Editor', and over 52 'Access Age' comments on bioethical issues — mostly in relation to the Right to Die with Dignity movement and the Victorian State Government's then controversial Medical Treatment Bill (since proclaimed as the *Medical Treatment Act* 1988). These articles, letters and comments featured the views of doctors, lawyers, philosophers, theologians, sociologists — even groups such as the Right to Life movement — and, not least, the public at large (Johnstone 1988b, p. 8).

Superficially, it appears that the media in this instance made a stringent effort to present a balanced view on the issues under discussion. On closer inspection, however, it is clear that quite the reverse is true. For example, of the 127 or so items published, none (with the exception of a short 52-word 'Access Age' comment) seriously attempts to represent the views of nurses; yet nurses comprise the largest single body of health providers in the health care system. The term 'nurse' has generally been used (particularly by television media) in relation to the 'emotional' aspect of the moral dilemma or problem being discussed rather than the intellectual or rational aspect. In some instances, the term 'nurse' has been loosely used in relation to the 'team' that is caring for a given patient — with acknowledgment being given more as a token gesture than as a serious recognition of the troubling dilemmas that nurses face in professional health care practice. In the 52-word comment that did appear, the author referred to an AIDS update article that had been recently printed in *The Age* and criticised the article for its 'glaring omission' of the contribution made by nurses in caring for AIDS patients (Mathews 1988, p. 12).

Editorial bias can also be found in individual newspaper reports and articles. For example, in an interesting newspaper article by Michael Pirrie (1987, p. 11), headed 'A disabled baby's right to live', the nursing perspective on the ethical issues under discussion was once again ignored. An analysis of the key terms used in this article is revealing: for example, the terms 'doctor', 'medical profession' and 'medical staff' are collectively mentioned at least fourteen times; the terms 'parents', 'family members', 'grandparents' and 'mother' are collectively mentioned at least eleven times; the terms 'medical treatment', 'treatment', 'medical care', 'medical practice', 'medical decisions' and 'medical technology' are collectively mentioned at least nine times; and the terms 'lawyers', 'judges' and 'the courts' are collectively mentioned at least three times. The term 'nurse', surprisingly, is mentioned only once, and the term 'nursing care' is not mentioned at all. The omission is extraordinary, given that nurses are involved twenty-four hours a day in caring for severely disabled newborns, and are inevitably concerned with the many moral problems that arise in this area.

In the same article, the views of five medical doctors, two judges, one other legal source, one philosopher and one sociologist are quoted. No parents or nurses are quoted.

The article also reported on a recommendation to set up a State advisory committee:

> to set broad guidelines for those involved in caring for deformed babies, as well as to review difficult cases to be certain that the interests of the infant, as well as parents and medical staff are given proper weight.
>
> (Pirrie 1987, p. 11)

On the basis of this newspaper report, readers might well assume that nurses have no moral interests at stake in dilemmatic situations involving the care and treatment of disabled newborns, let alone an active care role. Such thinking would be quite mistaken; in these and similar situations, nurses do have significant moral interests at stake — interests that are just as deserving of protection as are the interests of babies, parents and medical staff (Johnstone 1988c).

In fairness to *The Age*, it has reported on papers given by nurses at nursing ethics conferences, although not without constraint. A comprehensive report written by Ingrid Svendsen (1987) on two papers presented at a nursing ethics conference held at Monash University entitled 'The role of the nurse: doctors' handmaiden, patients' advocate or what?' was relegated to page 21 of the paper.

Almost a year later, a well written and accurate report by Peter Schumpeter (1988) on a controversial paper on Not For Resuscitation orders presented at another nursing ethics conference was printed in *The Age,* but in the first edition only, and again on page 21. It is significant that the first edition generally goes to country areas only; copies are not generally kept on file. Only copies of the second or later editions are kept, which effectively means that the report has been lost to history. Another report, written by Philip McIntosh (1988), one of *The Age's* medical reporters, featured a very controversial paper presented by a nurse at the second South-East Asian Regional Nurses Conference at Dallas Brooks Hall on 12 May 1988. Interestingly, the report was not published in *The Age,* as might be expected, but in the *Australian Dr Weekly* — complete with a major front-page headline and photograph!

Significantly, the past decade has seen little change in media attitudes and biases against representing a substantive nursing perspective on important and controversial bioethical issues. An instructive example of this can be found in the media coverage given to a survey conducted by Kuhse and Singer (1992) exploring nurses' attitudes and practices in regard to euthanasia. In an unusual and extraordinary act of attentiveness, both the electronic and print media reported widely on the survey results, which were published initially in the *Australian Nurses Journal.* What made this particular instance of media attention so unusual is that, in the past, the media have demonstrated a great antipathy towards reporting on issues of specific concern and importance to the nursing profession. Even now, it is most unusual for the media to report on an article published in the *Australian Nurses Journal* and, what is more, to give it front-page headlines (see, for example, Magazanik 1992a, p. 1). Why then were nurses around the State not 'jumping for joy' at this unprecedented media attention?

The short answer is that, as in the past, the media fell far short of representing a realistic or complete nursing perspective on the issue being debated, and, as in the past, ended up marginalising rather than according authority to a nursing point of view. Further, at the time, many nurses felt that, whatever else the media debate was being motivated by, it was not a genuine concern for exploring and making public the many problems nurses have to deal with when caring for people who might otherwise be considered candidates for euthanasia. They even believed that the nursing profession was being used to further the ends of the pro-euthanasia lobby. Some nurses also regarded the media coverage of the survey as being grossly irresponsible on account of its failure to take into consideration public perceptions of, and the realities of, the role of nurses in pain assessment and management. What is not widely known is that the media coverage given to the euthanasia survey caused some patients considerable anxiety about whether or not to trust their nurses, and even, in some instances, resulted in patients refusing responsibly prescribed and needed narcotic analgesia which would otherwise have been administered by their attending nurses. This, in turn, caused the nurses involved to suffer considerable and unnecessary distress. Other nurses were just plain angry, and responded by arguing that the original survey, which involved the views of just 943 nurses (just over 1 per cent of nurses holding practising certificates in Victoria), was not representative of the 82 280 nurses who held practising certificates in Victoria, and therefore could not be relied on (see, for example, Cotterhill 1992, p. 4; Millership 1992, p. 4; Monkivitch 1992, p. 12; Muirden et al. 1992, p. 12; O'Connor 1992, p. 4).

In several respects, the nurses' anger and concerns were justified. Consider the following: on 2 March 1992, *The Age* carried the front-page headline: 'Nurses back euthanasia, survey finds' (Magazanik 1992a, p. 1); on the same day, the *Herald-Sun* carried the more provocative headline **'NURSES ADMIT DEATH ROLE'** (p. 3). The next day, 3 March, the *Herald-Sun* carried another provocative headline: 'Nurses death aid "no shock"' (Gartland 1992, p. 5); *The Age*, meanwhile, carried the more subdued headline: 'Nurses in call for euthanasia inquiry' (Bock 1992, p. 6). On 4 March 1992, *The Age* carried another article headed 'When death is part of the quality of life', in which the views of four experienced nurses were reported in an informative and thought-provoking manner (Magazanik 1992b, p. 3). As the days passed, however, the nursing voice and perspective paled into insignificance as others with 'more authority' added their voices to the growing media debate on the nature of euthanasia, the circumstances in which it should or should not be permitted, and the need for the law to reflect community opinion on the matter. Significantly, most of these others (doctors, lawyers, politicians, philosophers, clergymen, and members of the Right to Life movement) all failed to place their comments in the context of nursing care, and, more specifically, failed to identify and address the very real problem of the unfair burden that nurses often have to carry when caring for people who are living lives characterised by intolerable suffering, or who are dying, or both (*The Age*, 5 March 1992, p. 3; Magazanik 1992c, 1992d, 1992e; Tighe 1992, p. 10; Syme 1992, p. 10; Briggs and McDonald 1992, p. 12; Skene 1992).

A good example of the extent to which the plight of nurses was overlooked in the media coverage of the survey can be found in the reported comments of Loane Skene, who was at that time the principal research officer of the now disbanded Victorian Law Reform Commission. Commenting on the need for law reform with regard to euthanasia and severely disabled newborns, Skene is reported to have said that 'doctors justifiably felt uncertain about their legal position when treating critically ill babies', and that:

there are lots of cases where doctors are required to do something that contravenes the letter of the law and there is a real risk that doctors might be charged with criminal offences for making those decisions.

(reported by Magazanik 1992e, p. 5)

Although nurses also harbour uncertainties about their legal position when caring for critically ill babies (and, it should be added, adults), and although there are many instances in which nurses are required (often by doctors) to do something that 'contravenes the letter of the law' (unconsented 'Not For Resuscitation' [NFR] orders being a case in point), no mention was made of this in the media reports covering Skene's comments. Further, although nurses are intimately involved in the care and treatment of sick babies, no nurse was quoted in the report; the views of a director of neonatology, the health minister, the president of the Victorian branch of the AMA, and the president of the Right to Life movement were, however, all quoted (Magazanik 1992e, p. 5). The initial media reports on the euthanasia issue began with nurses, but it was as though suddenly nurses no longer existed.

An important implication of nurses not being represented accurately or fairly, or being given a low media profile in bioethical debates, is, arguably, that it makes it easier for those in positions of power — and even for the community at large — to ignore the enormous moral burdens that nurses often face in health care domains. It may make it easier for those outside nursing to maintain and enforce the expectation that nurses will not question the morally troubling reality around them, nor speak out against any injustices and moral violations they witness. In short, it makes it easier to maintain the popular image of nurses as merely 'good women' who do not — and thus should not — have a code of ethics, much less a substantive moral position on bioethical issues.

A conference organiser's perspective

Until relatively recently, a nursing perspective was largely ignored by the organisers of 'interdisciplinary' bioethics conferences. If it was included, it was usually scheduled in an insignificant slot on the program. For example, at a 1987 conference on AIDS run by the Monash University Centre for Human Bioethics, the nurse speakers were programmed last, making it very difficult for them to make any sort of impact at the end of a very demanding day (Centre for Human Bioethics 1986).

The Centre for Human Bioethics 1988 conference on institutional ethics committees also did not provide for a substantive nursing perspective to be given, despite the obvious interest that the nursing profession has in the setting up and functioning of institutional ethics committees. A nurse did appear on the program, but her role amounted to nothing more than closing the conference. The Centre for Human Bioethics, however, has been very supportive of nurses exploring the issue of bioethics in relation to nursing practice. In fact, in 1987 the centre organised one of the first serious conferences in Victoria on ethical issues in nursing: 'The role of the nurse: doctors' handmaiden, patients' advocate, or what?' (Centre for Human Bioethics 1987a).

Another example of the extent to which the nursing perspective has been neglected in interdisciplinary bioethics conferences can be found in the program of the inaugural meeting of the Australian Summer School of Medicine, Science and Humanities (December 1988). The school chose as its theme 'Current topics in medical ethics', and focused on such topics as Not For Resuscitation orders, AIDS, clinical trials, and transplant surgery. (Why the notion of *medical ethics* rather than *bioethics* was used is a question worth considering.) Of the twenty or so panellists scheduled to participate in the school's inaugural program, only three were women and only two were nurses, both males. At least twelve were male medical doctors. In the light of these statistics, it is clear that the representation of doctors and nurses on the program was unbalanced. The faculty itself included a human rights commissioner, a professor of law and two doctors.

Although considerable progress has been made in regard to this issue, and nurses are now featuring more equitably on interdisciplinary bioethics conference programs in Australia, the views of philosophers, lawyers and doctors of medicine still tend to dominate, and still tend to be regarded as more authoritative than the views of nurses. An example of this can be found in the case of an interdisciplinary bioethics seminar held in 1991, at which a medical doctor, who was programmed to speak after an invited guest nurse speaker on the program, began his paper with these words: 'We all know Ms X [the guest nurse speaker] means well, but ...'. He then proceeded to denigrate and totally undermine a nursing perspective on the issue being addressed, which was 'The ethics and legal problems in resuscitation'. He concluded that resuscitation — and in particular the issue of 'Not For Resuscitation (NFR) — was a purely *medical* matter, and hence had 'absolutely nothing to do with ethics', or, indeed, with nurses (Johnstone 1994, pp. 258–9).

A legal perspective

The respect, or lack of it, paid by courts of law to nurses who have taken a strong moral stand on a matter involving their own individual nursing practice is an area worthy of some consideration.

One compelling example of how unsympathetic the courts can be to nurses who have been caught up in a morally troubling situation is the case of *Warthen v. Toms River Community Memorial Hospital* (1985).

This case involved a registered nurse who was dismissed from her employing hospital of eleven years for refusing to dialyse a terminally ill bilateral amputee patient. Warthen's refusal in this instance was based on what she cited as '"moral, medical and philosophical objections" to performing this procedure on the patient because the patient was terminally ill and ... the procedure was causing the patient additional complications' (*Warthen v. Toms River Community Memorial Hospital* 1985, p. 205).

Warthen had apparently dialysed the patient on two previous occasions. In both instances, however, the dialysis procedure had to be stopped because the patient suffered severe internal bleeding and cardiac arrest (*Warthen v. Toms River Community Memorial Hospital* 1985, p. 230). It was the complications of severe internal bleeding and cardiac arrest that she was referring to in her refusal. Her dismissal came when she refused to dialyse the patient for a third time.

Believing she had been wrongfully and unfairly dismissed, Warthen took her case to the Supreme Court, where she argued in her defence that the Code for Nurses of the American Nurses' Association (ANA) justified her refusal, since it essentially permitted nurses to refuse to participate in procedures to which they were personally opposed (Blum 1984, p. 50; *Warthen v. Toms River Community Memorial Hospital* 1985, p. 229).

The court did not find in her favour, however, and she lost her case. In making its final decision, the court made clear its position on a number of key points, three of which are relevant to this discussion.

1. An employee should not have the right to prevent his or her employer from pursuing its business because the employee perceives that a particular business decision violates the employee's personal morals, as distinguished from the recognized code of ethics of the employee's profession ... (p. 233).

2. [In support of the hospital's defence] it would be a virtual impossibility to administer a hospital if each nurse or member of the administration staff refused to carry out his or her duties based upon a personal private belief concerning the right to live ... (p. 234).

3. The position asserted by the plaintiff serves only the individual and the nurses' profession while leaving the public to wonder when and whether they will receive nursing care ... (p. 234).

(*Warthen v. Toms River Community Memorial Hospital* 1985)

There can be small doubt, given these comments, that the court had little regard for the nurse's conscientious objection to the tasks she was being compelled to perform. And there can also be little doubt that the court, in dismissing altogether the ANA Code for Nurses as an authoritative statement of public policy, had poor regard for the nursing profession's position on conscientious objection generally (Johnstone 1994, pp.251–67, 1988a).

In the past, nurses were frequently subjected to 'fair' dismissals on account of their refusing to participate in abortion and sterilisation procedures (Thompson and Thompson 1981; Muyskens 1982; Davis and Aroskar 1983; Clay 1987). Fortunately, however, this situation has changed markedly over the past twenty years; for the most part, American and English nurses are now legally permitted conscientiously to refuse in non-emergency situations to participate in abortion and sterilisation procedures. The difficulty remains, nevertheless, that while these nurses are legally permitted conscientiously to refuse to participate in abortion procedures, they are still not wholly permitted conscientiously to refuse to participate in other medical procedures that are morally contentious (not least the use and withdrawal of life-sustaining treatment, as occurred in the *Warthen* case). The difficulties faced by Australian nurses in this respect were highlighted in a recent front-page Melbourne newspaper article, in which it was claimed that nurses who are 'worried about the ethics of medical procedures such as organ transplants and abortions are facing the sack if they refuse to take part' (Miller 1988, p. 1). In another case, a New South Wales midwife was refused employment after she indicated to her prospective employer that she was conscientiously opposed to participating in abortion and sterilisation procedures because of her religious beliefs (Broekhuijse 1988, p. 13).

Unfortunately, there is a paucity of Australian and New Zealand legal examples of the kinds of difficulties that nurses might face in this area. Nevertheless, there is room to speculate that the attitude of Australian courts in regard to the legitimacy and status of professional nursing ethics, and the moral authority of nurses generally to question morally problematic medical or hospital practices, would probably be similar to that expressed in the *Warthen* case. Since this is a lengthy issue in its own right, and one which I have considered elsewhere (Johnstone 1994, pp.251–67), I shall say nothing further about it here.

A perspective from a National Commission of Inquiry

In 1987 New Zealand witnessed a national inquiry into what has become popularly referred to as the '"unfortunate experiment" at the National Women's Hospital'. The details of this inquiry and the 'unfortunate experiment' in question are well documented in the

Report of the Cervical Cancer Inquiry (prepared by the Committee of Inquiry into Allegations Concerning the Treatment of Cervical Cancer at National Women's Hospital and into Other Related Matters 1988), and in Sandra Coney's book *The unfortunate experiment* (1988). Nevertheless, there are aspects of this inquiry that are highly pertinent to our discussion here, and that are therefore worth considering at length.

The 'unfortunate experiment' began in 1958, under the direction of four National Women's Hospital doctors — one of whom, Dr Herbert Green, had once been described as 'one of the 25 outstanding physicians in the world' (Johns 1988, p. 9). The experiment, involving 948 women, sought to examine the invasive potential of carcinoma *in situ* (CIS) of the cervix. The experiment reached the public's attention when, in 1987, *Metro* magazine published an article by Sandra Coney and Phillida Bunkle in which allegations were made that not only had women with CIS been used as *unconsenting* subjects in a medical experiment, but also that, as a result of being a part of this experiment, some of these women had not had their condition adequately treated (claims which were to be fully vindicated by the inquiry's findings).

Initially, according to Coney, the article caused 'virtually no reaction', and both she and her co-author feared that the 'unfortunate experiment' had once again 'dropped into a hole' (Coney 1988, p. 71). The media would not take up the issue. One radio reporter stated that legal advice had been received to the effect 'if it was anything to do with doctors to keep away from it', while another newspaper reporter was told by the editor that it was 'too dangerous' (Coney 1988, p. 71). On top of this, as Coney wrote:

> No women's groups commented. Civil liberty groups were silent. Some individuals in the Cancer Society were supportive, but the society's executive contained a large number of doctors and they weren't sure they wanted to get involved. There was no one to quote.
>
> (Coney 1988, p. 72)

As a result of the efforts of some individual newspaper journalists and radio commentators, the information gradually filtered through to the public arena, and on 5 June 1987 the then Prime Minister of New Zealand, David Lange, announced that there would be a 'very rapid inquiry' (Coney 1988, p. 74). This 'rapid inquiry' was eventually to see the documentation of over two million sheets of evidence (*New Zealand Herald* 1988b).

As the inquiry got under way, the magnitude of what had happened began to be realised. It was not long before the public came fully to appreciate the extent to which the hospital and, more particularly, the doctors involved, had failed the women who had been unwitting participants in the 'unfortunate experiment' (*Report of the Cervical Cancer Inquiry* 1988, pp. 101, 210). The public also came to appreciate that not only had these women suffered unnecessarily but, in some cases, had also died unnecessarily, as was made evident by the inquiry's findings.

The 948 women used in the 'unfortunate experiment' had been divided into two groups. Those in group one (817 women) received treatment, while those in group two (131 women) received only 'limited' or no treatment. The outcome was that those in group two developed invasive carcinoma at the rate of 22 per cent, compared with only 1.5 per cent in group one, and had a mortality rate of 6 per cent, 5.5 per cent higher than that of group one (*Report of the Cervical Cancer Inquiry* 1988, p. 57; Coney 1988, pp. 14–15). Media reports also claimed that some women experienced as many as sixty hospital admissions and over fifty vaginal examinations — but received no treatment. As a *New Zealand Herald* article (1987a) reports, the women 'got more and more diagnoses but not always treatment, or treatment was left too late'.

As the inquiry progressed, the media began to reveal the disturbing details of other morally questionable medical practices that had been allowed to continue, unchecked, over the past twenty or so years. The *Waikato Times* (1987a), for example, revealed that '… the decision whether a patient received surgery or deep X-ray treatment in addition to radium was decided by the random process of tossing a coin'.

Two months later, the *New Zealand Herald* (1987b, p. 14) revealed that over 2200 newborn baby girls had been subjected to vaginal swabs at the National Women's Hospital without parental consent. It was also alleged that over two hundred fetal cervixes were collected from stillborn baby girls for histological studies — again without parental consent. One researcher is reported to have said that the samples were collected with 'a minimum of fuss and a maximum of discretion, but not with the knowledge of the mothers' (*New Zealand Herald* 1987e). It was also alleged that there was never any intention to get parental consent.

In the *Report of the Cervical Cancer Inquiry* it was later confirmed that not only had these babies been subjected to vaginal swabbing but that the swabbing had been done in vain. Judge Cartwright, the commissioner of the inquiry, explained that Dr Green, the chief researcher, had:

> lost interest in this trial after 200 babies had had smears taken. Unfortunately this decision not to continue the trial was not communicated to the nursing staff and the trial continued until smears had been taken from 2244 new-born babies.

... there was no system in place that ensured that the trial stopped ... an effective system for monitoring research and ensuring that unnecessary procedures are not conducted, should have been in place. If this had been so, then more than 2000 babies would not have been subjected to a useless and possibly damaging procedure.

(Report of the Cervical Cancer Inquiry 1988, p. 141*)

Most of the swabs were taken from newborn babies of Maori and Pacific Island women, as well as from unmarried mothers — in short, women who were least likely to be able to stand up for themselves (Coney 1988, p. 217). One nurse witness made the further claim that the 'babies of private patients were not swabbed', but that claim was contradicted by another witness (Coney 1988, p. 213).

Nurses, it seems, were actively involved in performing the swabbings. It is alleged that if mothers asked questions about the 'test', nurses would 'explain the test ... and reassure them' (Coney 1988, p. 213). Interestingly, none of the nurses involved gave evidence publicly, making it very difficult for the issue of informed consent to research to be discussed in full (Coney 1988, p. 213). Furthermore, one medical witness, Professor Dennis Bonham, allegedly attempted to discredit the evidence of a nurse witness on the overall matter by commenting that 'the remarks were out of character for the nurse concerned' (New Zealand Herald 1988a).

In the same inquiry, it was revealed that groups of medical students had been performing, and were still performing, vaginal examinations on anaesthetised women without consent. The National Women's Hospital was also alleged to have been allowing anaesthetised and unconsenting women to have intrauterine devices (IUDs) inserted and withdrawn, first by the duty surgeon as a demonstration, and then by attending postgraduate course doctors seeking educational experience (Report of the Cervical Cancer Inquiry 1988, pp. 190–1; Coney 1988, pp. 207–8). These examinations (also exposed in Australia at about the same time) were alleged to have been performed for over twenty years. Medical professors sought to justify this 'penetration without consent' (or 'rape' or 'indecent assault', as it is referred to in some circles) by arguing that 'in a teaching hospital the patients' rights had to be balanced against the need to teach' (Waikato Times 1987b). Other medical authorities claimed that women gave 'implied consent' to pelvic examination by medical students simply by attending a teaching hospital (Roberts 1987). At the inquiry, however, the practice was defended on the grounds that 'to teach a student with

---

* Quotations from this report are reprinted by permission of the Government Printing Office, Wellington, New Zealand.

a conscious patient will create tensions for the patient, hence the decision to examine under anaesthetic' (*Report of the Cervical Cancer Inquiry* 1988, p. 191).

Two pressing questions arise from this inquiry. First, why had vaginal examinations — not to mention insertion and withdrawal of IUDs — been performed on *unconsenting* anaesthetised women for more than twenty years without any public protest by represent-ative bodies of the nursing profession? Second, are we to understand that attending theatre nurses had no knowledge of these practices, or, if they did, that they failed to see them as morally objectionable and thus did not pass the information on to their professional representatives (Johnstone 1987, p. 19)?

The report on the inquiry offers interesting answers to these questions. In response to the first question, representatives of the nursing profession apparently tried to have the practices con-demned and stopped. The commissioner's findings on this matter are quoted here at length:

Teaching examination techniques on anaesthetised patients without their consent is not a new issue at National Women's Hospital. In 1978 the Nurses Society of New Zealand made rep-resentation to the Auckland Hospital Board condemning the practice. Their allegations concerned teaching sessions involving the insertion and removal of intra uterine contraceptive devices on patients under general anaesthetic for other purposes, without patient consent or knowledge. According to their evidence, no public comment was made by the Hospital Board as a result of the representations. The Nurses Society, however, published the matter and a newspaper article commented on the issue. Al-though a television interview was taped, it was never transmitted, apparently because of adverse reactions from a member of the Postgraduate [Medical] School.

(*Report of the Cervical Cancer Inquiry* 1988, p. 191)

In answering the first question, the commissioner's findings also partly answered the second question. In order for the Nurses Society of New Zealand to make its claim, it must have had reliable information, which presumably came from theatre nurses who were troubled by the practices they had been witnessing. Nevertheless, it is possible that there were instances in which it was genuinely difficult for theatre nurses to have a full grasp of the situation; for example, citing the evidence (given anonymously) of one theatre charge nurse, the commissioner explained:

unconscious patients were examined vaginally by up to four students. She [the nurse] *was not told whether the vaginal examination was part of that patient's treatment or not* [italics added]. Her concern centred on the possible discomfort the woman might experience later, and her anxiety that the patient's permission had not been sought. When she voiced her concerns, they were dismissed by her supervisor.

(*Report of the Cervical Cancer Inquiry* 1988, p. 191)

Nurses also apparently tried to take positive action in relation to other morally questionable practices. Coney showed, for example, that nurses had 'tried for eight months to find out from the Ethical Committee why they were expected to send pancreases from aborted foetuses [sic] for research, "to no avail". Finally, they simply stopped supplying the foetuses because they could not get anything in writing' (Coney 1988, p. 141).

That nurses were expected to collect and send fetal material to the hospital laboratory for research should come as no surprise. It is not uncommon for hospitals to regard aborted fetuses as 'hospital property' and thus as items to be treated as the hospital (or rather, its doctors) see fit. Aborted fetal tissue is often sent 'routinely' to the hospital laboratory for 'analysis'.

At one point during the inquiry, the commissioner noted that she had 'a big gap in her information'. This, she is reported to have said, was because 'she had not heard from any nurses'. The commissioner then proceeded to criticise nurses for having been 'less than brave in coming forward to give evidence at the inquiry' (*New Zealand Herald* 1987d).

One nurse who gave evidence at the inquiry reportedly responded to this criticism by alleging that the medical superintendent of the National Women's Hospital, Dr Collison, had sent out a memo to the effect that:

nurses currently employed by National Women's Hospital are advised not to go forward to the hearing, and it is in their hospital's best interests and their own interests that they do not take part in the hearing.

(*New Zealand Herald* 1987c)

The media went on to report that Dr Collison had denied these allegations, stating that the only memo she recalled sending out was one that 'reminded staff ... that it was an offence [under the Hospital Act concerning confidentiality of patient information] to disclose to anyone information concerning the condition or medical history of any patient' (*New Zealand Herald* 1987c).

Coney stated that the memo advised staff that, if they wished to give information at the inquiry, they should see Collison. One obvious implication of this directive was that any staff members presenting themselves to Collison would, of course, be identified. Collison, however, refused to accept that her memo 'had acted as a disincentive' (Coney 1988, p. 224).

The New Zealand Nurses Association had quite a different view on the matter from Collison, however. Coney wrote:

> The Nurses' Association said it had heard from several members that Collison's memo was 'interpreted as an instruction NOT to co-operate with the inquiry'. Two had given confidential interviews anonymously because of a very clearly expressed perception that their jobs would be in jeopardy or any future prospects for study hampered if they came out in the open.
>
> (Coney 1988, p. 224)

It was later revealed that the special authority given by the minister of health providing for the release of information to the inquiry had not been communicated to staff (Coney 1988, p. 224).

The outcome of the Cervical Cancer Inquiry in regard to the New Zealand nursing profession was not encouraging. Early nursing commentary on the whole affair was at the time less than satisfactory and not entirely optimistic. The New Zealand Nurses Association, for example, indulged in a little 'sigh of relief' that nurses were not implicated in any substantial way in the practices exposed. The professional officer of the New Zealand Nurses Association, Joy Bickley, commented:

> Minimal discussion of nurses in the report implies they played only a peripheral part in the matters investigated at the inquiry. But in general, Cartwright says the nursing staff at National Women's were 'highly praised' for the caring attitude to the women they looked after.
>
> (Bickley 1988, p. 15)

In fairness to Bickley, however, she lamented the report's grave reservations about the nurses' ability to defend the patients' rights and deplored the commissioner's comment that:

> Nurses, who most appropriately should be the advocates for the patient, feel sufficiently intimidated by the medical staff (who do not hire and fire them) that even today they fail or refuse to confront openly the issues arising from the 1988 trial.
>
> (Bickley 1988, p. 15)

In some respects, the commissioner's criticisms were well founded. In other respects, however, her findings reflected the malaise and inadequacy of a system that does not provide for the ethical views of nurses to be heard. Her report encouraged the 'side-lining of nursing' (to borrow from Bickley), and thus encouraged the non-involvement of nurses as independent and accountable practitioners. By not acknowledging or dealing with the constraining effect that doctors and hospital administrators have on nurses' ability to act morally, the commissioner in effect preserved the status quo, rather than challenged it. By not apportioning blame to those nurses who knew what was happening, but did nothing, the commissioner tended to reinforce the notion that nurses should be 'good women' (and be the vessels of 'caring attitudes'), but 'not have a code of ethics' and thus not be independently morally accountable to those who require care. Unless the problem of institutional constraints on nurses is confronted, and unless the issues of hegemonic power relations within health care institutions are addressed, the danger of a recurrence of 'unfortunate experiments', not to mention medical malpractice and negligence, will continue to prevail. As a point of interest, Dr Herbert Green, the chief researcher of the cervical cancer project, ultimately evaded charges of disgraceful conduct relating to his project on grounds that he was '"unfit mentally and physically" to face charges' (*Sun Herald* 17 June 1990, p. 168). However, Professor Bonham, who was head of the committee which approved the original project, and was also head of the department of obstetrics and gynaecology at the time the project was being carried out, is reported to have been found guilty by the New Zealand Medical Council of a 'total of six misconduct charges, including four of disgraceful conduct' (*Waikato Times*, 15 October 1990, p. 3; see also Coney 1990, pp. 201–45).

An historical perspective from Nazi Germany

The complicity of nurses in morally questionable medical acts and the side-lining of nurses by important inquiries into medical malpractice and criminal behaviour is not unique. An instructive historical example can be found by examining some notable events that occurred during the Nazi era in Germany during the 1930s and 1940s.

Nazi Germany witnessed the shameful involvement of doctors, nurses, psychiatrists, dentists and pharmacologists in Hitler's euthanasia, or 'medicalised killing', programs (Aly and Roth 1984; Lifton 1986; Proctor 1988; Lagnado and Dekel 1991; Steppe 1991, 1992; Caplan 1992). Nazi doctors quickly emerged as the guardians of what Lifton called the 'Nazi biomedical vision, which saw the mass murder of millions in the name of "healing" the racially "diseased" body of the German nation' (Lifton 1986).

Nazi doctors were primarily responsible for the administration of lethal injections to 'patients'. However, as the German nurse historian Hilde Steppe (1991) has pointed out, it is very clear that 'nurses followed orders and were [likewise] involved in all phases of the systematic annihilation of masses of people' (p. 29). In his remarkable book *The Nazi doctors*, Lifton (1986) suggests that nurses played a fundamental part in determining the necessary drug dosages for 'putting to sleep' those patients whose names had been placed on 'special lists' (p. 101). In instances where patients were not cooperative, nurses would 'reassure' them by explaining that the prescribed injections were simply for 'the treatment of their lung disease' or whatever other 'disease' they may have had (Lifton 1986, p. 101).

Where nurses were involved, they were generally ordered by attending Nazi doctors to administer lethal drug regimes:

> the chief doctor was expected to give orders to the head male nurse to kill male patients, and the head female nurse to do the same to female patients ... the orders were passed along by the head male and female nurses to the ward nurses, who carried them out.
>
> (Lifton 1986, pp. 100–1)

Steppe explains that, once the choice of patients to be killed had been made, their names were noted by the nurse in charge, and the patients:

> were brought to a room which was especially set aside for the purpose and were then killed with medication or an injection of air. The killing was to a large extent carried out by the nursing personnel.
>
> (Steppe 1991, p. 31)

Aly and Roth (1984) and Caplan (1992) also cite examples of nurse involvement in Nazi atrocities.

There is evidence to suggest that, if a doctor felt uneasy and could not perform a certain murderous act, the difficulty could be solved by ordering a nurse to administer a prescribed 'treatment'. In one case, when a doctor refused to send a pregnant woman to a gas chamber, the problem was 'resolved' by ordering a nurse to give the woman a lethal injection (Lifton 1986, pp. 64, 100).

Nurses were also both directly and indirectly involved in the killing of children. For example, midwives were required to report the births of disabled newborns to attending Nazi physicians (Aly and Roth 1984, p. 156). Consequently, many of the disabled newborns were marked for death or experimental research that invariably led to death (Lifton 1986, p. 52). As well, nurses working in select departments or institutions (euphemistically referred to as 'children's specialty departments' or 'therapeutic convalescent institutions') were involved in administering legally prescribed 'therapeutic regimes' to 'subnormal' or 'excitable' children who were 'completely idiotic [and who] could not be kept quiet with the normal dose of sedatives' (Lifton 1986, p. 54). These 'therapeutic regimes' included large and accumulatively lethal doses of luminal, followed by a morphine-scopolamine preparation. When children receiving these drugs eventually died, the cause of death was listed as 'a more or less ordinary disease such as pneumonia' (Lifton 1986, p. 55).

It is also now known that nurses played a fundamental role in preparing patients for death, and in some instances were especially chosen to be present in the death chambers. Their work consisted of helping to carry a patient's personal belongings to the gas chamber, helping patients to undress, accompanying them and generally helping them to calm down; some nurses even stayed to observe the actual gassing process (Steppe 1991, pp. 30–1). Commenting on the role of nurses working in psychiatric institutes, Steppe describes their involvement in the killing programs as follows:

> They packed up the personal belongings of the patient, gave identification numbers to the objects and to the patient, they accompanied the transport to an intermediate location or to the death site. They rode back to their workplace in the empty buses, and later said in court proceedings that they had given no thought to the question of what happened with their patients.
>
> (Steppe 1991, p. 29)

Some, however, gave considerable thought to what happened to their patients. In 1941, for instance, nurses were among those who celebrated the cremation of a ten-thousandth patient at a psychiatric hospital in Hadamar (Proctor 1992, p. 36).

It should be noted that not all nurses were willing accomplices to the workings of the Nazi biomedical machine; many acted under threat of death or imprisonment, or both (Steppe 1991, p. 35). Others courageously risked their lives to help patients escape from the institutions in which they were held. In one report a nurse blatantly refused to take part in the killings because she 'felt herself becoming "hysterical" from the mental strain' (Lifton 1986, p. 57). One nurse also cared for Jewish patients when they could not get needed medical or hospital treatment (Steppe 1991, p. 35). This included working secretly at night in a Jewish hospital at which she had been forbidden to work.

In another report, it is claimed that Catholic nurses refusing to participate in sterilisation procedures lost their jobs. Interestingly, these dissenting Catholic nurses were replaced by non-Catholic 'brown sisters', who belonged to the Nazi Order of Nurses. Koonz (1987) explains:

> These women with a crash course on Nazi doctrine and eugenics as well as basic nursing skills, took the jobs of registered nurses who had received a minimum of four years of formal education. The 'brown sisters' received lower pay than nurses and, perhaps more importantly, they brought Nazi beliefs to their clients.
>
> (Koonz 1987, p. 284)

An example of how strong these Brown Sisters' Nazi beliefs were can be found in the oath they swore on the completion of their training:

> I solemnly swear that I will be steadfastly faithful and obedient to Adolf Hitler, my Fuhrer. I promise to fulfil my duties, wherever I may be designated to work, faithfully and conscientiously as a national socialist nurse in the service of the national community, so help me God.
>
> (Archives Koblenz N S 37/1039, cited in Steppe 1991, p. 24)

As a point of interest, it appears that no nurse involved in the Nazi atrocities was barred from practising as a nurse (Steppe 1991, p. 18). Further, of those nurses who appeared in court to account for their Nazi activities, most were eventually acquitted, or, if found guilty, were released from prison after only a short time.

Curiously, formal literature on the subject (including publicly available literature on the Nuremberg trials) makes very little mention, if any, of nurses' participation in Nazi biomedical atrocities. Popular nursing history texts are also conspicuously silent on the subject. Moreover, neither the International Council of Nurses, the International Red Cross, the United Nations Information Centre, the United States National Archives nor the Melbourne Jewish Holocaust Centre has been able to provide useful information on either the involvement of nurses in Nazi biomedical practices or the postwar prosecution of nurses that might have taken place. There is an alleged incident where a registered nurse reportedly used a bed sheet to bind together the legs of a woman in the advanced stages of labour. Both the woman and her unborn child suffered enormously as a result of this single and barbaric act. Unfortunately, there appears to be no formal documentation of this incident, or any others like it. Thus the secrets of the past are likely to remain secrets, and the nursing profession, sadly, will remain deprived of an important historical lesson. Yet again, the image of nurses as merely 'good women' (viz, humble and obedient servants) and not having a code of ethics (which they did not have at that time [Kelly 1985, p. 207]) has been fully preserved. This stereo-typical view of nurses is proving very difficult to shift, as the following chapters show. Nevertheless, this should not preclude nurses from learning from the important historical lessons that the Nazi nurse question poses; as Hilde Steppe so succinctly puts it:

> We must never forget that nursing never takes place in a value free, neutral space but is always a socially significant force. This means we cannot simply observe what is taking place around us, but must also take a stand, take our responsibilities actively.

> (Steppe 1991, p. 36)

'Taking our responsibilities actively', in this instance, could begin by nurses identifying and comprehending the conditions that made it possible for their sister members of a 'caring' profession to engage in and support the atrocities they did. (See also Wikler and Barondess 1993; Caplan 1992.)

Biases and omissions in the *Encyclopedia of bioethics*

The Encyclopedia of bioethics, edited by Warren T. Reich (1978), is a standard international bioethics reference text. Developed with the support of the Kennedy Institute of Ethics at Georgetown Univers-ity, Washington DC, the complete unabridged volumes of this encyclopedia have given the Western world probably one of its most comprehensive and valuable literature resources in moral phil-osophy. Not only does it cover a broad range of issues in bioethics, but it does so from an impressive interdisciplinary, intercultural and international point of view.

Nevertheless, despite its comprehensiveness and outstanding list of contributors, the encyclopedia fails to do justice to a nursing perspective on bioethics. Examples of omissions and inadequacies can be found in the encyclopedia's preface, list of editorial advisory board members, list of contributors, index to contents and appendix of ethical codes.

The preface states that several editors from a number of schol-arly journals served both as advisory and critical reviewers of the encyclopedia project. Included are editors of scientific, theological, philosophical, psychological, medical, ethical and medical ethics journals. No nurse editors and no nursing journals are mentioned.

Of the sixty members of the editorial advisory board, most of the disciplines converging on bioethics are represented, but no profes-sors of nursing or lecturers in nursing are mentioned. Of these sixty members, only six are women.

The list of contributors rates a little better, but yields no grounds for optimism. Of the 285 contributors, only about 15 per cent are female. The 285 include, in substantial numbers, professors and associate professors of philosophy, religion and moral theology, medicine, surgery, psychiatry and law, as well as professors and associate professors of ethics, medical ethics, history of medicine, law and medicine, biology, behavioural studies and psychology, dentistry, sociology, humanities and English, economics, social demography, political science, oriental studies, anthropology and zoology. Numerous directors of organisations, research fellows and lecturers are also listed. Of these only *one* appears to be a nurse — Teresa Stanley, who is described as a Kennedy Nursing Faculty Fellow in Bioethics, Director, Division of Nursing, Incarnate Word College, San Antonio, Texas. Stanley wrote the only article devoted specifically to nursing. Nursing is mentioned specifically in only one other article, which appears last in the encyclopedia, entitled 'Women as health professionals'. This article, a historical account of women health professionals, is co-authored by two Harvard University associate professors of psychiatry, who are not nursing professionals.

The encyclopedia's editors claim that 'all manuscripts were thoroughly reviewed for appropriateness of scope, accuracy of content, and clarity of style'. In terms of scope and accuracy, a few points need to be considered in relation to Stanley's article.

Stanley (1978, p. 1138) points out that nurses in the United States began seriously to question ethical issues in nursing as early as 1900. One of the great pioneers of nursing ethics at that time was Isabel Hampton Robb who, in 1903, wrote *Nursing ethics for hospital and private use* — one of the first texts of its kind. By the 1930s and 1940s, ethics courses were a strong component in nursing curricula. Special courses in ethics were eventually deleted from nursing curricula, however. This did not go unnoticed by the 1976 Commission on the Teaching of Bioethics in the United States, which reported that 'ethics as an integral part of nursing education has been seriously overlooked' (Stanley 1978, p. 1138).

Stanley raises the issues of nursing education, the need for theory and knowledge-based practice, the moral significance of nursing, the special responsibility of the nursing profession to the community at large, and popular ethical concerns in nursing practice (including conflict in the nurse–doctor relationship, conscientious objection to abortion, informed consent, truth telling, nurse participation in ethics committees, and the ethical responsibilities of nurse researchers). Nevertheless, she cannot be expected to do justice to the issues she raises in the mere *nine pages* of her article. The space cannot compare with the overwhelming volume of other views given in the total of 1813 pages allocated for articles in the encyclopedia. Moreover, Stanley does not give an 'intercultural and international' perspective on the development of ethical concerns in nursing. Her article is presented entirely from a United

States perspective and gives the frank but misleading impression that this perspective accurately reflects the position of nursing worldwide.

Stanley omits the information that the International Council of Nurses (ICN) established the Ethics of Nursing Committee in 1933 to study and to collect data to formulate an international view on the ethical problems being encountered by nurse practitioners. The activities of this committee were delayed, partly because of World War II (Kelly 1985, p. 207). Nevertheless, it eventually formulated a code of conduct which was formally adopted in 1953, at a Grand Council meeting held in Brazil. A major revision of the 1965 version of this code was prompted rather forcefully by a group of Canadian student nurses who objected strongly to the statements in the code supporting 'nursing subservience to medicine' (Bergman 1973, p. 140). Their objections were formally presented to the ICN as well as to their national association representatives. The offending clause was eventually deleted. The ICN's current code of conduct is the legacy of these nursing students' initiative and foresight.

Stanley omits some other historical information. She states, for example, that 'there was no formal code of ethics to guide nursing practice in the early stages of the profession' (Stanley 1978, p. 1138). It is not clear whether this statement refers to universal or United States practice, but either way it is incorrect. In 1893, United States nurses had the Nightingale pledge, written by Lystra E. Gretter, superintendent of the school at Harper Hospital in Detroit (Kelly 1985, p. 44). This pledge had (and has) an ethical orientation, just like any other similar pledge, not least the celebrated Hippocratic Oath. Nursing codes or standards of care go back much further than this, however. There is evidence of formal standards of care existing in ancient India as early as 1000 BC (Smith and Lew 1968, p. 2). The author of this set of standards was the physician Charaka, who insisted, among other things, that those who care for the sick must be:

> of good behaviour, distinguished for purity; possessed of cleverness and skill; imbued with kindness; skilled in every service a patient may require; competent to cook food; skilled in bathing and washing the patient; rubbing and massaging the limb/s; lifting and assisting him to walk about; well skilled in the art of making beds; ready, patient and skilful in waiting upon one who is ailing and never unwilling to do anything that is ordered.
>
> (Smith and Lew 1968, p. 2)

It is fairly obvious that Charaka is not directing physicians in this instance, but those who *care* for the sick, notably, by modern-day interpretations, nurses.

The early Christian deaconesses and matrons (1–500 AD), the precursors of nursing as we know it today, conducted their activities in caring for the sick in strict accord with the moral demands of their religion. The early Christian 'golden rules' of 'do unto others' and 'love thy neighbour' that they rigorously observed prevail to this day — even in the more rationalistic and secular moralities. (Consider, for example, Kant's famous 'categorical imperative', which holds that people should only act on those principles that would be good for everybody to follow; and more recently the increasing attention being given to the sentiments of love and care as moral principles of conduct.) The deaconesses endeavoured to practise strictly the Corporal Works of Mercy (the formalisation of which stood as a kind of code) and to care and provide compassionately for those who were suffering. These Corporal Works of Mercy obligated the deaconesses:

- to feed the hungry;
- to give water to the thirsty;
- to clothe the naked;
- to visit the imprisoned;
- to shelter the homeless;
- to care for the sick;
- to bury the dead.

(Dolan et al. 1983, p. 45)

It might be objected here that the Corporal Works of Mercy are not an ethical code as such. However, if analysed from the perspective of a care-based ethic, as opposed to an ethic based on rational moral principles, the Corporal Works of Mercy are clearly as much an embodiment of a moral (prescriptive) code of conduct as is any other code specifying prescriptive rules of conduct.

The deaconesses and matrons successfully established the principles of selfless devotion and self-sacrificing and altruistic commitment to caring for the sick — principles that still have a firm grip on the nursing subconscious mind. There is also evidence that early Roman women caring for the sick were formally expected to have 'literacy, anatomic understanding, a sense of patient responsibility, and ethical concerns, particularly about confidentiality' (Nadelson and Notman 1978, p. 1713).

The most surprising omission in the Stanley article is Florence Nightingale's contribution to nursing ethics. As Olga Kanitsaki has observed, in many respects Nightingale was the first modern nurse ethicist (personal communication). Benefiting from a liberal arts education, Nightingale firmly believed that nurse leaders 'must be just and candid, looking at both sides, not moved by entreaties or by likes and dislikes but only by justice and always being reasonable' (cited in Barritt 1973, p. 18). Nightingale also urged nurses to be chaste, sober, honest, truthful, trustworthy, discreet, kind, benevolent, duty bound, and respectful of patient autonomy (Kelly 1985, p. 34). Nightingale emphasised that nursing had a moral influence (Barritt 1973, p. 29), and her writings and work all reflect the resolve and commitment she had to transforming nursing into a moral profession — one that was fully accountable to the community and that was able to prevent human beings from suffering unnecessarily.

Nightingale has often been blamed for having established the principle of 'blind obedience to physicians' and thus for establishing nursing as a docile and subservient profession — the source of many of our modern-day professional and moral problems. However, in many respects this blame is unfair. Although she had a profound respect for 'the rules' and for the 'principle of obedience', she was very aware that rules could be restrictive, that regulations 'were usually made by men who were incapable of devising suitable regulations for women', and that nurses required an 'obedience of intelligence, not obedience of slavery' (Barritt 1973, pp. 18, 19, 34; Johnstone 1994, p. 55). Nightingale believed that devotion and obedience might well be fine qualities in a porter and 'might even do for a horse' (Woodham-Smith 1964, p. 262). They would not do for a nurse, however, and would render her little more than a servant and, thereby, a professional failure (Nightingale 1970 edn, p. 75). She also firmly believed that nursing education and nursing practice should be controlled by nurses, and rejected the authority of doctors and hospital administrators over these domains. Her deeds and her writings stand as testimony that she most certainly did not believe that nurses should be 'blind obedient slaves'.

Stanley's article makes an important contribution to the encyclopedia's consideration of a nursing perspective on bioethics. However, the encyclopedia's shortcomings in presenting a full nursing perspective on bioethics are very apparent.

A brief analysis of the encyclopedia's index is also revealing. Subject titles beginning with the terms 'nurse' and 'nursing' have a total of five listings, with an additional 26 subheadings. Of these only two pertain to ethics — the subheadings 'nursing ethics for hospital and private use (Robb)' and 'ethics committees and', both of which refer to Stanley's article. This compares very poorly with the subject titles beginning with the terms 'medical', 'medicine' and 'physician', which receive approximately fifty listings, with an additional 314 subheadings. Within the subheadings, forty feature ethical considerations ranging from the history of medical ethics to medical codes of conduct. Unlike the nursing listings, these listings offer a cross-cultural, historical and international perspective, and include views from the Arab nations, Eastern and Western European countries, Latin America, North America, China and Japan. Both ancient and modern views are given. Stanley's account of nursing pales into insignificance next to this impressive profile of medicine. Also of significance is the fact that the subtitles feature the physician-nurse relationship, but do not include the nurse-physician one. Strike action by physicians is cited, but not strike action by nurses.

There is one further comment to be made, and this pertains to the encyclopedia's appendix entitled 'Codes and statements related to medical ethics' (pp. 1731–1815), in which the ICN 1973 Code for Nurses and the American Nurses' Association 1976 Code for Nurses are reprinted. The inclusion of these codes is commendable. Nevertheless, a number of observations remain to be made. First, it is philosophically objectionable that all codes included in this appendix (including non-nursing and non-medical codes such as those of the American Chiropractic Association, and those of osteopathic, pharmacological, psychiatric, psychological, and dental associations) are subsumed under 'medical ethics', rather than held to be codes in their own right. It is conceptually questionable to treat medical ethics as synonymous with bioethics, health care ethics or nursing ethics. The table of contents to this appendix introduces the codes as 'Codes of the health-care professions' (p. 1723), which is quite acceptable, and gives each of the four sections an appropriate heading.

A second feature of this appendix is that over fourteen medical codes are included, together with another six related to the ethics of medical research. This total of twenty codes (which includes, among others, the ancient codes of Greece, India, Syria, and Persia, and the modern codes of the USA, the USSR and the World Medical Association) completely overpowers nursing's almost imperceptible two codes. The inherent bias here speaks for itself. The medical codes are certainly worthy of inclusion, but the appendix is the poorer for not including some of nursing's older codes, not to mention other international nursing codes (see, for example, Sawyer 1989; Viens 1989). I have been told informally that the *Encyclopedia of bioethics* is being revised. At this stage, however, it seems that the status quo will be preserved, and that discussion on the distinctive field of professional nursing ethics will not be expanded beyond the encyclopedia's present parameters.

Issues and recommendations

The cases and examples discussed so far are instructive in that they poignantly illustrate how recorders of history, leaders of the community and the community at large have not yet come to grips with the moral significance of nursing practice, the nurse–patient relationship and the difficulties that many nurses face in delivering morally and legally responsible (and accountable) nursing care.

It is tempting to regard the poor understanding of the moral nature of nursing practice and the nurse–patient relationship as being simply matters of blameless ignorance and even historically conditioned naivety. Such a position is neither persuasive nor compelling, however. There is a very strong case for arguing that the exclusion of, or lack of attention to, a nursing perspective on bioethical and related issues at interdisciplinary conferences, in the media, in legal inquiries, and in medical and community areas generally, is not the product of ignorance or naivety alone. It is also the product of powerful attitudes and beliefs about the 'inside' knowledge nurses have in relation to bioethical issues arising in health care domains, and about whether nurses should be permitted to disclose this knowledge. Nurses know the truth and have the ability to tell it faithfully — given the right circumstances. Possibly there is even jealousy, to borrow from Henrietta Bolton (1898, p. 511), 'of seeing what they [the "scientific" establishment] consider their own field invaded'.

The suppression of unwanted and unpalatable truths and the holding of misplaced jealousies can hardly be the ingredients for a competent, wise and balanced bioethical debate. They are certainly not the ingredients for a constructive and productive debate. The first step, then, is to make visible the lived experiences of all involved, and to show that there is really nothing to be feared, at least not by those who have moral integrity. The second step is to show that bioethics is a field that belongs to everybody (including lay people, as well as philosophers, doctors, lawyers, nurses, other allied health workers, and, not least, the community at large), and is thus a field in which participation by all concerned is something to be encouraged, not something to be jealous of.

Many doctors, philosophers, lawyers and other members of the community already endorse an interdisciplinary, multi-paradigmatic, cooperative and contextual approach to bioethics. These people are already making a sincere attempt to include a nursing perspective on the many bioethical issues in health care and political domains. They have, fortunately, already contributed a great deal towards achieving a more morally tolerable clinical reality for patients and health professionals alike. Unfortunately, these 'agents of change' are not always supported in their endeavours, and may even be obstructed by those who fear losing their control of an otherwise self-contained situation and the power they have enjoyed in that situation.

Doctors, philosophers, lawyers, and other members of the community who are working to bring about the moral reforms in health care domains that are so urgently needed, need to be supported and assisted. The nursing profession is one group that can support and assist them, and can do so in a very powerful and fruitful way. For nurses to be able to do this, however, and for nurses to be able to contribute meaningfully to the debates that are likely to arise in relation to reforms being made, they must have at least a working knowledge of the issues at stake and of the moral language and differing viewpoints necessary for debating them. They must also have the freedom to contribute, and must not need to fear institutional or legal censure for doing so. There must also be a personal and professional commitment to bringing about positive change and moral reforms in nursing practice and health care generally. It is to the discussion of the issues, and the moral language and differing viewpoints needed for debating them, and to inspiring change, that the following chapters of this book give attention.

References

Aly, G. and Roth, K. (1984). The legalization of mercy killings in medical and nursing institutions in Nazi Germany from 1938 until 1941: a commented documentation *International Journal of Law and Psychiatry* 7, pp. 145–63.

Barritt, E. R. (1973). Florence Nightingale's values and modern nursing education. *Nursing Forum* 12 (1), pp. 7–47.

Beauchamp, T. L. and Childress, J. F. (1989). *Principles of biomedical ethics*, 3rd edn. Oxford University Press, New York.

Bergman, R. (1973). Ethics — concepts and practice. *International Nursing Review* 20 (5), pp. 140–2.

Bickley, J. (1988). What the cervical cancer inquiry report means for nurses. *New Zealand Nursing Journal* 81 (9), pp. 14–15.

Blum, J. D. (1984). The code of nurses and wrongful discharge. *Nursing Forum* 21, pp. 149–51.

Bock, A. (1992). Nurses in call for euthanasia inquiry. *The Age*, 3 March, p. 6.

Bolton, H. (1898). Women in science. *Popular Science Monthly* 53, pp. 506–11 (cited in M. Alic, *Hypatia's heritage*, Women's Press, London, 1986).

Bridges, D. C. (1968). 'International Nursing Review' past, present — and progress? *International Nursing Review* 15 (1), pp. 9–17.

Briggs, P. and McDonald, B. (1992). 'Straw Men' in the euthanasia debate. *The Age*, 24 March, p. 12.

Broekhuijse, P. (1988). Nurse loses job over abortion. *Sunday Telegraph* (Sydney), 21 February, p. 13.

Caplan, A. (ed.) (1992). *When medicine went mad: bioethics and the holocaust.* Humana Press, Totowa, New Jersey.

Centre for Human Bioethics (1986). *Proceedings of the conference, 'AIDS: Social Policy, Ethics and Law'.* Centre for Human Bioethics, Monash University, Melbourne.

Centre for Human Bioethics (1987). *Proceedings of the conference, 'The Role of the Nurse: Doctors' Handmaiden, Patients' Advocate, or What?* Centre for Human Bioethics, Monash University, Melbourne.

Centre for Human Bioethics (1987). *Proceedings of the conference, 'IVF: the Current Debate'.* Centre for Human Bioethics, Monash University, Melbourne.

Clay, T. (1987). *Nurses: power and politics.* Heinemann Nursing, London.

Coney, S. (1988). *The unfortunate experiment*. Penguin Books, Auckland, New Zealand.

Coney, S. (1990). *Out of the frying pan: inflammatory writing 1972–89*. Penguin Books, Auckland, NZ.

Coney, S. and Bunkle, P. (1987). An 'unfortunate experiment' at National Women's. *Metro*, June, pp. 47–65.

Cotterhill, D. (1992). Views not representative. *Australian Nurses Journal* 21 (10), p. 4.

Coulter, C. (1987). Women, infertility and IVF. In *Proceedings of the conference, 'IVF: the Current Debate'*. Centre for Human Bioethics, Monash University, Melbourne, pp. 156–68.

Davis, A. J. and Aroskar, M. A. (1983). *Ethical dilemmas and nursing practice*, 2nd edn. Appleton-Century-Crofts, Norwalk, Connecticut.

Dock, L. L. (1900). Ethics — or a code of ethics? In L.L. Dock, *Short papers on nursing subjects*. M. Louise Longeway, New York.

Dolan, J. A., Fitzpatrick, M. L. and Herrmann, E. K. (1983). *Nursing in society: an historical perspective*, 15th edn. W. B. Saunders, Philadelphia.

Gartland, S. (1992). Nurses death aid 'no shock'. *Herald-Sun*, 3 March, p. 5.

Johns, G. (1988). The commanding presence of George Herbert Green. *New Zealand Herald*, 6 August, p. 9.

Johnstone, M.-J. (1987). Nursing and professional ethics. In *Proceedings of the conference, 'The Role of the Nurse: Doctor's Handmaiden, Patients' Advocate or What?'* Centre for Human Bioethics, Monash University, Melbourne.

Johnstone, M.-J. (1988a). Law, professional ethics and the problem of conflict with personal values. *International Journal of Nursing Studies* 25 (2), pp. 147–57.

Johnstone, M.-J. (1988b). A critical bioethical issue. *Australian Nurses Journal* 18 (1), p. 8.

Johnstone, M.-J. (1988c). Ethical issues in neonatal nursing. Paper presented at the conference 'Storking the Future', Monash Medical Centre, 27 August, Melbourne.

Johnstone, M.-J. (1994). *Nursing and the injustices of the law*. W. B. Saunders/Baillière Tindall, Sydney.

Kelly, L. Y. (1985). *Dimensions of professional nursing*, 5th edn. Macmillan Publishing, New York.

Koonz, C. (1987). *Mothers in the Fatherland: women, the family and Nazi politics*. St Martin's Press, New York.

Kuhse, H. and Singer, P. (1992). Euthanasia: a survey of nurses' attitudes and practices. *Australian Nurses Journal* 21 (9), pp. 21–2.

Lagnado, L. and Dekel, S. (1991). *Children of the flames: Dr Josef Mengele and the untold story of the twins of Auschwitz*. Sidgwick & Jackson, London.

Lifton, R. J. (1986). *The Nazi doctors: a study of the psychology of evil*. Macmillan, London.

McIntosh, P. (1988). Nurses must be more aggressive. *Australian Dr Weekly*, 10 June, pp. 1, 10.

Magazanik, M. (1992a). Nurses back euthanasia, survey finds. *The Age*, 2 March, p. 1.

Magazanik, M. (1992b). When death is part of the quality of life. *The Age*, 4 March, p. 3.

Magazanik, P. (1992c). Euthanasia should be legal, says clergyman. *The Age*, 5 March, p. 3.

Magazanik, P. (1992d). Euthanasia law is unrealistic: doctor. *The Age*, 5 June, p. 1.

Magazanik, P. (1992e). Law Commission supports reform on treatment of sick babies. *The Age*, 6 June, p. 5.

Mathews, S. (1988). Nurses overlooked. *The Age*, 24 March, p. 12.

Miller, C. (1988). Transplant row: nurses fear sack. *Herald* (Melbourne), 18 July, p. 1.

Millership, R. (1992). A better way. *Australian Nurses Journal* 21 (10), p. 4.

Monkivitch, A. (1992). Euthanasia result not accurate. *The Age*, 5 March, p. 12.

Muirden, N., Jackson, K., Pisasale, M., Williams, B., Bingham, J. and Evans, B. (1992). A survey among palliative care nurses would give differing view. *The Age*, 10 March, p. 12.

Muyskens, J. L. (1982). *Moral problems in nursing: a philosophical investigation.* Rowman & Littlefield, Totowa, New Jersey.

Nadelson, C. C. and Notman, M. T. (1978). Women as health professionals. In Reich (ed.), *Encyclopedia of bioethics,* pp. 1713–20.

New Zealand Herald (1987a). Cancer cases quoted. 12 August, p. 13.

New Zealand Herald (1987b). 'Absolutely appalled' over tests. 12 November, p. 14.

New Zealand Herald (1987c). Dr Collison denies imposing staff gag. 18 November.

New Zealand Herald (1987d). Inquiry judge seeks more nurses' views. 3 December.

New Zealand Herald (1987e). Consent 'not asked' for samples. 10 December.

New Zealand Herald (1988a). Swabbed girls 'often Maoris and Islanders'. 20 January.

New Zealand Herald (1988b). Dr Green 'Did not treat all cases'. 28 January, p. 3.

Nightingale, F. (1970 edn). *Notes on nursing.* Duckworth, London. (First published 1859 by Harrison & Sons.)

Nursing Times (1990). Nurses obliged to lie to cancer patients. 86 (28), 11 July, p. 9.

O'Connor, M. (1992). Representative sample? *Australian Nurses Journal* 21 (10) May, p. 4.

Pirrie, M. (1987). A disabled baby's right to live. *The Age*, 28 April, p. 11.

Proctor, R. (1988). *Racial hygiene: medicine under the Nazis.* Harvard University Press, Cambridge, Mass.

Proctor, R. (1992). Nazi biomedical politics. In Caplan (ed.), *When medicine went mad: bioethics and the holocaust,* pp. 23–42.

Reich, W. T. (ed.) (1978). *Encyclopedia of bioethics.* The Free Press, New York.

Report of the Cervical Cancer Inquiry (1988). Prepared by the Committee of Inquiry into Allegations Concerning the Treatment of Cervical Cancer at National Women's Hospital and into Other Related Matters. Government Printing Office, Auckland, New Zealand.

Report of the Study of Professional Issues in Nursing (1988). Health Department (Vic.), Melbourne.

Robb, I. H. (1903). *Nursing ethics for hospital and private use.* J. B. Savage, Cleveland.

Roberts, J. (1987). Women not told of intimate checks. *Sunday Star* (Auckland), 26 September.

Sanders, K. (1988). Obeying doctor's orders: professional accountability. In *Proceedings of 'Nursing Law and Ethics'. First Victorian State Conference. Theme: 'Matters of Life and Death',* School of Nursing, Phillip Institute of Technology, Melbourne.

Sawyer, L. M. (1989). Nursing code of ethics: an international comparison. *International Nursing Review* 36 (5), pp. 145–8.

Schumpeter, P. (1988). No-resuscitation rules are unclear: lecturer. *The Age,* 1 October, p. 21.

Skene, L. (1992). Doctor ending baby's pain should not face risk of jail. *The Age,* 9 June, p. 12.

Smith, W. B. and Lew, Y. L. (1968). *Nursing care of the patient.* Dymock, Sydney.

Stanley, T. (1978). Nursing. In Reich (ed.), *Encyclopedia of bioethics,* pp. 1138–46.

Steppe, H. (1991). Nursing in the Third Reich. *History of Nursing Journal* 3 (4), pp. 21–37.

Steppe, H. (1992). Nursing in Nazi Germany. *Victorian Journal of Nursing Research* 14 (6), pp. 744–53.

Sun-Herald (1990). Medically unfit. 17 June, p. 168.

Svendsen, I. (1987). Lecturer calls for code of nursing conduct, *The Age,* 17 November, p. 21.

Syme, R. (1992). A missing voice in euthanasia debate. *The Age,* 21 March, p. 10.

The Age (1992). Editorial — The law and the right to die. 5 March, p. 13.

Thompson, J. B. and Thompson, H. O. (1981). *Ethics in nursing.* Macmillan, New York.

Tighe, M. (1992). Slippery slope to killing patients. *The Age,* 21 March, p. 10.

Viens, D. C. (1989). A history of nursing's code of ethics. *Nursing Outlook* 37 (1), pp. 45–9.

Waikato Times (1987a). Patient recall: decision later. 1 September.

Waikato Times (1987b). Rape by medical students? 18 September.

Waikato Times (1990), Ethical guidelines underway. 15 October, p. 3.

Warthen v. Toms River Community Memorial Hospital, Superior Court of New Jersey, AD, 8/1/85–14/2/85. In *Atlantic Reporter,* 2nd Series, New Jersey, pp. 229–34.

Wikler, D. and Barondess, J. (1993). Boethics and anti-bioethics in light of Nazi medicine: what must we remember? *Kennedy Institute of Ethics Journal* 3 (1), pp. 39–55.

Woodham-Smith, C. (1964). *Florence Nightingale 1820–1910.* Collins Fontana, London.

Yarling, R. R. and McElmurry, B. J. (1986). The moral foundation of nursing. *Advances in Nursing Science* 8 (2), pp. 63–73.

Chapter

2

What is ethics?

In HIS CELEBRATED WORK *Contemporary moral philosophy*, G. J. Warnock warned that:

> When we talk about 'morals' we do not all know what we mean; what moral problems, moral principles, moral judgments are is not a matter so clear that it can be passed over as simple datum. We must discover when we would say, and when we would not, that an issue is a moral issue, and why: and if, as is more than likely, disagreements should come to light even at this stage, we could at least discriminate and investigate what reasonably tenable alternative positions there may be.
>
> (Warnock 1967, p. 75)

The terms 'ethics', 'morality', 'rights', 'duties', 'obligations', 'moral principles', 'moral rules', 'morally right', 'morally wrong', 'moral theory', to name some, are all commonly used in ethical discourse. Nurses, like others, may use some of these terms when discussing life events and situations which are perceived as having a moral dimension. Whether nurses use these terms correctly, however, is another matter. For example, there is a popular tendency by nurses (including some nurse authors) to draw a firm but erroneous distinction between ethics and morality (see, for example, Kelly 1985). Many see 'morality' as involving more a personal or private set of values, in contrast with 'ethics', which is seen as involving a more formalised, public and universal set of values. Another common error (see also Fagin 1975) is to regard the terms 'rights' and 'responsibilities' or 'duties' as being synonymous, and thus able to be used interchangeably. An example of this is found in the International Council of Nurses (ICN) position statement on the 'rights and duties of nurses', adopted at the ICN's Council of National Representatives meeting in Brazil in June 1983: 'Nurses have a *right* [italics added] to practise within the code of ethics and nursing legislation' (Keireini 1983, p. 4). When we later examine the nature of rights and duties, it will become clear that the term 'right' in this example should, in fact, read 'duty'. Not surprisingly, the incorrect use of fundamental ethical terms and concepts has led to a certain degree of confusion in nursing ethics discourse. This is particularly evident in literature discussing the supposed role of the nurse as a patient's advocate. It has also caused confusion about and misunderstanding of a nursing perspective on bioethics generally; the language and grammar of ethics has probably been misunderstood as much by doctors, lawyers, the media, theologians and other members of the community as by nurses. One unfortunate consequence of this distortion in communication has been (and in many respects continues to be) an inability of people in health care domains to achieve tolerable and peaceable solutions to many moral problems plaguing both them and the health care arena as a whole.

The need to understand clearly the moral language and grammar used in moral discourse is made explicit by the contemporary English philosopher, Richard Hare:

> in a world in which the problems of conduct become every day more complex and tormenting, there is a great need for an understanding of the language in which these problems are posed and answered. For confusion about our moral language leads, not merely to theoretical muddles, but to needless practical perplexities.

> (Hare 1964, pp. 1–2)

These words are as relevant and as important for nurses as they are for the community of academic philosophers for whom Hare wrote. Nursing is just as vulnerable to the 'theoretical muddles' and 'needless practical perplexities' that flow from a confusion about moral language as are other disciplines engaged in the business of ethics. It is to clearing up some of the confusion surrounding the selection, interpretation, and use of moral language, and the concepts they import, that this chapter now turns.

Understanding moral language

The need for a common moral language

In order to be able to discuss bioethics in a meaningful way, it is important, first, to share a common and working knowledge and understanding of the fundamental ethical terms that are central to ethical discourse and thought. In other words, unless nurses use the same moral language and grammar as others, little hope remains for either agreement or disagreement being reached on

what is considered a competing moral view (i.e. a genuine difference of moral opinion), much less on what is considered a morally
right or wrong course of action. For example, if two dissenting
parties do not share a common conception about human rights and
what these entail, they cannot even begin to debate the conditions
under which a violation of human rights might be morally wrong or
morally permissible. If those engaged in bioethical debate do not
use a common moral language, then they risk spending a lifetime
arguing fruitlessly at cross-purposes and engaging in endless
human misunderstanding. In this respect the philosophical adage
that 'there must be agreement before there can be disagreement' is
by no means trivial.

A second ingredient critical to any meaningful bioethical discussion is the use of clearly articulated, substantiated and
mutually agreed upon *definitions* of ethical terms and concepts.
This is necessary for at least two reasons. First, ethical definitions
have an important role to play in evaluating moral disagreements
and in commenting on how these might be best resolved. Second,
ethical definitions are themselves 'ethically "loaded" with moral pre-
suppositions, and therefore ... may need to be backed up by appeal
to moral principles and an examination of specific instances'
(Walton 1980, p. 16).

Consider, for example, the philosophical notion of 'person',
which in mainstream Western moral philosophy relies very heavily
on rational criteria and, to some extent, sentience (i.e. the capacity
to feel and to experience sensations). The philosophical definition of
'person' (usually distinguished from the notion of 'human being')
has an important bearing on deciding the moral permissibility of,
for example, abortion, fetal tissue transplants, or the use of live-
born anencephalic babies or brain-dead human beings as organ
donors. In this instance, a philosophically defined notion of 'person'
(together with its ethical 'loading') could make all the difference in
the world between, say, a doctor being deemed, in the case of organ
transplantation, to have 'committed murder' as opposed to having
merely 'harvested organs', a notion that itself is designed to sound
value neutral. In the same way, a mother could be deemed to have
'committed infanticide' as opposed to having merely 'got rid of the
unwanted products of conception' in the case of abortion. A philosophical definition of 'person' could also determine which medical
procedures nurses could be morally and reasonably expected to
assist with — for example, organ transplants, abortions and
experimental research procedures.

The important lesson to be learned here is that unless ethical
definitions are scrupulously formulated, given, and revised, moral
language will be in danger of corrupting and/or distorting sound
and purposeful bioethical debate, rather than contributing reliably
and constructively to it. Poorly or inappropriately defined ethical

terms and concepts can also seriously impinge upon and limit the moral imagination, and not least the moral options and choices that might otherwise be apprehended, contemplated and chosen in the face of moral adversity (Johnstone 1988). The notion of 'quality of life' is a good example. Many writers on bioethics assume that when a life ceases to be 'independent' it has diminished worth. In such instances, euthanasia might be considered a right and proper course of action to take. Here the ethically loaded notion of 'dependence' imparts a sense of permissibility of the euthanasia option and limits any thought of, say, pursuing a rehabilitation option. It also overrides any thought of the possibility that for some people 'dependence' may be quite irrelevant to the notion of a worthwhile life. Kanitsaki (1989, 1993, 1994), for example, makes it abundantly clear that in some traditional cultural groups, familial and friendly relationships are characteristically *collective and interdependent,* and thus any thought of *individual independence* is quite irrelevant to the assessment of 'a life worth living' .

The limiting effects of language on the moral imagination will be demonstrated more thoroughly as the discussions in this book are advanced. It remains the task here to identify and define the ethical terms and concepts that are most commonly used in bioethical discourse, and with which nurses must become familiar if they are to make a meaningful contribution to the bioethics debate.

What is ethics?

It is appropriate to begin the task of defining commonly used ethical terms and concepts by first examining the terms 'ethics' and 'morality' themselves. Contrary to popular nursing opinion, there is no philosophically significant difference between the terms 'ethics' and 'morality' (Ladd 1978, p. 400). If a distinction is to be drawn between these two terms it is one that is based on etymological grounds, with 'ethics' coming from the ancient Greek *ethikos* (originally meaning 'pertaining to custom or habit'), and 'morality' coming from the Latin *moralitas* (also originally meaning 'custom' or 'habit'). This means, of course, that it is not incorrect to use the terms interchangeably, as many philosophers in fact do, and as is done here. With respect to deciding which terms should be used in ethical discourse (i.e. whether to use the term 'ethics' or the term 'morality'), this is very much a matter of personal preference rather than of rigorous philosophical debate. Of course, contemporary definitions of the terms ethics and morality are far more sophisticated than those given earlier of 'custom' or 'habit'.

What is bioethics?

The term 'bioethics', from Greek *bios*, meaning 'life', means ordinary ethics applied to the 'bio-realm' (Clouser 1978, p. 150). The 'bio-realm' in this instance is to be distinguished from the 'medical realm' or 'nursing realm', which refer to more particular, although related, realms of facts, values, beliefs and concerns.

Bioethics, in essence, is a subclass of ethics, which, in turn, is a branch of philosophy. Medical ethics and nursing ethics, on the other hand, are distinctive specialised fields of inquiry naturally born of the practices of medicine and nursing respectively. Although the facts and concerns of these two disciplines overlap in many areas, they are ideologically separate in their endeavours, and it would be conceptually incorrect to treat them as being synonymous. Some authors have suggested that nursing ethics is merely a 'subcategory of medical ethics' (see, for example, Veatch 1985; Veatch and Fry 1987). However, from the definition given earlier, it is quite apparent that these concepts are distinct — that bioethics, biomedical ethics and medical ethics are most definitely not one and the same thing. The generic use of the term 'medical' is misleading, and serves to promote the hegemony of the medical profession in this area. At best medical ethics is merely a sub-category of bioethics, as is nursing ethics (Johnstone 1987b).

In considering bioethics and its relation to medical ethics and nursing ethics, it needs to be understood that 'medicine', 'nursing' and 'health' are quite distinct concepts, as are the notions of 'medical care', 'nursing care' and 'health care'. To hold 'medicine' as paradigmatic of 'health' is, as Kleinman (1980, p. 37) correctly points out, 'ethnocentric and reductionistic', or, to borrow from Barnard 1988, 'medicocentric'. 'Health' involves a holistic concept of well-being, in contrast with the notion of the mere reduction or absence of disease (Eberst 1984; Boddy 1985; Newman 1986; Nordenfelt 1987). As well, the social reality is that 'health care' can be and is provided by entities other than 'scientific professionals' such as doctors; health care is also provided by folk healers and by lay (or popular) healers and care givers (most of whom are women who are not paid for their 'labour of love' (Waring 1988; Rowland 1988; Abel and Nelson 1990). In this tripartite model of health care (namely scientific professionals, folk healers, and lay healers and care givers), scientific health professionals comprise only a very small percentage of health care deliverers. Chrisman (1981), for example, cites an American study on this issue:

> ... only 10 to 20 per cent of the people who are sick at a particular time consult a scientific health professional about the health problem ... only about 1 to 2 per cent of those who consult a physician are hospitalized ... . Most of the invisible majority (the 70 to 90 per cent who do not seek professional care) receive help with health problems from other people.
>
> (Chrisman 1981, p. 38)

The 'other people' in this instance include lay healers and care givers, notably mothers, grandmothers, sisters, friends, spouses, and so on, and folk healers, notably herbalists, masseurs and the like (Sax 1984; Abel and Nelson 1990). Practitioners such as chiropractors and osteopaths used to be classified as folk healers; more recently, however, they have begun to adopt the characteristics of 'scientific health professionals' (for example, formalised education modes, the use of diagnostic technology such as X-ray machines, wearing conventional 'doctors' white coats'), and thus no longer fall so neatly under the 'folk healer' category.

The implication of these observations is that the practice of medicine and the medico-moral point of view are in fact minority considerations in the broader domain of bioethics — a point that is poorly understood even in modern moral philosophy, as evidenced by the medical bias of the *Encyclopedia of bioethics* (Reich 1978) discussed in the previous chapter. The implications of this for nursing and the question of nursing ethics generally will become increasingly apparent in the ensuing chapters. Meanwhile, there remains the task of answering the question: what is ethics?

Modern moral philosophy and its view of ethics

Western moral philosophy has its origins in ancient Greece, and to date has been strongly influenced by the ancient Greek philosophers Socrates (born 469 BC), Plato (born 428 BC) and Aristotle (born 384 BC). The works of these early philosophers saw to it that ethics was firmly established as a branch of philosophical inquiry which sought rational clarification and justification of the basic assumptions and beliefs that people have about what is to be considered morally acceptable and morally unacceptable behaviour. This early mode of ethical inquiry asked people to question why they considered a particular act either right or wrong, and further, whether their judgments were correct. This view of ethics has been a lasting one, and is as relevant to defining the nature of modern moral philosophy as it is to defining ancient moral philosophy.

Ethics, as a critically reflective activity, remains fundamentally concerned with the systematic examination of the moral life and 'is designed to illuminate what we ought to do by asking us to consider and reconsider our ordinary actions, judgments and justifications' (Beauchamp and Childress 1983, p.xii).

In conducting its examinations of the moral life, ethical inquiry concerns itself not so much with how the world is, but rather with how it *ought* to be. In other words, ethics is not concerned with merely *describing* the world (although a description of the world would of course be helpful to its discourse), but rather in *prescribing* how it should be. Its prescriptions are given through critically reflective guiding principles of conduct which are popularly, although controversially, regarded as *universal* (i.e., applying to all persons equally throughout space and time) and *overriding* (i.e., they may override all other considerations which might otherwise influence the choice a person actually makes — notions that will be examined further in the following three chapters). In this respect, then, ethics may be rather simplistically described as a complex system of prescriptive principles of conduct which, when critically applied, override all other considerations that might have had some bearing on the choices made and the actions taken in a given situation. Ethics in this sense is sometimes referred to as 'systematic ethics'.

The term 'systematic ethics' is therefore to be firmly distinguished here from 'common-sense ethics' or 'common-sense morality' as it is usually referred to. Common-sense morality, by contrast, is a system of rules which have largely been derived from considerations of habit, custom, convention, tradition and the like, and which are thought to be binding for no other reason or justification than that they have always been so (Weber 1964, p. 60). In short, as Singer (1979, p. 4) comments, it is 'the morality accepted by most people without systematic thought'. In deciding moral problems, appeal is made not to critically reflective moral principles of conduct, but to the dictates of habit, custom, convention, tradition and so forth. For example, given the dictates of common-sense morality, the question 'What should I do?' would probably be answered with something like: 'You should do what has always been done ...', or 'You should do what you have always done in the past ...', or 'Do what everyone else has done in the past ...' Here decisions are made on grounds of what is likely to preserve the status quo rather than challenge it. While common-sense morality has its place in the social schema, it is never regarded as supplying the ultimate principles of moral conduct, or as having ultimate moral authority in deciding complex moral matters. One reason for this is that it simply lacks the force of a more reliable and sound critically reflective moral schema.

What ethics is not

Now that we have come some way in discovering what ethics is, it would be useful to give some attention to what ethics is not. It is important in this debate to distinguish ethics from 'legal' law (i.e. law referred to in this text in the legal sense as distinct from moral law), a code of conduct or ethics, hospital etiquette, hospital policy, public opinion, following the orders of a superior, or even mere 'gut response' on the supposed rightness or wrongness of a given act. If nurses fail to distinguish ethics from these, they not only risk failing to prevent moral errors and harms from occurring in health care domains, but may actually cause them to occur.

1. LEGAL LAW

Ethics and legal law overlap in significant ways, but they are nevertheless quite distinct from one another. This distinction becomes particularly clear in instances where what the law may require in a given situation, ethics might equally reject, and vice versa. Consider, for example, the issue of active voluntary euthanasia and the plight of patients suffering intractable and intolerable pain who request euthanasia as a 'treatment' option. Current Australian legal law prohibits voluntary active euthanasia (Lanham 1993). As the law stands, it is quite clear that any nurse or doctor who administers a lethal injection to a patient with the sole intention of bringing about that patient's death would probably be charged with murder. The fact that such an act was demonstrably in accordance with the patient's rational wishes would not be a legitimate defence. Regardless of the benevolence and voluntariness of an act of euthanasia, it would still be deemed by law as illegal, and thereby *legally wrong*. This legal wrongness, however, is in no way synonymous with moral wrongness. Consider the following.

Secular moral law (the essence of which is discussed in greater detail in chapter 3) essentially requires that people be respected as rational and autonomous choosers, and further that the rational preferences of persons be maximised. This requirement holds even in instances where a person's individual preferences might be considered mistaken or foolish by others. Moral law also requires that otherwise avoidable harm (such as the needless suffering of intractable and intolerable pain) should be prevented where this can be done without sacrificing other important moral interests. Returning to our euthanasia example, it soon becomes clear that an application of moral law (or, more particularly, moral principles) in this instance would probably permit the administration of a lethal injection to a suffering patient who has rationally requested it. Not only would moral law permit such an act; it would most likely demand it to be done. Given the benevolence and voluntariness of the act, it would be deemed as having accorded with moral law and thereby as being *morally right*.

Other compelling examples illuminating the difference between law and morality can be found by considering the laws enforced during war time (such as those upheld by the Nazi regime), and the laws used to enforce apartheid (such as those upheld in early North America, and now in South Africa). The legal laws of the Nazis and of the apartheid-supporting regimes, although iniquitous, still stand as constituting valid *legal* law (Hart 1958). We would presumably want to resist condoning the *morality* of these laws, however.

Law and ethics are quite separate action-guiding systems, and care must be taken to distinguish between them. Making this distinction may not only help to prevent moral errors, but may also enforce moral and intellectual honesty about the undesirability of morally iniquitous law (Hart 1958). Further, if we do not make this distinction we will not have an independent value system from which to judge the moral acceptability or unacceptability of valid legal law. For instance, if morality were not distinct from legal law, we could not judge certain laws (e.g. Nazi laws) to be morally iniquitous.

The question remains, however, of how the distinction between law and ethics can be made, and, equally important, what the essential differences are between a legal decision and a moral/ethical decision, and, indeed, a clinical decision.*

A very traditional view of law is that it is the command or order of a sovereign (for example, a government) backed by a threat or sanction (for example, punishment) (Hart 1961). For instance, governments in the Western world have formulated laws which command their citizens to pay taxes; if the citizens in question fail to pay their taxes, they can expect to be punished in some way, such as by being fined or even sent to prison. The mere fact that they have not complied with the command — in essence, have broken the law — would probably be deemed sufficient justification for a sanction or punishment to be directed against them. Although this view of law does not capture its more political nature (see, for example, Kairys 1982; Thornton 1990; Fineman and Thomadsen 1991; Johnstone 1994b), it is nevertheless sufficient for the purposes of this discussion in regard to distinguishing between law and ethics.

Accepting the above view of law, there is a fundamental sense in which the concept 'legal decision' as it is used colloquially by nurses probably refers to a type of decision that is made on the basis of what is required or prohibited by law — together with a desire to avoid a legal sanction or punishment for non-compliance. In this respect, the notion 'legal decision' is probably more aptly described as a 'legally defensive' decision. Consider the following example. A nurse who regards voluntary euthanasia as morally justified in cases of intolerable and intractable suffering may nevertheless decline a patient's considered request for assistance to die in order to avoid any risk of receiving the penalty that would almost certainly be applied for murder should her actions be dis-

---

* The following discussion of these distinctions is drawn from Johnstone 1994a.

covered. In this instance, the nurse's decision not to comply with the patient's request could be described as a 'legal decision' rather than a moral or clinical decision, and also as being 'legally defensive'. This is because her decision was influenced predominantly by considering the legal consequences of complying with the patient's request, rather than the moral or clinical consequences of doing so.

The question remains, however, of how a legal decision differs from an ethical decision. As is discussed more fully in the following chapter, ethics can be defined as a system of overriding rules and principles which function by specifying that certain behaviours are either required, prohibited or permitted. These principles are chosen autonomously on the basis of critical reflection, and are backed by autonomous moral reason (generally recognised in moral philosophy as the central organising principle of morality) and/or by feelings of guilt, shame, moral remorse and the like which operate as kinds of moral sanctions. For example, we may choose autonomously to follow a moral principle which demands truth telling; if we fail to tell the truth in a given situation, we may then reason the act to be wrong and/or experience feelings of guilt, shame or moral remorse accordingly. Unlike what happens in instances involving a breach of legal law, however, we are not generally 'punished' for lying — for example, by being fined or sent to prison — unless, of course, our lying entails an outright act of perjury in a court of law.

Accepting this view of ethics, it is probably true to say that the concept 'ethical decision', as it is used colloquially in health care contexts, refers to a type of decision which is guided by certain prescriptive and proscriptive moral principles of conduct (rather than by punitive legal laws) and a desire to achieve a given moral end. Thus, a doctor or a nurse tempted to tell a lie to either a colleague or a patient may choose instead to tell the truth in order to achieve some predicted overriding moral benefit and thereby also preserve her or his integrity as a morally autonomous person (as distinct from, say, a law-abiding citizen).

In light of these simplistic views on law and ethics, what is the essential nature of nursing and medicine in this decision-making schema? Primarily, nursing and medicine involve the skilful practice and application of tested principles or applied science and care to prevent, diagnose, alleviate or cure disease, illness and sickness and restore a person's health and sense of well-being; the practices of nursing and medicine are backed by legal and professional sanctions. For example, doctors and nurses can be found financially liable for negligence, and can be deregistered for professional misconduct, or even for civil misconduct unbefitting a professional person (see, for example, Pyne 1981).

To say of a decision that it is a 'nursing decision' or a 'medical decision' in this context, however, is probably to say little more than that it has been made by a nurse or a doctor respectively, and is based on an established body of knowledge and 'reasonable' professional opinion on how this knowledge should or should not be applied in a clinical situation. For example, a doctor may venture the 'reasonable' medical opinion that if such and such a life-saving treatment is stopped the patient will surely die. Or a nurse may venture the 'reasonable' nursing opinion that if such and such a nursing care is not given the patient will suffer a particular type of harm. It must be understood here, however, that neither of the clinical opinions expressed in these instances is tantamount to expressing a valid moral judgment. For example, to say that a patient 'will die' if such and such a drug or other treatment (for example, surgery) is given or withheld says nothing about the moral permissibility or imperatives of giving or withholding the drug or other treatment in question. The morality of a given clinical act is not implicit in the act itself; this is something which can be determined only by independent moral analysis.

Given these rough comparisons, it can be seen that legal, ethical and clinical decisions can be readily distinguished from one another. What is also obvious is the enormous potential for the respective demands of each of these three types of decisions to come into conflict. For example, a medical decision not to resuscitate a patient in the event of a cardiac arrest (on the grounds that the patient's condition is 'medically hopeless') may be supported by an established body of medical opinion, but nevertheless be deemed morally unsound or even illegal, or both. For instance, the patient's autonomous wishes may not have been established before the medical decision was made, or the patient's legally valid consent may not have been obtained to withhold cardiopulmonary resuscitation (CPR) in the event of a cardiac arrest. Or, to take another example, a medical decision to continue treating a patient may accord with a 'reasonable body of medical opinion', be legal (as in cases where patients have been deemed rationally incompetent under a mental health act), yet be quite unethical if the patient has expressly stated a wish not to be treated, and if this expressed wish, contrary to popular medical opinion, is not 'irrational' (as happened in the John McEwan case, to be cited later in this text). We can also imagine cases where a medical decision to cease treatment accords with moral principles but may nevertheless invite legal censure — as in the case of withholding treatment from severely disabled newborns or severely brain-injured adults.

Although there is potential for conflict between ethical, legal and clinical decisions, it is not the case that these are always on a direct collision course; indeed, they may even be in full harmony with each other, as examples given later in this text show.

In drawing comparisons between legal, ethical and clinical decisions, there remains another crucial point to be observed: that it is conceptually incorrect to regard nursing or medical decisions per se as synonymous with either legal or moral decisions. This is not to say that we cannot meaningfully speak of nursing or medical decisions as being legally or morally correct or incorrect, as the case may be. On the contrary, it merely makes the point that, in asserting the legal or moral status of a given clinical (nursing or medical) decision, a judgment *independent* of the generally accepted scientific or indeed conventional standards of nursing or medicine must be made: in the case of ethics, the moral status of a clinical decision requires independent *philosophical/moral* analysis and judgment based on relevant ethical rules and principles; and in the case of law, the legal status of a clinical decision requires an independent *legal* analysis and judgment based on relevant legal rules and principles.

2. CODES OF ETHICS

In a little known but important essay entitled 'Ethics — or a code of ethics?', the distinguished American nurse Lavinia Dock challenged:

> What, exactly, could a Code of Ethics be?' [...] What are ethics and can they be codified? Do we aim at ethical exclusiveness and shall our ethical development be bounded or limited by a code? 'Code' suggests statutes, infringements, penalties, antagonisms. If we have the ethics, we will not need a code. The code is to regulate those who have no ethics, and in proportion as ethical principles are made a part of our natures and lives, our codes and restrictions will shrivel away and die the death of inanition.
>
> (Dock 1900, p. 37)

Dock goes on to explain that she is not advocating the total rejection of rules and regulations of professional conduct — to the contrary, particularly since such rules and regulations, as given in a code, could serve as helpful mechanisms 'to prop up the steps of those who are young in self-government or feeble in self-control' (p. 38). Rather, the issue was not to call codes of rules and regulations *ethics*, since, as she argued persuasively, there was a real risk that:

> If we call them ethics we may perhaps come to believe that they are all there is of ethics, and presently be worshipping the code rather than the thing — so unreasoning a reverence is there in

our souls for statutes, fines, and punishments; so exaggerated a notion of the potency of drafted laws; so strong a tendency to make rules the end and aim of life rather than simply conveniences, changeable contrivances.

(Dock 1900, p. 38)

Although written almost a century ago, Dock's visionary words are applicable today. And nurses around the world would be well advised to be cautious in their use of formally stated and adopted codes of ethics, and to be especially vigilant not to fall prey to 'worshipping the code' at the expense of *being* ethical — and not to fall into the trap of treating the prescriptions and proscriptions of a code as absolute, and as ends in themselves, rather than as prima facie guides to ethical professional conduct.

It has long been recognised that a professional code of ethics is an important hallmark of a profession (Goldman 1980; Bayles 1981; Johnstone 1986). Whether professional codes as such have succeeded in fulfilling their intended purpose of 'formulating the norms of professional ethics' (Bayles 1981, p. 25) and guiding ethical professional conduct is, however, another matter. Some have argued that codes of ethics have failed to ensure this; instead, codes of ethics have served to protect the interests of the professional group espousing them, rather than the interests of the client groups whom the professionals are supposed to be serving (Kultgen 1982, pp. 53–69, Beauchamp and Childress 1989, pp. 10–13).

Despite the demonstrable shortcomings of professional codes of ethics, it is evident that many professional codes of ethics (such as those included as appendixes to this text) have been written with the noble intention of guiding ethically just professional practice. What needs to be understood, however, is that even the most scrupulously formulated and well intended professional code of ethics is not without its limitations and, in the final analysis, may do little to either guide moral deliberation or ensure the realisation of morally just outcomes in morally problematic situations. In the case of the nursing profession, neither will following a code of ethics necessarily protect nurses when they are called upon to defend their actions, say, in a court or disciplinary hearing (see Johnstone 1994b, pp. 251–67).

In the noted case of *Warthen v. Toms River Community Memorial Hospital* (1985), for example, the court dismissed altogether the ANA Code for Nurses as an authoritative statement of public policy. And in a recent Australian case involving the alleged unfair dismissal of a registered nurse involved in a case of suspected child sexual abuse, the Deputy President of the Industrial Relations Commission of Victoria criticised and rejected the authority of the ICN (1973) *Code for Nurses*, which was referred to in defence of the nurse's actions in this area. Specifically, the Deputy President of the Commission criticised the ICN Code as being 'imprecise' and lacking the ability to provide 'clear guidance' in matters requiring fine discretionary professional judgment. He also pointed out that the 'code in its terms cannot stand alone' and must be considered in relation to the guidance which is also offered by the law (*In re alleged unfair dismissal of Ms K. Howden by the City of Whittlesea* 6/9/90). The fact that the ICN Code is widely accepted by professional nursing organisations around the world had little bearing on the Deputy President's views in this case. The legal status of the acclaimed *Code of Professional Practice* of the United Kingdom Central Council for Nursing, Midwifery and Health Visiting (1984) is also uncertain, its authority having been rejected by at least one court since its adoption in the early 1980s (Rea 1987, p. 534).

One question which arises here is that, if codes of ethics are problematic, and have only limited legal (and, it should be added, moral) authority, should nurses adopt them? The short answer to this question is, yes. The primary justification for this is that, despite their limitations, codes of ethics have an important role to play in the broader schema of professional nursing ethics in so far as they can provide a public statement on the kinds of moral standards and values that patients and the broader community can expect nurses to uphold, and against which nurses can be held publicly accountable. They can also inform those contemplating entering the profession of the kinds of values and standards which they will be expected to uphold, and which, if not upheld, could result in some sort of professional censure. For example, the ICN *Code for Nurses* makes explicit that a nurse's 'primary responsibility is to those people who require nursing care', and that, in providing care, the nurse will promote 'an environment in which the values, customs and spiritual beliefs of the individual are respected'. If people contemplating entering the profession of nursing are informed of these prescriptions, and do not agree with them, they will be in a better position to make an informed choice about whether to enter the profession.

The point remains, however, as already argued, that codes of ethics have only prima facie moral authority (that is, they may be overridden by other and stronger moral considerations), and hence can only guide, not mandate, moral conduct in particular situations. Further, as Seedhouse (1988, p. 65) points out, it is important to understand that a code cannot inform a nurse which principles to follow in a given situation, how to interpret chosen principles, how to choose between conflicting principles, or 'how to decide when it is most ethical to disregard the rules and deliberate instead as a unique and independent individual' as is sometimes required. Accepting this, and as the examples given in the following chapters show, it can be seen that no code of professional nursing ethics should be regarded as an authoritative statement of universal action guides. Rather, it should be regarded only as a statement of prima facie rules which may be helpful in guiding moral decision making in nursing care contexts, but which can be justly overridden by other and stronger moral considerations.

3. HOSPITAL OR PROFESSIONAL ETIQUETTE

Nothing could be more different from ethics than etiquette. Although both seek to guide behaviour and conduct, they do so in quite different ways and for quite different purposes. Ethics, for example, speaks to morally significant rights and wrongs, with behaviour being guided by critically reflective moral principles which seek to maximise the interests of all people equally. Etiquette, by contrast, speaks more to maintaining style and decorum, with behaviour being guided by the unreflective and arbitrary dictates of custom and convention. In application, etiquette paves the way for coordinated, consistent, predictable and, where possible, aesthetically pleasant practice and conduct, and serves only the interests of particular persons in particular circumstances (May 1983). As with legal law, what etiquette might demand in one situation, systematic ethics might reject, and vice versa.

The extent to which the notions of ethics and etiquette are confused in health care settings is well illustrated by the following cases — all of which, in varying degrees, emphasise the reluctance by health professionals (including nurses) to advise patients to seek a second medical opinion, in the mistaken belief that doing so would constitute a serious breach of ethics.

The first case (personal communication) involves a middle-aged woman suffering moderately severe retrosternal chest pain and shortness of breath who presented to the accident and emergency department of a large city hospital. The nursing staff admitted the woman into a cubicle equipped to deal with 'cardiac emergencies' and proceeded to perform an electrocardiograph (ECG). The ECG showed a number of cardiac arrhythmias, all of which were suggestive of an acute cardiac condition warranting immediate specialised medical and nursing care. Upon further questioning, it was revealed that the woman was also suffering a mild pain in her left arm (a pain she had 'never had before'), which is characteristic of cardiac disease. The pain improved, however, while she rested in the casualty department. Her past medical history indicated no known heart disease or any previous incidence of chest pain. This was the first time she had ever experienced such symptoms — symptoms which were indicative of significant underlying cardiac disease.

A first-year medical resident examined the woman and decided she should be admitted immediately into the coronary care unit for further cardiac monitoring and tests. As required by the hospital's admission policy, he contacted the registrar 'on call' to have his diagnosis confirmed and to arrange the woman's admission formally. Upon examining the patient, however, the registrar declined to admit her, since there were no 'cardiac beds' available in the hospital and he was not convinced that the ECG findings indicated a life-threatening cardiac condition. He discharged the woman, advising her to see her own general practitioner the following morning. He gave her a medical note and a prescription for an oral cardiac anti-arrhythmic agent.

The nursing staff were very concerned, as was the junior first-year medical resident. All felt the patient should have been seen by another doctor for a 'second opinion', but could not decide whether to advise the woman to go immediately to another hospital. After some twenty minutes of deliberation, the attending nursing supervisor concluded it would be 'unethical' to advise the patient to go to another hospital for a second examination. The nursing staff and junior doctor involved agreed. The patient walked out of the door and was not informed that it would be in her interests to seek a second medical opinion. At this hospital, it was not 'standard practice' to advise patients to seek second medical opinions; such actions were perceived as not conforming with established hospital etiquette.

The second case is taken from Wendy Carlton's *In our professional opinion* (1978), and concerns an eleven-year-old girl with Down's Syndrome who was two months past menarche. The girl was admitted to hospital for a cardiac catheterisation in order to assess whether she could withstand the stresses of a hysterectomy (and a general anaesthetic); the hysterectomy had been recommended as a contraceptive measure. When a third-year medical student sought an explanation for why the girl was being admitted for such an elaborate procedure (it was evident to him that an oral contraceptive would have been quite sufficient to deal with the problem), a senior doctor admitted, 'It's a long drive on a short punt' (Carlton 1978, p. 33). When asked whether the girl's parents had been informed of the risks of the procedure, the attending doctor replied 'that he had minimised the risk rather than refusing to do the procedure, because "it turns people off, and they go elsewhere to get it done"' (Carlton 1978, p. 33). Another doctor, however, was strongly against the idea of the girl having the hysterectomy. He argued that 'a tubal ligation at sixteen was a real possibility, but not a hysterectomy at eleven' (Carlton 1978, p. 33). Many involved in the case felt that the proposed procedures (i.e. the cardiac catheterisation and the hysterectomy) were unnecessary. Although the suggestion was made to contact the doctor who would be doing the cardiac catheterisation, 'the call was never made': '[No one] was willing to incur the probable wrath of Dr Fine [the attending physician], who would resist any criticism of his clinical judgment. The proposed phone call would be a violation of *professional etiquette* [italics added]' (Carlton 1978, p. 34).

The last case to be considered here concerns a woman who was advised by her surgeon to have a radical mastectomy for breast cancer (Johnstone 1987a). A domiciliary nurse involved in the care of this woman advised her to seek a second medical opinion, explaining that not all breast cancers warranted radical surgery, and that some conditions could be successfully treated by more conservative methods. Despite the fact that the woman's condition was indeed treatable by conservative methods (which the surgeon later admitted), the nurse was severely castigated by the surgeon in question — and by some of her nursing colleagues — and was criticised for being 'unethical'. The surgeon's response was: 'Yes, Mrs X would benefit from conservative treatment, but ...' (the 'but' implying he was a *surgeon* and was unable to offer a *medical* alternative). The patient did have a radical mastectomy. It is very clear that, contrary to popular criticism, and given a sound ethical analysis of this case, the nurse in question acted in a morally just way. Rather than breaching the demands of ethics, she had merely breached professional etiquette.

Etiquette has its place in the professional and health care arena; it is not without limits, however, and there is a great need to determine the boundaries within which it may and can be justly and defensibly applied. Unfortunately, as Blackburn (1984, p. 189) points out, people do 'often care more about etiquette, or reputation, or selfish advantage, than they do about morality'. The lesson to be learned here is that acting in accord with hospital or professional etiquette might sometimes be tantamount to acting unethically or immorally — or, in some instances, even illegally.

4. HOSPITAL OR INSTITUTIONAL POLICY

Hospital policy or institutional policy is often appealed to in order to legitimise a worker's actions and, in some cases, to settle a conflict of opinion about what course of action should be taken in a particular situation. In this respect, institutional or hospital policy plays an important practical role — it helps to coordinate 'the running of the system' and to make institutional practices consistent and predictable; nevertheless, it also paves the way for uncompromising control. Like legal law and etiquette, institutional policy can be morally iniquitous and in application can seriously conflict with the demands of ethics. The following case (taken from the author's personal observations) is a good example of how institutional policy can be at serious odds with ethics.

A twenty-year-old woman in advanced premature labour was admitted to the casualty department of a city hospital. She was of a traditional Maori background, married, and the pregnancy had been planned. This was her third premature labour. On the two previous occasions, she had spontaneously aborted at around twenty weeks' gestation. Her current pregnancy was also of approximately twenty weeks' gestation.

The obstetrics registrar was notified, but failed to appear before the young woman delivered her fully formed male fetus. The fetus was active upon delivery and was noted by nursing staff to have breathed, emitting a faint but audible high-pitched 'rasp' as it did so. In accordance with 'standard hospital procedure' the fetus was placed in a stainless steel kidney dish, taken immediately away from the mother's view, and placed, covered with a bed pan sheet, in the sluice room to die. The mother and her family, however, wanted to have 'the baby' near, not only to see it but more importantly to perform *karakia* (a kind of incantation or prayer), as stringently required by ancient Maori custom.*

Maori enrolled nurses working in the casualty department were greatly distressed by what was happening. As the mother and her family (one of whom was a *Tohunga*) were pleading to have the fetus returned, one of the Maori enrolled nurses went to the fetus in the sluice room 'to be with it, so that it would not die without knowing love'. Crying softly, she also admitted to a registered nurse involved in the case that she was going to offer a prayer 'for the child as he goes on his way ...'.

The doctor had, meanwhile, arrived in the department and examined the mother. He explained to her and her family that the fetus could not be released to them because 'tests had to be done on it'. He later explained to protesting nursing staff that fetuses delivered at the hospital were generally regarded as 'hospital property' and that it was 'hospital policy to send all aborted fetuses

---

* The Oxford scholar Makereti (otherwise known as Maggie Papakura), the first Maori scholar to publish a comprehensive ethnographic account of Maori life, offers an illuminating explanation of this custom. In her celebrated work *The Old-Time Maori*, first published in 1938, she wrote:

> A case of premature birth seldom happened in the old days, and when it did, was supposed to be caused by the mother's breaking the laws of tapu [taboo]. A *Tohunga* [priest] then had to perform a *karakia Takutaku* over the woman to send away the *wairua* (spirit) of the unformed child, which was supposed to fly about in space — or it might enter a *mokomoko* (lizard) — and do harm to living people. A *wairua* of this kind, having never been properly formed, would never know any feelings of affection or love, and so would only try to do harm ... to living men, women and children ...'

(pp. 121–2).

to the laboratory for analysis'. He also explained that the present case was particularly complicated because the fetus was of twenty weeks' gestation, and had breathed. It was therefore technically speaking a 'live birth', and thus an autopsy would have to be performed. This, he further claimed, was a legal requirement. Whether in fact this was correct was not known by those present at the time; informal sources have since indicated that autopsies cannot be performed without consent, and it is likely that the parents' claim to the fetus could have been legally upheld. Most of the registered nurses present nevertheless accepted the doctor's explanation and resigned themselves to 'hospital policy'.

One registered nurse, however, pressed the matter further and explained to the doctor that the 'hospital policy' in this instance was quite inappropriate given the situation at hand, and that to uphold the policy so rigidly stood to violate the Maori family's rights and interests. At the same time, the fetus had meanwhile been mistakenly submerged in the liquid preservative formalin and taken by a hospital orderly to the laboratory.

Fortunately, the doctor was sympathetic and sought to resolve the difficulties he perceived he would have with the hospital authorities by registering the fetus as being of less than twenty weeks' gestation, and as not having breathed. Nevertheless, the fetus was not retrieved from the laboratory for another twenty-four hours, by which time, sadly, considerable damage had already been done. The most the family and the *Tohunga* could now do was to try and appease the *wairua* through *karakia*, and to try and persuade it to travel without taking harm with it. The mother's single room was turned into a *marae* (meeting place) setting, and a *tangi* (funeral) commenced. This was an act of sheer desperation, and in part an attempt to explain to the *wairua* why the violation and act of cruelty had occurred. It was also to grieve for what they had lost, and what would be lost to them forever.

Upholding hospital policy in this case resulted in an unacceptable level of human suffering — suffering which could have been avoided by a more critically reflective approach to the situation. Had those present been more aware of their moral obligations to respect the wishes of the mother and her family, a morally tolerable outcome could have been achieved. Fortunately, as a result of this particular incident, the hospital policy was revised, making it much easier for Maori mothers to claim their spontaneously aborted fetuses.

This case demonstrates a situation where ethics is quite distinct from institutional policy, and where a review of ethical considerations may prompt reform of policy. It also shows how respect for hospital policy is not sufficient to ensure the realisation of morally desirable or morally tolerable outcomes.

5. PUBLIC OPINION OR THE VIEW OF THE MAJORITY

If ethics were merely a matter of public opinion or majority view, all we would have to do is conduct an opinion poll on a given practice or procedure; its results would suffice to confirm whether the practice or procedure in question was morally right or wrong. Polling would quickly reduce moral testing to a crude 'might is right' formula — a formula which history, for one thing, has shown to be overwhelmingly unreliable. For example, the 'might is right' formula witnessed the witch hunts of the fourteenth to the seventeenth centuries and the legal execution of many women who were killed by live burnings at the stake for alleged witchcraft (estimates range from less than a thousand to millions) (Ehrenreich and English 1973, 1979; Corea 1977, p. 23; Daly 1978, pp. 178–222; Achterberg 1991, p. 85; Hester 1992, pp. 128–30). It has witnessed the mass genocide of Jews, Cambodians, and, closer to home, Maoris and Australian Aborigines; it has witnessed abuses and lynchings of American blacks; and it has witnessed what Bellini (1987) calls the 'high tech holocaust'. Applied in health care contexts, the 'might is right' formula rightly causes feelings of intuitive unease. Consider the following examples.

In 1987, a Saulwick poll published in *The Age* indicated that an overwhelming majority of Australians (66 per cent) 'approved of abortion in some circumstances' (Stephens 1987, p. 5). In April 1989, three hundred thousand people demonstrated their public support of legal abortion by marching on Capitol Hill in Washington, United States (Wainer 1989, p. 4). If ethics were merely a matter of public opinion, in this instance we would clearly be committed to accepting the permissibility of abortion. If public opinion were to change, we would likewise be committed to accepting the impermissibility of abortion. A public opinion view of ethics, in this instance, could change a judgment on the rightness or wrongness of abortion from one day to the next.

To take another example, in 1988 Kuhse and Singer published the results of their research project surveying medical opinion on active voluntary euthanasia. Their findings indicated that 'a clear majority of those who responded to the questionnaire support active voluntary euthanasia and that many doctors have provided active help in dying' (Kuhse and Singer 1988, p. 623). If the majority view were to reign as the overriding moral view in this instance, doctors would be committed to support and practise active voluntary euthanasia until such time as the majority view changed.

A public opinion or majority view of ethics is open to serious objection. On a philosophical level, it violates a formal and necessary requirement for sound moral judgments, notably the requirement for *internal consistency* (Kuhse 1987, p. 25). Its findings are capricious, and thus morally unreliable. As well as this, on a more pragmatic level, there is the distasteful possibility that public opinion might be mistaken or wrong or misguided — particularly where public opinion has been manipulated by pressure groups or minorities (Brandt 1959, p. 59), or by the media, as occurred in the much publicised Chamberlain murder case in Australia, or by collective denial, as has occurred in cases of domestic and child abuse (Herman 1992). There is also, of course, the risk of opinion polls being fraudulent. As one woman wrote in a letter to the editor of *The Age:*

> If I felt strongly enough about the issue at hand [television phone-in polls] I could have spent the evening by my phone and, with the simple touch of one button, registered votes almost continuously without anyone being any the wiser to my hundreds and possibly thousands of votes ...
>
> ... Unfortunately many people never question the validity of opinion polls and instead take them at face value. I suspect that many think they represent general opinion, otherwise why conduct them.
>
> (Romanin 1988, p. 12)

It is not being denied here that public opinion is an important and relevant fact which should be taken into account when deciding what is right. On the contrary, public opinion which reliably indicates a certain view on a given matter might well be a useful tool in guiding beneficial social policy and law reforms. However, public opinion is not infallible in matters of morality and mere *common acceptance* does not imply validity (Brandt 1959, p. 57). The moral rightness or wrongness of an act can be decided only by sound critical reflection, not merely by public opinion or 'collective desire' or 'collective preference'.

6. FOLLOWING THE ORDERS OF A SUPERIOR

Modern Western moral thinking relies heavily on the notion of rationality, and in particular on rational persons autonomously and freely choosing the moral principles they are going to commit themselves to, and are going to rely upon for guiding their moral actions and decisions. In this respect (and see also chapter 3) it is autonomous reason that stands as a person's supreme moral authority. By this account, it can be seen that following the moral commands or authority of another is quite incompatible with the notion of autonomous moral thinking and acting. Moreover, it paves the way for the abdication of moral responsibility and accountability. Superiors have superiors, and these superiors have still more superiors. A hierarchical system of authority may mean in practice that, because everyone is accountable for a given action, it is difficult or impossible to decide who is to be held ultimately accountable (Barry 1982, p. 13).

A classic example of this occurred at Waikato Hospital, New Zealand, in 1982. The incident in question involved a twenty-eight-year-old woman who died after being given an incorrectly prescribed dose of morphine. At the coronial inquiry into her death, it was revealed that the charge nurse who administered the 50-milligram intramuscular dose of morphine did so on the insistence of the prescribing 'doctor' (who was in fact a final-year medical student from Australia). The prescribing 'doctor' in turn insisted that she 'did not prescribe the morphine, but simply passed on [the covering registrar's] prescription for the nurse to administer' (*Waikato Times* 1984b, p. 3). The medical registrar, in turn, claimed that he had worked from eight in the morning on Saturday to midday Sunday, and had only had four hours' sleep during that time — implying that 'the system' was to blame. The medical consultant under whom the registrar was working meanwhile stated that 'if he was asked' he would not regard the duties of the medical student as being 'those of a house surgeon' (the New Zealand term for medical resident) — implying that his registrar was ultimately responsible (*Waikato Times* 1984a, p. 1). The medical superintendent, in turn, stated that the registrar 'should have been in charge of prescribing narcotics' (*Waikato Times* 1984a, p. 1), while the Waikato Hospital Board suggested that 'no one person be blamed for the overdose' (*Waikato Times* 1984b, p. 3).

The coroner concluded that it would be quite 'unfair, unkind and not based on the evidence' to blame the medical student who prescribed the morphine for the woman's death. On the basis of the coroner's overall findings, the police did not press charges.

Admittedly this case emphasises more the issues of legal responsibility and accountability than those of moral responsibility. Legal and moral responsibility and accountability, however, travel a common path, as made evident by the much noted *Bormann defence*, named after Martin Bormann, third deputy under the Nazi regime of World War II, who argued in defence of his involvement in wartime atrocities that he was 'just following orders' (Barry 1982, p. 13). This kind of defence is a convenient 'moral cop-out' for those who have no sense of moral accountability, or a poorly developed sense, and who ordinarily try to justify their behaviour as Bormann did: 'I was told to do it'; 'I was expected to do it'; 'I was just doing my job'; 'That's how things operate around here'; and so forth (Barry 1982, p. 13).

The outcome of the 1945–46 Nuremberg trials made it abundantly clear that a plea of following the orders of one's superiors was not to hold as a legitimate defence in the eyes of the law. Such a precedent had already been well established for nurses as early as 1929, however, with the successful prosecution in the Philippines of a newly graduated nurse by the name of Lorenza Somera, who was found guilty of manslaughter, sentenced to a year in prison, and fined one thousand pesos because she had followed a physician's incorrect drug order (Grennan 1930). In court it was proved that the physician had ordered the drug, that Somera had verified it, and that the physician had administered the injection. But, as Winslow (1984) writes, 'the physician was acquitted and Somera found guilty because she failed to *question* the orders'. The case stunned nurses around the world. A campaign of protest was organised, and Somera was given a conditional pardon before serving a day of her sentence.

In an institutional setting, it is very easy to rationalise moral 'unaccountability':

> So many people, even institutions, can get involved at so many levels that moral buck-passing can become the order of the day. The blind pursuit of prestige and profits also blurs moral accountability. And most important, the intense pressure to keep one's job and to secure promotions can be used to justify almost anything. The point is that working within an organization provides easy excuses for abdicating personal moral account-ability for decisions and actions.
>
> (Barry 1982, p. 13)

One way of avoiding this abdication is to draw a firm distinction between ethics and following the orders of a superior, and to recognise that moral demands are always the overriding consider-ation, irrespective of a superior's orders. (This point is explored further in chapter 13 when conscientious objection is discussed.)

7. 'GUT RESPONSE'

A 'gut response' thesis of ethics holds that, if a person 'feels good' about a given act, the act in question is morally right. Conversely, if a person 'feels bad' about a given act, the act in question is morally wrong. This thesis is hardly tenable in a world comprised of diverse groups of people who have diverse preferences and feelings. Such a thesis would be wholly unhelpful in a situation where all the people involved had quite different feelings, and thus quite different views on what was morally right and morally wrong. There would probably be no satisfactory answer to the questions of *whose* feelings should count in a given situation, and *whose* feelings should be regarded as being ultimately correct.

It is not being suggested here that 'gut feelings' have no role to play in ethics or ethical decision making. Rather, it is being claimed that they do not have an *ultimate* role to play. At best the role of gut feelings is complementary to reasoned morality; at worst gut feelings alone may have no role at all. The issue of 'gut feelings' and intuition in moral thinking is explored more fully in chapter 3.

What is the task of ethics?

In considering what ethics is, and what it is not, it is also important to have some understanding of what exactly ethics is attempting to achieve; in short, what is the task of ethics?

In identifying and exploring the task of ethics, it is necessary to give a brief historical overview of the development of Western moral thinking. The task of ethics has been the subject of rigorous philosophical debate for almost two and a half thousand years. In the Platonic dialogues, for example, we are told that the ultimate task of morality is to find out 'how best to live' or, in other words, how to lead 'the good life' and enjoy supreme well-being (Allen 1966, pp. 57–255). For the British philosopher Thomas Hobbes (1588–1679), the task of morality is a little different: notably, to find a device that will ensure mutual agreement and cooperation among each of society's members. It was Hobbes' view that, without such a device, the prospects of human survival would at best be slim (Hobbes 1968 edn, p. 205).

Hobbes' concerns were echoed almost a century later by the Scottish philosopher David Hume (1711–76), who insisted, among other things, that morality was a subject of supreme interest since its decisions had the very peace of society firmly at stake (Hume 1888 edn, p. 455). Like Hobbes, Hume recognised that the human mind was more than capable of courting the undesirable qualities of 'avarice, ambition, cruelty [and] selfishness'; and, like Hobbes, he recognised that society's hope for peace depended very much on the formulation of certain rules of conduct (Hume 1888 edn, pp. 494–6). These rules of conduct need to be developed and enforced precisely because people fail to pursue the public interest 'naturally, and with a hearty affection' (Hume 1888 edn, p. 496).

The influential German philosopher, Immanuel Kant (1724–1804) took a slightly different view from his predecessors. Unlike Hobbes and Hume, he saw the task of ethics (or rather, moral philosophy) as being 'to seek out and establish the supreme principle of morality' (Kant 1972 edn, p. 57). Like those before him, Kant recognised that persons were vulnerable to being 'affected ... by so many inclinations and lacked the power to conduct their life in accordance with practical reason' (Kant 1972 edn, p. 55). Kant went on to argue that as long as the 'ultimate norm for correct moral judgment' is lacking, morals themselves will be vulnerable to corruption.

Kant's overall investigation succeeded in providing a supreme, although not uncontroversial, principle of morality for guiding human actions. This principle took the form of a *categorical imperative* which essentially commands that rational autonomous choosers should 'act only on that maxim through which you can at the same time will that it should become universal law' (Kant 1972 edn, p. 84). His final analysis made clear that the influences of self-interest and/or of individual 'feelings, impulses and inclinations' could have no place in a schema of sound morality (Kant 1972 edn, p. 84). If rational agents are to act morally, they must act in strict accordance with the dictates of rational moral law.

The moral law was seen by Kant as providing ultimate, overriding principles of conduct and ones which all rational agents ought to respect. He was optimistic that if all rational persons lived absolutely by the moral law then they could hope to live in a world (or rather 'a kingdom', as he called it) where rational agents would be respected as ends in themselves and not as the mere means to the ends of others (Kant 1972 edn, p. 96).

The influential views of Plato, Hobbes, Hume and Kant concerning the task of ethics continue to have force in modern moral philosophy. For example, the Australian philosopher John Mackie (born in Sydney in 1917) argues that so-called 'limited sympathies' exist as a profound threat to what might otherwise be regarded as the 'good life' (Mackie 1977, p. 108).* Mackie echoes the view that if an all-enduring and decent (harmonious) life is to be secured, the problem of limited sympathies needs to be counteracted. The only way this can be done is by finding something which will coordinate and marry together individual and differing choices of action. In other words, what is needed is a device which could act as a kind of 'invisible chain' keeping together many sorts of 'useful agreements' (Mackie 1977, pp. 116, 118).

The solution for Mackie lies squarely at the feet of morality, which he interprets as:

> a system of a particular sort of constraints on conduct — ones whose central task is to protect the interests of persons other than the agent and present themselves to an agent as checks on his [sic] natural inclinations or spontaneous tendencies to act.
>
> (Mackie 1977, p. 106)

Mackie argues further that a morality applied appropriately is a morality which will help to facilitate the realisation of the overall well-being of people. In order for morality to work in this way, however, it must have at its core the vital component 'humane disposition' (Mackie 1977, p. 194). A humane disposition in this

---

* Quotations from J. L. Mackie (1977), *Ethics: inventing right and wrong*, Penguin Books, Harmondsworth, Middlesex, are reproduced by permission of Penguin Books Ltd.

instance is that which 'naturally manifests itself in hostility to and disgust at cruelty, and in sympathy with pain and suffering whenever they occur' (p. 194). People who are of humane disposition, suggests Mackie, 'cannot be callous and indifferent, let alone actively cruel either toward permanently defective human beings or toward non-human animals' (p. 194).

The English philosopher Richard Hare also views the task of ethics in terms of imposing stringent requirements on persons to act in morally just ways. On this, Hare argues that:

> Morality compels us to accommodate ourselves to the preferences of others, and this has the effect that when we are thinking morally and doing it rationally we shall all prefer the same moral prescriptions about matters which affect other people ...
>
> (Hare 1981, p. 228)

Hare ultimately advocates morality as a form of compelling 'rational universal prescriptivism', and concludes (in somewhat Kantian terms) that 'moral reason leaves us with our freedom, but constrains us to respect the freedom of others, and to combine with them in exercising it' (Hare 1981, p. 228).

The notion that the task of ethics is to supply a system of ultimate, overriding principles of conduct is also supported by the contemporary American philosopher Stephen Ross (1972, p. 283), who argues that the goal of morality is 'to reach a common set of moral ideals which everyone can follow' or, rather, to 'seek principles of conduct which everyone can live by'. According to Ross, moral principles are needed to regulate our moral decisions and to help settle competing alternatives. Moral principles remind us of our overriding duties to others and of the merits of morally principled action. Principles of morality also lend people 'tools' which can be used to deal appropriately and effectively with moral crises and dilemmas in both everyday and special (e.g. professional) worlds. They remind us that, without secure, ultimate and overriding rules of conduct, people may find it all too easy to abdicate their moral responsibilities and to commit atrocities (the My Lai massacre during the Vietnam War is a poignant example of how unclear and unstable rules of conduct can contribute significantly to the realisation of atrocious human behaviour [see in particular Peers 1979, p. 33; Bilton and Sim 1992; Kelman and Hamilton 1989]).

More recently, the contemporary American philosophers David Gauthier, Tom Beauchamp and James Childress, John Rawls, and H. Tristram Engelhardt Jr have described the task of modern moral philosophy in similar terms again. Gauthier (1986, p. 6), for example, sees the task of ethics as to validate the conception of morality 'as a set of rational, impartial constraints on the pursuit of individual interest', and to adjudicate cases in which there are conflicts of interest. Beauchamp and Childress, on the other hand, suggest that the task of ethics is to supply an 'ideal code consisting of a set of rules that guide the members of a society to maximize intrinsic value' (1983, p. 40). And Rawls (1971) describes the task of ethics as that of developing a way of ordering interests. The most refreshing of all views, however, comes from Engelhardt (1986), who sees the task of ethics as searching for common grounds to bind rational individuals in a peaceable community — in short, to achieve peaceable bonds among persons. He also sees the task of ethics as being that which:

> aspires to provide a logic for a pluralism of beliefs, a common view of a good life that can transcend particular communities, professions, legal jurisdictions, and religions, but whose grounds for authenticity are immanent to the secular world.
>
> (Engelhardt 1986, p. 26)

Towards achieving peaceable outcomes

In light of the views considered so far, it can be seen that the task of ethics is a complex and complicated one. Nevertheless, it is a worthwhile task, and, if successful, promises a great deal for the world at large, not to mention for health care domains. Its attempts to achieve peaceable bonds among people, and to assist in securing agreement among people of different world views, are by no means trivial and afford an optimism which might otherwise not be felt if we were all left to our own devices and to pursue our own unconstrained self-interest. It is to the content of moral thinking, and to showing how ethics might succeed in fulfilling its difficult task, that the next chapter now turns.

References

Abel, E. K. and Nelson, M. K. (eds) (1990). *Circles of care: work and identity in women's lives*. State University of New York Press, Albany.

Achterberg, J. (1990). *Woman as healer*. Rider (imprint of Random Century Group), London.

Allen, R. E . (ed.) (1966). *Greek philosophy: Thales to Aristotle*. The Free Press, MacMillan, New York, pp. 57–255.

Barnard, D. (1988). 'Ship? What ship? I thought I was going to the doctor!': patient-centred perspectives on the health care team. In N. M. P. King, L. R. Churchill and A.W. Cross, *Physician as captain of the ship*, D. Reidel, Dordrecht, pp. 89–111.

Barry, V. (1982). *Moral aspects of health care*. Wadsworth, Belmont, California.

Bayles, M. D. (1981). *Professional ethics*. Wadsworth, Belmont, California.

Beauchamp, T. L. and Childress, J. F. (1983). *Principles of biomedical ethics*, 2nd edn. Oxford University Press, New York.

Beauchamp, T. L. and Childress, J. F. (1989). *Principles of biomedical ethics,* 3nd edn. Oxford University Press, New York.

Bellini, J. (1987). *High tech holocaust.* Greenhouse Publications, Richmond, Victoria.

Bilton, M. and Sim, K. (1992). *Four hours in My Lai: a war crime and its aftermath.* Viking, London.

Blackburn, S. (1984). *Spreading the word.* Clarendon Press, Oxford.

Boddy, J. (ed.) (1985). *Health: perspectives and practices.* The Dunmore Press, Palmerston North, New Zealand.

Brandt, R. (1959). *Ethical theory.* Prentice Hall, Englewood Cliffs, New Jersey (see in particular chapter 4, 'The use of authority in ethics').

Carlton, W. (1978). '*In our professional opinion ...': the primacy of clinical judgment over moral choice.* University of Notre Dame Press, Notre Dame.

Chrisman, N. J. (1981). Nursing in the context of social and cultural systems. In P. Mitchell and A. Loustau, *Concepts basic to nursing,* McGraw-Hill, New York, pp. 37–52.

Clouser, K. Danner (1978). Bioethics. In Reich, *Encyclopedia of bioethics,* pp. 115–27.

Corea, G. (1977). *The hidden malpractice: how American medicine treats women as patients and professionals.* William Morrow & Company, New York.

Daly, M. (1978). *Gyn/Ecology.* The Women's Press, London.

Dock, L. L. (1900). Ethics — or a Code of Ethics? In L. L. Dock, *Short papers on nursing subjects,* M. Louise Longeway, New York, pp. 37–56 (p. 57 missing).

Eberst, R. M. (1984). Defining health: a multidimensional model. *JOSH* 54 (3), March, pp. 99–104.

Ehrenreich, B. and English, D. (1973). *Witches, midwives, and nurses: a history of women healers.* The Feminist Press, Old Westbury, New York.

Ehrenreich, B. and English, D. (1979). *For her own good: 150 years of the experts' advice to women.* Pluto Press, London.

Engelhardt, H. Tristram Jr (1986). *The foundations of bioethics.* Oxford University Press, New York.

Fagin, C. M. (1975). Nurses' rights. *American Journal of Nursing* 75 (1), pp. 82–5.

Fineman, M. A. and Thomadsen, N. S. (eds) (1991). *At the boundaries of law: feminism and legal theory.* Routledge, New York and London.

Gauthier, D. P. (1986). *Morals by agreement.* Clarendon Press, Oxford.

Grennan, E. (1930). The Somera case. *International Nursing Review* 5, December/January, pp. 325–33.

Goldman, A. H. (1980). *The moral foundations of professional ethics.* Rowman & Littlefield, Totowa, New Jersey.

Hare, R. M. (1964). *The language of morals.* Oxford University Press, Oxford.

Hare, R. M. (1981). *Moral thinking.* Clarendon Press, Oxford.

Hart, H. L. A. (1958). Positivism and the separation of law and morals. *Harvard Law Review* 71 (1–4) pp. 593–629.

Hart, H. L. A. (1961). *The concept of law.* Oxford University Press (Clarendon Law Series), Oxford.

Herman, J. L. (1992). *Trauma and recovery.* Basic Books, New York.

Hester, M. (1992). *Lewd women and wicked witches: a 'study of the dynamics of male domination'.* Routledge, London and New York.

Hobbes, T. (1968 edn). *Leviathan* (reprinted from 1651 edn, with notes by C. B. MacPherson). Penguin Books, Harmondsworth, Middlesex.

Hume, D. (1888 edn). *Treatise of human nature* (edited by L. A. Selby-Bigge). Oxford University Press, London.

In re alleged unfair dismissal of Ms K. Howden by the City of Whittlesea 6/9/90 (Case No 90/3672, Decision D90/1933) IRCV (unreported)).

Johnstone, M.-J. (1986). *Professional ethics and the problems of conflict with ordinary morality.* Minor thesis completed in partial fulfilment of the requirements for the Master's Preliminary (Philosophy), Monash University, Melbourne.

Johnstone, M.-J. (1987a). Professional ethics in nursing: a philosophical analysis. *Australian Journal of Advanced Nursing* 4 (3), pp. 12–21.

Johnstone, M.-J. (1987b). Nursing and professional ethics. *Proceedings of the conference 'The Role of the Nurse: Doctors' Handmaiden, Patients' Advocate or What?',* Centre for Human Bioethics, Monash University, Melbourne.

Johnstone, M.-J. (1988). Ethical issues in planning rehabilitation in patients with advanced cancer. Paper presented at seminar, 'Rehabilitation in patients with advanced cancer — a contradiction in terms?', College of Nursing, Australia, in conjunction with Victorian Association of Hospice Care Programs, Melbourne, 17 October.

Johnstone, M.-J. (1994a). Ethical aspects. In J. Romanini and J. Daly, *Critical care nursing: Australian perspectives,* W. B. Saunders/Baillière Tindall, Sydney.

Johnstone, M.-J. (1994b). *Nursing and the injustices of the law.* W. B. Saunders/Baillière Tindall, Sydney.

Kairys, D. (ed.) (1982). *The politics of law: a progressive critique.* Pantheon Books, New York.

Kanitsaki, O. (1988). Cancer and informed consent: a cultural perspective. Paper presented at seminar, 'Controversial Ethical Issues in Patients with Cancer', Heidelberg Repatriation General Hospital, Melbourne, 13 October.

Kanitsaki, O. (1989). Crosscultural sensitivity in palliative care. In P. Hodder and A. Turney (eds), *The creative options of palliative care,* Pandora, Sydney, pp. 13–19.

Kanitsaki, O. (1993). Transcultural human care: its challenge to and critique of professional nursing care. In D. A. Gaut, *A global agenda for caring,* National League for Nursing Press, New York, pp. 19–45.

Kanitsaki, O. (1994). Cultural and linguistic diversity. In J. Romanini and J. Daly, *Critical care nursing: Australian perspectives,* W. B. Saunders/Baillière Tindall, Sydney.

Kant, I. (1972 edn). *The moral law* (translated by H. J. Paton). Hutchinson, London.

Keireini, E. (1983). International Council of Nurses, Council of National Representatives Meeting, Brasilia, Brazil, 6–10 June 1983. *New Zealand Nursing Journal* 76 (9), pp. 3–9.

Kelly, L. Y. (1985). *Dimensions of professional nursing,* 5th edn. Macmillan, New York.

Kelman, H. C. and Hamilton, V. L. (1989). *Crimes of obedience.* Yale University Press, New Haven and London.

Kleinman, A. (1980). *Patients and healers in the context of culture.* University of California Press, Berkeley, Los Angeles.

Kuhse, H. (1987). *The sanctity-of-life doctrine in medicine: a critique.* Clarendon Press, Oxford.

Kuhse, H. and Singer, P. (1988). Doctors' practices and attitudes regarding voluntary euthanasia. *Medical Journal of Australia* 148 (June 20), pp. 623–7.

Kultgen, J. (1982). The ideological use of professional codes. *Business and Professional Ethics Journal* 1 (3), Spring, pp. 53–69.

Ladd, J. (1978). The task of ethics. In Reich, *Encyclopedia of bioethics,* pp. 400–7.

Lanham, D. (1993). *Taming death by law.* Longman Professional, Melbourne.

Mackie, J. L. (1977). *Ethics: inventing right and wrong.* Penguin Books, Harmondsworth, Middlesex.

Makereti (1986). *The old-time Maori.* New Women's Press, Auckland, New Zealand.

May, W. F. (1983). Code and covenant or philanthropy and contract? In S. Gorovitz, R. Macklin, A. L. Jameton, J. M. O'Connor and S. Sherwin (eds), *Moral problems in medicine,* 2nd edn. Prentice Hall, Englewood Cliffs, New Jersey, pp. 83–99.

Newman, M. A. (1986). *Health as expanding consciousness.* C. V. Mosby, St Louis, Missouri.

Nordenfelt, L. (1987). *On the nature of health.* D. Reidel, Dordrecht.

Peers, Lt Gen. W. R. (1979). *The My Lai Inquiry.* W. W. Norton, New York.

Pyne, R. H. (1981). *Professional discipline in nursing: theory and practice.* Blackwell Scientific Publications, Oxford.

Rawls, J. (1971). *A theory of justice.* Oxford University Press, Oxford.

Rea, K. (1987). Negligence. *Nursing. The Add-on Journal of Clinical Nursing* 3 (14), pp. 533–6.

Reich, W. T. (ed.) (1978). *Encyclopedia of bioethics.* The Free Press, New York.

Romanin, S. (1988). TV telephone poll was unsatisfactory. *The Age,* 11 February, p. 12.

Ross, S. D. (1972). *Moral decision: an introduction to ethics.* Freeman, Cooper & Company, San Francisco, California.

Rowland, R. (1988). *Woman herself: a transdisciplinary perspective on women's identity.* Oxford University Press, Melbourne.

Sax, S. (1984). *A strife of interests: politics and policies in Australian health services.* George Allen & Unwin, Sydney.

Seedhouse, D. (1988). *Ethics: the heart of health care.* John Wiley & Sons, Chichester.

Singer, P. (1979). *Practical ethics.* Cambridge University Press, Cambridge.

Stephens, P. (1987). Tolerance of abortion is much wider now. *The Age,* 7 December, p. 5.

Thornton, M. (1990). *The liberal promise: anti-discrimination legislation in Australia.* Oxford University Press, Melbourne.

United Kingdom Central Council for Nursing, Midwifery and Health Visiting [UKCC] (1984). *Code of Professional Conduct for the Nurse, Midwife and Health Visitor,* 2nd edn. UKCC, London.

Veatch, R. M. (1985). Nursing ethics, physician ethics and medical ethics. *Bioethics Reporter* 6 (7), pp. 381–3.

Veatch, R. M. and Fry, S. T. (1987). *Case studies in nursing ethics.* J. B. Lippincott Company, Philadelphia.

Waikato Times (1984a). Waikato Hospital chief says: morphine off limits to trainee. 16 February, p. 1.

Waikato Times (1984b). Police to lay no charges. 11 July, p. 1.

Wainer, J. (1989). Report on the pro-abortion march in Washington. *Alive and WEL* (May), pp. 4–5.

Walton D. N. (1980). The ethical force of definitions. *Journal of Medical Ethics* 6, pp. 16–18.

Waring, M. (1988). *Counting for nothing: what men value and what women are worth.* Allen & Unwin, Port Nicholson Press, Wellington (NZ).

Warnock G. J. (1967). *Contemporary moral philosophy.* Macmillan Education, Basingstoke, UK.

Warthen v. Toms River Community Memorial Hospital 488 A 2d 229 (NJ Super AD 1985).

Weber, M. (1964). *The theory of social and economic organisation.* The Free Press, New York.

Winslow, G. R. (1984). From loyalty to advocacy: a new metaphor for nursing. *Hastings Center Report* 14 (3), June, pp. 32–40.

Chapter

3

Western moral philosophy

Its modes, theories and conclusions

OUR STUDY OF BIOETHICS would be less than complete if it did not include some discussion on the ethical theories that have emerged from Western philosophical thinking.

Not everybody has been in agreement with the idea of a general (universal) moral theory which would deal with particular ethical problems; some have seen a need for moral theories which apply only to particular fields, as in the case of medical ethics (Gert 1984, p. 532); and others have argued that ethics is — and can only ever be — culturally derived and relativistic (Stout 1988; Cortese 1990; Leininger 1990; Singer 1991; Elliott 1992). The problem of 'difficult cases', however, made the argument to abandon the more parochial and particular forms of ethics much more compelling — at least for health professionals. It became a matter of urgency to find and adopt a more general moral theory which would cover all cases.

In considering moral issues and problems in nursing practice, and in determining morally appropriate decisions and actions, there are at least four different and competing types of theory which can be appealed to. The first two types include the 'parent' theories of *deontological ethics* and *teleological* or *consequentialist* ethics. These 'parent' theories in turn have given rise to a number of competing subtheories. Neither of these theories is free of controversy, however, and they have been the focus of intense philosophical debate since their inception. Some consider deontological theories enlightening and persuasive, while others find them thoroughly objectionable, and even oppressive. Similar objections or supporting arguments are made for teleological or consequentialist theories. Still others find neither type of theory persuasive, and have sought to condemn both on grounds of untenability and implausibility (for example, the case of moral sceptics and ethical nihilists), or for being unworkable (for example, the case of moral pragmatists).

The third type of ethical theory which may be appealed to is contemporary *feminist moral theory*. I have chosen to address this type of theory separately in chapter 4, for three main reasons. First, feminist moral theory itself claims to be ideologically opposed to and incompatible with many of the features of a 'classical' or 'rationalistic' (masculinist) approach to Western philosophical and moral thinking. Second, the features of feminist moral theory differ significantly from those of the more classical moral perspectives; the theory does therefore deserve to be considered as a distinctive moral theory in its own right, and not merely as an emerging sub-category of mainstream (malestream) Western moral philosophy. Feminist moral theory has much to contribute to the development of a substantive ethic (and bioethic), and must be permitted to do so independently of any classic philosophical mode that might otherwise be imposed on it. My third reason for treating feminist moral theory separately is that it has much to offer the development of a holistic nursing philosophy, and not least to the philosophical basis of the nurse–patient relationship. It also has much to contribute to the development of a substantive philosophical professional nursing ethic — as, I hope, the discussion in chapter 4 will make evident.

The fourth and final type of ethical theory or approach which can be appealed to is *transcultural ethics*. Since this perspective warrants attention in its own right, it is considered in chapter 5, following the discussion of feminist moral philosophy in chapter 4.

The purpose of this book is not to discuss these theories at length (or the arguments and counterarguments against them) but to identify the development of Western moral thinking, its strengths and weaknesses, and to illuminate the direction (or directions) in which it is going, and to consider possible alternative directions. It is important for nurses to have some understanding of different and competing moral theories and the respective position each theory asserts, as these have some bearing on the frameworks nurses might later adopt for deciding ethical issues in the course of their work. If nurses are to make a wise and informed choice in this instance, they need to have the full picture of what each theory has to say, and has to offer.

Deontological theories

'Deontology' comes from the Greek *deon*, meaning 'duty', and *logos*, meaning 'discourse'. As an ethical theory, deontology takes 'duty' to be the basis of morality and holds roughly that some acts are obligatory regardless of their consequences. A number of important views derive from deontological ethics, including the theological, rationalistic, emotivist and intuitionist views, and the view offered by social contract theory. All these views raise interesting ethical questions for nurses.

1. Theological ethics

Classic deontological theory has its origins in religious ethics, and relies heavily on the idea of 'divine command'. It emphasises the moral imperative of obeying God because 'he [sic] knows what is best for us, and what is best for us is to obey him [sic]' (MacIntyre 1966, p. 111). To disobey God would be to become estranged from him [sic], and to risk denying ourselves the fruits of heaven. The ideal life is one marked by 'obedience to the will of God', regardless of one's own individual plans and desires.

For classic deontologists, it is God's command that determines whether something is to be regarded as morally right and good, and God's forbidding that determines whether it is to be considered wrong and bad. If God commands 'thou shalt not kill', 'thou shalt not steal', 'thou shalt love thy father and mother as thyself', and the like, then conduct that upholds or accords with these commands is right 'because and only because it is commanded by God' (Frankena 1973, p. 28).

This view is convenient, because it readily supplies concrete answers to otherwise complex problems. It is nevertheless problematic on a number of counts. First, it presumes the existence of God. The atheist (someone who has no sustained belief in the existence of God) would view God's supposed commands as having no content — as being 'fictitious' — and therefore totally lacking in terms of supplying compelling reasons for behaving in a 'divinely ordained' way. Atheist nurses working in a religious hospital (say, a Catholic or Jewish hospital) may find little if any consolation in any religious dogma put forward to justify certain moral–medical decisions made in the clinical setting. This also applies to atheist patients who might be admitted into a religious hospital for care.

A second problem here concerns the ethical limitations on God's omnipotence (Mackie 1962). If God is all-powerful, it follows that God has the capacity to create evil. This has important implications for the argument (generally raised in criticisms of a theological view of ethics) that, if God commands certain unjust and cruel acts, it follows that believers are committed to viewing such acts as morally right, good and obligatory. Believers might object, however, that, since God is all good, God is incapable of being cruel and would never command evil acts. While this is an interesting objection, it does little to rescue the thesis of God's being omnipotent. What is left seems to be the incompatible and logically contradictory thesis that God is both omnipotent (all-powerful and able to bring about all things — including evil) and not omnipotent (not all-powerful, and unable to bring about all things — especially evil) at the same time. A further, related, concern is raised by Socrates in Plato's *Euthyphro*: 'Is that which is holy loved by the gods because it is holy, or is it holy because it is loved by the gods?' (Allen 1966, p. 67). This famous Socratic dialogue questions the possibility of there being a superior reality that exists even above God. If such a reality does exist, God's supposed omnipotence and omnipresence are immediately thrown into serious question.

A third difficulty with the theological perspective is the problem of how mere mortals could possibly know whether God's commands are right or wrong (Frankena 1973, p. 29). This gives rise to one of two possibilities — either morality is totally arbitrary (we act morally simply because God commands us to), or it is intrinsically self-interested (we act morally simply to avoid God's wrath) — both of which stand to condemn a systematic and critically reflective morality and all that it stands for.

A more practical difficulty relates to the problem of how to reconcile differing theological views and interpretations of God's commands. For example, how is the Catholic view on the sanctity of life (which would, among other things, probably condone the administration of a blood transfusion in a medically urgent but possibly life-saving situation) to be reconciled with the Jehovah's Witness view on the sanctity of God's commands (which are held to include a prohibition against the administration of a blood transfusion in the same situation)? Again, how is the Christian Science view on the sanctity of faith (which would be likely to prohibit the use of material cures such as drugs) to be reconciled with the Jewish view (Musgrave 1987, pp. 183, 186) on the sanctity of life (which would be likely to condone the use of life-saving drugs)?

These questions belong properly to theological discourse, and cannot be considered here. Nevertheless, they raise some important questions for nurses, for example:

1. Can nurses validly claim a right to conscientiously object to assisting with or performing certain morally contentious (but legal) medical procedures on the basis of personally held religious beliefs, and if so, under what conditions?

2. To what extent are nurses bound to conduct their practice in a way that respects the religious beliefs of others?

3. Are nurses absolutely bound to respect the religious beliefs of others in situations where doing so would be likely to entail a violation of their (the nurses') personal moral values?

These questions are explored further in later chapters.

2. Rationalism

The theological or Judaeo-Christian view of deontology has been significantly modified under the influence of the famous German philosopher, Immanuel Kant (1734–1804). Kant's views to this day are a major influence on the development of Western moral thinking.

For Kant, the supreme principle of morality is 'reason', whose ultimate end is 'good will'. Reason is free (autonomous) to formulate moral law and to determine just what is to count as being an overriding moral duty. Kant held duty to be that which is done for its own sake — for its own intrinsic moral worth — and 'not for the results it attains or seeks to attain' (Kant 1972 edn, p. 20). Just what is to count as one's duty is determined by appealing to some formal (reasoned) principle or 'maxim'. In choosing such a maxim, however, we must take care not to choose something which serves merely to uphold our own individual interests or to satisfy our own unruly desires. Indeed, Kant went on to assert that it is precisely because of our human weaknesses (especially our inclinations towards satisfying our own desires and interests) that the maxim we adopt must have the characteristics of being a universally valid 'law' — that is, something which 'commands or compels obedience' (Kant 1972 edn, p. 21), and which is binding on all persons equally.

Kant's solution to the problem of establishing a universally valid law comes in his formulation of what he called the 'categorical imperative', which states: 'Act only on that maxim through which you can at the same time will that it should become universal law' (Kant 1972 edn, p. 29). What this maxim or formal principle essentially demands is that we should only act in accord with a given principle or set of principles if we can, *at the same time*, reasonably *will* that it should become binding on all others throughout space and time. For example, if we are to adopt, and act, in accord with a principle that, let's say, permits our lying to others, then we are committed to accepting that all others are permitted to lie to us in return. If, in adopting this principle, however, we do not accept that others should be permitted to lie to us, then we are prohibited from adopting it, since, in adopting or acting on the maxim in question, we 'cannot at the same time will that it should become universal law' (Kant 1972 edn, p. 29). As a point of interest, there are striking similarities between the demands of Kant's 'categorical imperative' and those of the Christian command to 'do unto others as we would have done unto ourselves', loosely referred to in moral philosophy as the 'golden rule'.

In summary, Kant believed that moral considerations are always overriding ones. Thus, in situations where a number of considerations are competing (for instance, between practical, economic, political, emotional, moral and cultural considerations), it is always the moral considerations which should 'win out', so to speak. For example, if a nurse is in the position of having to decide whether to risk losing his or her job (a practical consideration) by exposing the unethical conduct of a superior (a moral consideration), it is the moral consideration which is, according to Kant's view, the weightier of the two; the nurse, by this analysis, should expose the superior. Whether losing one's job is a purely practical consideration devoid of any moral content, however, is another matter.

As well as holding that moral considerations should always override non-moral considerations, Kant maintained that moral imperatives (as based on universal moral law) are by their very nature unconditional, absolute and inescapable. This means that moral imperatives, or duties in this instance, are both overriding and binding *regardless of their consequences*. Therefore we, as rational autonomous moral choosers, cannot escape the demands which a moral imperative may place upon us; the bottom line, given a Kantian deontology, is that we are absolutely required and therefore compelled to fulfil our moral duties. By this view, morally decent persons are those who fulfil their duties and who are not distracted by self-interested or practical considerations; morally indecent persons, on the other hand, are those who shirk or abandon their moral duties — probably in favour of other considerations such as the pursuit of material self-interest and pleasure.

Moral considerations and moral duties will be explored more fully as we go on to discuss the bioethical issues specific to grass-roots nursing practice. In particular, two important questions will be considered:

1. Does a nurse always have a duty to care for a patient who has been assigned to her or his care in instances where other non-moral considerations have an important bearing on the situation at hand?

2. Can superiors, all things considered, decently order or compel a nurse to perform a task or an act which would otherwise stand to violate that nurse's reasoned or critical moral judgment?

3. Emotivism

For the emotivist, a moral statement is nothing more than an expression of emotion or an expression of attitude for or against things (Harmon 1977, p. 30; McNaughton 1988, pp. 24–7). Moral statements, by this view, can never be meaningfully judged as either true or false. At best they can only be deemed appropriate or inappropriate, genuine or fraudulent, justified or unjustified, rational or irrational, and the like (Frankena 1973, p. 107; Flew 1979, p. 104).

One of philosophy's most powerful advocates of emotivism was the Scottish philosopher David Hume (1711–76), who maintained, among other things, that 'reason is, and ought only to be, the slave of the passions and can never pretend to any other office than to serve and obey them' (Hume 1888 edn, p. 415).

Hume utterly rejected reason or science as having ultimate moral authority, arguing that these things are nothing more than the 'comparing of ideas and the discovery of their relations' (Hume 1888 edn, p. 466). He regarded reason as 'utterly impotent' (p. 457) in moral domains and said that it is 'perfectly inert, and can never either prevent or produce any action or affection' (p. 458). The only power reason has, in Hume's conceptual framework, is to shape beliefs — and, even then, beliefs cannot be relied upon to move one to action, unless they are relevant to the satisfaction of some passion, desire or need (Harmon 1977, p. 5).

The question remains, how does Hume's ontology capture the making of moral judgments? In essence, Hume's morality is something to be 'properly felt' rather than 'rationally judged', with goods and evils being known simply by particular sensations of pleasure and pain (Hume 1888 edn, p. 470). He argued:

Nothing can be more real, or concern us more, than our own sentiments of pleasure and uneasiness; and if these be favourable to virtue, and unfavourable to vice, no more can be requisite to the regulation of our conduct and behaviour.

(Hume 1888 edn, p. 469)

In summary, the Humean account of morality sees the sensations of pleasure as distinguishing that which is virtuous, and the sensations of pain or uneasiness as distinguishing that which is vicious. If something appears either virtuous or vicious, there is no reason to doubt that appearance — the sentiment just 'stands on its own', so to speak. In this respect, to quote the famous Humean quip, ''Tis not contrary to reason to prefer the destruction of the whole world to the scratching of my finger' (Hume 1888 edn, p. 416).

One of philosophy's most sophisticated exponents of emotivism is the twentieth-century United States philosopher Charles Stevenson (born 1908). Stevenson argued that all moral statements are essentially an attempt to persuade others to share one's own attitudes about the rightness or wrongness of certain acts. He explained that to call something 'good' is to create an influence; that is, to try and influence the other person to have a 'pro-attitude' towards it. For instance, if we were to say to someone 'the use of brain-dead babies as organ donors is always morally wrong or bad', we would not only be expressing our own dislike of and hostility towards this practice, but would also be trying to make the listener share that dislike and hostility. Likewise, if we were to say to a person something along the lines of 'euthanasia in medically hopeless cases is good', we would not only be expressing our own preference and support for euthanasia, but would also be trying to make the listener share that attitude.

Stevenson thought that the persuasive effect of ethical terms, in so far as their ability to direct attitudes is concerned, derives from what he called 'a characteristic and subtle kind of emotive meaning':

> The emotive meaning of a word is the power that the word acquires, on account of its history in emotional situations, to evoke or directly express attitudes, as distinct from describing or designating them.
>
> (Stevenson 1944, p. 33)

The lesson here (contrary to the rationalist thesis) is that 'ethical terms cannot be taken as fully comparable to scientific ones' (Stevenson 1944, p. 36); we must pay careful attention to the emotive meanings of the terms we use, and must distinguish their evaluative function from their descriptive function.

Emotivism has been heavily criticised on a number of counts. In particular it has been criticised for its exclusion of rationality from moral arguments and for its failure to distinguish serious moral arguments from irrational or non-rational propaganda. Stevenson's views are particularly vulnerable to the objection that not all moral statements are instances of trying to persuade others to share one's personal point of view. For example, we may talk with someone who already shares our views and wish merely to reach a private decision. Harmon (1977, pp. 39–40) offers the more scathing criticism that emotivism is trivial and is not much different from simple common sense! The role of feelings in moral thinking will be raised again in chapter 4 in the discussion on feminist moral theory.

4. Intuitionism

Like other moral theories, intuitionism has a long and respectable history, pre-dating even Plato. Simply put, the thesis of moral intuitionism holds that moral principles and moral judgments are known to be true simply by intuition. For example, if a moral intuitionist were asked whether abortion is wrong, the reply would probably be: 'I just know it is', with the truth of this judgment taken as being more or less self-evident and thus not requiring any form of rational justification. Like emotivism, intuitionism totally rejects reason as having ultimate moral authority (Frankena 1973, pp. 102–5), and claims intuition as being the 'prime avenue to truth' (Goldberg 1983, p. 17).

The question remains, how does intuitionism *actually* determine the moral rightness or wrongness of a particular act? The short answer is that it determines the intrinsic good or bad nature of a given act, which in turn derives from the properties of that act — whether they are intrinsically good or bad. For example, an intuitionist might claim that the wilful act of leaving an innocent road-accident victim to die needlessly has the self-evident property of wrongness, whereas the thoughtful act of assisting and resuscitating an innocent road-accident victim and thereby preventing a needless and untimely death has the self-evident property of goodness.

The process of knowing by intuition the rightness or wrongness of an action goes something like this: first, properties making the act in question right or wrong must be determined. These properties in turn are classified as being either 'prima facie right' (i.e., the 'rightness' of the properties may be overridden by stronger moral properties) or 'wrong, all things considered' (i.e., in light of other morally significant considerations, and when these considerations have been weighed up against each other, the act is wrong) (Baier 1978a, p. 415). For example, resuscitating an innocent road-accident victim may be regarded as 'prima facie right' where other stronger moral considerations do not impinge (for example, the rescuer may risk her or his own life in the attempt to resuscitate or save the victim); whereas leaving the innocent accident victim to die needlessly might be regarded as 'wrong all things considered' (for example, when the rescuer is regarded as well qualified to instigate life-saving measures, and would be likely to succeed in the attempt, but is in too much of a hurry to stop, having promised to meet friends for a social dinner).

The second step involves determining the relative weight of given properties and deciding which imposes the more stringent of duties on a person to act. Once it has been decided which of the duties in question is the more stringent, the 'final duty', or 'duty, all things considered', can be established (Baier 1978a, p. 415). For example, once it is determined that the duty to save an innocent road accident victim's life is more stringent than the duty to fulfil one's promise to friends to share a social meal with them, so too is it established that saving the life of the innocent road accident victim is the 'final duty' or 'duty, all things considered'. How do we know this is our final duty, it might be asked? The answer? We 'just know', it is 'self-evident', and that is all there is to say on the matter.

Moral intuitionism is considered by many philosophers to be implausible. They have severely criticised intuitionism on the grounds that it is misleading; that it fails to answer important moral questions; that it is unable to define and analyse the properties to which ethical terms refer; that it lacks objectivity; that it fails to provide a theory of moral motivation (i.e., what motivates people to do morally good acts); that it fails to provide a convincing theory of moral justification; and, more seriously, that it cannot be relied upon to resolve moral conflict (Warnock 1967; Frankena 1973; Rawls 1971; Swanton 1987; Baier 1978a).

These criticisms may well be deserved, but they should not be taken as implying that intuition itself has no role whatsoever to play in moral or other forms of reasoning. Such a conclusion would represent a troubling loss to the bioethical debate and, not least, to the development of a substantive moral theory generally.

Intuition, reassuringly, has not been totally lost to mainstream contemporary moral thinking. In his book *Moral thinking*, Richard Hare (1981) puts intuition back on the road to philosophical respectability. Although Hare completely rejects intuition as the basis of moral thinking, and rejects its independent ability to resolve moral conflict, he nevertheless accepts that 'the intuitive level of moral thinking certainly exists and is (humanly speaking) an essential part of the whole structure' (Hare 1981, p. 210).

Hare basically argues that neither intuition nor reason is adequate on its own to deal effectively with moral problems. A sounder or more complete approach to moral thinking, he suggests, would be to admit a kind of 'collaborative relationship' between these two faculties and to cease viewing them as being necessary opponents:

> Let us be clear, first of all, that critical and intuitive moral thinking are not rival procedures, as much of the dispute between utilitarians and intuitionists seem to suppose. They are elements in a common structure, each with its parts to play.
>
> (Hare 1981, p. 44)

Admittedly, Hare views intuition in somewhat rationalistic terms. He regards intuition essentially as being comprised of prima facie moral principles which have been selected by critical thinking or reason (Hare 1981, pp. 49–50). This might lead anti-rationalists to be somewhat suspicious of his supposedly enlightened account of moral thinking. However, it should not detract from the worth of Hare's thesis or the significant contribution it can make to the development of a more progressive and flexible moral theory, one which can be more readily accepted by nursing philosophy. It is worth noting here that nursing professionals are now recognising formally the role that intuition plays in expert nursing practice and in making expert clinical judgments (Rew 1987; Rew and Barrow 1987; Benner and Tanner 1987; Miller and Rew 1989). This view has been rather forcefully articulated by the American nurse theorist Patricia Benner (1984), who speaks of intuition in terms of its being the beginning rules and formulas of practice, which has essentially moved to an unconscious level or 'gone underground' (p. 37). It can be seen that Benner's thesis is not incompatible with Hare's views on the subject.

Psychologists are also stressing the importance of intuition in our everyday practical and working lives, and the need to enhance it if we are to make better rational decisions. Goldberg (1983, p. 33) argues that intuition is very much a part of reason, and in fact plays a crucial role in aiding the reasoning process itself. Intuition does this by feeding and stimulating rational thought and then by evaluating its products. If a reason or a thought does not 'feel' right, the reasoner or thinker simply switches tracks. Goldberg even makes the radical suggestion that 'reason is merely slow intuition' (p. 37), and that intuition has a particularly important role to play when dealing with problems which are too complex to be solved by rational analysis (p. 23). Goldberg's thesis, again, is not incompatible with Hare's views, but his prescriptions are more fruitful. What is needed, concludes Goldberg, is:

> a balance and a recognition of the intricate, mutually enhancing relationship between intuition and rationality. We need not just more intuition but better intuition. We need not only to trust it but to make it more trustworthy. And at the same time we need sharp, discriminating rationality.
>
> (Goldberg 1983, p. 28)

Regardless of the classic objections raised against intuition, it has its place both in our moral thinking and in our everyday lives (see also Vaughan 1979). (It also has an important place in substantive nursing ethics, as is discussed in chapter 6.) As Urmson (1975, p. 119) correctly points out, intuition is needed to weigh up the 'plurality of primary moral reasons for action', something which, in his view, is no cause for either surprise or distress. Why is this? The answer is that the need for an intuitive weighing up of a plurality of moral reasons is 'not an irrational anomaly but our ordinary predicament with regard to reasons in most fields' (Urmson 1975, p. 119).

5. Social contract theory

A social contract view of ethics holds actions to be right or wrong on the basis of whether they conform to or violate the terms of the social contract between the individual and the state. Early social contract theorists argued that the individual should form an agreement with the state (or given ruling power) to surrender freely

certain liberties in return for the advantages of an orderly, beneficial and well governed society. Remnants of this crude contract-
arian approach can be found even today in many aspects of social
living. For example, by observing the road rules, we surrender
certain personal liberties in the hope of receiving safe road-driving
conditions in return. If people did not agree to follow the road laws
governing which side of the road to drive on, acceptable rates of
speed, behaviour at intersections, safe blood alcohol limits, and so
on, chaos and death would result (and do result, as the nation's
appalling road toll each year makes evident).

Remnants of crude contractarianism can also be found in the
social contract view of professionalism, which argues, roughly, that
if society wishes to receive well organised and skilful professional
services, it must be prepared to relinquish a certain degree of
autonomy and grant professionals special privileges of autonomy
and power in return. In exchange for these privileges, professionals
perform certain tasks and carry out certain duties that would not
be expected of them were they acting as 'ordinary' persons (Newton
1981). By surrendering a portion of its liberty and autonomy,
society can look forward in return to its interests being served by
these all-powerful and autonomous professionals. If its interests
are not served, and the professionals in question do not deliver the
organised and skilful services they promised to deliver (as in the
case of strike action), they may be deemed to have violated the
terms of their 'social contract' and thus may be justly censured (for
example, by being deregistered, charged with legal negligence,
fined).

Whatever the nature of the social contract, what emerges is the
classic position that the surrendering individuals become bound by
the political and social contracts into which they enter, and can be
justly censured for breaching their terms and conditions. Here the
contract forms the very basis of obligation and determines the
standard by which right and wrong actions, justice and injustice,
are to be measured (Hobbes 1968 edn; Locke 1947 edn; Hume 1947
edn; Rousseau 1947 edn).

Recent contract theory, however, takes quite a different view
from this classical position. It holds, for example, that right and
wrong actions, justice and injustice, are determined by the 'cooperative maximisation of good'. This maximisation of good is
achieved by all rational people choosing impartially (i.e., from
behind a strictly hypothetical and decontextualised 'veil of
ignorance') to adopt universal moral principles and to apply these
in a way that ensures that no other person is unfairly disadvantaged. Individual interests are secured not by political or social
bargaining (as in the case of classical contractarianism), but by a
procedural principle of justice whose judgments seek to provide
'the most appropriate moral basis for a democratic society' (Rawls

1971, p. viii). Rawls, an influential proponent of contemporary social contract theory, explains that the contract, which 'implies a certain level of abstraction', emphasises social cooperation and ensures the distribution of advantages only to those who do their 'fair share' (Rawls 1971, p. 16). The principle of justice works meanwhile to regulate further agreements between cooperating individuals (Rawls 1971, p. 11). Although it is beyond the scope of this text to consider Rawls' thesis in detail, and the many criticisms raised against it, some important questions raised by his notion of choosing from a hypothetical and decontextualised position are touched upon in chapters 4 and 5.

Rights and duties

Central to deontological ethics are the terms 'rights' and 'duties'. Nurses, like others, use these terms frequently — and may or may not use them correctly in each instance. The distinctions to be made between these is a matter warranting some in-depth attention.

RIGHTS

Moral rights (to be distinguished here from legal rights, institutional rights, civil rights, etc.) generally entail claims about some special entitlement or interest which ought, for moral reasons, to be protected. The kinds of interests for which protection might be sought include, for example, life, freedom, happiness, privacy, self-determination, fair treatment and bodily integrity. The language used in asserting rights typically involves expressions such as: 'I have a right to ...', 'It is your right to ...', 'They have a right to ...', and so on.

There is no single thesis of moral rights. The following is a brief overview of better known theories concerning the existence of moral rights and the conditions under which they can be validly claimed.

1.   Based on natural law and divine command

Natural rights theory argues that certain entitlements are simply 'built into' the universe like the laws of gravity, and as such are neither the products of human invention nor the constructs of other moral theories (Martin and Nickel 1980). A variation of this thesis is that natural rights have been divinely ordained for *all* human beings. From both these points of view, since the laws of nature and the ordinances of God apply equally to all human beings, it follows that all human beings, young and old, male and female, unconditionally have natural rights.

Objections to this account of moral rights derive from those raised against a theological account of morality generally. For example, if it were shown that God did not exist, or that natural law did not exist, this account of moral rights would immediately collapse because its very foundation had been pulled out from underneath it. Another objection rests on the problem that natural rights essentially defy scientific verification.

2. Based on common humanity

Another popular natural rights thesis is that all human beings have rights simply by virtue of being 'human' and 'equal'. What is critical to this thesis is the notion that 'being human' is something over which we have no control; that is, we cannot choose to be either human or not human (Martin and Nickel 1980). In this sense, then, we can be said to enjoy a 'common humanity', a notion which Leah Curtin (1986) explores in her treatment of advocacy. This view of rights is vulnerable to the objection that not all human rights are natural rights. The human right to education, which is contingent on the availability of educational resources, is an example of a human right which is not a natural right. Likewise the rights to health care, legal representation and so on are human rights but not natural rights.

3. Based on rationality

A Kantian thesis of natural rights holds rationality as being the sole basis upon which a right's claim can be made. In other words, only those people who are capable of rational, autonomous thought are entitled to claim moral rights. One disturbing consequence of this thesis is that any human being (or non-human being, for that matter) who is unable to reason is not regarded as having moral status. Such a view clearly excludes infants, brain-dead and intellectually disabled persons from having a just claim to moral rights. We have evidence even today that a Kantian account of moral rights is not only alive and well in an academic sense, but also unashamedly in a practical sense. (Consider, for example, the use of brain-dead persons as organ donors, and, more recently, the suggestion that live-born anencephalic babies and fetuses should be used as organ donors [Meinke 1989; Gillam 1989; Sanders and Moore 1991].)

4. Based on interests

The contemporary philosopher Joel Feinberg offers quite a different theory of moral rights. He argues that, in order for an entity to be able to claim rights meaningfully, that entity must have interests (Feinberg 1979). To have interests, the entity must be capable of being either benefited or harmed. In order to be either benefited or harmed, one must be able to experience pleasure and pain. In short, unless one has sentience one cannot have interests, and thus cannot be either benefited or harmed, and therefore cannot make claims.

This theory of moral rights can be expressed diagramatically as shown in figure 3.1.

It can be seen that by this view it would be nonsense to assert, for example, that a rock has rights. Why? Because a rock does not have sentience and therefore cannot, strictly speaking, be benefited or harmed, and thus cannot meaningfully be said to have interests and hence rights. Those who *value rocks* (for example, conservationists, geologists, rock collectors) might be benefited or harmed by what happens to a rock, but it is not meaningful, philosophically speaking, to assert that a rock per se has rights. In contrast, any entity which can be shown to have sentience (that is, the capacity to experience pleasure or suffer pain) would, by this view, be entitled to be respected as having rights. Given this, it is clear that we can, for example, assert meaningfully that entities such as dolphins, puppies, kittens, horses, demented people and babies have moral rights.

Like Bentham, the founding father of utilitarianism, Feinberg sees the capacity to suffer, not reason, as the ultimate basis upon which a person's interest claims become the focus of moral action.

One shortcoming of this view is that agents must be able to represent their own interests. Feinberg (1979, p. 595) argues that, if agents cannot represent their own interests, they have no more rights than 'redwood trees and rosebushes'. Unhappily, the 'human vegetable', it seems, is no better off under an interests-based thesis of moral rights than it is under a thesis based on reason.

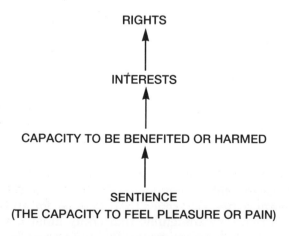

RIGHTS

↑

INTERESTS

↑

CAPACITY TO BE BENEFITED OR HARMED

↑

SENTIENCE
(THE CAPACITY TO FEEL PLEASURE OR PAIN)

Figure 3.1 Feinberg's theory of moral rights.

DIFFERENT TYPES OF RIGHTS

When speaking of moral rights, it is important to distinguish three different types which can be claimed: notably, inalienable, absolute and prima facie rights.

1. Inalienable rights

An inalienable right is one which cannot be transferred under any circumstances. For example, if we accept the right to life as being an inalienable right, we are committed to accepting that it cannot be transferred to someone else or for some other cause under any circumstances. According to this view, sacrificing one's life either in suicide, martyrdom, or in an act of supreme altruism (for example, a mother sacrificing her life for her child) would be condemned as morally wrong. Of course, we may ask the question whether the right to life is an inalienable right.

2. Absolute rights

An absolute right, by contrast, is a right which cannot be over ridden under any circumstances. For example, if we take the right to life as being absolute, we would be bound to respect it *whatever the cost*. By this view, *any* wilful taking of life, whether through war, self-defence, abortion, capital punishment, or any other act, would be morally wrong. Again the question arises whether the right to life really is an absolute right.

3. Prima facie rights

A prima facie right (from the Latin *primus,* meaning 'first', and *facies,* meaning 'face') is a right which may be overridden by stronger moral claims. For example, a patient's right to privacy may be overridden by the right to life in a cardiac arrest situation where the patient's body is exposed during the resuscitation procedure. In such an emergency, it would be silly for a well meaning but thoroughly misguided ethicist to insist that the patient's right to privacy should be upheld.

Some argue against the notion of prima facie rights by saying that if a right can be overridden it does not exist. Against such a criticism, Martin and Nickel (1980) comment:

> to describe a right as Prima Facie is to say something about its weight but not about its scope or conditions of possession ... Overridence depends on whether the case of conflict is central to the values that the right serves to protect or whether it is a marginal case and thus can be expected in all cases without great loss to those values.

(Martin and Nickel 1980, pp. 172–4)

MAKING A RIGHTS CLAIM

Having a right usually entails that another has a corresponding duty to respect that right. As Feinberg (1978, p. 1508) explains, when people assert their moral rights, they assert a kind of 'moral power' over us which we feel constrained to respect. Where claims have a special convincing force they have a coercive effect on our judgments, which in turn make us feel driven to both acknowledge and support the interest claims being made as being genuine rights claims.

Rights which entail a corresponding duty are typically referred to as 'claims rights'. These rights can be either positive or negative, and can entail either a positive or a negative rights claim. Positive rights claims generally entail a correlative duty *to act* or *to do*, in contrast with a negative rights claim which generally entails a correlative duty *to omit* or *to refrain* (Feinberg 1978, p. 1509). For example, if a patient claims a right not to be harmed, this claim imposes a negative duty on an attending nurse to refrain from acts which may cause harm. On the other hand, if a patient claims a right to be benefited in some way, such as by having an intolerable pain state relieved, this imposes a duty on an attending nurse to perform the positive act of promptly administering an effective analgesic. If a person's rights claims are not upheld, or are infringed or violated in some way, that person generally feels wronged or feels a serious injustice has been done.

PROBLEMS WITH RIGHTS CLAIMS

In discussing rights it is important to keep in mind at least four central problems that can arise when dealing with rights claims. First, rights and interests can compete and conflict with one another. For example, a patient's right to life could seriously compete or conflict with another patient's right to life in a situation involving scarce medical resources; or a nurse's conscientious refusal to assist with an abortion procedure could conflict with a patient's right to have an abortion and to receive care following the procedure. In such instances there may be no easy solution to the conflict of interests at hand.

Second, it may be difficult to establish the extent to which a person's rights claim entails a correlative duty. For example, if someone claims a right to life, who or what has the corresponding duty to respond to that claim? Does it fall to the health professional, or to family, friends, the hospital, the state, or another body? There may be no satisfactory answer to this question.

Third, there may be disagreement about which entities have rights. For example, some might rigorously argue that brain-dead people, anencephalic babies, the intellectually impaired and babies do not have moral rights, while others might just as rigorously argue that they do. Again there may be no happy solution to this type of disagreement.

Fourth, it may be very difficult to try and satisfy the rights claims of all people equally. For instance, if there is a genuine lack of resources, it may be impossible to satisfy all rights claims. Again, we are left, unhappily, with an unresolved moral problem.

The issue of moral rights is an important one for nurses — particularly as the issue relates to patients' rights and the patients' rights movement. As this is an enormous issue on its own, it is considered separately in chapter 7.

CORRELATIVE MORAL DUTIES

A moral duty (to be distinguished here from a legal duty, a civil duty, a professional duty, and so on) is an action which a person ought to do. In other words, it is a task or an action which a person is bound to perform for moral reasons. Bear in mind that a person can be bound to perform tasks for other reasons, such as legal reasons in the case of legal duties. In a rights view of morality, a moral reason is supplied by a correlative rights claim. This contrasts with a teleological ethical theory, in which duties are generated by respect for or consideration of some predicted moral consequence which ought to be furthered or upheld. Language used in identifying duties typically involves expressions such as: 'I have a duty to ...', 'You have a duty to ...', 'They have a duty to ...', and so on. The critical task for moral agents is to decide just what one's duty is. This, of course, is contingent on correctly determining what is to count as an overriding moral reason for doing something or, as in the case of rights, correctly determining whether a given rights claim is genuine, and, further, whether the agent does in fact have a duty correlative to the claim in question.

The notion of moral duties is examined further in the discussion on teleological theory in the second section of this chapter. Before moving on to consider teleological moral theory, the important task remains of clearing up once and for all the confusion which many nurses seem to have about their own rights and duties in relation to caring for patients. Consider, for example, a situation involving an abortion procedure. A nurse could reasonably claim either a *right* to refuse to participate in the abortion procedure or a *duty* to refuse. What is important here is to distinguish the basis upon which each claim might rest. If a nurse claims the right to refuse, this is fundamentally a claim involving the protection of the nurse's *own* interests (as opposed to the interests of the patient). The nurse might, for instance, have a religious-based conscientious objection to abortion and assert an entitlement to practise the tenets of that faith. A refusal based on a duty claim is significantly different, however. In this instance, the refusal is based more on the consideration of *another's* interests; that is, the interests of the patient or the fetus. Here the duty to refuse would derive from the broader moral duty to, say, prevent harm or to preserve life.

By this brief account it can be seen that to use the terms 'rights' and 'duties' interchangeably is not only incorrect, but thoroughly misleading. When nurses speak of their *right* to, say, care for a patient in such and such a way, it is quite possible they are really asserting that they have a *duty* to care for the patient in that way. This is just another example of an area where nurses need to clear up their use of moral language.

Applying deontological theory

Deontological theory can be applied to making moral decisions either by the separate evaluation of a given act (act-deontology) or by an appeal to general rules (rule-deontology).

Act-deontology requires agents to make separate evaluations on their own when making moral decisions, rather than appealing to a general system of rules. This approach emphasises the individual *situation* as being the ultimate guide on how to respond, and accepts that 'circumstances alter cases' (Fletcher 1966, p. 29). In the words of the Christian ethicist Dietrich Bonhoeffer (executed for his part in the assassination attempt on Hitler):

> The question of good is posed and is decided in the midst of each definite, yet unconcluded, unique and transient situation of our lives, in the midst of our living relationships with men [sic], things, institutions and powers, in other words in the midst of our human existence.

> (cited in Fletcher 1966, p. 33)

It can be seen that an act-deontological approach could, if taken to its extreme, commit one to conclusions which would not ordinarily be accepted. For example, act-deontology could even permit murder, as Bonhoeffer's actions against Hitler make plain.

This approach requires the agent to be very careful to get an accurate assessment of the situation before making a decision. The rightness of the decision, in the final analysis, depends very much on the correctness of the facts gathered in that situation, and the correct interpretation of those facts. Apart from the facts of the situation, act-deontology offers no other guiding criteria or principles in moral decision making (Frankena 1973, p. 23). This approach is sometimes referred to as 'situation ethics' (Fletcher 1966).

Rule-deontology, by contrast, requires agents to mediate their decisions by appealing to a system of general rules. This approach takes absolutely no account of the situation at hand; the general rules are to be followed regardless of the facts at hand. For example, if agents subscribe to rule-deontology and thereby accept the general rule 'always tell the truth', they would be compelled to tell the truth even in situations where a harmful consequence would follow from the truth-telling act (Frankena 1973, p. 17). Critics argue that rule-deontology, like act-deontology, could commit one to conclusions which ordinarily would not be accepted. The rule-deontologist's seeming over-reliance on rules has been criticised by modern philosophers as unmitigated 'superstitious rule worship' (Smart and Williams 1973, p. 6).

This discussion of deontological views is by no means exhaustive or conclusive, and much more remains to be said on them. This, however, is a task for philosophical texts, not nursing texts. Nevertheless, what has been presented so far provides an important theoretical background to a major theoretical movement in ethics, and begins to paint a backdrop against which other ethical theories can be compared and contrasted. This consideration of deontological ethics marks an important step towards critical moral thinking. The next step involves the discussion of another major, and competing, ethical theory: namely, teleological, or consequentialist, ethical theory.

Teleological theories

Teleological ethics (from the Greek *telos,* meaning 'end', and *logos,* meaning 'word') refers to a group of ethical theories which differ from and compete with deontological ethics. In essence, teleology denies everything that deontology asserts — or at least almost everything. By this view, and in contrast with deontological ethics, actions are judged good or bad, right or wrong, on the basis of the *consequences* they produce. Disputes in teleological ethics generally centre on issues such as: What is to be regarded as a moral good? Whose good should be promoted? What kinds of guidance can a moral theory provide for persons deliberating about what should be done in a given situation? (Baier 1978b, p. 417).

Responses to the question 'what is good?' have ranged from the achievement of mere happiness and the satisfaction of desires (monistic goods), through to the acquisition of knowledge for its own sake, freedom, dignity, and so on (pluralistic goods). The good life quickly translates into a life characterised by monistic and/or pluralistic goods — whichever is thought to hold.

Of equal importance has been the philosophical debate surrounding the questions 'whose good should be promoted?' or 'whose good should count?' — questions which plague even the most practical of worlds. The debate has raised four possibilities:

ethical egoism, ethical elitism, ethical parochialism, and ethical universalism (Baier 1978b; Frankena 1973).

Ethical egoism holds that people should do only that which will promote their own greatest good (Frankena 1973, p. 15). If, for example, going out to dinner with friends is perceived as being a greater good than stopping at the scene of an accident to render life-saving measures to an unknown accident victim, the ethical egoist would probably decide to drive past the accident and continue on to the restaurant.

Ethical elitism, on the other hand, holds that only the good of the elite should be maximised. By this view, the interests of those who are 'less gifted' should be set aside in favour of those who have a better chance of achieving 'perfection' or excellence (Baier 1978b). A good example of this is the distribution of more resources to the elite or 'hard' sciences such as medicine, than to the 'less sophisticated' or 'softer' sciences such as nursing.

Ethical parochialism, by contrast, serves only the good of an individual's appropriate 'in-group'. The 'in-group' may be, for example, the individual's relevant profession, or else the family, circle of friends, class, gender, religion, political party, social club, or cultural group. Some professional codes of conduct are examples of 'ethical parochialism', particularly where these stand to serve more the interests of the professional group than the interests of those whom the professional group is supposed to be serving (the community at large and the individuals comprising it).

Ethical universalism, the fourth possibility, essentially demands that the good of all humankind must be given equal consideration, and that human interests should all be treated equally. Ethical universalism is generally regarded as being more acceptable than the limited approaches of ethical egoism, ethical elitism and ethical parochialism, since its outcomes are more just and more defensible. Utilitarianism is popularly regarded as one of the more compelling theories of ethical universalism, in that it promotes the 'greatest good for the greatest number' (Frankena 1973, p. 15). Before considering this theory, however, one or two comments should be made about a teleological account of moral duties.

Moral duties and teleological theory

As already mentioned, a moral duty is an action which a person is bound, for moral reasons, to perform. From a teleological perspective, duties generally derive from the consideration of some predicted moral consequence that ought to be furthered or upheld. It might be argued, for instance, that one has a stringent moral duty to prevent otherwise avoidable harmful consequences from occurring where this can be done without sacrificing other important moral interests (Singer 1979a). Given this teleological maxim, if a person's action stands to prevent a particular harmful consequence from occurring, that person is duty-bound to perform that action, provided other important moral interests are not sacrificed in the process. An off-duty nurse, for example, could be said to be duty-bound to render life-saving care at the scene of a road accident, regardless of any inconvenience this might cause (mere *inconvenience* is not generally regarded as a morally significant consideration). If the life of the nurse were put at risk, however, the moral duty to render assistance would not be so clear cut.

Duties are primarily concerned with avoiding intolerable results; they are thought to provide the basic requirements that may be universally demanded in an effort to achieve a 'tolerable basis of social life' (Urmson 1969, p. 73). They also work 'to secure reliability, a state of affairs in which people can reasonably expect others to behave in some ways and not in others' (Williams 1985, p. 187). If a duty fails to avoid an intolerable result, there is room for questioning whether in fact it was a duty in the first place (Urmson, 1969). It might also be argued that if a duty can be overridden (for example, where there appears to be a conflict of duties) it is not a duty at all; we have merely mistakenly thought that it was (Hare 1981, p. 26). On the other hand, it might be replied that just because a duty can be overridden this does not mean 'it was not a duty in the first place' but only that it was a 'prima facie duty'. There is nothing philosophically wrong in holding that duties can be prima facie in nature (Ross 1930, p. 19).

Moral obligations

The notion of moral duty is related to the notion of moral 'obligation' (a notion that also finds usage in deontological moral discourse). The language of obligations is very similar to the language of duties, and typically involves expressions like: 'I have an obligation to ...', 'You have an obligation to ...', 'We have an obligation to ...', 'They have an obligation to ...', and so on. Although many philosophers treat the terms 'duties' and 'obligations' synonymously, an important and useful distinction can be drawn between them, which rests on the differing moral strengths each notion has, rather than on a difference in their essential moral nature. Duties are regarded as having a stronger force than obligations, or, to put this another way, duties are more morally compelling than are obligations. Dworkin (1977, pp. 48–9), an influential exponent of this distinction, gives the example that it is one thing to say a person has an obligation to give to a charity, but it is quite another to say that person has a duty to do so. While it would be 'good' if someone made a charitable donation, it would be erroneous to suggest a moral compulsion to do so. To a limited extent, Dworkin's thesis helps to alleviate the tension created by the problem of supposed conflicting duties.

The concept of obligation and its distinctiveness from duty has interesting and important implications for nurses, particularly in relation to the issue of following a doctor's or a superior's orders. For instance, it may well be that nurses have an *obligation* to follow a doctor's or a superior's orders, but it is far from clear that they always have a *duty* to do so, either morally or legally. In fact, if a doctor's or a superior's orders are 'dubious', a nurse has both a legal and a moral duty to question such orders. In some cases, the nurse may even have a duty to refuse to follow a given order when such an order is 'unreasonable', 'unlawful' or 'likely to cause otherwise avoidable harm'.

Utilitarianism

As mentioned earlier, utilitarianism is thought to be the more generally persuasive of the teleological theories on the grounds of its ethical universalism. Utilitarianism involves a principle which concerns itself more with the general welfare of people than the particular welfare of individuals, and is generally contrasted with a rights view of ethics. In other words, utilitarianism views the world not in terms of certain individual rights which people may or may not have, but in terms of people's collective and overall interests.

A broad view of utilitarianism is persuasive in that it promotes a universal point of view: that is, that one person's interests cannot count as being superior to the interests of another just because they are personal interests (Singer 1979b, p. 12). For example, I cannot claim that my interests count more than your interests *just because they are my interests*.

Modern utilitarianism was founded by the English philosopher Jeremy Bentham (1748–1832). Bentham's utility thesis holds that actions should be judged right or wrong on the basis of whether they tend to promote pleasure (and happiness) and diminish pain (and unhappiness) and, more specifically, whether they tend to maximise the balance of good over bad (Bentham 1962 edn, p. 34).

Bentham held the principle of utility to apply equally to the private actions of individuals and to the public actions of government, and he took great pains to elaborate the principle's relevance to legal, political, educational and social institutions. One troubling aspect of his thesis, however, is that it is thoroughly tainted with ethical egoism. Bentham insisted, for example, that the key to maximising the community's interests is to maximise the individual's interests. He essentially saw the community as a 'fictitious body', and community interests as nothing more than 'the sum interests of the several members who comprise it' (Bentham 1962 edn, p. 35).

The influence of the British philosopher John Stuart Mill (1806–73), who was the son of the Scottish philosopher James Mill (1773–1836), saw a major modification of Bentham's thesis. Mill was much more specific in his treatment of what he called the 'greatest happiness principle', and was quite adamant that the ultimate standard of utility is not the individual's 'own greatest happiness, but the greatest amount of happiness altogether' (1962b edn, p. 262).

Mill stressed that utilitarianism was quite distinct from mere ethical egoism (i.e. the promotion of one's own pleasure and happiness *only*), and in fact argued that in some instances individuals might even have a duty to sacrifice their own greatest good for the good of others (1962b edn, p. 268). He also advanced the notion that people should be striving to act cooperatively with one another and 'proposing to themselves a collective, not an individual interest as the aim ... of their action' (Mill 1962b edn, p. 285). Once people form a collective interest, suggested Mill, they are more inclined to view the interests of others as their own.

Although Mill essentially embraced a more cooperative and collective view of morality, he nevertheless upheld the sovereignty of the individual, individual independence and freedom of choice (1962a edn, p. 135). He generally considered rational persons as the best judges of their own best interests and entitled to make mistakes. However, he did recognise that in some instances a person's liberty of action may be justly interfered with. The first instance is where a given individual is incapable of exercising an informed choice, as in the case of children or other persons who lack the 'maturity of their faculties' (1962a edn, p. 135). The second instance is when an individual's conduct stands to hurt others or stands to 'affect prejudicially the interests of others', in which case both society and the law would have a prima facie case for interfering with a person's liberty of action, and possibly even for punishing that person (1962a edn, pp. 136, 205).

For Mill, the principle of utility is the ultimate source of moral obligation. Utility can and should be used to decide between competing demands: its application may be difficult, argued Mill (1962b edn, p. 277), but it is better than no principle at all!

The works of Bentham and Mill sought to simplify ethics by providing one universally applicable principle by which all moral judgments should be made. Utility proved to be such a principle. As well as having philosophical appeal, the principle had the attraction of being democratic, and secular; that is, it could be upheld independently of any prevailing religious dogma or moral theology. Despite its appeal, however, classical utilitarianism has sustained heavy criticism on several grounds, some of which are:

: difficulties likely to be encountered in reliably
:dicting the consequences of given actions;

.e time-consuming nature of utilitarian calculations and
analyses;

- the risk of making mistakes in predicting and calculating
the moral worth of outcomes;

- difficulties likely to be encountered in accurately trying to
measure pleasure, happiness, pain and unhappiness;

- The problem of sacrificing individual interests to the whole.

RECENT UTILITARIAN THEORY

Bentham's and Mill's hedonistic account of utility no longer has
currency in modern moral thinking, although, as a word of caution,
some nurse authors persist in advocating the 'greatest happiness
principle' as having supreme merit in nursing ethics and nursing
models of moral decision making. The main reason for abandoning
hedonistic utilitarianism has been its inadequacy to determine
right action 'objectively'. The major alternative approach is 'preference utilitarianism', which views the maximisation of individual
preferences as being of intrinsic value, rather than the maximisation of hedonistic pleasures or hedonistic states of affairs. As
Beauchamp and Childress observe, 'what is intrinsically valuable is
what individuals prefer to obtain, and utility is thus translated into
the satisfaction of those needs and desires that individuals choose
to satisfy' (Beauchamp and Childress 1989, p. 28).

By this view, preference utilitarianism as a moral theory translates into the demand that we ought in all circumstances to
produce the greatest possible balance of 'value over disvalue' for all
persons affected (Beauchamp and Childress 1989, p. 29). In other
words, we ought in all circumstances to produce the greatest
possible balance of individuals satisfying their preferences over
individuals not satisfying their preferences. The problem of individuals asserting 'unacceptable' desires or preferences is overcome
by the claim that our common sense and past experience will be
enough to distinguish unacceptable desires which can be excluded
'on more general utilitarian grounds' (Beauchamp and Childress
1989, p. 29).

On the whole, preference utilitarianism is considered more satisfying, since its calculations are easier to work out. For instance, it
takes little more than basic 'common sense and careful deliberation' to determine an individual's preferences; it would take
considerably more to determine an individual's internal experiences of pleasure and pain, if, indeed, these things can be determined at all.

APPLYING UTILITARIAN THEORY

As with deontological moral theory, utilitarian theory can be applied either by separate evaluation of a given act (act-utilitarian-ism), or by an appeal to general rules (rule-utilitarianism). Each approach places different demands on the deliberating agent.

Act-utilitarianism demands that the deliberator considers the moral consequences of *each particular* act under scrutiny. The rightness or wrongness of the act in question is ultimately determined by the total goodness and badness of its particular consequences; that is, whether it alone maximises or minimises intrinsic value (Smart and Williams 1973, p. 4). Consider, for example, the case of a nurse involved in the care of the seriously injured motor vehicle accident victim whose neurological prognosis is uncertain. A person applying act-utilitarianism would, in this case, ask what good or bad consequences would result from *this particular* motor accident victim being resuscitated at all costs? The ultimate answer will depend on whether such an act in this particular case results in the maximisation of value over disvalue. Act-utilitarianism, like act-deontology, has been severely criticised on much the same grounds: that it would commit an agent to unacceptable conclusions and may permit acts which ordinarily would not be permitted, such as lying or sacrificing innocent life.

Rule-utilitarianism, on the other hand, demands that the deliberator considers the moral consequences of generally observ-ing a rule. In the example of the nurse involved in the care of a seriously injured motor accident victim, rule-utilitarianism would require the nurse to ask what good or bad consequences would result from the general rule that all motor accident victims with uncertain neurological prognoses must be resuscitated rigorously. The ultimate answer depends on whether *as a general rule* the unconstrained resuscitation of all accident victims results in the maximisation of value over disvalue. Rule-utilitarianism has also been the subject of much criticism, with objectors arguing that it too could commit the deliberator to accept otherwise unacceptable conclusions such as lying or sacrificing innocent life. Another criticism is that rule-utilitarianism collapses into act-utilitarianism once the 'best consequences' are adhered to (Smart and Williams 1973).

Which theory to choose?

It is beyond the scope of this text to consider utilitarianism and the many objections raised against it in the depth that is warranted. As with the discussion on ethical deontology, however, the views and points raised here stand as an important beginning to a critical approach to bioethics in nursing. There remains the troubling question, meanwhile, of which theory nurses should choose in dealing with moral problems in the workplace?

For all the philosophical debate that has been generated about the acceptability and reliability of both deontological and teleological ethical theories, it is just possible that it ultimately makes very little difference which theory is chosen. While these different theories emphasise different moral reflections and justifications, it is nevertheless possible that these differences may have been over-emphasised (Beauchamp and Childress 1989, pp. 44–7). One wonders, for example, just what the difference is between deontology and utilitarianism, given that both aim to prevent intolerable outcomes from occurring. Engelhardt (1986) makes the radical suggestion that the two theories are two sides of the same coin: moral principles are accepted deontologically and applied consequentially. Some feminist moral theorists make the even more radical claim that the theories of Western moral philosophy should be abandoned altogether (see chapter 4).

Moral principles and moral rules

In completing our discussion of classical moral theory, we need to examine what gives moral theories their substance or their 'guts', and so we turn to moral principles and rules. Like the theories under which they operate, moral principles and moral rules are subject to philosophical controversy. Nevertheless, they have an important role to play in guiding moral behaviour and moral decision making, as will become clearer in the chapters to follow. What, then, are some of the popular moral principles which people appeal to when attempting to solve moral problems? How do we know the difference between moral principles and moral rules as prescriptive action guides? The following sections attempt to answer these questions briefly.

Moral principles

General standards of conduct which make up an ethical system are known as moral principles. To say that a principle is 'moral' is merely to assert that it is a behaviour guide which 'entails particular imperatives' (Harrison 1954, p. 115).

Moral principles function by specifying that some type of action or conduct is either prohibited, required, or permitted in certain circumstances (Solomon 1978, p. 408). As I have pointed out elsewhere (Johnstone 1990, p. 1.30) an action or decision is generally considered morally right or good when it accords with a given relevant moral principle, and morally wrong or bad when it does not. To illustrate how this works, consider the action of making a measurement using a ruler. If the line you have drawn measures the desired length of, say, 12 cm — as measured against your ruler — you would judge the length as 'correct'. If, however, the line you have drawn is only 10 cm long — not the desired 12 cm — you would judge the length to be 'incorrect'. By analogy, principles also function like rulers, in so far as they provide a standard against which something (in this case, actions) can be measured. For example, if an action fails to 'measure up' to the ultimate standards set by a given principle, we would judge the action to be 'incorrect' or, more specifically, morally wrong. If, however, an action fully measures up to the ultimate standards set by a given principle, we would judge the action to be 'correct' or morally right. So far, so good. The next question is: what are these moral principles against which actions can be measured?

Moral principles commonly used in bioethical discussions include the principles of autonomy, non-maleficence, beneficence, and justice. It is to examining the content, prescriptive force and application of these principles that this discussion now turns.

1. AUTONOMY

The term 'autonomy' comes from the Greek *autos* (meaning 'self') and *nomos* (meaning 'rule', 'governance' or 'law'). When the concept of autonomy is used in moral discourse, what is commonly being referred to is a person's ability to make or to exercise self-determining choice — literally, 'self-governing'. Included here is the additional notion of 'respect for persons'; that is, of treating or respecting persons as ends in themselves, as dignified and rational autonomous choosers, and not as the mere means (objects or tools) to the ends of others (Kant 1972 edn; Benn 1971). The principle of autonomy, however, is a little different, and is eloquently formulated by Beauchamp and Walters (1982) as follows:

> Insofar as an autonomous agent's actions *do not infringe on the autonomous actions of others* [italics added], that person should be free to perform whatever action he or she wishes (presumably even if it involves considerable risk to himself or herself and even if others consider the action to be foolish).
>
> (Beauchamp and Walters 1982, p. 27)

What this basically means is that people should be free to choose and entitled to act on their preferences *provided* their decisions and actions do not stand to violate, or impinge on, the significant moral interests of others.

Both the concept and the principle of autonomy have important implications for nursing practice. For example, if autonomy is to be taken seriously by nurses, nursing practice must truly respect patients as dignified human beings capable of deciding what is to count as being in their own best interests — even if what they decide is considered by others (including nurses) to be 'foolish'. In short, nurses must allow patients to participate in decision making concerning their care. Given this, it soon becomes clear that the whole practice of 'negotiated patient goals' and 'negotiated patient care' as advocated by contemporary nursing philosophy is thoroughly rooted in the moral principle of autonomy, and the derived duty to respect persons as autonomous moral choosers. It is not derived merely from a concept of 'acceptable professional nursing practice'.

In application, the principle of autonomy would judge as being morally objectionable and condemnable any act which unjustly prevents rational and autonomous persons from deciding what is to count as being in their own best interests. The kinds of act which might come in for criticism here include, for example:

- treating patients without their consent;
- treating patients without giving them all the relevant information necessary for making an informed and intelligent choice;
- telling patients 'white lies' (such as telling a patient that 'the operation went well', meaning that there were no intra-operative or post-operative complications, but, in fact, a large inoperable malignant tumour was found);
- withholding information from patients when they have expressed a reflective choice to receive it;
- forcing information upon patients when they have expressed a reflective choice not to receive it;
- forcing nurses to act against their reasoned moral judgments or conscience.

It should be noted, however, that while the moral principle of autonomy is very helpful in guiding ethically just practices in health care contexts, it is not entirely unproblematic. Indeed, its uncritical and culturally inappropriate application in some contexts may, in fact, inadvertently cause rather than prevent significant moral harms to patients, for reasons which are considered in chapters 4 and 5.

2. NON-MALEFICENCE

The principle of non-maleficence ('above all, do no harm') entails a stringent duty not to injure others. In discussing the essential nature of this principle, Beauchamp and Childress (1989, p. 121) argue that it is important to distinguish 'non-maleficence' from 'beneficence' ('above all, do good'), so as not to obscure other important distinctions which might be made in ordinary moral discourse. They contend that the duty 'not to injure others' is both distinct from and more stringent than the duty required by the principle of beneficence to take 'positive steps to benefit someone'. They argue that:

> our duty not to push someone who cannot swim into deep water seems stronger than our duty to rescue someone who has accidentally strayed into deep water. It is also morally imperative for us to take substantial risks with our safety in many cases in order not to endanger others, but it is less obvious that even moderate risks are morally required to benefit others.
>
> (Beauchamp and Childress 1989, p. 122)

Perhaps a more relevant example here might be that we have a comparatively strong duty not to force a colleague to work (or even to 'rescue' a colleague from working) in an area or care for a patient where that person has sound and just moral or personal reasons for refusing to do so; we may even risk censure by arguing with a nurse supervisor or superior against sending our colleague to the contentious area. We would obviously not have such a strong duty to come to the aid of colleagues who were refusing an assignment just because they 'did not like it' or 'wished to go off to the beach instead'.

This principle in application would be likely to condemn any act which unjustly injures a person or causes them to suffer an otherwise avoidable harm.

3. BENEFICENCE

As already briefly mentioned, the principle of beneficence demands 'above all, do good'. When applied, the principle of beneficence requires both the 'provision of benefits' (preventing and removing harm/doing good), and 'a balancing of benefits and harms', which is a version of utility (Beauchamp and Childress 1989, pp. 194–5). According to Beauchamp and Childress, a person (X) has a duty of beneficence towards another (Y):

> if each of the following conditions is satisfied and X is aware of all the relevant facts: (1) Y is at risk of significant loss or damage; (2) X's action is needed (singly or in concert with others) to prevent this loss; (3) X's action (singly or in concert with others) has a high probability of preventing it; (4) X's actions would not present significant risks, costs, or burdens to X; and (5) the benefit that Y can be expected to gain outweighs any harms, costs, or burdens that X is likely to incur.
>
> (Beauchamp and Childress 1989, p 201)

They go on to suggest that it is only when these conditions are satisfied that a person's 'general duty of beneficence' becomes a 'specific duty of beneficence' toward another given individual.

The principle stands to have an interesting and useful application in nursing practice. Consider the following case (personal communication; names have been changed).

Mrs Jones, a Jehovah's Witness, is admitted to an intensive care unit in a terminal condition, suffering from advanced hepatitis B and severe liver failure. She has a slow internal haemorrhage and is only semiconscious. Before her alteration in consciousness she had given her doctors a written statement specifically requesting that she not be given a blood transfusion under any circumstances. Upon her arrival in the unit, however, the attending doctor prescribes a unit of blood and requests that it be given immediately. Mrs Jones' husband and children are all present and, upon overhearing the doctor's request, become very upset. Mr Jones approaches the doctor and asks that his wife not be given the blood transfusion. He reminds the doctor that Mrs Jones has made explicit her wish not to have a blood transfusion under any circumstances. Nurse Smith, the registered nurse caring for Mrs Jones, hears the discussion and has to make a decision whether or not to intervene on her patient's behalf. In making her decision, Nurse Smith might appeal to the principle of beneficence in the following manner:

1. Mrs Jones, a terminally ill Jehovah's Witness, is at risk of suffering a significant loss (a violation of her spiritual values and beliefs) if she is given the prescribed blood transfusion.

2. Action by Nurse Smith, the attending nurse, is needed to prevent Mrs Jones from experiencing the loss in question.

3. Nurse Smith's action of refusing to administer the prescribed transfusion would probably prevent Mrs Jones' loss.

4. Nurse Smith's action will not present a significant risk to her (for example, she will not lose her job).

5. The benefits gained by Mrs Jones outweigh any harms Nurse Smith is likely to suffer (given that Nurse Smith autonomously chooses to uphold Mrs Jones' interests, and does not stand to suffer any morally significant consequences of her actions).

In this particular case the nurse refused to give the transfusion which had been prescribed. When the doctor insisted that it be given, the nurse pointed out that the transfusion would probably be of no benefit to Mrs Jones, as she was clearly in the end stages of her disease — to put it bluntly, 'she was dying'. Nurse Smith then suggested to the doctor that perhaps he would prefer to administer the transfusion himself. Interestingly, the doctor declined this invitation, and the transfusion was not given. Mrs Jones died a short while later, without having to experience a needless violation of her expressed wishes, values and beliefs.

In summary, by this principle, an act which does not bestow benefits on people, or which fails to address an imbalance of harms over benefits, could rightly be condemned.

4. JUSTICE

The principle of justice (its nature and content), unlike the principles above, is not so amenable to definition or quantification. As a point of interest, questions concerning what justice is and what its origins are have occupied the minds of philosophers for nearly three thousand years, and to this day remain the subject of intensive philosophical debate (MacIntyre 1988; Solomon and Murphy 1990). Significantly, the end result of this great philosophical debate has not been the development of an exquisitely refined universal theory of justice, but the development of a range of rival theories of justice — and, it should be added, a range of competing underlying rationalities supporting each of these respective theories (MacIntyre 1988). Different conceptions of justice have included: justice as revenge (retributive justice — for example, 'an eye for an eye'); justice as mercy (Christian ethics); justice as harmony in the soul and harmony in the state (Pythagorean ethics, 600 BC–1 AD); justice as equality ('equals must be treated equally, and unequals unequally'); justice as an equal distribution of benefits and burdens (distributive justice); justice as what is deserved ('each according to one's merit or worth'); and justice as love (Rawls 1971; Outka 1972; MacIntyre 1985, 1988; Waithe 1987; Beauchamp and Childress 1989; Solomon and Murphy 1990; Singer 1991).

Given these different conceptions of justice, the problem arises of what, if any, conception of justice nurses should adopt? While it is beyond the scope of this text to answer this question in depth, there is nevertheless room to advocate at least two senses of justice which nurses might find helpful: (1) justice as fairness; and (2) justice as the equal distribution of benefits and burdens (Beauchamp and Childress 1989, p. 256). It is these two senses of justice which will now be considered.

Justice as fairness finds interpretation in terms of 'what is deserved'. Here, it can be said that: 'One acts justly toward a person when that person has given what is due or owed, and thus what he and she deserves and can legitimately claim' (Beauchamp and Childress 1989, p. 257).

If someone deserved such and such, justice is done when that person receives such and such. Here, 'such and such' may be something which is either positive (a reward) or negative (a punishment). This view relies very heavily on an 'intuitive' sense of justice. For example, we may 'feel' it is unjust to punish or censure someone for a harm they did not cause, or not to punish someone for a harm they did deliberately cause. Likewise we may feel that it is unjust to reward someone for an accomplishment to which they contributed nothing, and yet not reward someone who contributed a great deal.

We do not need to look far in nursing practice to find sobering examples of where the principle of justice as fairness has been violated. Consider cases where nurses have been subjected to severe legal and professional censure on the basis of mistakes made by doctors (Johnstone, 1994). The Somera case of 1929, cited in chapter 2, involving a nurse who was fined and sentenced to prison after following an incorrect medical order, stands as an important example here (Grennan 1930). While it may well have been 'fair' that Somera was censured for her part in the administration of an incorrectly prescribed drug, it was hardly 'fair' that the doctor — who prescribed the drug, checked it with Somera, and administered it — was acquitted.

Other less dramatic examples involve cases where nurses have gained promotion or have secured employment on the basis of their claiming credit for the work of either their peers or their subordinates; at the other end of the continuum, some nurses have been denied promotion or employment because their superior has ignored, or refused for whatever reasons to recognise, significant professional achievements the nurse applicant has in fact made. The story of 'Sally Trihard', a registered nurse who had difficulty getting a job because of a past difference of professional opinion with a charge nurse, is a case in point (Johnstone 1987, p. 41; see also 'A costly misjudgment', p. 3).

How, then, might we make choices on this view of justice? One possible approach which has received widespread attention is that discussed by the contemporary philosopher John Rawls, briefly mentioned earlier in this chapter. He argues, for example, that if parties are to exercise truly just or fair choices, they must choose from a hypothetically 'neutral' position, or from a position of what he describes as being 'behind the veil of ignorance' (Rawls 1971, p. 12). From such a position he argues:

> no one knows his [sic] place in society, his [sic] class position or social status, nor does any one know his [sic] fortune in the distribution of natural assets and abilities, his [sic] intelligence,

strength, and the like … [T]his ensures that no one is advantaged or disadvantaged in the choice of principles by the outcome of natural chance or the contingency of social circumstances. Since all are similarly situated and no one is able to design principles to favor his [sic] particular condition, the principles of justice are the result of a fair agreement or bargain.

(Rawls 1971, p. 12)

While Rawls' view is problematic (for instance, it is open to serious question whether, in fact, all choosers are or could ever be 'similarly situated', as he assumes), it is nevertheless persuasive, particularly when considered in the light of broader philosophical demands which emphasise among other things that moral choice and judgment should be exercised from a position of impartiality and objectivity. Whether in fact human beings are ever capable of exercising truly impartial and 'objective' choices — indeed, of choosing from behind that veil of ignorance — is a matter of great controversy, however. Despite its weaknesses, Rawls' justice theory helps us to come to terms with the notion of fairness and how it might be used in real life situations. It also alerts us to some of the potential difficulties of trying to determine and apply an uncontentious view of justice.

A second sense in which justice can be used is that pertaining to 'distributive justice'; that is, an equal distribution of benefits and harms. By this view, all people are required to bear an equal share of their society's burdens and benefits. Such a view admits that all persons must have equal claims to liberty and opportunity, but in a way that is compatible with the claims of others. As well as this, there must be equal access (and opportunity to gain access) to positions of authority and power, and there must be an equal distribution of wealth and income. The only morally acceptable exception to this would be if an 'unequal distribution would work to everyone's advantage' (Beauchamp and Childress 1989, p. 269); or where an unequal distribution of benefits would be necessary so as to 'maximize the minimum level of primary goods in order to protect vital interests in potentially damaging or disastrous contexts' (Beauchamp and Childress 1989, p. 269). Simply put, inequalities in distributing benefits and primary goods are 'just' as long as this results in the least well off (that is, those who are already disadvantaged unfairly) achieving a decent minimum level of well-being (that is, being advantaged by the benefits which have been conferred unequally). Given this view, 'injustice' finds interpretation as 'simply inequalities that are not to the benefit of all' (Rawls 1971, pp. 60–1).

As with the fairness sense of justice discussed earlier, we do not need to look far to find sobering examples in nursing where the principle of distributive justice has been violated. In many cases, nurses have had to (and continue to) bear unequal and intolerable burdens on account of certain inequities in the distribution of scarce health care resources. For example, historically nurses have had to endure poor and unsafe working conditions with a maximum of responsibility and a minimum of financial or personal reward (Johnstone 1994). Indeed, the historic 1986 nurses' strike for fifty days in the State of Victoria (Australia) was largely a protest by nurses against the decline in their work conditions and in standards of patient care, against heavy and diverse workloads, and against the tardy government response to their log of claims. (The issue of strike action by nurses is discussed in greater depth in chapter 13.)

Another example illustrates that to deny the principle of distributive justice may have an immediate practical effect. Nurses can perhaps be forgiven for feeling a powerful sense of injustice when a new piece of costly medical equipment or a considerable quantity of pharmaceutical supplies is purchased, while at the same time basic items of critical use in safe patient care and management are apparently lacking. In such a situation it is ludicrous to allocate a considerable portion of a hospital budget to, say, antibiotics, but to cut back on the supply of items such as sterile surgical scissors and forceps — both of which are basic items necessary for aseptic wound packing and management. Of course, this equipment will help to avoid unnecessary and prolonged wound infection, and thus avoid the likelihood of the patient having to endure (unjustly) a prolonged stay in hospital.

In considering the fairness and the distributive senses of justice, it is instructive to note that both uphold two common minimal principles: formal equality ('equals must be treated equally, and unequals must be treated unequally'); and a mixture of autonomy and beneficence ('we all ought to bear certain burdens, usually of a minimal sort, for the common good') (Beauchamp and Childress 1989, pp. 256–306).

In calculating the balance or distribution of harms and benefits, the notions of comparative and non-comparative justice are commonly used. Justice is 'comparative' when what a person deserves can be determined only by balancing the competing claims of others against the person's own claims (Beauchamp and Childress 1989, pp. 256–306). For example, whether a nurse qualifies for a job or a promotion will depend largely on the competing claims of the other applicants. If the other applicants are more qualified and more experienced, it seems reasonable to hold that they are more 'deserving' of the position being offered. Justice is 'non-comparative', on the other hand, when 'desert is judged by standards independent of the claims of others (Beauchamp and Childress 1989, pp. 256–306). For example, a nurse who is guilty of breaching acceptable professional standards of conduct deserves to be censured, or even deregistered, if the breach of conduct warrants such an action; a nurse who is innocent of professional misconduct, however, does not deserve to be censured or deregistered.

(See Beauchamp and Childress [1989, pp. 256–75] for a brief but comprehensive overview of the principle of formal justice; the material principles of justice; utilitarian, libertarian and egalitarian theories of justice; and the 'fair opportunity rule'.)

Moral rules

Like moral principles, moral rules also have a place in making up a general overriding and prescriptive action-guiding system. And, like moral principles, moral rules function by specifying that some type of action or conduct is either prohibited, required or permitted (Solomon 1978, pp. 408–9). What distinguishes a moral rule from a moral principle is its structure and nature. Moral principles, for instance, tend to be regarded as the very essence of morality, and the bases or the 'parent' forms from which general moral truths (in so far as these can be determined) are derived. In application, moral principles incline more toward a general focus. Consider, for example, the broad moral principle of 'autonomy'. In general, the principle demands that rational persons should be respected as autonomous choosers, capable of judging what is in their own best interests. As such, rational persons should be free to act as they wish provided their actions do not violate the moral interests of others.

Moral rules, on the other hand, stand as being merely derivative of morality's essence and basis and, in application, are much more particular in their focus. Although it is difficult to draw a firm distinction between moral rules and moral principles, it is generally recognised that moral rules have different force, sanctioning power, conditions of existence, scope of application, and level of concreteness from moral principles (Solomon 1978). An example of a moral rule would be the demand, say, to 'always tell the truth' or 'never tell a lie'. Thus, if a patient asks an attending health care professional a question concerning a diagnosis and proposed treatment, the health care professional could be said to be obliged to give the information the patient has requested. The apparent 'obligation' here finds its force not just from the moral rule 'always tell the truth', but from the moral principle of autonomy which demands that rational people be respected as autonomous choosers, and be given the information required to make an informed and intelligent choice. In order for a particular moral rule (or set of moral rules) to be justified, it must be fully derived from and reducible to established parent principles of morality.

In summary, moral rules derive from moral principles, and as such have only prima facie force (i.e., they can be overridden by stronger moral claims). Given their prima facie nature, moral rules cannot override the moral principles from which they have been derived. To accept that they could would be to suggest, somewhat paradoxically, that derived rules could meaningfully conflict with parent principles — which, of course, is absurd. The question of moral rules is an important one for nurses, particularly as it relates to the broader issue of professional codes of conduct, an issue that will become clearer in the following chapters.

References

Allen, R. E. (ed.) (1966). *Greek philosophy: Thales to Aristotle*. The Free Press, New York.

A costly misjudgment. Anonymous (1988). *Australian Nurses Journal* 17 (6), December/January, p. 3.

Baier, K. (1978a). Deontological theories. In Reich (1978), pp. 413–17.

Baier, K. 1978b). Teleological theories. In Reich (1978), pp. 417–21.

Beauchamp, T. L. and Childress, J. F. (1989). *Principles of biomedical ethics*, 3rd edn. Oxford University Press, New York.

Beauchamp, T. L. and Walters, L. (eds) (1982). *Contemporary issues in bioethics*, 2nd edn. Wadsworth, Belmont, California.

Benn, S. I. (1971). Privacy, freedom, and respect for persons. *Nomos* 13 (J. R. Pennock and J. W. Chapman (eds) American Society for Political and Legal Philosophy: Privacy, Artherton Press, New York), pp. 1–21.

Benner, P. (1984). *From novice to expert: excellence and power in clinical nursing practice*. Addison-Wesley, Nursing Division, Menlo Park, California.

Benner, P. and Tanner, C. (1987). Clinical judgment: how expert nurses use intuition. *American Journal of Nursing* 87 (1), January, pp. 23–31.

Bentham, J. (1962 edn). An introduction to the principles of morals and legislation (reprinted from 1789 edition). In Warnock 1962, pp. 33–77.

Cortese, A. (1990). *Ethnic ethics: the restructuring of moral theory*. State University of New York Press, Albany.

Curtin, L. L. (1986). The nurse as advocate: a philosophical foundation for nursing. In P. Chinn (ed.), *Ethical issues in nursing*, Aspen System, Rockville, Maryland, pp. 11–20.

Dworkin, R. (1977). *Taking rights seriously*. Duckworth, London.

Elliott, C. (1992). Where ethics comes from and what to do about it. *Hastings Center Report* 22 (4), pp. 28–35.

Engelhardt, H. Tristram Jr (1986). *The foundations of bioethics*. Oxford University Press, New York.

Feinberg, J. (1978). Rights. In Reich (1978), pp. 1507–11.

Feinberg, J. (1979). The rights of animals and unborn generations. In R. A. Wasserstrom (ed.), *Today's moral problems*, Macmillan, New York, pp. 581–601.

Fletcher, J. (1966). *Situation ethics*. SCM Press, Bloomsbury Street, London.

Flew, A. (ed.) (1979). *A dictionary of philosophy*. Pan Books, London.

Frankena, W. K. (1973). *Ethics*, 2nd edn. Prentice Hall, Englewood Cliffs, New Jersey.

Gert, B. (1984). Moral theory and applied ethics. *The Monist* 67 (4), October, pp. 532–48.

Gillam, L. (ed.) (1989). *Proceedings of the conference 'The Fetus as Tissue Donor: Use or Abuse?'* Centre for Human Bioethics, Monash University, Melbourne.

Goldberg, p. (1983). *The intuitive edge.* Jeremy Tarcher, Los Angeles.

Grennan, E. (1930). The Somera case. *International Nursing Review* 5 (December/January), pp. 325–33.

Hare, R. M. (1981). *Moral thinking: its levels, method and point.* Clarendon Press, Oxford.

Harmon, G. (1977). *The nature of morality.* Oxford University Press, New York.

Harrison, J. (1954). When is a principle a moral principle? *Aristotelian Society,* supplementary vol. 28, July 9–11, pp. 111–34.

Hobbes, T. (1968 edn). *Leviathan* (reprinted from 1651 edition with notes by C. B. Macpherson). Pelican Books, Harmondsworth, Middlesex.

Hume, D. (1888 edn). *A treatise of human nature.* Clarendon Press, Oxford.

Hume, D. (1947 edn). Of the original contract (reprinted from 1748 edition). In Sir Ernest Barker, *Social contract,* Oxford University Press, London, pp. 209–36.

Johnstone, M.-J. (1987). Ethics in focus. *Australian Nurses Journal* 17 (3), September, pp. 41–2.

Johnstone, M.-J. (1990). *Ethics and nursing: Module 601E — An external course for registered nurses.* Royal College of Nursing, Australia, Melbourne.

Johnstone, M.-J. (1994). *Nursing and the injustices of the law.* W. B. Saunders/Baillière Tindall, Sydney.

Kant, I. (1972 edn). *The moral law* (translated by H. J. Paton). Hutchinson University Library, London.

Leininger, M. (1990). Culture: the conspicuous missing link to understand ethical and moral dimensions of human care. In M. Leininger (ed.), *Ethical and moral dimensions of care,* Wayne State University Press, Detroit, pp. 49–66.

Locke, J. (1947 edn). An essay concerning the true, original extent and end of civil government (reprinted from 1690 edition). In Sir Ernest Barker, *Social contract,* Oxford University Press, London. pp. 3–206.

MacIntyre, A. (1966). *A short history of ethics.* Routledge & Kegan Paul, London.

MacIntyre, A. (1985). *After virtue: a study in moral theory,* 2nd edn. Duckworth, London.

MacIntyre, A. 1988). *Whose justice? Which rationality?* Duckworth, London.

Mackie, J. L. (1962). Omnipotence. *Sophia* 1 (2), July, pp. 14–25.

McNaughton, D. (1988). *Moral vision: an introduction to ethics.* Basil Blackwell, Oxford.

Martin, R. and Nickel, J. W. (1980). Recent work on the concepts of rights. *American Philosophical Quarterly* 17 (3), July, pp. 165–80.

Meinke, S. A. (1989). *Anencephalic infants as potential organ sources: ethical and legal issues: Scope Notes 12.* Kennedy Institute of Ethics, Georgetown University, Washington DC.

Mill, J. S. (1962a edn). On liberty (reprinted from 1859 edn). In Warnock 1962, pp. 126–250.

Mill, J. S. (1962b edn). Utilitarianism (reprinted from 1861 edn). In Warnock 1962, pp. 251–342.

Miller, V. G. and Rew, L. (1989). Analysis and intuition: the need for both in nursing education. *Journal of Nursing Education* 28 (2), February, pp. 84–6.

Musgrave, C. F. (1987). The ethical and legal implications of hospice care. *Cancer Nursing* 10 (4), pp. 183–9.

Newton, L. (1981). Lawgiving for professional life: reflections on the place of the professional code. *Business and Professional Ethics Journal* 1 (1), pp. 41–53.

Outka, G. (1972). *Agape: an ethical analysis.* Yale University Press, New Haven and London.

Plato (1966 edn). Euthyphro. In Allen 1966, pp. 59–74.

Rawls, J. (1971). *A theory of justice.* Oxford University Press, Oxford.

Reich, W. T. (ed.) (1978). *Encyclopedia of bioethics.* The Free Press, New York.

Rew, L. (1987). Nursing intuition: too powerful and too valuable to ignore. *Nursing 87* 17 (7), July, pp. 43–5.

Rew, L. and Barrow, E. M. (1987). Intuition: a neglected hallmark of nursing knowledge. *Advances in Nursing Science* 10 (1), pp. 49–62.

Ross, W. D. (1930). *The right and the good.* Clarendon Press, Oxford.

Rousseau, J.-J. (1947 edn). The social contract (reprinted from 1762 edition). In Sir Ernest Barker, *Social contract,* Oxford University Press, London, pp. 239–440.

Sanders, K. and Moore, B. (eds) (1991). *Anencephalics, infants and brain death treatment options and the issue of organ donation. Proceedings of Consensus Development Conference.* Law Reform Commission of Victoria, Royal Children's Hospital, Melbourne, and Australian Association of Paediatric Teaching Centres, Melbourne.

Singer, P. (1979a). Famine, affluence, and morality. In R. A. Wasserstrom (ed.), *Today's moral problems,* Macmillan, New York, pp. 561–72.

Singer, P. (1979b). *Practical ethics.* Cambridge University Press, Cambridge.

Singer, P. (ed.) (1991). *A companion to ethics.* Basil Blackwell, Oxford.

Smart, J. J. C. and Williams, B. (1973). *Utilitarianism: for and against.* Cambridge University Press, Cambridge.

Solomon, R. C. and Murphy, M. C. (eds) (1990). *What is justice? Classic and contemporary readings.* Oxford University Press, New York.

Solomon, W. D. (1978). Rules and principles. In Reich (1978), pp. 407–12.

Stevenson, C. L. (1944). *Ethics and language.* Yale University Press, New Haven.

Stout, J. (1988). *Ethics after Babel: the languages of morals and their discontents.* Beacon Press, Boston.

Swanton, C. (1987). The rationality of ethical intuitionism. *Australasian Journal of Philosophy* 65 (2), June, pp. 172–81.

Urmson, J. O. (1958). Saints and heroes. First published in A. I. Melden (ed.), *Essays in moral philosophy,* University of Washington Press, pp. 198–216; reprinted in J. Feinberg, *Moral concepts,* Oxford University Press, Oxford, pp. 60–73.

Urmson, J. O. (1975). A defence of intuitionism. *Proceedings of the Aristotelian Society* 65, pp. 111–19.

Vaughan, F. E. (1979). *Awakening intuition.* Anchor Books/Doubleday, New York.

Waithe, M. E. (ed.) (1987). *A history of women philosophers. Volume 1: 600 BC–500 AD.* Martinus Nijhoff, Dordrecht.

Warnock, G. J. (1967). *Contemporary moral philosophy.* Macmillan Education, Houndmills, Basingstoke, Hampshire.

Warnock, M. (ed.) (1962). *Utilitarianism.* Fontana Library/Collins, London.

Williams, B. (1985). *Ethics and the limits of philosophy.* Fontana and Collins, London.

Chapter

4

Feminist moral philosophy

IN THE INTRODUCTION TO the previous chapter, on Western moral philosophy, it was averred that not everyone was in agreement that there is a universal moral theory which could be appealed to by everyone for dealing with particular problems in specific and clearly demarcated contexts. The reasons for this disagreement are complex and varied, and have generated a substantial body of literature. Some have even rejected altogether the adequacy of mainstream Western moral thinking, arguing, among other things, that: (1) it is too abstract to have much currency in the practical world of everyday affairs; (2) it pays too much attention to upholding abstract rules and principles, rather than promoting quality relationships between people; and (3) it has tended to privilege the interests and concerns of white middle-class able-bodied heterosexual males at the expense of those deemed 'other', and hence inferior — for example, women, people of non-English-speaking and culturally diverse backgrounds, disabled people, and so on.

Critical to this debate have been the challenges posed by feminist moral theory and transcultural ethics. This and the following chapter briefly examine the nature and content of these two theoretical perspectives, and present a rudimentary overview of their respective critiques of mainstream Western moral thinking.

Feminist moral theory

Feminist moral theory is probably regarded by more conservative philosophers as not having a bona fide place in modern moral philosophy at all. However, such academic opinion is not only poorly informed, but wholly unhelpful to the development of a substantive contemporary bioethics debate — and, indeed, to moral theory generally.

A gender bias in philosophy is well recognised. Popular philosophy texts and standard reference texts (for example, encyclopedias and dictionaries of philosophy) make little reference, and in most instances none, to the philosophical contributions of women. This absence was highlighted some years ago by a seemingly trivial incident. In 1987 Dr Lynda Burns, an academic at Melbourne University, entered a 'Philosophy's Greatest Hits' competition, run by the university's philosophy department. Her entry was disqualified, because none of the female philosophers she named were in the required sources — specifically, the *Encyclopedia of philosophy* or the index of *Modern philosophical writings* (Hutton 1987, p. 20).

Another example of bias involved a female registered nurse who had successfully completed a first degree majoring in philosophy (with straight 'A' passes and the university prize for philosophy in her third year), and who transferred to another university to continue her studies. On her first visit to the philosophy department of the new university at which she was intending to study, and with which she had already been in contact by correspondence, a senior lecturer (male) approached her, inquiring: 'Who are you?' After she introduced herself, the lecturer exclaimed: 'Oh yes. I've heard about you. The *nurse* ...', and without another word abruptly walked off! Later she learned that this same lecturer had been overheard lamenting the increase in the number of female students enrolling in philosophy courses and declaring that it would mark the demise of philosophy as a sound and respectable discipline.

The contributions of women to philosophy

Contrary to popular impressions, and despite the lack of visible evidence in standard philosophy texts, the contributions made by women to philosophy — and to moral philosophy in particular — have been substantial, with some of the earliest recorded contributions dating back to the early and late Pythagorean cults of the sixth century BC to the first century AD. The moral theories developed by the Pythagorean mothers share a number of similarities with each other, in particular their emphasis on kindness, friendship, compassion, harmony, justice, care, wisdom, and the recognition of obligations incurred in immediate relationships (Waithe 1987, 1989a, 1989b, 1991).

The early Pythagorean philosopher Theano I emphasised the principle of *harmonia* (harmony) and the existence of a principled and harmonious universe. Immoral acts, by her view, are at serious odds with the principle of *harmonia* and stand to contribute to disorder and discord — in particular of the otherwise orderly and harmonious universe.

Theano saw women as those who bear the major responsibility for maintaining order, harmony and justice in the state. Her reasoning on this typically reflects Greek culture, both past and present. For Theano, the family or the home is a microcosm of the state: women's responsibility for maintaining harmony and order in the home extends to the maintenance of harmony and justice in the state. This responsibility is not merely 'natural', but requires a critically reflective approach. As Theano said, 'It is better to be on a runaway horse than to be a woman who does not reflect' (cited in Waithe 1987, p. 15).

Another accomplished personage during this period was Arete of Cyrene (fourth century BC). This remarkable figure succeeded her father as head of the Cyrenaic School of Philosophy. It is recorded that she taught natural science, moral philosophy and ethics for over thirty-five years and wrote at least forty books, including treatises on Socrates. It is also believed that she taught over a hundred and ten philosophers. On Arete's tomb is an epitaph calling her 'the splendour of Greece' with 'the beauty of Helen [of Troy], the virtue of Thirma, the pen of Aristippus, the soul of Socrates, and the tongue of Homer' (cited in Alec 1986, p. 26).

Following close in these women's footsteps was the ingenious Aesara of Lucania, a late Pythagorean who generated a comprehensive (familiar and intuitive) natural law theory of morality. Like Theano, Aesara saw the family as playing an important part in defining moral obligations. Her natural law theory views moral law as applying on three levels: individual or private, familial (one which emphasises the family), and social. These three levels are all characterised by the moral virtues of love, as defined in terms of compassion for others, kindliness, self-esteem, and a justice that is fair and considerate of special needs and concerns, including 'extenuating circumstances and reasons for non-compliance' (an individualistic sense of justice) (Waithe 1987, p. 23).

Another influential Pythagorean mother was Perictone I, who actively encouraged women to philosophise and to seek the virtues of justice and courage (Waithe 1987, p. 32). She had little regard for the 'ideal theories' of morality (theories which sought to prescribe how the world ought to be), emphasising instead theories which were well grounded in pragmatism and the social reality into which one is inescapably born. She insisted that the principle of harmonia was one that should be applied in the actual and concrete circumstances of life — the here and now — and not in the decontextualised, hypothetical and ideal fantasies of the imagination (Waithe 1987, p. 35).

Women have made important contributions to philosophy and moral philosophy in other eras as well, although, as Waithe (1987) makes plain, these contributions continue to be ignored in the 'standard' philosophical texts. In fact, as Waithe notes in her introduction, the accomplishments of over one hundred women philosophers have been omitted from the standard philosophical reference works and histories of philosophy (see also Waithe 1989a, 1991).

In fifteenth-century Italy an academic by the name of Dorotea Bocchi succeeded her father as professor of medicine and moral philosophy at the University of Bologna (Alec 1986, p. 58). In seventeenth-century Germany, Elizabeth of Bohemia (1618–80), a close friend, colleague and confidante of the French philosopher Descartes, lectured in Cartesian philosophy at the University of Heidelberg (Alec 1986, p. 9). Descartes later dedicated his *Principles of philosophy* (1644) to her. In eighteenth-century England, Mary Wollstonecraft wrote the acclaimed *A vindication of the rights of woman* (1792), the first serious work on the subject. This book was later published in 1929 in an edition also featuring John Stuart Mill's *The subjection of women*, an essay written some sixty years earlier. Wollstonecraft believed that, if inequalities in society were to be eliminated, distinctions drawn on the basis of wealth, class and gender would have to be abolished.

Mill's essay on the subjection of women, although an enlightening and provocative study, is rarely, if ever, considered seriously in philosophy courses. Mill's essays *Utilitarianism* and *On liberty* regularly feature on reading lists for philosophy courses, but *The subjection of women* is conspicuous by its absence. Its radical position favouring the emancipation of women may account for this omission. Mill argues in *The subjection of women* that male power (the success of which derives from its professed benevolence) is the instrument of female oppression. He writes:

> ... power holds a smoother language, and whomsoever it oppresses, always pretends to do so for their own good: accordingly, when anything is forbidden to women, it is thought necessary to say, and desirable to believe, that they are incapable of doing it, and that they depart from their real path of success and happiness when they aspire to it.
>
> (Mill 1929 edn, p. 266)

(It should be noted here that *The subjection of women* and other pro-women essays written by Mill benefited from the influence of his wife and probable collaborator, Harriet Taylor. Spender [1988, p. 188] writes, for example, that *The subjection of women* would probably not have been written without Harriet Taylor's influence, and, by Mill's own admission, certainly would not have taken the form that it did without her — and later her daughter's — collaboration.)

Mill's words are as profound today as they were in 1869, and hold particular relevance for nurses. Consider how often nurses are told that they are incapable of moral thinking; or that if they pursue academic learning they will not be 'good practical nurses', or will be 'unhappy' in their profession, or even, as one doctor is reported as saying, 'won't be able to nurse' at all (Webb 1988; Wertheimer 1990).

This brief historical overview shows that contemporary feminist moral theory is the product of an eventful and respectable history (or rather *her*story), not of some 'fringe lunacy' recently invented, as some perhaps have believed. (For further commentary on the contribution of women to philosophy, see Waithe 1989a, 1991; McAlister 1989.) The rise and development of contemporary feminist moral philosophy and its relevance to nursing are now discussed as part of this historical framework.

Keeping off Theano's 'runaway horse'

Modern feminist moral theory argues, among other things, that a profound and, in some respects, irreconcilable difference exists between male and female moral thinking. It further contends that (white) male moral thinking has come to dominate Western moral philosophy, to the extent that the interests and sufferings of women have been rendered irrelevant and invisible (Mullet 1988, p. 109; see also Tronto 1993; Cole and Coultrap-McQuin 1992; Frazer et al. 1992; Holmes and Purdy 1992; Sherwin 1992; Card 1991; Porter 1991; Brabeck 1989; Hoagland 1988; Kittay and Meyers 1987). As a result, modern moral philosophy is incomplete and inadequate and therefore incapable of supplying the world with a substantive moral theory on how best to conduct its affairs. Further to this, feminists argue, modern moral philosophy, contrary to its claims, has not succeeded in supplying a sound, reliable and universal moral theory. At best, it has only given the world a system of *competing and different theories*, each of which offers a different view of life, a different set of action-guiding principles, and a different style of moral decision making (Parsons 1986, p. 82). The failure of modern moral philosophy in this respect, together with its unfruitful preoccupation with attempting to find rational explanations for the nature of moral language and the logic of moral thinking, has led some feminist critics to accuse modern moral philosophy of being little more than 'a pale shadow of its former self' (Parsons 1986, p. 76).

The task of modern feminist moral theory is twofold: first, to function as a moral critique; and, second, to operate as a 'substantive radical moral theory' (Morgan 1988, p. 161). As a moral critique, the task of feminist moral theory is fourfold: first, to examine critically supposedly empirically grounded theories of human nature, particularly those which exclude women and other 'non-rational' beings; second, to generate new paradigms of moral thinking; third, to distinguish what constitutes a genuine moral dilemma in the concrete circumstances of life; and fourth to 'discover and render visible the hidden moral domains of women's lives while establishing women's claim to the full human spectrum of moral action and character, whether good or evil' (Morgan 1988, p. 161).

As a substantive radical moral theory, on the other hand, feminist ethics aims to challenge 'the model of the moral subject as an autonomous, detached, rational subject, often seeing this hypermasculinist ideal of the moral self as both psychologically and morally flawed' (Morgan 1988, p. 161). This model is replaced, in feminist theory, with a more pluralistic model of morality, and one which literally incorporates 'a sense of moral imagination, moral empathy, and moral feeling into an integrated, other-connected self' (Morgan 1988, p. 162).

Feminist moral theorists conclude that, unless the gender imbalance in modern moral thinking is redressed, and unless the 'genuine womanly virtues' are placed firmly back on the hypothetical 'moral map', the moral outlook for the world is bleak. Not only are the welfare and survival of women at stake in this instance, but the welfare and survival of all humankind. On this, Carol Gilligan (1987) concludes:

> The promise in joining women and moral theory lies in the fact that human survival, in the late twentieth century, may depend less on formal agreement than on human connection.

> (Gilligan 1987, p. 32)

Despite the persuasiveness of the feminist theorists' claims, some questions remain. Are there significant differences between male and female moral thinking? Is Western moral philosophy nothing more than a collective of male-gender-specific ideologies? If so, has this been seriously detrimental to the formulation and development of a reliable and substantive moral theory? It is to answering these questions that this chapter now turns.

The supposed difference between male and female thinking

The supposed difference between male and female thinking has been given considerable attention in philosophy by many notable male 'authorities', including the ancient Greek philosopher Aristotle (384–22 BC), the moral theologian and scholastic philosopher

Thomas Aquinas (1225–74), the French political and educational philosopher Jean-Jacques Rousseau (1712–78), and the German philosopher Immanuel Kant (1724–1804).

Aristotle's writings clearly depict women as both rationally and morally inferior to men, and thus lacking any form of moral authority. In *Politics* (1957 edn), for example, Aristotle argued (or rather assumed, since he did not, in fact, put forward any systematic argument to support his position) that the male 'is more fitted to rule than the female, unless conditions are quite contrary to nature' (1259a37) and that, as head of the household, the male is rightly the source of virtue in his wife, children and slaves (1259b18–1260b24). The source of male virtue is thought to be the rational element of the soul, which, while present, in the female is 'ineffective' (1259b32). Aristotle required women to have virtue (especially the virtue of silence!), but only in so far as this is required by her master (or husband, as the case may be) to fulfil her function; even then, she is expected to have only little if any 'intellectual appreciation of its [virtue's] nature and reasons' (1259b32). As Morgan (1988) observes on this passage in *Politics*, 'the most that a woman can aspire to, from a moral point of view, is to be aligned with a fully developed man of moral integrity, and to obey his commands silently' (p. 148).

In *Ethics*, Aristotle (1976 edn, pp. 269, 276) again emphasised the moral differences between males and females, and the superiority of male virtues. Women are portrayed as congenitally defective in virtue (Aristotle 1976 edn, p. 243), while a man of even modest rational competence is regarded as still being able to 'conduct himself virtuously' (Aristotle 1976 edn, p. 334). To be governed by the senses, in Aristotle's view, is to be utterly 'brutish' (Aristotle 1976 edn, p. 328) or, worse, 'incontinent'.

Aquinas, a thirteenth-century moral theologian and scholastic philosopher, also regarded women as being rationally and morally inferior to men. He argued:

> As regards the individual nature, woman is defective and misbegotten, for the active force in the male seed tends to the production of a perfect likeness in the masculine sex.
>
> (cited in Morgan 1988 edn, p. 148)

Aquinas argued that women lacked the 'discretion of reason' and could only achieve, at best, moral mediocrity when and if they were in positions of authority. For this reason, Aquinas considered that women should be rightly denied 'full moral and religious personhood as priests' (Morgan 1988, p. 148).

Rousseau (1911 edn, pp. 321, 325), like many of his colleagues, also held women to be morally different and inferior to men. In the celebrated *Emile*, women are expected not 'to complain of the in-equalities of manmade laws', while men are expected not to regard their laws as 'equally binding' on both sexes (Rousseau 1911 edn, p. 324). A husband who is faithless to his wife is merely wrong, while a wife who is faithless to her husband is positively evil, since 'she destroys the family and breaks the bonds of nature' (p. 324). (It is worth considering the parallels that could be drawn here with nursing: if a male doctor is 'faithless' to a female nurse and, for example, lowers her reputation in the eyes of a patient or colleague, or gives an incorrect medical order, he is 'merely wrong'; if a female nurse is 'faithless' to a male doctor, she is 'positively evil' and could be successfully sued for defamation or negligence, imprisoned, fined or deregistered [see also Johnstone 1994].) If a woman were to usurp the rights of a man, she would succeed only in asserting her inferiority (Rousseau 1911 edn, p. 327). Superiority of women, meanwhile, can only be achieved through obedience (p. 335), a logic difficult to follow. (Compare this with the notion of the supremely 'good' nurse being the supremely 'obedient' nurse [Johnstone 1994, chapters 5 and 6].) In terms of developing morality, Rousseau claimed that a woman should merely observe the world and discover by her observations 'an experimental morality'; a man, on the other hand, should use his reason and reduce the experimental morality of women into a system (Rousseau 1911 edn, p. 350). The underlying reasons for this are, of course, that women are not capable of theoretical reasoning or of shaping a systematic morality. Only men should undertake this task. (Again, in drawing parallels to nursing today, nurses are supposed merely to 'observe' and collect data, while the doctor puts it all together and makes the diagnosis — a practice regarded by many in the medical profession as a doctor's overriding prerogative in all medical, moral and even nursing matters [Johnstone 1994, chapters 6 and 7].)

The last philosopher to be considered here is Immanuel Kant. Like his predecessors, Kant saw women as incapable of theoretical reasoning, arguing that 'women's morality should essentially be one of sentiment, governed by irrational moral feelings of aversion and beauty' (cited in Morgan 1988, p. 149). Kant's moral scheme of things is one based firmly on rationality. By denying the rational capabilities of women, Kant succeeded in excluding them from any substantial involvement in the development of moral discourse and the moral life.

The views of these philosophers and others like them have been overwhelmingly influential both inside and outside moral philosophy. Outside moral philosophy, for example, women are still regarded as being rationally inferior to men and emotionally fickle, and thus quite unsuitable for positions of authority (Pateman 1989; Lloyd 1984; Jaggar 1983; McMillan 1982). Evidence of this can be found in the under-representation of women in government, business management, professorial chairs and the traditional professions, not to mention in positions of religious leadership. (Australia has only just seen the ordination of women as priests [see, for example Porter 1989].) As well, the 'anatomy is destiny' ethos of Freudianism and neo-Freudianism is still influential, as are the imprisoning labels of insanity that this ethos ascribed to social and cultural nonconformity (Chesler 1972; Ussher 1991).

Inside moral philosophy, on the other hand, gender dualism in moral thinking continues to be rigorously debated. Male moral thinking is described in terms of rational constructs and abstract moral principles, such as those of autonomy and justice; female moral thinking is described more in terms of non-rational constructs, notably feelings of care, empathy, compassion, love, sympathy and friendship.

The supposed gender dualism in moral thinking has received particular attention over the past few years, initially because of the celebrated Kohlberg–Gilligan debate. Lawrence Kohlberg, an internationally renowned moral developmental theorist, is credited with having laid the foundations of modern moral psychology (Flanagan and Jackson 1987, p. 622). His views have been influential on the development of moral education programs — including those in some United States schools of nursing (Berkowitz 1982; Bridston 1982). Carol Gilligan, Kohlberg's former collaborator, challenged the validity of Kohlberg's research and entered into a strenuous public debate, as a result of which Kohlberg modified some of his claims.

Kohlberg's theory is based on empirical research. It asserts that there are culturally universal stages of moral development through which moral reasoning progresses. The ultimate level, stage 6, embodies a Rawlsian ideal of justice, and represents the highest stage of moral development. Kohlberg (1981, p. 123) maintains that his research shows that there are 'no important differences in development of moral thinking between Catholics, Protestants, Jews, Buddhists, Moslems, and atheists'. Research carried out in third-world countries, including Mexico and Taiwan, indicated the same six stages of development, except that their progress was 'slower' (Kohlberg 1981, p. 23).

The six moral development stages identified by Kohlberg (1981, pp. 409–12) are summarised as follows:

Stage 1. *Punishment and obedience*: an egocentric view of the world, judging actions in terms of physical consequences rather than in terms of the psychological interests of others.

Stage 2. *Individual instrumental purpose and exchange*: a concrete individualistic perspective which takes into account the actor's pragmatic needs and instrumental intentions; conflicting interests and needs can be met through instrumental exchange of services or good will, or by fair dealing; the agent recognises that others have personal interests to pursue.

Stage 3. *Mutual interpersonal expectations, relationships, and conformity*: the perspective of individual relationships to other individuals, including the shared feelings, expectations, concerns, loyalties and trusts in these relationships; what is right is determined by what is expected by people who are close in the relationship, or by what is expected of someone in a particular role — e.g., as brother, sister, or friend.

Stage 4. *Social system and conscience maintenance*: the perspective of 'the system', which judges actions on the basis of whether they conform to societal requirements and values, and other social conventions serving social order.

Stage 5. *Prior rights and social contract or utility*: a view of the individual as an objective, rational and impartial spectator who is aware of values and rights which exist prior to 'social attachment and contracts'; right is seen in terms of upholding basic rights, values and social contracts.

Stage 6. *Universal ethical principles*: a view of the world in terms of a higher order or transcendent morality, assuming that all humanity should follow universal ethical principles (in particular, the universal principle of justice); right is judged on the basis of whether actions accord with universal moral principles.

Stages 1 to 4 of Kohlberg's moral development levels do not involve principled reasoning and are regarded as the *lower levels* of moral development; agents who achieve these levels of development are regarded as morally undeveloped and morally immature. Stages 5 and 6, on the other hand, involve principled reasoning and are therefore regarded as the higher levels of moral development; agents who achieve these levels, in particular stage 6, are regarded as being morally developed and morally mature.

Berkowitz, an associate professor of psychology, was quick to embrace Kohlberg's theory to assess the moral development of nurses and to recommend educational strategies accordingly. Berkowitz argues that nurses should not be taught to be 'Kantian moralists', since it is 'unlikely' they could develop such a level of moral thinking. He contends that nurses could possibly reach Kohlberg's stage 3 of moral development, or even stage 4 (or at least progress towards it), but no more. Berkowitz concludes that 'nursing ethics curricula should therefore be tailored to initiate and consolidate stages 3 and 4 not ... stages 5 and 6' (1982, p. 38).

The comprehensiveness and reliability of Kohlberg's 'empirically based' moral development theory became the subject of much criticism, however, when his former collaborator, Carol Gilligan, revealed a major design fault in Kohlberg's moral judgment research, namely 'the use of all-male samples as the empirical basis for theory construction' (Gilligan 1987, p. 21). Kohlberg had in fact studied the same group of seventy-five boys at three-year intervals for a total of fifteen years, following them from early adolescence through to young manhood; he later generalised his findings to apply to females, which (predictably) showed females to be morally 'undeveloped' and 'immature' (Kohlberg 1981, p. 115; Gilligan 1987).

Upon realising that Kohlberg's research had not examined girls and women, Gilligan condemned it as inherently biased, pointing out that it could hardly be taken as 'representative' of human experience. (Mistaking the masculine bias as universally representative has been dubbed 'phallocentrism' in some circles [Braidotti 1986, p. 48].) On the basis of her own observations and research into the apparent gender differences between male and female moral reasoning, Gilligan also argued that, by eliminating women from the research samples, Kohlberg had eliminated a 'care focus' in moral reasoning, a principal ingredient in women's moral thinking (Gilligan 1987, 1982).

Irrespective of Gilligan's criticisms, Kohlberg's findings have essentially reinforced the popular myth that 'rationality' and reasoning by abstract principle are morally supreme, while 'feelings' or 'sentiment' are morally inferior. At least one author has defended Kohlberg and voiced scathing criticisms against Gilligan, claiming that Gilligan herself appeals to the same rational principles she has condemned in Kohlberg's analysis, and that her own theoretical stages of moral development are not very different from Kohlberg's (Broughton 1983). Another critic claims that 'looking more closely at Gilligan's research it is hard not to see there a methodology designed to exaggerate difference and to disregard similarity between men and women' (Segal 1987, p. 147). Nevertheless, the implications of Kohlberg's moral development theory are far-reaching: those (usually women) who base their moral judgments on non-rational considerations (for example, sentiment, care, friendship) inevitably emerge as 'morally undeveloped' and thus 'morally immature', while those (usually men) who base their judgments on rational and universal ethical principles emerge as 'morally developed' and 'morally mature'. Women, once again, are portrayed as being incapable of authoritative moral reasoning.

Kohlberg accepted some of Gilligan's criticisms and eventually modified his claims, as already mentioned. He acknowledged the presence of a care perspective in people's 'higher order' moral thinking (Gilligan 1987, p. 22), although he maintained that an ethic of *agape* (Greek for 'love') 'still must rely on the stage 6 fairness principles to resolve justice problems' (Kohlberg 1981, p. 354). Gilligan's own research, meanwhile, suggests that, while a significant proportion (69 per cent) of both women *and* men can incline towards a dominant but alternating *care and justice* perspective in their moral reasoning, women are more inclined to include a 'care focus' in moral reasoning, and therefore that, if women are eliminated from a research sample, the 'care focus' will 'virtually disappear' (Gilligan 1987, p. 25).

Kohlberg's theory has also been criticised on more conventional philosophical grounds. Nicolayev and Phillips (1979), for example, have criticised his reliance on a dominant conception of morality and the connection he makes with a theory of increasing moral adequacy. They point out that there are many different ways of thinking about morality and about how different people should act in particular moral situations. How people view and think about moral issues is 'not necessarily committed to a developmental orientation, much less to the view that there are clear-cut stages of development' (Nicolayev and Phillips 1979, p. 232). They argue that there is absolutely nothing to suggest why Kohlberg's stage 6 of moral development should be considered superior to stage 5, stage 4, stage 3, stage 2, or stage 1 for that matter. A moral justification based on a principle of care could easily be just as compelling as a moral justification based on a principle of rational justice.

Crittenden (1979) has also been highly critical of Kohlberg's thesis. He openly disputes Kohlberg's account of justice and, in particular, its equation with morality. He contends that one of the major weaknesses of Kohlberg's position is his reliance on and endorsement of the views of 'certain distinguished ethical theorists' rather than on his own 'systematic exposition' (Crittenden 1979, p. 251). One unfortunate consequence of this debate for Kohlberg is that his account of justice is vulnerable to exactly the same criticisms as have already been made against the justice theorists he supports. Crittenden (1979, p. 259) has also disparaged Kohlberg's defence of what by all accounts is merely a 'particular moral system dominated by an interpretation of justice'. He further points out that there is nothing arbitrary or logically inconsistent in holding 'a plurality of ultimate moral principles' (Crittenden 1979, p. 258), something that Kohlberg's theory (and, in particular, its principle of justice-as-morality) seems to negate. In short, Kohlberg's theory of moral development wobbles on its inadequate account of the moral terms and concepts it inherently relies on, using interpretations that have been the subject of intense philosophical controversy, and that are by no means accepted as universally true. One important implication, of course, is that if the central moral concepts of Kohlberg's theory of moral development are not universally true, how can his theory itself be plausibly regarded as being universally true?

The hypothetical versus the real

Western moral philosophy, in its present form, is unequivocally based on rationality, and in particular on critically reflective or 'reasoned' abstract principles of conduct. Proponents of rationality fervently argue that reason is value-neutral or objective (unlike feelings, which are value-laden and subjective), and therefore stands supreme as an enlightened authority on how best to live and how best to conduct one's behaviour in a world of competing self-interest. The *individual*, in so far as he (and, less frequently, she) is capable of functioning as a self-governing or law-making 'agent', is the centre of moral endeavour and is free to pursue self-interest, constrained only by the 'significant moral interests of others'. The individual — or rather, *the agent*, as 'he' is now referred to — emerges as the objective and impartial spectator or 'ideal observer', choosing from behind a Rawlsian 'veil of ignorance'. Paradoxically, self-interest becomes interpreted as upholding the interests of others, which, in turn, reduces back to self-interest. In his celebrated essay *Utilitarianism*, Mill told us, for example, that if we maximise the general welfare, our own welfare will be enhanced in the process; the contemporary philosophers Rawls (1971) and Gauthier (1986) argue along similar lines.

Under the guidance of critically reflective moral principles, the person who was once an important member of a familial group, sharing the experiences, pains, joys, decisions and responsibilities of that group, is transformed into a solitary agent, operating alone towards achieving some ideal hypothetical good (Mullett 1988). Moral problems are no longer constructed in terms of care, responsibility and personal relationships, but in terms of abstract rights and duties and principles of conduct (Gilligan 1982). For example, the problem of a grief-stricken parent weeping over the brain death of an only son injured in a recent car accident is reconstructed into a detached and hypothetical problem of serving some ideal greater good. The parent is expected to be stoically and heroically detached from the parent–son relationship, and to consent to the son's vital organs being 'retrieved' or 'harvested' for transplantation into the worn-out body of some unknown other person. Coupled with this, the parent is supposed to feel virtuous for consenting to the desecration of that son's body and to feel guilty if consent is not given. Another example concerns the problem of whether a young and unsuspecting wife should be told that her husband has AIDS. The problem is not constructed in terms of 'care' for her as a person and as someone who is at risk of being seriously hurt, but is reconstructed in the rather abstract terms of an attending doctor being bound by the 'rational' principle of confidentiality, said to be 'implicit' in the professional relationship the doctor has with the patient, the AIDS infected husband. In this case, the attending doctor does not tell the unsuspecting wife of her husband's fatal diagnosis, even though the doctor knows that the couple have an active sex life and are planning a child. The doctor refuses to breach confidentiality because the patient specifically requests that his wife not be told of his AIDS diagnosis.

Sissela Bok (1980) cites a similar case, which occurred in 1904, where a physician refused to warn a prospective victim that her fiancé was a syphilitic, thereby risking both her and her offspring being exposed to the disease. Commenting on the case, the physician wrote:

> A single word [...] would save her from this terrible fate, yet the physician is fettered hand and foot by his cast-iron code, his tongue is silenced, he cannot lift a finger or utter a word to prevent this catastrophe.

> (Bok 1980, p. 147)

Modern moral philosophy argues that the moral sentiments of sympathy, compassion, care and similar feelings are quite irrelevant to the moral worth of an action. The moral worth of an action is something that can be decided only by appealing to sound critically reflective and universal moral principles, not mere sentiments. Even if an agent 'feels' bad, he must follow the dictates of reason; in short, he must free himself from the corrupting influences of the passions and discover through reason alone the blinding ideals of truth. If a man is to prove his moral integrity, he must act on reason alone — even if this means sacrificing those he loves. A classic example is the 'Abraham myth', discussed later in this chapter (Gilligan 1982, p. 104; Noddings 1984, pp. 40–6).

In many respects, feminist moral theory is the antithesis of mainstream Western moral theory; in other respects, it stands as its happy companion — bearing in mind that not all moral philosophy falls under the same 'umbrella', so to speak. For example, the celebrated works of Bernard Williams (1972; 1981; 1985), Alasdair MacIntyre (1985), and Lawrence Blum (1980), three contemporary male moral philosophers, all seriously challenge the adequacy and reliability of contemporary moral philosophy. Each of these philosophers suggests that modern moral philosophy is in a state of crisis and that a radical new direction in moral thinking is required if this crisis is to be overcome. Admittedly, neither Williams nor MacIntyre nor Blum suggests that feminist moral theory indicates the direction needed. Nevertheless, their views give significant support to a feminist critique of modern moral thinking, and, like feminist moral philosophy itself, stand to make a valuable contribution to the development of a more substantive moral theory generally. The moral views of the Austrian-born philosopher

Ludwig Wittgenstein (1889–1951) are also enlightening, and, although not directly suggesting that modern moral philosophy is in crisis, nevertheless recommend a radical change in moral thinking. The views of these philosophers are briefly considered shortly.

Feminist moral theory's critique of modern moral philosophy basically examines the nature of rationality and its supposed supremacy as a moral guide, denies the sovereignty of the individual and the acceptability of the pursuit of self-interest, and resists the demands of abstract rules and principles. It has also sought to emphasise interdependent relationships (particularly those involving family and friends), to promote the values of sharing, empathy, nurture and caring, and to stress the importance of context and situational demands (Grimshaw 1986, p. 203; Walker 1992, p. 165). As well, feminist moral theory argues that a substantive moral theory or ethic is one that should be well grounded in the 'concrete circumstances of life' and not the 'detached fantasies of the hypothetical ideal' (Perictone I, cited in Waithe 1987, p. 35; see also Harding and Hintikka 1983; Grimshaw 1986; Kittay and Meyers 1987; Code et al. 1988; Gatens 1986; Braidotti 1986; Noddings 1984; Andolsen et al. 1987; Hoagland 1988; Brabeck 1989; Porter 1991; Card 1991; Sherwin 1992; Holmes and Purdy 1992; Frazer et al. 1992; Cole and Coultrap-McQuin 1992; Tronto 1993). Provocative questions are raised about the reliability of a value-neutral account of rationality, and about why *reason* should be regarded as having any more authority in moral thinking than the moral sentiments of, for example, empathy, compassion, sympathy, kindness, friendliness or caring.

Moulton (1983), a feminist scholar, gives a persuasive account of how the notion of value-free reasoning has been thoroughly rejected in respectable scientific circles. She points out that there is now widespread recognition that the paradigms of beliefs about methodology and evaluation, acceptable methods of inquiry, and notions of scientific good — for example, of *good* questions to ask; *satisfying* theories to follow; questions that are *felt to be more important* — *all* import value orientations, and are subject to change. She is careful to point out that this now accepted value-laden account of reasoning does not mean that scientific theories or paradigms descendent of reason are 'irrational or not worth studying', but that 'there is no simple universal characterisation of good scientific reasoning' (Moulton 1983, p. 152; see also Harding 1987, 1991; Code 1991). This implies that 'objective' scientific reasoning is really no more 'objective' than the subjectivity with which it has been chosen (Gatens 1986, p. 25; Rich 1979, p. 207; Jaggar 1983, p. 360).

The next step in Moulton's thesis is to argue that criticisms of the value-neutral account of reasoning in science apply equally to the value-neutral account of reasoning in philosophy (Moulton 1983, p. 152). The weak link in the supposed objective and value-free chain of Western philosophical thinking can be found in its paradigm of reasoning, notably the 'adversary paradigm', as Moulton calls it, which sees 'an unimpassioned debate between "adversaries" who try to defend their own views against counter examples and produce counter examples to opposing views' (Moulton 1983, p. 153).

The adversary method supposedly ensures that only the 'best' of philosophical theses survive, bestowing upon them in the process of public scrutiny the supreme seal of approval — notably, the stamp of 'proven objectivity'. On this philosophical presumption, Moulton makes the rhetorical point:

> since there is no way to determine with certainty what is good and what is bad philosophy, the Adversary Method is the best there is. If one wants philosophy to be objective, one should prefer the Adversary Method to other, more subjective, forms of evaluation which would give preferential treatment to some claims by not submitting them to extreme adversarial tests.

> (Moulton 1983, p. 153)

Moulton convincingly rejects the adversary paradigm by pointing out that what is wrong with its method is not just its role as *a* paradigm, but its role as *the* paradigm of philosophical reasoning. If it were merely one among many methods which philosophy could employ, 'there might be nothing worth objecting to except that conditions of hostility are not likely to elicit the best reasoning' (Moulton 1983, p. 153). But, as Moulton argues, 'when it *dominates* [italics added] the methodology and evaluation of philosophy, it restricts and misrepresents what philosophic reasoning is' (p. 153).

There are other, non-adversarial, modes of evaluating, reasoning about and discussing philosophy, but philosophers do not seem to recognise these. Neither has philosophy learned from its philosophical father, Socrates, whose method of philosophical reasoning encouraged dialogue and discussion, and carefully resisted ridiculing speakers who held opposing views (Moulton 1983, p. 156). For his academic style and approach to philosophy (an approach that I have found very successful even in the teaching of non-philosophical clinical nursing subjects), Socrates has been described in the Platonic dialogues as the 'wisest man on earth'. As Moulton points out, as a playful and helpful teacher, Socrates' aim 'is not to rebut, it is to show people how to think for themselves' (p. 157).

Moulton concludes that the adversary paradigm of philosophical reasoning has presented the world with distorted images about 'what sorts of positions are worthy of attention', and has fallen prey to the world view of the hypothetical adversary who fundamentally ignores the 'positions which make more valuable or interesting claims' (p. 158). The pessimism of Moulton leaves the lasting impression that perhaps modern moral philosophy as it has been commonly portrayed really has failed at its most basic task: to guide us as the 'lovers or friends of wisdom' to discover the truth about the world in which we live and how best to live the good life in that world.

Gibson (1976), a philosophy scholar, also launches a scathing critique on the value-neutral account of rationality. Her thesis argues that rationality cannot escape the influences of the social patterns and institutions around it, and that a value-neutral account of rationality is quite inadequate for dealing with this fact. She concludes that at best rationality should be regarded as a *value*, rather than as a *property* which all normal people have (Gibson 1976, p. 193). Gatens (1986) argues along similar lines, saying that the male desire for objectivity (philosophy's sacred cow) 'is itself a subjective drive and this subjective drive throws into question the objectivity that many philosophers claim for their accounts' (Gatens 1986, p. 25).

Parsons (1986) formulates an imaginative and interesting critique on rationality and on what she sees as the rise and rule of 'rational imperialism'. Citing Mary Midgley's *Beast and man* (1980), Parsons points out that Western thinking on human nature has been 'hampered by dualistic thinking regarding our nature which has not allowed us to appreciate the fullness or complexity of both our inheritance and our possibilities' (Parsons 1986, p. 85). Referring to Midgley's views, Parsons (1986, p. 86) contends that, if reason is to occupy a fruitful position in our moral thinking, it should not be viewed 'as a colonial oppressor ordering the natives to behave in ways which have been designated for them extraneously, but rather as a "clever integrater"'. The real task of moral reasoning, Parsons suggests, is not to determine our human potential and desires, but to help us assess, organise, and express these more effectively. If moral reasoning is to fulfil its task, it needs to be viewed as a complex and interdependent concept, not a simple and independent one.

Another important philosophical notion to be criticised by feminist moral theory is the notion of the *individual agent* operating as a lone decision maker in a hypothetical world comprised of philosophical fantasies about ideal moral truths. Important questions are raised concerning why modern moral philosophy has tended to neglect the intermediate region of family relations and relations of friendship which otherwise exist between the rationally self-interested agent and the collectively interested universal others (Held 1987, p. 117). Indeed, why has it also neglected the significant phenomena of caring, concern and sympathy which people feel for those with whom they have personal and closely entwined relationships?

Perhaps one of the most disturbing things about modern moral philosophy's neglect of the family and personal relations is that it appears to have been deliberate. Lloyd (1984, p. 75), for example, points out that the pride of classical philosophy derives from its success in achieving 'complete detachment from the complexities and participation of ordinary living'. This pride inevitably extended to classical moral philosophy, which has come to prize the self-conscious ethical life as being closely associated with 'breaking away from the family' (the family, of course, is regarded as being closely allied with 'particularity') (Lloyd 1984, p. 92). The need to 'break from the family' and to surrender the 'private' domain of domesticity for the 'public' domain of higher-order activities is well documented in both ancient and modern philosophical literature.

In part 4, book 3 ('Guardians and auxiliaries') of the celebrated *Republic,* Plato advocated that the state's rulers and auxiliaries must live a life of 'austere simplicity, without private property or family life'. And in part 6, book 5 ('Women and the family'), Plato advocated that women should receive the same physical and intellectual education as men — including being trained for war. This egalitarian view of the role of women is not without a price, however, as we shall soon see. Plato went on to assert that 'if men and women are to lead the same lives, the family must be abolished'. In its place would come the setting up of state nurseries which would be filled with the babies born of 'breeding rituals'. Plato saw the advantages of this system as being twofold:

> first, that it makes it possible to breed good citizens, and second, that it gets rid of the distracting loyalties, affections and interests of the family system.
>
> (Plato, 1955 edn, p. 211)

The influence of 'anti-family' sentiment is more subtle in later works, but is nevertheless there. John Stuart Mill, for example, advocated individual liberty, but failed to consider that the liberty he spoke of was not even a remote possibility for the women of his society, who were grounded by the responsibilities of children, household management and, dare it be said, philosophising husbands (a point made abundantly clear in Midgley and Hughes' interesting book *Women's choices* [1983]). More recently, Richard Hare (1981, p. 27), in *Moral thinking,* uses a provocative example in which he appears to adopt the position that breaking a promise to his children (for example, that he would take them on a picnic) is less odious than disappointing a lifelong friend who arrives unexpectedly from overseas and wishes to be shown around the Oxford colleges. After engaging in an elaborate philosophical argument on the philosophy of moral language, Hare concludes that breaking the promise he has made to his children (and thereby hurtfully disappointing them) is a matter only of *regret*, not of *moral remorse* (Hare 1981, p. 28). Thus the apparent conflict of duties raised by the unexpected visit of his overseas friend is rendered not to be a conflict at all. Hare therefore feels free to show his friend around the Oxford colleges without a flicker of remorse for the disappointment he has caused his children and without offering any acceptable alternatives to cancelling the picnic. (Another disturbing feature about Hare's position here is that it is so readily accepted by the philosophers who read it.)

This 'breaking away from the family' and being freed from the 'distracting loyalties of family life' has been legitimised by the doctrine of decontextualisation. This doctrine holds, roughly, that if moral choices are to be *objective* (popularly regarded as one of the minimum requirements of sound moral decision making) they should be made from the position of an 'impartial spectator' or, to borrow again from Rawls, from behind 'a veil of ignorance'. In other words, the decision maker must transcend the boundaries otherwise imposed by context, and choose from a universal, objective, impartial and unbiased point of view, notably one guided by sound rational and universal moral principles. Since it is doubtful whether any chooser could successfully transcend his or her context, the doctrine of decontextualisation is less than compelling, however. Anthropologists, historians, political scientists, sociologists, psychologists, and, more recently, some philosophers, have made it abundantly clear that we are overwhelmingly the products of our culture and history in the broadest sense, irrespective of any prevailing ideal theory of morality (see, in particular, Marshall 1992; Elliott 1992; Singer 1991; Cortese 1990; de Bono 1990; Leininger 1990a, 1990b; Stout 1988). The notion that an individual (abstract agent, or otherwise) could genuinely operate in a value-void is quite implausible.

Even admitting the behavioural guiding force of rational moral principles does little to rescue the doctrine. As Grimshaw (1986) points out:

> principles *invite* contextualisation of judgements, consideration of the particular. To have principles is not to be inclined to ignore complexity; it is quite compatible with recognising that the judgement one made in a particular situation was so specific to that situation that other apparently similar situations might require a different one.

> (Grimshaw 1986, p. 208)

Neither does the doctrine of decontextualisation's promise of securing sound moral judgments stand to rescue it — a promise of which feminist moral theory is rightly suspicious. Gilligan (1987), for example, warns that decontextualisation, and the detachment from self and others it advocates, 'breeds moral blindness' and an intolerable indifference to the needs of others (p. 24). It advances an ethic that 'has become principled at the expense of care' (Gilligan 1982, p. 105), and that, by blinding itself to the actual harms of particular individuals, fails altogether in fulfilling its task. There is no better example of this than that supplied by the Abraham myth, referred to earlier. In this classical myth, the biblical character Abraham is prepared to sacrifice the life of his son for the principle of supreme truth (God) and as a demonstration of his integrity to the principles of his faith (Gilligan 1982, p. 104; Noddings 1984, pp. 404–6). Abraham's actions in this myth stand in stark contrast to those of the lowly woman who comes before King Solomon and refuses to sacrifice the life of her son, even for the principle of truth, and demonstrates her care by relinquishing the child to the other woman who has falsely claimed to be the boy's mother. Joining Gilligan in her selection of this example, Virginia Held (1987) exclaims:

> A number of feminists have independently declared their rejection of the Abraham myth. We do not approve the sacrifice of children out of religious duty. Perhaps, for those capable of giving birth, reasons to value the actual life of the born will, in general, seem to be better than reasons justifying the sacrifice of such life. This may reflect an accordance of priority to caring for particular others over abstract principle.
>
> (Held 1987, p. 126)

The principle of care, placed entirely in context, offers modern moral philosophy a new and vital direction of inquiry.

Feminist moral theory does not altogether reject modern moral philosophy, or the moral principles derived from it. It merely asks that the products of modern moral philosophy be examined more thoroughly and its demands applied more cautiously and caringly. In other words, feminist moral theory is not about 'getting rid of morality', but about deciding 'which rules we will have' (Midgley 1980, p. 299), how and by whom they should be interpreted, and when they should be applied. Neither is feminist moral theory about splitting morality into gender-linked categories; such a split would be not only 'irrational' (Midgley 1980, p. 355), but a great waste of 'human potential', and would result in the narrowing of everyone's life. Nothing positive is to be achieved by having the world hopelessly divided.

Gilligan (1987) reminds us that *all* human relations are, at some stage, characterised by equality and attachment, inequality and detachment, and therefore *everyone* is vulnerable to oppression and abandonment. This risk of oppression and abandonment, if nothing else, calls for a comprehensive behaviour guide — something which probably neither a rational principle of justice nor a feminist moral principle of care can supply on its own. What is needed are the moral principles of *both* justice and care, with each constraining the authority of the other (Flanagan and Jackson 1987, p. 635), or, more to the point, *each* being viewed as 'essential elements of morally right actions' (the Pythagoreans, for example, held that for an act to be moral it needed to be *both* just *and* caring) (Waithe 1989b, p. 5).

Feminist moral philosophy has yet to articulate a coherent and substantive moral theory. (For an instructive overview of diverse feminist perspectives in moral thinking, see Robb 1985.) Principles such as care, compassion, empathy, kindness, friendship and sympathy have been identified as valid components of a substantive moral theory, but have not as yet been sufficiently articulated, or integrated, to form an independent and substantive ethical theory as such. Similarly, modern moral philosophy has yet to develop a substantive moral theory capable of directing human activity on to a path of harmonious order.

Whatever its weaknesses, feminist moral theory has provided the basis upon which a substantive moral theory can begin to be constructed — a theory which takes into account the 'concrete circumstances of life', which resists giving more weight than is due to the abstract principles of a rationally constructed morality, and which fully recognises the dangers of a 'particular perspective' creating and forcing unnecessary and destructive dichotomies (Katzenstein and Laitin, 1987, p. 264). It is a theory which recognises the strengths of both women's and men's moral perceptions. The strength of women's moral perceptions, in this instance:

> lies in the refusal of detachment and depersonalisation, and insistence on making connections that can lead to seeing the person killed in war or living in poverty as someone's son or father or brother or sister, or mother, or daughter or friend.
>
> (Gilligan 1987, p. 32)

The strength of men's perceptions, on the other hand, lies in commitment to promoting true human welfare, questioning basic assumptions, refusing to be blinded by false ideals, and rediscovering the wisdom of their Socratic forefather.

If there is an ultimate lesson to be learned from feminist moral theory, it is this: it is not enough to just *have* a morality or a reliable moral theory; there must also be *care for* and *concern about* how it will operate, and what it will achieve, viz, its outcomes. Morality is precisely about caring for what happens in the domain of human living (Cole and Coultrap-McQuin 1992; Hoagland 1988; Fisher and Tronto 1990; Brabeck 1989; Baier 1985; Noddings 1984). Any moral system which fails to care is a system of which all decent human beings should rightly be suspicious.

Many issues have still to be addressed by feminist moral philosophy. Its pragmatic grounding has yet to confront the reality of a world which culturally values individuality, autonomy and reason; which, rightly or wrongly, has condoned the disintegration of the extended family; and which is beginning to condone the disintegration of the nuclear family. It also has yet to persuade those thoroughly indoctrinated with the faith of Western moral philosophy that philosophy has failed at its most basic task: 'to question one's basic assumptions thereby to discover the truth' (Waithe 1987), a situation made overwhelmingly evident by the consistent exclusion of women from centuries of philosophical debate and philosophy's history. More importantly, it remains the task both of feminist moral theorists and the dominant and powerful leaders of masculinist modern moral thinking to integrate the contributions of women successfully with those made by men, and vice versa. Moral philosophy will be all the richer and more substantial for it.

New directions in male moral thinking

In *Beyond good and evil*, Nietzsche (1972 edn) declares that morality is nothing but 'a protracted audacious forgery' (p. 291). He is even less complimentary about the philosopher, describing him (sic) as a 'creature' around whom 'snarling quarrelling, discord and uncanniness is always going on' (p. 292), and who 'often runs away from itself, is often afraid of itself — but which is too inquisitive not to keep "coming to itself" again ...' (p. 292).

Some feminist moral theorists would undoubtedly feel vindicated by these passages. Feminist moral theory is not alone in its concern about the reliability and adequacy of modern moral philosophy and its methods, theories and conclusions. A number of internationally reputed male moral philosophers share this concern, which indicates that in some respects feminist criticism of 'male' philosophy and moral philosophy has not always been fair. Some of these male philosophers, past and present, have unrelentingly pursued a course of 'moral radicalism', although their works have been aggressively criticised by philosophical peers, or simply ignored or dismissed as 'insignificant' or 'too trivial' to be worthy of attention. (Mill's *The subjection of women* is a case in point, as is the dismissal of some existential philosophy.) Of course, we should reject modern moral philosophy only on the basis of the philosophy itself, not because it is merely 'male'; to dismiss 'male' philosophical thought would be as capricious as the historical dismissal of 'female' philosophical thought has been. One form of chauvinism does not answer another, and neither is it the answer to the development of a substantive moral theory.

The English philosopher Bernard Williams (born 1929) has written several books in which he discusses the crisis of modern moral philosophy and the need for a radical new direction in moral thinking. Among other things, he argues that philosophical questions take far too much for granted and that some moral theories 'may well turn out to be mere prejudices' (Williams 1985, p. 117).

In advancing his discussion, Williams challenges the assumptions of Kantian philosophy — in particular, that reason or rationality has supreme moral authority and is the basis of sound moral theory, and, second, that abstraction and decontextualisation of the individual is necessary in order to arrive at objective moral truths (Williams 1985, pp. 17, 28). In his critique of a Kantian approach to morality, Williams (1985, p. 17) argues that the assumption about rationality in ethics is 'at once very powerful and utterly baseless', and that its widespread acceptance is more a product of 'unblinking habit' than of reflective inquiry. He also takes the provocative step of condemning the Kantian abstraction of the individual as being both absurd and dangerous. The absurdity here derives from the ridiculousness of the abstract agent trying to 'model precisely the moral choice of a concrete agent' on the basis of what the concrete agent would choose had he (sic) made 'the kinds of abstractions from his [sic] actual personality, situation and relations which the Kantian picture of moral experience requires' (Williams 1981, p. 3). The danger of the Kantian abstraction, on the other hand, derives from its total misrepresentation of the issues at stake, distracting attention from moral responsibility in the process (Williams 1981, p. 19). Williams points out that just who acts in a given situation has enormous bearing on determining responsibility; by abstracting the individual and decontextualising the abstracted individual's actions, responsibility may become diffused (p. 4). Williams argues forcefully in favour of contextualisation, pointing out that, unless people have 'enough substance or conviction' in their lives, nothing will bind their allegiance to life itself (the pessimistic consequences of this being glaringly obvious). He writes:

> Life has to have substance if anything is to have sense, including adherence to the impartial system; but if it has substance, then it cannot grant supreme importance to the impartial system, and that system's hold on it will be, at the limit, insecure.

> (Williams 1981, p. 18)

The cultural, historical, social, political and religious reality of a particular ethical life is crucial to any ethical analysis of it, and to any ethical theory that might be generated for it. Williams suggests that, if modern moral philosophy persists in disregarding these variables, it does so at its own peril — whether philosophers wish to admit it or not, morality is not an invention of philosophy, but an outlook on life, of which almost all of us are a part (Williams 1985, p. 174).

Ethics for Williams is more than a matter of decision; it is also a matter of agreeing what to decide (1985, p. 170). We then have to go through an elaborate process of selecting and contrasting moral and factual knowledge, and then assimilating them (Williams 1972, p. 48). This process, however, also fundamentally involves 'caring about what happens' and not abandoning this care just because 'someone else disagrees with you' (Williams 1972, p. 48). Williams, like so many feminist moral theorists, views care as the fundamental and crucial common denominator of ethical and factual knowledge. To abandon care is to abandon morality, and to doom human welfare and survival. Since this is a supremely irrational outcome, there is room to suggest a very strong sense in which the sentiment of care is not the antithesis of rationality, but rather its counterpart.

The British philosopher Alasdair MacIntyre (1985, p. 256), a contemporary of Bernard Williams, also warns that modern moral philosophy 'is in a state of grave disorder'. This disorder, he suggests, is largely the product of barren armchair philosophy (MacIntyre 1985, p. ix), of misleading and betraying moral language (p. 4), and of a blind reliance on ideas that have claimed false independence from the cultural, social and historical milieus in which they have been generated (MacIntyre 1985, p. 11).

Like Williams, MacIntyre rejects the view of rationality as having supreme moral authority, and as offering a convincing escape from emotivism; that is, the view that moral utterances are really expressions of emotion and individual preferences. In his critique of rational morality and its activities, MacIntyre (1985, p. 9) raises the provocative question: 'What is it about rational argument which is so important that it is the nearly universal appearance assumed by those who engage in moral conflict?'. His short answer to this is that there is nothing compelling or important about it at all. If anything, the rational paradigm of moral argument is uncomfortably aligned with a 'disquieting private arbitrariness' (MacIntyre 1985, p. 8). What appears to be a 'rational' approach is not a rational approach at all, at least not in the genuine 'critically reflective' sense. Philosophical opponents enter into moral debates with their minds already firmly made up. Their lack of unassailable criteria to convince their opponents inevitably sees what should be an instructive and enlightening debate reduced to nothing more than a battleground characterised by dogmatic assertions and counter-assertions (MacIntyre 1985, p. 8). Small wonder, MacIntyre ponders, that 'we become defensive and therefore shrill' in our public arguments.

The conclusion of MacIntyre's philosophy is pessimistic. He warns that we have entered a 'new dark age', and one which, unlike other dark ages, is *already* governed by the barbarians. This predicament, he argues, is every bit the product of our diminished moral consciousness and our failure to construct local forms of community 'within which civility and the intellectual and moral life can be sustained' (MacIntyre 1985, p. 263).

The theme of diminished moral consciousness is one also advanced by the contemporary philosopher Lawrence Blum. In *Friendship, altruism and morality*, Blum (1980) writes that modern Anglo-American moral philosophy has paid appallingly little attention to the moral emotions of sympathy, compassion and human concern, and to friendship 'as a context in which these emotions play a fundamental role' (p. 1). He writes further that the Anglo-American tradition within moral philosophy has not only ignored these moral emotions but has positively militated against their having 'any substantial role in the moral life' (p. 1).

Blum goes on to argue that the moral emotions such as sympathy, compassion, friendship and altruism are just as valid, just as reliable, and have just as an important role to play in moral life as do rational constructs such as moral duty, impartiality, fairness or consistency. On this point, Blum (1980, p. 55) notes that 'impartiality, fairness, and justice are personal virtues, but they are merely some virtues among others. They are not definitive of moral virtue altogether'.

The ultimate finding of Blum's thesis is not just that moral emotions have a place in the moral scheme of things, but that it is *good* to have them. That is, being sympathetic, being compassionate, being friendly, being altruistic, and being concerned about other people are all *morally good* things to be. And, as moral behaviour guides, they are no less reliable and no more vulnerable to the corrupting influence of 'negative moods' than is a rationally inspired sense of duty (Blum 1980, p. 29).

Blum's presentation of a dynamic moral life resting firmly on a sustained concern for the well-being of others offers some hope of escaping MacIntyre's 'new dark age' and the tyranny of Kantian barbarians. The realisation of this hope, however, altogether depends on how enlightened people (and philosophers!) are prepared to allow their moral consciousness to become, and just how prepared they are to modify their attitudes and admit that possibly they have, after all, been mistaken in their beliefs.

Other modern moral philosophers are also beginning to change their attitudes and are beginning to refer and appeal to the moral emotions in their moral monologues. Engelhardt (1986, p. 71), for example, speaks of morality as 'a reciprocal web of sympathies'. Richard Hare (1981, p. 73) concedes that our moral thinking will be less than complete, and will even be faulty, if we do not 'put ourselves in the place of somebody who is suffering'. He also concedes that principles of altruism might, on occasion, be chosen as a means of keeping 'us away from the more seductive vice of selfishness', a view originally advanced by the great patriarch Aristotle (Hare 1981, p. 129).

One of the most dynamic radical views on ethics comes from the sensitive but controversial interpretation by James Edwards (1982) of the moral views of the famous and influential Austrian-born philosopher Ludwig Wittgenstein (1889–1951). Wittgenstein viewed the moral life not as something that can be reduced to abstract rules and principles, or deduced from some general theory, but as something which can only be achieved by upholding a transcendent *ethic of love* and by *actually living* 'a life devoted to direct action in service to others' (Edwards 1982, p. 228). Ethics is not a scientific curiosity, nor anything to do with a scientific approach to dealing with the problems of human conduct (Edwards 1982, p. 234). Rather, it is a matter of profound humanism, characterised by deep sensibility and interconnectedness with the real concrete world and the real living and breathing human beings in that world. To treat morality as 'a set of obstacles to be surmounted, or as a maze to be run, or as a set of tasks to be fulfilled, or as a set of decisions to be computed and taken' is to render it 'a sort of technical, even technologised problem', something which is truly horrible (Edwards 1982, p. 238).

Edwards (1982, p. 98) argues that Wittgenstein held that theory had nothing to offer ethical reflection and in fact impeded the development of moral sensitivities and human understanding. For example, if we become obsessed with rational representations of the moral life and devote all our energies to rational reflection, we will quite simply lose sight of important human concerns and will not have the energy to 'love thy neighbour'. Instead of helping us to get on with the business of 'loving thy neighbour', reflection distracts our attention from this and plunges us into a total and fruitless preoccupation with questions such as: 'But *who is* our neighbour?' (Edwards 1982, p. 228). By the time we come anywhere near to an answer, if we come near to one at all, our neighbour will have long gone. The love of neighbours requires actual deeds, not fruitless theoretical reflection, and it requires 'that we abandon the global for the local, the abstract for the concrete, the willful for the self-effacing' (Edwards 1982, p. 243). In short, love of neighbours requires a life devoted to the service of others.

Ethics is, in a Wittgensteinian sense, a commensurate of sound human understanding. To gain this sound understanding, however, we need to 'deliteralise' our perceptions of the world (Edwards 1982, p. 214). To achieve this deliteralisation of our perceptions of the world, we need to disengage from our *idolatrous worship* of naive realism and refrain from taking our rational representations of the world as being *the* realities themselves and allowing these, like idols, to govern our life and practices. If we do not disengage from this 'idolatrous dogmatism', as Edwards calls it, then we risk 'a debilitating loss of moral energy or the collapse of ethical sensibility into an arbitrary willing' (Edwards 1982, p. 223).

Interestingly, Wittgenstein (originally an engineer by profession) despised professional philosophy, and felt oppressed and conscientiously troubled by his own career as a professional philosopher (Malcolm 1958, p. 62; Edwards 1982, p. 228). He apparently broke away from philosophy, and returned only because 'he felt that he could again do creative work' (Von Wright 1958, p. 12). Wittgenstein basically believed that philosophy had 'therapeutic value' in that it could work to deliteralise our perceptions of the world in much the same way that poetry and the poetic image 'can help us to see through what we ordinarily see'; in other words, philosophy, like poetry, 'is a way of deliteralising and thus expanding our perceptions' (Edwards 1982, p. 213). Just as the poet can help us to see an image that we might ordinarily fail to see in our usual way of perceiving the world, so too does philosophy. Once we have experienced 'deliteralisation', and the perceptual expansion that comes with it, we will learn that the world is 'much richer than our everyday conceptions of it' and 'we can never be so complacent in our ordinary ways of seeing, feeling, and acting' (Edwards 1982, p. 213). Philosophy, like poetry, can help us to go beyond the 'cage of language', as Wittgenstein (1965, p. 12) called it, and beyond our naive thought-representations of the world, to a more meaningful experience of life. Thus, when a person complains of a 'broken heart', we know, thanks to our expanded perceptions, that it is not a cardiologist who is needed, but the hand of human love and understanding.

Wittgenstein's academic life at Cambridge University was not typical of a professor of philosophy. He dissuaded his favourite students from becoming professional philosophers, declined professional association with philosophers, sought no wide recognition for his work (and in fact was greatly distressed that his work had emerged as virtually 'gospel' in philosophical circles), and resigned his chair of philosophy at an early opportunity (Malcolm 1958; Von Wright 1958; Edwards 1982). Interestingly, Wittgenstein was profoundly influenced by the works of Leo Tolstoy and sought to live the Tolstoyan ethic of 'love of neighbour, especially the poor and untutored; rejection of personal wealth and affectation; pursuit of simplicity' (Edwards 1982, p. 245). He gave away his large patrimony, lived and dressed frugally, spent six years teaching in the peasant schools of Lower Austria, worked as a gardener's assistant in a monastery, and, during the war, worked as a hospital orderly and laboratory assistant. Edwards (1982, p. 76) also recounts the touching story of how Wittgenstein repaired the steam engine of a wool factory and, in lieu of payment, directed the owners to distribute woollen cloth to the needy children of the village.

Edwards's rather saintly portrait of Wittgenstein, however, may not be altogether accurate. Other biographers describe Wittgenstein as a man of harsh and even violent temperament, and as someone who had enormous difficulty getting on with people; even his friends feared him and found it a great strain being with him (Von Wright 1958; Malcolm 1958). There is even some suggestion that he left teaching in the peasant schools of Lower Austria because of interpersonal conflict (Von Wright 1958, p. 10).

Whatever Wittgenstein's personal life was, he has undoubtedly left a valuable philosophical legacy. Drengson (1985) describes Wittgenstein's contribution to modern moral philosophy in this way:

> [he] sought to change sensibilities and engender a healthy human understanding. He offered not a theory, but a way of being in the world, not just another way of seeing, but a way of acting and appreciating, an attitude ...

> (Drengson 1985, p. 131)

The lesson of Wittgenstein's ethics is the reminder that what is crucial in ethical reflection 'is the quality of attention that comprises it'; as Edwards concludes:

> In reflecting upon the formulation and application of the ethical terms, principles and judgments of a person or culture, we can discriminate care from carelessness, patience from haste, scruple from self-interest, courage from fear, and the like; and these qualities of attention are just what is at issue.

> (Edwards 1982, p. 249)

The ultimate lesson, though, is that it is people who matter, not things, and it is the love of people that directs the moral life, not the love of abstract and decontextualised principles.

Issues and recommendations

The parallels between feminist moral theory and modern nursing philosophy are striking. Both emphasise the principle of care, and both are acutely aware of the dangers of enforced and hierarchicised dichotomies such as fact and value; reason and non-reason (for example, intuition, emotion, sentiment); thinking and feeling; objectivity and subjectivity; independent individual operating in isolation and interdependent individual engaged in cooperative relationships; scientific (professional) distance and personal involvement; context dependence and context independence; rational justice and human care; self-interest and other interest; abstract objective agent and 'flesh and blood' human being. Even more significant, however, is that both feminist moral theory and modern nursing philosophy are firmly grounded in pragmatics — in 'the concrete circumstances of life' and in the full knowledge of the capacity that human beings have to suffer, to be hurt, to be abused and to bleed.

The parallels between modern moral philosophy and scientific reductionistic medicine are also striking. Both have traditionally respected abstract detachment, and the need to separate the private realm of being from the public realm of being. Medicine's so-called 'professional distancing' from the particular world views and lived experiences of its patients is remarkably similar to modern moral philosophy's distancing from context and its reliance on the supposed fail-safe process of abstraction and appeal to the hypothetical. Both seek to flee 'the corrupting influences of the passions', and worship rationality as a supreme behaviour guide; and both have used the doctrine of rationality to exclude women from their respective domains. (See, for example, Mary Roth Walsh's *Doctors wanted: no women need apply* [1977].)

Perhaps even more instructive are the striking parallels that can be drawn between modern moral philosophy's narcissistic preoccupation with its own abilities and activities, teasing out the logic of moral language, and building moral theories on what constitutes the good life, and scientific reductionistic medicine's preoccupation with its own abilities and activities, teasing out the bio-logic of medical language and the 'inner-logic of the doctor–patient relationship' (Daniels 1984, p. 348), and building medical theories on what constitutes quality of life and what medicine should and should not do in order to achieve this. In matters of life and death, it can be seen that the relationship between masculinist moral philosophy and medicine is almost symbiotic in nature.

If there is a poignant lesson to be learned by drawing these parallels, it is this: nursing needs to be very cautious in its adoption of modern moral philosophy and the model of bioethics it presently offers. To embrace uncritically a scientific rationalistic and reductionistic model of bioethics in nursing would be akin to adopting a scientific reductionistic model of health, a model that is now recognised as being incompatible with modern nursing's holistic health philosophy.

Nursing has a well articulated philosophy of care. This articulation is largely due to the celebrated works of a number of influential nurse theorists, including Madeleine Leininger (1988, 1991), Jean Watson (1985a, 1985b); Sister M. Simone Roach (1987); Patricia Benner and Judith Wrubel (1989); and many others (see, for example, Gaut 1992; Brown et al. 1992; Chinn 1991; Bishop and Scudder 1991; Gaut and Leininger 1991; Leininger and Watson 1990). Nursing also has a well articulated ethic of care, with *care* being recognised increasingly as the moral foundation, ideal and imperative of nursing (Watson 1985a, 1985b; Carper 1986; Roach 1987; Fry 1988a, 1988b, 1989a, 1989b; Twomey 1989; Klimek 1990, Leininger 1990a; Leininger and Watson 1990; Cooper 1991; Benner 1984).

While it might be objected here that nursing's articulation of care is incomplete and inadequate, this need not be problematic. One reason for this is that, in the ultimate analysis, it may be that care cannot be defined adequately or quantified. Indeed, there is considerable room to suggest that, like the concept of 'the good', the concept of care is simple, unanalysable and indefinable. Even if it is conceded that care can be defined, in terms of, say, compassion, sympathy and empathy, this does little to enlighten our rational understanding of it; all that defining care in these terms does is to define it in terms of a string of *other sentiments* about which we know equally little, and which may also be simple, unanalysable and indefinable.

Perhaps we have yet to learn, and be satisfied with the fact, that there are some things in life which just cannot be rationally explained or articulated, as G. E. Moore (1903) eventually discovered in his attempts to define 'the good'. Even reason itself concedes that some things just cannot be adequately defined including, paradoxically, reason itself. As the Pan *Dictionary of philosophy* (1979, p. 300) instructs, 'We have no independent road to acquaintance with the Goddess Reason' (note the female gender attached to the notion of reason here!).

Care cannot occur in the abstract (Carper 1986, p. 4). Neither is it something to be controlled, coerced or even rationalised: to do these things to care would be, to borrow from Benner (1984, p. 170), 'to do violence to it'. Rather, care occurs in the very real and 'concrete circumstances of life', and it occurs spontaneously and with deep human feeling. It also epitomises the bridging of dichotomies, in this instance between fact (practice) and value (attitude).

The task confronting nursing at this time is not to articulate its philosophy of care better than it has already done, nor to define precisely the concept of care itself (this may not be possible), but to make *care* (as it has been articulated to date) more visible as something to be valued both as a virtue and as a principle. By fulfilling this task, nursing will come closer to succeeding not only in developing a profession capable of practising morally, but also in making an invaluable contribution to the development of a sound feminist moral theory and in turn a substantive moral theory generally.

In pursuing the development of a substantive bioethic, nursing must reject the tradition of the destructive dichotomies that have dominated Western philosophical thought and scientific medicine and are now threatening to dominate nursing. Further, nursing must recognise that the 'hypothetical ought' has little currency in a world of real people, who are constrained by real circumstances, and who have the capacity both to hurt and be hurt and to suffer at a level which even the most creative and fertile of imaginations can fail to comprehend fully.

It is not being suggested here that nursing should abandon the lessons of modern moral philosophy; indeed, moral principles and moral language are needed to adjudicate rationality (Moulton 1983), to secure some reliability about what people can reasonably expect from each other (Williams 1985), to help order our value priorities, to remind us not to be capricious (Held 1987, p. 119), and to produce some stability in the interpersonal relations we have with people who otherwise have no personal connection with us (Flanagan and Jackson 1987, p. 633). The importance of this discussion is to suggest that nursing needs to be cautious in its adoption and rejection of competing ethical theories. Moreover, nursing needs to be better informed about the development of a substantive moral theory and what it (nursing) can and should contribute to it.

MacIntyre's 'new dark age' governed by barbarians and Nietzsche's 'trembling creatures' all warn of the urgent need for a radical new direction in moral thinking. The direction this moral thinking should take is clear. It must strive to:

- rediscover the principle of *harmonia,* so well articulated by the ancient Pythagoreans, which, in their hands, once promised an achievable *balance* in the world of human affairs and a harmonisation of diversity;

- construct a theory which is firmly based and shaped by practice, viz. the concrete circumstances of life;

- recognise the importance of shared lived experience, context, and the significance of interdependency;

- bridge the yawning gulf that has emerged between, for example, fact and value, objectivity and subjectivity, reason and non-reason, public and private;

- recognise the biases of its own tradition and be prepared to admit that its findings might sometimes be mistaken;

- recognise the relation of the individual to the group, and the shared responsibility all group members have for each other, as well as for achieving a broader spectrum of human welfare and survival;

- accept that there are some things that cannot be rationalised and objectively defined, and that some of our most decent human acts might be beyond rational explanation — such as those performed out of love and friendship. To think of acts performed out of love and friendship in terms of abstract principle or duty is, to quote Williams (1981, p. 18), to think 'one thought too many'.

Nurses are in an excellent position to contribute to the development of a substantive and integrated bioethic. All that remains, now, is for them actually to do it — and to do it competently and without delay.

References

Alec, M. (1986). *Hypatia's heritage*. The Women's Press, London.

Andolsen, B. Hilkert, Gudorf, C. E. and Pellauer, M. D. (eds) (1987). *Women's consciousness, women's conscience*. Harper & Row, San Francisco (first published by Winston Press, 1985).

Aristotle (1957 edn). *The politics*. Penguin Books, Harmondsworth, Middlesex.

Aristotle (1976 edn). *Ethics*. Penguin Books, Harmondsworth, Middlesex.

Baier, A. (1985). *Postures of the mind: essays on mind and morals*. Methuen, London. Chapter 6: Caring about caring: a reply to Frankfurt.

Benner, P. (1984). *From novice to expert*. Addison-Wesley, Menlo Park, California.

Benner, P. and Wrubel, J. (1989). *The primacy of caring*. Addison-Wesley, Menlo Park, California.

Berkowitz, M. (1982). The role of discussion in ethics training. *Topics in Clinical Nursing* 4 (1), April, pp. 33–48.

Bishop, A. H. and Scudder, J. R. (1991). *Nursing: the practice of caring*. National League for Nursing Press, New York.

Blum, L. (1980). *Friendship, altruism and morality*. Routledge & Kegan Paul, London.

Bok, S. (1980). *Lying: moral choice in public and private life*. Quartet Books, London.

Brabeck, M. M. (ed.) (1989). *Who cares? Theory, research, and educational implications of the ethic of care*. Praeger, New York.

Braidotti, R. (1986). Ethics revisited: Women and/in philosophy. In C. Pateman and E. Gross (eds) (1986), *Feminist challenges*, Allen & Unwin, Sydney.

Bridston, E. (1982). An educational strategy for enhancement of moral–ethical decision making. *Topics in Clinical Nursing* 4 (1), April, pp. 57–65.

Broughton, J. M. (1983). Women's rationality and men's virtues: a critique of gender dualism in Gilligan's theory of moral development. *Social Research* 50 (3), Autumn, pp. 597–642.

Brown, J. M., Kitson, A. L. and McKnight, T. J. (1992). *Challenges in caring: explorations in nursing and ethics.* Chapman & Hall, London.

Card, C. (ed.) (1991). *Feminist ethics.* University of Kansas Press, Lawrence, Kansas.

Carper, B. (1986). The ethics of caring. In P. Chinn (ed.), *Ethical issues in nursing,* Aspen Systems, Rockville, Maryland.

Chesler, P. (1972). *Women and madness.* Avon Books, New York.

Chinn, P. L. (ed.) (1991). *Anthology on caring.* National League for Nursing Press, New York.

Code, L. (1991). *What can she know? Feminist theory and the construction of knowledge.* Cornell University Press, Ithaca and London.

Code, L., Mullett, S. and Overall, C. (eds) (1988). *Feminist perspectives: philosophical essays on methods and morals.* University of Toronto Press, Toronto.

Cole, E. B. and Coultrap-McQuin, S. (eds) (1992). *Explorations in feminist ethics: theory and practice.* Indiana University Press, Bloomington and Indianapolis.

Cooper, M. C. (1991). Principle-orientated ethics and the ethic of care: a creative tension. *Advances in Nursing Science* 14 (2), pp. 22–31.

Cortese, A. (1990). *Ethnic ethics: the restructuring of moral theory.* State University of New York Press, Albany.

Crittenden, B. (1979). The limitations of morality as justice in Kohlberg's theory. In D. B. Cochrane, C. M. Hamm and A. C. Kazepides (eds), *The domain of moral education,* Paulist Press, New York, pp. 251–66.

Daniels, N. (1984). Understanding physician power: a review of the social transformation of American medicine. *Philosophy and Public Affairs* 13 (4), Fall, pp. 347–57.

de Bono, E. (1990). *I am right — you are wrong.* Penguin, London.

Drengson, A. R. (1985). Critical notice. *Canadian Journal of Philosophy* 15 (1), March, pp. 111–31.

Edwards, J. C. (1982). *Ethics without philosophy: Wittgenstein and the moral life.* University Presses of Florida, Tampa.

Elliott, C. (1992). Where ethics comes from and what to do about it. *Hastings Center Report* 22 (4), pp. 28–35.

Engelhardt, H. Tristram Jr (1986). *The foundations of bioethics.* Oxford University Press, New York.

Fisher, B. and Tronto, J. (1990). Toward a feminist theory of caring. In E. K. Abel and M. K. Nelson (eds), *Circles of care, work and identity in women's lives.* State University of New York Press, Albany, pp. 35–62.

Flanagan, O. and Jackson, K. (1987). Justice, care, and gender: the Kohlberg–Gilligan debate revisited. *Ethics* 97, April, pp. 622–37.

Frazer, E., Hornsby, J. and Lovibond, S. (eds) (1992). *Ethics: a feminist reader.* Blackwell, Oxford.

Fry, S. (1988a). The ethic of caring: can it survive in nursing? *Nursing Outlook* 36 (1), p. 48.

Fry, S. (1988b). Response to 'Virtue, ethics, caring and nursing'. *Scholarly Inquiry for Nursing Practice: An International Journal* 2 (2), pp. 97–101.

Fry, S. (1989a). Toward a theory of nursing ethics. *Advances in Nursing Science* 11 (4), pp. 9–22.

Fry, S. (1989b). The role of caring in a theory of nursing ethics. *Hypatia* 4 (2). Reprinted in Holmes and Purdy 1992, pp. 93–106.

Gatens, M. (1986). Feminism, philosophy and riddles without answers. In C. O. Pateman and E. Gross (eds), *Feminist challenges*, Allen & Unwin, Sydney, pp. 13–29.

Gaut, D. A. (ed.) (1992). *The presence of caring in nursing*. National League for Nursing Press, New York.

Gaut, D. A. and Leininger, M. M. (eds) (1991). *Caring: the compassionate healer*. National League for Nursing Press, New York.

Gauthier, D. (1986). *Morals by agreement*. Clarendon Press, Oxford.

Gibson, M. (1976). Rationality. *Philosophy and Public Affairs* 6 (3), pp. 193–225.

Gilligan, C. (1982). *In a different voice: psychological theory and women's development*. Harvard University Press, Cambridge, Mass. (See in particular chapter 3, 'Concepts of self and morality'.)

Gilligan, C. (1987). Moral orientation and moral development. In Kittay and Meyers 1987, pp. 19–33.

Grimshaw, J. (1986). *Feminist philosophers*. Wheatsheaf Books, Brighton, Sussex.

Harding, S. (ed.) (1987). *Feminism and methodology: social science issues*. Indiana University Press, Bloomington and Indianapolis, and Open University Press, Milton Keynes.

Harding, S. (ed.) (1991). *Whose Science? Whose knowledge? Thinking from women's lives*. Open University Press, Milton Keynes.

Harding, S. and Hintikka, M. B. (eds) (1983). *Discovering reality*. D. Reidel, Dordrecht.

Hare, R. M. (1981). *Moral thinking*. Clarendon Press, Oxford.

Held, V. (1987). Feminism and moral theory. In Kittay and Meyers 1987, pp. 111–28.

Hoagland, S. L. (1988). *Lesbian ethics: toward new value*. Institute of Lesbian Studies, Palo Alto, California.

Holmes, H. B. and Purdy, L. M. (eds) (1992). *Feminist perspectives in medical ethics*. Indiana University Press, Bloomington and Indianapolis.

Hutton, B. (1987). The oft-forgotten grandmothers of Western philosophy. *The Age*, 23 September, p. 20.

Jaggar, A. M. (1983). *Feminist politics and human nature*. Rowman & Allanheld, Totowa, New Jersey.

Johnstone, M.-J. (1994). *Nursing and the injustices of the law*. W. B. Saunders/Baillière Tindall, Sydney.

Katzenstein, M. F. and Laitin, D. D. (1987). Politics, feminism, and the ethics of caring. In Kittay and Meyers 1987, pp. 261–81.

Kittay, E. F. and Meyers, D. T. (eds) (1987). *Women and moral theory*. Rowman & Littlefield, Totowa, New Jersey.

Klimek, M. (1990). Virtue, ethics, and care: developing the personal dimension of caring in nursing education. In Leininger and Watson 1990, pp. 177–87.

Kohlberg, L. (1981). The *philosophy of moral development: moral stages and the idea of justice*. Harper & Row, San Francisco.

Leininger, M. M. (ed.) (1988). *Care: the essence of nursing and health*, Wayne State University Press, Detroit.

Leininger, M. M. (ed.) (1990a). *Ethical and moral dimensions of care*. Wayne State University Press, Detroit.

Leininger, M. M. (1990b). Culture: the conspicuous missing link to understand ethical and moral dimensions of human care. In Leininger 1990, pp. 49–66.

Leininger, M. M. (ed.) (1991). *Culture care diversity and universality: a theory of nursing*. National League for Nursing Press, New York.

Leininger, M. M. and Watson, J. (eds) (1990). *The caring imperative in education*. National League for Nursing Press, New York.

Lloyd, G. (1984). *The man of reason: 'male' and 'female' in Western philosophy*, Methuen, London.

McAlister, L. Lopez (ed.) (1989). *Hypatia*. Special issue 4 (1), Spring, *The history of women in philosophy*.

MacIntyre, A. (1985). *After virtue: a study in moral theory*. Duckworth, London.

McMillan, C. (1982). *Women, reason and nature: some philosophical problems with feminism*. Princeton University Press, Princeton, New Jersey.

Malcolm, N. (1958). *Ludwig Wittgenstein: a memoir*. Oxford University Press, London.

Marshall, P.A. (1992). Anthropology and bioethics. *Medical Anthropology Quarterly* 6 (1), pp. 49–73.

Midgley, M. (1980). *Beast and man*. Methuen, London.

Midgley, M. and Hughes, J. (1983). *Women's choices*. Weidenfeld & Nicolson, London.

Mill, J. S. (1929 edn). The subjection of women. In M. Wollstonecraft, *A vindication of the rights of woman*, and J. S. Mill, *The subjection of women*, Everyman's Library, London, pp. 219–317.

Morgan, K. P. (1988). Women and moral madness. In Code et al. 1988, pp. 146–67.

Moore, G. E. (1903). *Principia ethica*. Cambridge University Press, London.

Moulton, J. (1983). A paradigm of philosophy: the adversary method. In Harding and Hintikka 1983, pp. 149–64.

Mullett, S. (1988). Shifting perspectives: a new approach to ethics. In Code et al. 1988, pp. 109–26.

Nicolayev, J. and Phillips, D. C. (1979). On assessing Kohlberg's stage theory of moral development. In D. B. Cochrane, C. M. Hamm and A. C. Kazepides (eds), *The domain of moral education*, Paulist Press, New York, pp. 231–50.

Nietzsche, F. (1972 edn). *Beyond good and evil*. Penguin Books, Harmondsworth, Middlesex.

Noddings, N. (1984). *Caring: a feminine approach to ethics and moral education*. University of California Press, Berkeley.

Parsons, S. (1986). Feminism and moral reasoning. *Australasian Journal of Philosophy*. Supplement to vol. 64, June, pp. 75–90.

Pateman, C. (1989). *The disorder of woman*. Polity Press, Cambridge.

Plato (1955 edn). *The Republic*. Penguin Classics, Harmondsworth, Middlesex.

Porter, E. (1991). *Women and moral identity*. Allen & Unwin, Sydney.

Porter, M. (1989). *Women in the church: the great ordination debate in Australia*. Penguin Books, Ringwood, Victoria.

Rawls, J. (1971). *A theory of justice*. Oxford University Press, Oxford.

Rich, A. (1979). *On lies, secrets and silence: selected prose 1966–1978*. Virago Press, London.

Roach, Sister M. Simone (1987). *The human act of caring: a blueprint for the health professions*. Canadian Hospital Association, Ottawa, Ontario.

Robb, C. S. (1985). A framework for feminist ethics. In Andolsen et al. 1987, pp. 211–33.

Rousseau, J.-J. (1911 edn). *Emile*. Everyman's Library, London.

Segal, L. (1987). *Is the future female? Troubled thoughts on contemporary feminism*. Virago Press, London.

Sherwin, S. (1992). *No longer patient: feminist ethics and health care*. Temple University Press, Philadelphia.

Singer, P. (ed.) (1991). *A companion to ethics*. Basil Blackwell, Oxford.

Spender, D. (1988). *Women of ideas, and what men have done to them*. Pandora Press, London (first published by Routledge & Kegan Paul, 1982). (See in particular essay on Harriet Taylor [1807–58], pp. 184–96.)

Stout, J. (1988). *Ethics after Babel: the languages of morals and their discontents*. Beacon Press, Boston.

Tronto, J. C. (1993). *Moral boundaries: a political argument for an ethic of care.* Routledge, New York/London.

Twomey, J. G. (1989). Analysis of the claim to distinct nursing ethics: normative and nonnormative approaches. *Advances in Nursing Science,* 11 (3), pp. 25–32.

Ussher, J. (1991). *Women's madness: misogyny or mental illness?* Harvester/ Wheatsheaf, New York.

Von Wright, G. H. (1958). Biographical sketch. In Malcolm 1958.

Waithe, M. E. (ed.) (1987). *A history of women philosophers.* Volume I: *Ancient women philosophers, 600 BC–500 AD,* Martinus Nijhoff, Dordrecht.

Waithe, M. E. (ed.) (1989a). *A history of women philosophers.* Volume II: *Medieval, Renaissance and Enlightenment women philosophers, AD 500–1600.* Kluwer Academic Publishers, Dordrecht.

Waithe, M. E. (1989b). Twenty-three hundred years of women philosophers: toward a gender indifferentiated moral theory. In Brabeck 1989, pp. 3–18.

Waithe, M. E. (ed.) (1991). *A history of women philosophers.* Volume III: *Modern women philosophers, 1600–1900.* Kluwer Academic Publishers, Dordrecht.

Walker, M. U. (1992). Moral understanding: alternative 'epistemology' for a feminist ethics. In Cole and Coultrap-McQuin 1992, pp. 165–75.

Walsh, M. Roth (1977). *'Doctors wanted: no women need apply' — Sexual barriers in the medical profession, 1935–1975.* Yale University Press, New Haven and London.

Watson, J. (1985a). *Nursing: the philosophy and science of caring.* Colorado Associated University Press, Boulder, Colorado.

Watson, J. (1985b). *Nursing: human science and human care: a theory of nursing.* Appleton-Century-Crofts, Norwalk, Connecticut.

Webb, S. (1988). Is the hospital system sick? *Sunday Examiner,* Tasmania, 19 June, p. 6.

Wertheimer, M. (1990). Separate roles for doctors and nurses need to be recognised. *Medicine* 2 (7), 16 April, p. 11.

Williams, B. (1972). *Morality: an introduction to ethics.* Cambridge University Press, Cambridge.

Williams, B. (1981). *Moral luck.* Cambridge University Press, Cambridge.

Williams, B. (1985). *Ethics and the limits of philosophy.* Fontana/Collins, London.

Wittgenstein, L. (1965 edn). A lecture on ethics. *Philosophical Review* 74, January, pp. 3–12.

Wollstonecraft, M. (1929 edn). *A vindication of the rights of woman.* In M. Wollstonecraft, *A vindication of the rights of woman,* and J. S. Mill, *The subjection of women,* Everyman's Library, London, pp. 3–215.

Chapter

5

Transcultural ethics

In THIS TEXT the discussion of the theoretical underpinnings of our moral thinking in nursing would not be complete without some reference to and acknowledgment of the cultural specificity, or the (Anglo-American) 'ethnocentrism', of the moral perspectives being presented here as it bears upon the topics chosen, the questions asked, and the type of moral thinking used to consider these.

It is no coincidence that most of the issues considered and the views expressed in this text reflect the dominant cultural Western (Anglo-American) philosophical traditions that have constructed and informed them (hence the reference to *Western* moral thinking and philosophy throughout this text). And it is no coincidence either that even the previous chapter, which has as its focus a brief overview and examination of contemporary feminist moral theory's powerful critique of mainstream (malestream) bioethics, is also *ethnocentric*, having been informed by the now substantial body of Anglo-American feminist literature on the subject of ethics and moral conduct. One important reason why this ethnocentricism is not coincidental is that the discipline of ethics, as being considered here, is a product of the cultural (social and historical) context from which it has emerged.

Given this, it can be seen that ethics (and its derivatives) can be described appropriately as having been 'culturally constructed' (Cortese 1990, p. 1) and that dominant views suggesting the *naturality, objectivity, rationality* and *universality* of established Western ethical thinking (its theories and principles) are not only misleading but false. (For a comprehensive and critical discussion of whether ethics is a human invention or a naturally occurring material fact interwoven into the fabric of the observable world, see McNaughton 1988; Brink 1989; Dancy 1993). Indeed, it is evident that, contrary to the dominant views of mainstream Anglo-American moral philosophers, *culture exists logically prior to ethics, not the other way around.* To reject this view is to risk corrupting rather than preserving the integrity of our moral thinking, and, in the ultimate analysis, to undermine our ability to *be* moral in a world which is unequivocally multicultural in nature and outlook. To insist on upholding an ethnocentric and imperialist 'universal' world view of ethics would be not only to pervert morality and all that it has been constructed to protect, but to threaten the survival of morality itself, for reasons that will be considered shortly.

Leininger (1990), an American leader in transcultural nursing, has made the important claim that 'culture has been the critical and conspicuously missing dimension in the study and practice of ethical and moral [sic] dimensions of human care' (p. 49). She has also criticised nurse ethicists for their failure to recognise the important and significant role that culture plays in guiding moral judgments and behaviour in human care contexts; and she contends further that some nurse ethicists have even 'deliberately avoided' the concept of culture altogether, preferring instead to assume the universality of the ethical principles, codes and standards of human conduct that have become so prevalent in mainstream nursing ethics discourse (Leininger 1990, p. 51). Leininger concludes that, if nurses are to provide appropriate ethical care to individuals, families and groups of different cultural backgrounds, they must have knowledge of and the ability to uphold sensitively the culturally based moral values of the people for whom they care (Leininger 1990, p. 52). On this point, she states:

> most assuredly, the evolving discipline of nursing needs an epistemic ethical and moral [sic] knowledge base that takes into account cultural differences and similarities in order to provide knowledgeable and accurate judgements that are congruent with clients' values and lifeways.
>
> (Leininger 1990, pp. 52–3).

Without this knowledge base, Leininger contends, it is not possible for nurses to make the 'right' decisions or to provide the 'right' (ethical) human care when planning and implementing nursing care (Leininger 1990, p. 64).

Questions remain, however: What is culture? and, further, What is culture's relationship to and role in ethics generally, and nursing ethics in particular? It is to briefly answering these questions that this discussion now turns.

Culture and its relationship to ethics

Culture is an extremely complex concept, and one that has been defined, interpreted and analysed from a variety of disciplinary perspectives (see, for example, Mead 1955; Sorokin 1957; Kluckholn 1962; Spindler 1974; Beals 1979; Bullivant 1981, 1984;

Wuthnow et al. 1984; Fieldhouse 1986; Williams 1989; Helman 1990; Leininger 1991; Midgley 1991a; Kanitsaki 1993, 1994). Not surprisingly, this has seen the emergence of a number of rival theories and viewpoints on what culture is, and on what its relationship to and role in human affairs is or should be (Kanitsaki 1992, p. 5). Even anthropologists do not agree about how culture should be defined, interpreted and analysed (Kanitsaki 1989a, p. 11). Nevertheless, there is some agreement among scholars that culture is a human invention and one which is critical for human survival and the development of human potential (Kanitsaki 1989a, p. 11).

What then is culture? As already stated, culture has been defined, interpreted and analysed in a variety of ways. Cohen, for example, argues that:

> culture is made up of the energy systems, the objective and specific artifacts, the organizations of social relations, the modes of thought, the ideologies, and the total range of customary behaviour that are transmitted from one generation to another by a social group and that enables it to maintain life in a particular habitat.
>
> (Cohen 1968, p. 1)

Bullivant argues along similar lines, adding to the description of culture that it is something which:

> can be thought of as the knowledge and conceptions embodied in symbolic and non-symbolic communication modes about the technology and skills, customary behaviours, values, beliefs, and attitudes, a society has evolved from its historical past, and progressively modifies and augments to give meaning to and cope with the present and anticipated future problems of its existence.
>
> (Bullivant 1981, p. 19)

A more accessible description of culture, however, and one which is very helpful to this discussion, comes from an Australian leader in transcultural nursing, Olga Kanitsaki. Kanitsaki describes culture as follows:

> Culture includes a particular people's beliefs, value orientations and value systems, which give meaning, logic, worth and significance to their existence and experience in relation to both the universe and other human beings. These value orientations, value systems and beliefs in turn shape customs and traditions, prescribe and proscribe behaviour, determine the structure of social institutions and power relations, and identify and prescribe

social relations, modes and rules of communication, *moral order* [emphasis added], and, indeed, the whole spirit and web of meaning and purpose of a given group in a particular place and time. Culture thus reflects the shared history, traditions, achievements, struggles for survival and lived experiences of a particular people. Its influence extends over politics, economics, the development and use of technology, the boundaries and meaning of class, the determination of gender roles, and so on.

(Kanitsaki 1994, p. 95)

Unfortunately, it is beyond the scope of this text to discuss the concept of culture at the level and depth it warrants, and its consideration must be left for another time. Nevertheless, there is room to emphasise the point that, regardless of the competing theories on what culture is, it is clear that it (culture) plays a fundamental and critical role in shaping people's values, beliefs, perceptions and knowledge about the world within which they live, that it influences people's behaviour and generally gives logic and meaning to a whole way of life in that world, and that it ultimately provides the 'blueprint' for their (human) survival in that world (Kanitsaki 1992, p. 5). It is also clear that culture's relationship to and role in ethics (including its relationship to the theoretical underpinnings and practical application of ethics) cannot be plausibly denied. One does not have to be a distinguished cultural anthropologist to recognise and accept the critical link between culture and people's moral values, beliefs, perceptions and knowledge of what constitutes morally right and wrong conduct. As Mary Midgley points out, the 'communication explosion' has meant, among other things, that:

virtually everybody, even in quite remote corners of the world, now grows up with the background knowledge that there are many ways of life deeply different from their own — a kind of knowledge which once used to be quite rare.

(Midgley 1991a, p. 72).

Similarly, nearly all of us know that there are in the world many people whose moral values and beliefs are radically different from our own (Midgley 1991a, p. 72). And we also know that in any one society there is likely to be a diversity of valid moral schemas (moral pluralism), and that this has created the possibility for, and the actuality of, irreconcilable moral disagreements, examples of which are given throughout this text (Elliott 1992, p. 32). Questions arising here include: What, if any, is the best way to respond to the problematic of moral pluralism? and, more specifically: How should nurses respond to the challenge of what can be appropriately referred to as transcultural ethics? It is to briefly answering these questions that this discussion now turns.

The nature and implications of transcultural ethics

It is not the purpose of this text to advance a substantive theory of transcultural ethics or to provide an in-depth study of the ethical concepts, theories and practices of different cultural groups. Such a task is beyond our present scope, and requires much more space than it is possible to provide here. (See, meanwhile, Cortese 1990; Leininger 1990; Singer 1991; Midgley 1991a; Elliott 1992; Marshall 1992.) Nevertheless, it is important to have some understanding of the nature and implications of transcultural ethics (a form of ethical pluralism), and of how nurses might respond better to the challenges it poses.

One central point that needs to be thoroughly understood is that, while all societies have some sort of moral system for guiding and evaluating the conduct of their members, the moral constructs of one culture (in this case, for example, Western moral philosophy) cannot always be applied appropriately or reliably to another culture — at least not without some modification (Silberbauer 1991, p. 15). Further, language usage alone, and the difficulties encountered in reaching accurate culturally thick (rich) translations of accepted moral terms and concepts, may even make meaningful moral discourse across cultures impossible (Stout 1988). These points have, however, been largely overlooked by Western moral philosophers, who have tended to support an imperialist model of morality — that is, that their way of moral knowing and thinking is not only superior but 'right', and is thus something to be applied (read imposed) universally on to others whose moral systems they have judged to be inferior — even 'savage' (Midgley 1991a, p. 78).

As already argued, this is an inadequate and fraudulent approach to moral thinking and conduct, and one which should be questioned. Nevertheless, this does not mean that Western moral philosophy itself should be abandoned. To the contrary — its rich traditions offer us important insights into our own culture-specific moral values and beliefs about how to be moral beings. We must, however, pay much greater attention to the influences of the primary organising principle of morality, namely, culture; and we need to recognise that, while it is true that all cultures have some 'priority rules', or principles for arbitrating between conflicting obligations and duties, just what these rules and principles are, how they are defined and interpreted, when they will be applied, and who ultimately applies them (and to what end) will, contrary to an imperialist model of ethics, vary across — and even within — different cultures (Midgley 1991b, p. 11). In short, morality will be expressed differently cross-culturally.

An interesting example of the different ways in which morality can be expressed cross-culturally or even intra-culturally can be found in the case of small-scale and large-scale societies. In small-scale or traditional societies, for example, morality tends to be viewed as a *process* — as a means to an end — and is expressed through *the quality of relationships* (characterised by upholding values such as friendship, loyalty to kin, empathy, altruism, familial trust, and so on), rather than a deontological adherence to abstract principles. Silberbauer explains:

> Morality is less of an end in itself but is seen more clearly as a set of orientations for establishing and maintaining the health of relationships. Morality, then, is a means to a desired, enjoyed end.
>
> (Silberbauer 1991, p. 27)

This view is in sharp contrast to that upheld by large-scale (non-traditional or industrialised) societies, in which relationships are less proximate, less intense and less significant, both at the individual and the societal level. Here morality is viewed as an end in itself rather than as a means to an end, and is expressed by *adherence to rules* (viz, adjudicating the conduct between strangers) rather than by and in the quality of relationships per se. On this point, Silberbauer explains:

> Morality certainly provides a set of orientations and thus helps to create and maintain coherent expectations of behaviour, but operates *impersonally* in that there is not the same capacity for negotiation. Morality thus tends to be valued more as an end in itself and less as a means to an end [emphasis added].
>
> (Silberbauer, p. 27)

To illustrate the different ways in which small-scale and large-scale societies might each express their different moralities, Silberbauer (1991) uses the simple example of the relationship between a bus-conductor and a passenger. He suggests that, in large-scale societies, where relationships tend to be 'single-purpose and impersonal', the relationship between a bus-conductor and a passenger would be of limited importance, and would probably manifest itself quite differently than it would in a small-scale society, where relationships were more proximate, multi-purpose and personal. He points out:

how different it would be if the conductor were also my sister-in-law, near neighbour and the daughter of my father's golfing partner — I would never dare to tender anything other than the correct fare. In a small-scale society every fellow member whom I encounter in my day is likely to be connected to me by a comparable, or even more complex web of strands, each of which must be maintained in its appropriate alignment and tension lest all the others become tangled. My father's missed putts or my inconsiderate use of a motor-mower at daybreak will necessitate very diplomatic behaviour on the bus, or a long walk to work and a dismal dinner on my return.

(Silberbauer 1991, p. 14)

A less masculinist and more relevant example here can be found in the comparison of nurses working in large city-based university teaching hospitals with those who work in small, close-knit 'outback' country communities. It has been my experience that nurses working in small (rural) 'outback' country communities (where 'everyone is known to everyone') are far more vulnerable to putting local community members 'off side' by offending an individual member of that community than are nurses working in large city-based university teaching hospitals. In this instance, we could speculate that nurses working in small country-based community nursing care settings might put more weight on *preserving the quality of relationships* in that community than on *upholding abstract moral principles*. Conversely, nurses working in large and impersonal communities may put greater emphasis on upholding abstract principles of conduct than on preserving the quality of relationships with 'strangers' whom they are unlikely to encounter more than once during their working lives.

Bear in mind, however, that this is only an example, being used here to help clarify Silberbauer's point. In reality it is likely that nurses express morality both as a process (as a means to an end) and as an end in itself. Whether this is so, and the extent to which it is so (that is, where the balance lies), may depend ultimately on the nature of the context they are in — whether it is characterised by personal or impersonal relationships. When it is considered that it is not contradictory to view the maintenance of quality relationships as an important moral end in itself (not just a means to an end), there is room to suggest that the distinction Silberbauer makes may, in the final analysis, be overstated.

Despite this observation, Silberbauer is correct to point out that abstract moral principles do not always have currency in some cultural or social groups, and that, even if there do exist some commonly accepted standards of moral conduct, we cannot assume that these standards will be expressed or applied uniformly across, or even within, different cultural groups. A good example of this can be found in the wide and popular acceptance of the moral principles of autonomy, non-maleficence, beneficence and justice, which are considered in chapter 3. These principles are referred to and used widely in mainstream bioethics discourse (see in particular Beauchamp and Childress 1989), and are viewed popularly as 'self-standing conceptual systems by which we can impose some sort of order upon ethical problems' (Elliott 1992, p. 29). But, as Elliott correctly points out, what proponents of this view tend to overlook is that

> in reality, ethics does not stand apart. It is one thread in the fabric of a society, and it is intertwined with others. Ethical concepts are tied to a society's customs, manners, traditions, institutions — all of the concepts that structure and inform the ways in which a member of that society deals with the world.
>
> (Elliott 1992, p. 29)

He goes on to warn that, if people forget this inextricable link between ethics and culture:

> we are in danger of leaving the world of genuine moral experience for the world of moral fiction — a simplified, hypothetical creation suited less for practical difficulties than for intellectual convenience.
>
> (Elliott 1992, p. 29)

A poignant example of the inaccuracy and fraud of viewing moral principles as self-standing conceptual systems rather than as ethical concepts tied to a particular tradition (culture) can be seen in the way in which the principle of autonomy tends to be interpreted and applied in professional health care contexts. As stated in chapter 3, the concept of autonomy refers to an individual's *independent* and *self-contained* ability to decide. As a principle, autonomy prescribes that an *individual's rational preferences* ought to be respected even if we do not agree with them — and even if others consider them foolish — provided they do not interfere with or harm prejudicially the significant moral interests of others.

At first glance, this articulation of the concept and principle of autonomy appears unproblematic. And it is probably true that most nurses familiarising themselves with the moral nature and application of the principle of autonomy value the 'right' to make their own self-determining choices, and would probably feel a strong sense of outrage if their considered wishes were overridden arbitrarily by another. They may also share a strong conviction that patients should always be informed about their diagnoses, and about the details of their proposed treatment and care, and that it would be a gross violation of patients' rights not to accept or facilitate patients' self-determining choices regarding their own care and treatment options. In most cases, this position would probably be a demonstrably justifiable one to take. It would, however, be a grave mistake to accept the concept and principle of autonomy (as articulated above) as holding *universally*. Consider the following.

Earlier in this text, it was pointed out that definitions of ethical terms and concepts can be 'ethically loaded', and hence can themselves be an important influence on how a moral debate or analysis might be conducted and what the outcomes of a given debate or analysis might be. This is true even (or perhaps especially) in the case of moral principles — the moral principle of autonomy being a case in point. It will be noted, for example, that even the definition of the concept and principle of autonomy reflects the dominant cultural values of the highly individualised large-scale Western Anglo-American culture from which it has arisen (Marshall 1992). Of particular importance to this discussion are the italicised terms *individual's, independent, self-contained*. Here the ethical loading clearly rests on respecting individualism, independence, and isolation (insulation) from one's social connectedness. For people who hold these values, this ethical loading is not a major problem. But for people who do *not* hold or share these values — who may, for instance, subscribe to the values of collectiveness, interdependence, and social connectedness (context) — it is open to serious question whether the concept and principle of autonomy as popularly defined in mainstream bioethics discourse could, or indeed should, be given any currency in mediating the relationships, and the responsibilities within those relationships, of people who do not subscribe to the values embraced by autonomy as described.

To illustrate the kinds of moral problems that can arise as a result of applying the principle of autonomy in an abstract, universal and context-independent way rather than in a substantive, context-dependent, culture-specific way, consider the case of Mr G (taken from Johnstone and Kanitsaki 1991). Mr G, an elderly Greek who spoke no English, was admitted to hospital for investigations, and was later diagnosed as having cancer of the lung. Mr G had a number of other health problems, including a mildly debilitating hemiplegia — although he could move about with assistance. Before his admission into hospital, Mr G was totally dependent on and cared for by his family.

When radiological and laboratory tests confirmed the provisional medical diagnosis of a malignant lung tumour, Mr G's physician arranged for an interpreter to come to the ward and through him informed Mr G directly that he had cancer of the lung. In this instance, it was the physician's personal policy to be candid with his patients, and inform them according to what he judged to be 'their right to know and be informed', as prescribed by the moral principle of autonomy. Unfortunately, in this case, although well intended, the physician's approach was culturally inappropriate, and had the undesirable moral consequence of causing the patient and his family otherwise avoidable suffering (Johnstone and Kanitsaki 1991).

A mainstream ethical analysis of the physician's actions in this case would probably support the view that informing the patient of his cancer diagnosis was a 'morally right' thing to do. And, interestingly, when I present this case to students (nursing and medical students alike), most contend that the physician's actions were not only morally correct but *praiseworthy*, given the reluctance by many doctors to be candid with their patients about diagnostic, care and treatment matters of this nature.

From a cultural perspective, however, the physican's actions can be shown to be not only mistaken but morally harmful, for reasons that will now be explained. In this case it would have been more culturally appropriate and morally beneficial had the physician communicated the cancer diagnosis to the patient's *family* rather than to the patient himself (see also Kanitsaki 1993, 1994). This is because, as Johnstone and Kanitsaki point out, during a health crisis, patients like Mr G who are of a traditional (rural, small-scale societal) cultural background, tend to prefer

> the close involvement of their family and value the supportive, protective and therapeutic role that the family can and does play when one of its members is ill or suffering [...]. Indeed, the involvement of the patient's family is an essential and integral part of the therapeutic relationship and of the process required to uphold the patient's best interests.
>
> (Johnstone and Kanitsaki 1991, p. 280)

By not recognising the protective authority of Mr G's family to decide '*if, when, how and by whom* the diagnoses should be disclosed to Mr G', the physician inadvertently 'pointed the bone' at his patient and thereby undermined rather than promoted Mr G's autonomy. The reasons for this are complicated, but important. Kanitsaki (1989a) explains that for many rurally based Greeks who emigrated to Australia during the 1950s and 1960s, the very word 'cancer' carries a whole range of negative connotations and thus is something never to be mentioned, since to do so would be to risk stimulating the *nocebo phenomenon*. The *nocebo phenomenon* (from the Latinate *noceo*, 'I hurt', and the Greek *nosis*, 'disease') is defined by Helman (1990, p. 257) as 'the negative effect on health of beliefs and expectations — and therefore the exact reverse of the "placebo" phenomenon' (see also Dossey 1982, 1991; Weil 1983; Chopra 1989; Moyers 1993). Kanitsaki (1989a, p. 46) explains that during the 1950s and 1960s, rural Greece had virtually no hospitals, and that if people required treatment for serious illness they would have to travel great distances to the nearest cities. She goes on to point out that, because of this, as well as because of a scepticism about scientific medicine's ability to treat diseases effectively, people from rural areas would seek hospital treatment only as a last resort. As Kanitsaki explains:

> the reluctance to frequent doctors and hospitals was exacerbated by a general dislike of hospitals, rumours about the lack of nursing care and unkind nursing staff, and a fear of cities generally. Pressures of local work demands, a lack of economic resources, and the probability of having to travel alone and thus without the protection, support, and physical presence of the family, also militated against scientific medical services being used by rural community members.
>
> (Kanitsaki 1989a, p. 47)

As a result of this reluctance — and, indeed, inability — to access scientific medical services, many people suffering from cancer-related illness did not receive the optimal treatment available, and as a result frequently died painful and agonising deaths (Kanitsaki 1989a). And it is the memories of these kinds of cancer-related deaths that many rural Greek immigrants have brought with them to Australia. Kanitsaki (personal communication) explains that many Greek immigrants of this class simply do not have any experiential knowledge of, or even a conception of, the kind of treatment and care that is available in Australia today; thus, even mentioning the word 'cancer' is sufficient to trigger in ill persons an overwhelming sense of hopelessness which ultimately finds its expression in their losing their will to live. Under these circumstances, to tell such patients, 'You've got cancer' — no matter how benevolent the intention in doing so — would probably be sufficient to trigger the nocebo phenomenon, resulting ultimately in the ill person's premature death (Kanitsaki, personal communication).

The way to avoid this disastrous situation is for the patient to be spared the information likely to stimulate the nocebo phenomenon, and for the patient's family to be respected as having the authority to decide — in the moral interests and for the well being of their sick loved one — *whether, when, where, how and by whom* information about the diagnosis of a serious illness and poor prognosis will be given (Kanitsaki, personal communication). A major *moral* motivation for this, Kanitsaki (personal communication) explains, is to avoid undermining the sick person's hope (about getting better and being able to go on living a meaningful life), and thereby to maximise the person's ability to continue making important life-interested choices; that is, to maximise the person's autonomy. Interestingly, recently published research has shown that, even in contemporary Greek society, truth telling about a diagnosis of serious life-threatening illness is still viewed by many rural Greeks as something 'undesirable', on the grounds that it could undermine hope and the will to live (Dalla-Vorgia et al. 1992).

It should be noted that this moral world-view is not held exclusively by Greeks of rural or traditional cultural backgrounds. The following anecdote shows that people of other traditional cultural backgrounds also believe that in some circumstances patients should not be told that they have a serious life-threatening illness, and that to do so would be sufficient to trigger the nocebo phenomenon. The case concerns an elderly non-English-speaking Italian man who, like Mr G, had emigrated to Australia in the 1950s. He was admitted to hospital for tests which later confirmed a cancer diagnosis. Although the man's family explicitly requested that their father not be given any information about the test results if they were positive, an interpreter was called in their absence and the man was told of his cancer diagnosis and poor prognosis. This information caused the man to become extremely distressed and, as his son commented later, 'the life just went out of his eyes and we knew he would die very soon'. The son, who was Australian-born and a qualified pharmacist, decided in consultation with the rest of his family to remedy the situation. This he did by contacting Italian friends who worked as doctors at the hospital where his father was a patient and arranging for all his father's tests to be repeated. His friends agreed to explain to his father that the tests needed to be repeated because 'there had been a terrible mistake' and that 'his earlier tests results had got mixed up with someone else's'. They later returned to tell the man that his tests showed he in fact did *not* have cancer. The son explained that his father was told he still needed medical treatment, but that he would 'be all right'. Ultimately, the family took their father home and cared for him. He continued to live beyond the time limit suggested by his poor prognosis and, in fact, was still alive at the time the anecdote was being shared. The son attributed this to the fact that they were able to convince their father all was not hopeless, which in turn had the effect of restoring his will to live. In short, the son's actions reversed his father's sense of hopelessness, and thus promoted rather than undermined his father's autonomy.

Interestingly, when I have shared this anecdote with students, many are appalled at the blatant deception that was employed in this case. Others, however, notably those whose parents are from rural Greece or Italy, have expressed enormous relief at the insights this and other cases like it have given them. One postgraduate nursing student, for example, commented:

> I've always felt that if either of my parents should get cancer they should be told their diagnosis. But when speaking of this issue, my mother — who is Italian — has always insisted, 'No! You must not allow that to happen'. My Australian side of me tells me it is wrong not to tell them. But now I can see it would be wrong *to tell* them, and that my mother is right. I can live with this now. It is such an enormous relief. I am no longer in a dilemma. Thank you.

(personal communication)

The comments of this student are included here because, among other things, they demonstrate the very practical help that adopting a cultural view of ethics can offer; they help to support the view that, by tying ethical views to the cultural traditions that inform them, we will be in a much better position to embrace morality as an experience rather than as an abstraction (Marshall 1992, pp. 53–7), and to avoid falling prey to the unhelpful, idle fantasies of moral fiction which, as Elliott (1992, p. 2) suggests, are suited more to the purposes of intellectual convenience than to resolving genuine practical difficulties in the concrete circumstances of life. The student's comments and, indeed, the anecdotes themselves also show, to borrow from Cortese (1990, p. 157) that 'relationships [...] are the essence of life and morality', and that to view morality simply as conceptions of abstract reified rational principles is 'to remove us from the real world in which we live, and separate us from real people whom we love' (Cortese 1990, p. 157). The lesson to be learned here is that, unless we embrace morality as an experience rather than as an abstraction, what we will end up with is only a concept of morality and not morality itself. And, borrowing again from Cortese (1990), unless we have a 'deep sense of relationship, we may have a conceptualisation of the highest level of justice, but we will not be moral (p. 158) — the point being that without relationships, justice — morality — 'contains no system of checks and balances. It becomes primarily an end in itself without regard to the purpose of morality' (Cortese 1990, p. 158).

Although only the principle of autonomy has been considered here, the other principles considered in chapter 3 (non-maleficence, beneficence and justice) could all be examined along similar lines. We could, for example, ask in regard to each of these principles: from whose perspective are these principles to be meaningfully and appropriately defined, interpreted, analysed and applied? In the case of non-maleficence, for instance, meaningful questions can be asked about what constitutes a 'harm' in a given culturally constructed clinical context? By whose standards and cultural perspectives is the notion of harm to be measured and evaluated? Likewise for the principles of beneficence and justice.

Where then does this leave the role of moral principles and culturally different moral schemas in our nursing ethics discourse? In answering this question, it might be useful at this point to consider the problematic of diversity or pluralism in moral values and moral world views.

Moral diversity and the challenge of moral pluralism

Earlier, it was asserted that the world in which we now live has become unequivocally multicultural in nature and outlook, and that this has brought with it a diversity or pluralism of moral values and beliefs. Some fear that this diversity or pluralism of values may be 'the barrier to agreement' (Elliott 1992, p. 32), and, hence, the catalyst to producing a world hopelessly divided by radical and destructive moral disagreement. Others reject moral pluralism outright on the grounds that, in their view, it is 'just another name for confusion' (Stout 1988, p. 1). Moral diversity need not lead to destructive disagreement, however, nor to blinding confusion. Indeed, as is well recognised within the discipline of moral philosophy, moral disagreement has historically been the beginning and the refinement of moral thinking, not its end or disintegration (see also Stout 1988; Benhabib and Dallmayr 1990). Further, as Mary Midgley correctly points out, 'nobody is infallible; and for that reason many different points of view are needed' (Midgley 1991a, p. 83).

What must also be recognised and understood here is that a diversity of values and beliefs is the key to morality's survival; it prompts critical reflection, rather than uncritical acceptance, and in so doing invites constant revision and creative refinement. Moral diversity also helps to ensure that no one moral point of view dominates; in short, it helps to prevent what might otherwise be termed 'moral fascism'. Meanwhile, its emphasis on understanding difference rather than striving for uniformity will help to ensure that the moral systems we end up embracing will be of a nature that is truly responsive to the lived realities and experiences of all human beings, not merely those of a select few whose positions of power have enabled them to manipulate morality into a tool for repressing unwanted truths and legitimating further the authority of moral imperialists who would impose their values on others as a means of maintaining rather than challenging their cultural hegemony.

The lesson for nurses is, I believe, that moral diversity is not something to be feared, but something to be embraced as a means of challenging our complacent thinking about the moral world we live in, and of improving our understanding of and ability to experience both ourselves and others as moral beings who have a mutual interest in living a worthwhile and meaningful life. Further, whether we wish to admit it or not, as Elliott argues persuasively:

> Moral disagreement will be with us as long as there is disagreement about what way of life is best for human beings. It is not at all obvious that this is a question that is answerable, even in principle. There may be no best life, only better and worse lives. And if morality is tied to a form of life, then it is a mistake to think that we can eliminate moral differences without eliminating the differences in cultures, and in individuals, to which morality is tied.
>
> (Elliott 1992, p. 35)

Elliott goes on to make the important point that:

> Though the biological characteristics humans share will mean that some lives, and some features of lives, are necessarily good or bad for human beings, there is no compelling reason, universally applicable, for adopting any one particular sort of life over all others — even if we had the choice, which we do not. For this reason, we should expect diversity in the sort of lives that people live, as well as the moral differences that inevitably follow.
>
> (Elliott 1992, p. 35)

Issues and recommendations

Transcultural ethics, like feminist ethics, recognises the problematic of genuine moral problems in human life being 'confronted as abstraction rather than experiential realities' (Marshall 1992, p. 52), and affirms that, if moral abstractions are to count for anything, they must be brought 'back to earth' (Stout 1988, p. 8). It also recognises the inability of abstract and decontextualised moral thinking to provide concrete answers to complex questions concerning human pain and suffering, intense and sometimes conflicting human emotions, ambivalent and ambiguous human relationships, and, not least, differing cultural world-views about the value and meaning of life — all of which often (too often) have to be dealt with in the face of overwhelming uncertainty, the unpredictability of probable outcomes (positive and negative), fallible modes of communication, and the fallibilities of decision-makers (Stout 1988; Cortese 1990; Marshall 1992; Elliott 1992).

Unlike other moral critiques, however, transcultural ethics offers an optimistic outlook. Its suggestion that acceptance of and achieving a harmony of moral diversity offer the key to sustaining the existence and purpose of morality provides an important basis upon which we can all develop, not just our moral thinking and sensibilities, but our ability to actually *be* moral in a world characterised by diverse and competing valid world-views. This is not merely compromise, as some might believe, or even tolerance the blinded eye of an indiscriminate mind (see Wolff et al. 1969; Midgley 1991a). Nor is it confusion. Rather, it is celebration. In particular, it is the celebration of the 'other' as different, but not inferior or fallacious or superstitious — as having something worthwhile to share, not as being something worthless to be marginalised, trivialised and ignored. If we accept this, we will all be in a much better position to judge what is really unethical as opposed to being merely disliked; what is truly wrong, as opposed to being merely unfamiliar and strange; and what is really confusion as opposed to simple misunderstanding of another's moral language with which we are not familiar (Stout 1988). This insight is, among other things, what we stand to gain by embracing a diversity of moral values and beliefs as being the beginning of morality and not its end.

In conclusion, I should like to list a number of questions nurses ought to ask when making moral decisions about the nursing care of people from diverse cultural backgrounds. Borrowing from Kanitsaki:

- Is my understanding of this person's values and value systems such that it entitles me to override her or his family's requests or instructions?

- Can I by way of a third party (such as an interpreter) really ensure that my interventions will result in benefits not harms to that person?

- Are my values and frame of reference the only ones which warrant overrding consideration in this relationship?

- How do I know my judgments in this relationship are morally and culturally appropriate? In short, how do I know I am right?

(Kanitsaki 1989b, p. 70)

By asking these and similar questions, and by seeking the 'right' answers to them, nurses will demonstrate successfully that they are able to embrace morality as something more than a set of abstract self-standing principles, and that in the ultimate analysis it is people and relationships that count — not a blind deference to rules, which, when stripped of their cultural content and context, become little more than intellectual curiosities empowered by arbitrary will, incapable of responding to the lived realities and needs of human beings who have been born into circumstances which are very often beyond their control. Embracing this approach will also remind us that:

> any theory of ethics is, in the end, only as plausible as the complete picture of the world of which it forms a part.

> (McNaughton 1988, p. 41)

References

Beals, A. R. (1979). *Culture in process.* Holt, Rinehart & Winston, New York.

Beauchamp, T. L. and Childress, J. F. (1989). *Principles of biomedical ethics,* 3rd edn. Oxford University Press, New York.

Benhabib, S. and Dallmayr, F. (eds) (1990). *The communicative ethics controversy.* MIT Press, Cambridge, Mass.

Brink, D. O. (1989). *Moral realism and the foundations of ethics.* Cambridge University Press, Cambridge.

Bullivant, B. M. (1981). *Race, ethnicity and curriculum.* Macmillan, Melbourne.

Bullivant, B. M. (1984). *Pluralism, cultural maintenance and evolution.* Bank House, Clevedon, Avon.

Chopra, D. (1989). *Quantum healing.* Bantam Books, New York.

Cohen, Y. A. (1968). *Man in adaptation: the cultural present.* Aldine, Chicago.

Cortese, A. (1990). *Ethnic ethics: the restructuring of moral theory.* State University of New York Press, Albany.

Dalla-Vorgia, P., Katsouyanni, K., Garanis, T. N., Touloumi, G., Drogari, P. and Koutselinis, A. (1992). Attitudes of a Mediterranean population to the truth-telling issue. *Journal of Medical Ethics* 18 (2), pp. 67–74.

Dancy, J. (1993). *Moral reasons.* Blackwell, Oxford, UK and Cambridge, USA.

Dossey, L. (1982). *Space, time and medicine.* New Science Library, Boston, Mass.

Dossey, L. (1991). *Meaning and medicine.* Bantam Books, New York.

Elliott, C. (1992). Where ethics comes from and what to do about it. *Hastings Center Report* 22 (4), pp. 28–35.

Fieldhouse, P. (1986). *Food and nutrition: customs and culture.* Croom Helm, London.

Helman, C. (1990). *Culture, health and illness.* Wright, London.

Johnstone, M.-J. and Kanitsaki, O. (1991). Some moral implications of cultural and linguistic diversity in health care. *Bioethics News* 10 (2), pp. 22–32.

Kanitsaki, O. (1989a). Health–illness–suffering experiences of a sample of Greek-born members of 12 Greek–Australian families living in Melbourne. Minor thesis completed in partial fulfilment of the requirements for the Degree of Master of Educational Studies, Faculty of Education, Monash University, Melbourne.

Kanitsaki, O. (1989b). Cross-cultural sensitivity in palliative care. In P. Hodder and A. Turley (eds), *The creative option of palliative care: a manual for health professionals,* Melbourne City Mission, Melbourne, pp. 68–71.

Kanitsaki, O. (1992). Meeting the challenge of patients' rights: a transcultural perspective. *Proceedings of Fourth Victorian State Conference on Nursing Law and Ethics: 'Meeting the challenge of patients rights — issues for the 1990s'*, held Dallas Brooks Hall, 20 November. Faculty of Nursing, RMIT, Bundoora, Melbourne.

Kanitsaki, O. (1993). Transcultural human care: its challenge and critique of professional nursing care. In D. Gaut (ed.), *A global agenda for caring.* National League for Nursing Press, New York, pp. 19–45.

Kanitsaki, O. (1994). Cultural and linguistic diversity. In J. Romanini and J. Daly (eds), *Critical care nursing: Australian perspectives*, W. B. Saunders/Baillière Tindall, Sydney.

Kluckhohn, C. (1962). *Culture and behavior.* The Free Press, New York.

Leininger, M. (1990). Culture: the conspicuous missing link to understand ethical and moral dimensions of human care. In M. Leininger (ed.), *Ethical and moral dimensions of care*, Wayne State University Press, Detroit, pp. 49–66.

Leininger, M. (ed.) (1991). *Culture care diversity and universality: a theory of nursing.* National League for Nursing Press, New York.

McNaughton, D. (1988). *Moral vision: an introduction to ethics.* Basil Blackwell, Oxford.

Marshall, P. A. (1992). Anthropology and bioethics. *Medical Anthropology Quarterly* 6 (1), pp. 49–73.

Mead, M. (1955). *Cultural patterns and technical change.* Mentor Books, New York.

Midgley, M. (1991a). *Can't we make moral judgements?* The Bristol Press, Bristol.

Midgley, M. (1991b). The origins of ethics. In Singer 1991, pp. 3–13.

Moyers, B. (1993). *Healing and the mind.* Doubleday, New York.

Silberbauer, G. (1991). Ethics in small-scale societies. In Singer 1991, pp. 14–28.

Singer, P. (ed). (1991). *A companion to ethics.* Basil Blackwell, Cambridge, Mass.

Sorokin, P. (1957). *Social and cultural dynamics.* Extending Horizons. Books–Porter Sargent, Boston.

Spindler, G. D. (1974). *Education and cultural process: towards an anthropology of education.* Holt, Rinehart & Winston, New York.

Stout, J. (1988). *Ethics after Babel: the languages of morals and their discontents.* Beacon Press, Boston.

Weil, A. (1983). *Health and healing: understanding conventional and alternative medicine.* Houghton Mifflin, Boston.

Williams, R. (1989). *Resources of hope: culture, democracy, socialism.* Verso, London.

Wolff, R. P., Moore, B. and Marcuse, H. (1969). *A critique of pure tolerance.* Beacon Press, Boston.

Wuthnow, R., Hunter, J. D., Bergesen, A. and Kurzweil, E. (1984). *Cultural analysis.* Routledge & Kegan Paul, London.

Chapter

6

Identifying and resolving
moral problems

N<small>URSES, LIKE DOCTORS AND OTHER</small> health professionals, encounter many moral problems in the course of their everyday professional practice. These problems are not merely *hypothetical* (that is, involving only imaginary people in imaginary circumstances), but are overwhelmingly real. They involve real people, with real feelings, in real circumstances, who are more often than not faced with very real threats to their moral well-being. Attempts by nurses to deal with moral problems appropriately and effectively are often plagued by difficulties, however. Some of these difficulties involve general unpreparedness of both nurses and others to deal with morally troubling situations, moral blindness, moral indifference, amoralism, moral complacency and moral fanaticism. Other major difficulties include moral disagreement, and, of course, the proverbial moral dilemma (a much discussed problem in nursing ethics literature).

As discussed earlier, there are those who believe that nurses should keep clear of the domain of moral problems (as if nurses can wilfully do this); there are others who believe, quite simply, that nurses just do not face any moral problems in nursing practice, or, if they do, that the problems are never more than trivial. Such views, however, are not only misguided and naive, but are also irresponsible, abusive and oppressive.

What needs to be firmly understood here, as is repeatedly emphasised in the chapters to follow, is that the nurse–patient relationship is a morally significant one, and is bound by the same ultimate moral standards as is any doctor–patient relationship or any other health professional–patient relationship. Thus a nurse who is confronted by a moral problem in the course of caring for a patient is just as bound as any other health professional to respond in a morally appropriate way. Why? Quite simply, because a nurse's failure to respond appropriately in a morally troubling situation might not only result in a concomitant failure to prevent an otherwise avoidable moral harm, but may even cause it to occur.

In order to deal with moral problems appropriately and effectively, nurses need to know, first, what a moral problem is and how to recognise it; and, second, how and where a solution might be found. It is to answering these questions that this chapter now turns.

Types of moral problems

As with other ethical terms and concepts, nurses and other health professionals tend to misunderstand and misuse the terms 'moral problem', 'moral dilemma' and the like. An example of this can be found in the Victorian State Government's 1988 *Report of the study of professional issues in nursing*. In chapter 4 of this report, in which specific attention is given to ethical issues in nursing practice, the terms 'ethical dilemma' and 'ethical problem' tend to be treated synonymously. However, while an ethical dilemma might well pose an 'ethical problem', it is not always the case that an ethical problem poses an 'ethical dilemma' per se. It is also evident that the author has little appreciation that not all 'dilemmas' or 'problems' encountered in the workplace are necessarily moral in nature. They may, for example, be problems of a somewhat practical nature involving poor communication, misunderstanding, personality conflict, ignorance of factual knowledge, ignorance of the law, inadequate institutional policy, or misinterpretation of institutional policy — problems that could be settled simply by clarifying certain information, improving communication or reformulating policies, rather than by rigorous philosophical debate.

Moral problems can emerge in many forms: they can be of a somewhat 'unglamorous' nature, as in cases involving a decision about whether to restrain a happily demented elderly person who keeps wandering unaided from her bed and risks debilitating injury if she falls; or they can be of a somewhat 'exotic' nature, as in cases involving abortion, organ transplantation and experimental medicine. Our concern in this chapter, however, is not with these more practical and secondary bioethical problems but with the more fundamental and primary problems of how bioethical issues are perceived (i.e. whether they are perceived correctly, if at all), and how bioethical problems are dealt with (i.e. whether they are dealt with appropriately and effectively, or whether they are simply dismissed as being too difficult, and not dealt with at all).

Unfortunately, it is beyond the scope of this text to give the discussion that is warranted to the issue of identifying and resolving moral problems. Nevertheless, it is hoped that the following discussion will help to clarify and rectify some of the common misconceptions nurses have had about what moral problems are and how they might be best dealt with.

1. Moral unpreparedness

The first type of moral problem to be considered here is that of general 'unpreparedness' to deal appropriately and effectively with morally troubling situations. What invariably happens here is that a nurse or other health professional enters into a situation without being sufficiently prepared to deal with the moral complexities of that situation; that is, the nurse may lack the necessary moral knowledge, attitude or vocabulary. When eventually faced with a particular moral problem, the nurse acts in bad faith by pretending that the situation at hand is one which can be handled 'with one's given moral apparatus' (Lemmon 1987, p. 112). The room for moral error here, needless to say, is very considerable.

To illustrate the seriousness of moral unpreparedness, consider the analogous situation of clinical unpreparedness. A nurse who is not educated in the complexities of, say, intensive care nursing, but who is nevertheless sent to 'help out' and care for a ventilated patient in intensive care, would not only be inadequate in this role, but could even be potentially dangerous. Such a nurse would not have the learned skills necessary to detect the subtle changes in a sedated patient's condition — changes indicating, for example, the need for more sedation, or the need to perform tracheal suctioning, or the need to increase the tidal volume of air flow or oxygen administration. Neither would this nurse be able to distinguish the many different alarms that can go off on the high-tech equipment being used to give full life support to the patient, or to detect any malfunctioning of this sophisticated equipment. Without these skills, a nurse working in intensive care would be likely to place the life and well-being of the patient at serious risk. The argument of the seriousness of unpreparedness also applies to the complexities of sound ethical reasoning and ethical health care practice generally. Such a nurse, left to deal with a morally troubling situation, would not only be inadequate in that role, but, as the intensive care example shows, any 'action' could be potentially hazardous. Without the learned moral skills necessary to detect moral problems and to resolve them in a sound, reliable and defensible manner, an unprepared nurse, no matter how well intentioned, could fail to correctly detect moral hazards in the workplace, and therefore fail to act or respond in a way that would prevent a moral calamity from occurring.

The kinds of moral calamities or near calamities that can occur as a result of nurses' (and doctors', and other allied health professionals') moral unpreparedness to deal appropriately and effectively with moral problems in professional practice are well illustrated by the numerous anecdotal case studies and other factual legal case studies discussed in both nursing and bioethical literature. The 'unfortunate experiment' at Auckland's National Women's Hospital, discussed in chapter 1, is an important example here. The moral unpreparedness of nurses and doctors alike resulted in an unchecked violation of patients' rights for over twenty years. Some women have been left permanently scarred — both emotionally and physically — as a result of this experiment; and still other women have needlessly lost their lives. Had the doctors and nurses witnessing the 'unfortunate experiment' been better prepared to deal with the moral complexities involved, the moral calamity that followed could have been prevented.

An important Australian example of the kind of moral calamity that can occur as a consequence of nurses' and others' moral unpreparedness to respond effectively to moral problems in health care contexts can be found in the human tragedy involving Sydney's Chelmsford Private Hospital. In this case, many people were left permanently damaged and scarred — some even died — as a result of receiving deep sleep therapy (DST) prescribed by Dr Harry Bailey, a consultant psychiatrist, who later suicided in connection with the scandal that was eventually uncovered (Bromberger and Fife-Yeomans 1991; Rice 1988). It is now known that approximately a thousand patients were 'treated' with DST at this hospital. It is also known, as revealed as early as 1977 by the current affairs television program '60 Minutes', that many of these patients did not receive the standard of care and treatment they were entitled to receive. Among other things — including the deaths of seven people between 1974 and 1977 — the '60 Minutes' program revealed that 'recognised standard precautions for the safety of patients were not taken; and that patients received the treatment without their consent' (Bromberger and Fife-Yeomans 1991, p. 142). In the Chelmsford Royal Commission that was eventually established in 1988 to 'examine the provision of Deep Sleep Therapy and the administration of Chelmsford Private Hospital', it was confirmed that:

> The signature of some [consent] forms were obtained by fraud and deceit. Some were signed by people whose judgement was compromised by drugs. Some patients were even woken up from their DST [Deep Sleep Therapy] treatment to complete their authorisation. Other patients were treated contrary to their express wishes and some were treated despite the fact they had specifically refused the treatment.
>
> (Commissioner Slattery, cited in Bromberger and Fife-Yeomans 1991, p. 171)

Nursing care was also seriously substandard. In one notable case, the nursing care had been so negligent that a patient developed severe decubitus ulcers between her knees, which became 'glued' together as though they had been skin-grafted. The former patient recalled:

> I was having hallucinations about a lot of coloured ribbons and trying to climb out through them finding the world again. I woke up in a bath tub and two nurses were bathing me. I felt really dirty. One of the nurses said, 'My God, look at her knees.' I looked down and they were joined together. The nurses gently pulled them apart.
>
> (Bromberger and Fife-Yeomans 1991, p. 94)

Bromberger and Fife-Yeomans (1991, p. 94) comment that the patient 'still retains the scars on the inside of her knees'.

Another example of the substandard nursing care that was provided (or more to the point, *not* provided) can be found in the experiences of another patient, Barry Hart, outlined in the following statement read to the New South Wales Parliament in 1984:

> Basic, common-sense nursing practice was ignored. Patients were sedated for ten days and given no exercise during this period. They were incontinent of faeces and urine most of the time and were left lying incontinent of faeces until they woke up.
>
> There was no attempt to maintain a fluid balance. Patients wet the bed and remained lying in the urine until the sheets were changed. The staff made an approximation of whether the patients were actually passing urine (i.e. a fluid output) by seeing how wet the bed was.
>
> (cited in Rice 1988, p. 47)

One of the troubling things about the whole Chelmsford scandal is that rumours about Dr Bailey's unscrupulous practices had been circulating for years, yet nothing was done about it (Bromberger and Fife-Yeomans 1991, p. 176). Equally disturbing is the fact that it was not until 1988 — twenty-four years after the investigated death of the first 'deep sleep' patient, and only after 'treatment' had led to the deaths of twenty-four patients — that a Royal Commission was set up to investigate the allegations concerning the blatant patient abuse that was subsequently proved to have occurred at Chelmsford Private Hospital (Bromberger and Fife-Yeomans 1991, p. 162). Significantly, in the Royal Commission of Inquiry that was conducted, and in the report on its findings, it was revealed that between 1963 and 1979 only *two* nurses took action in an attempt to expose the unscrupulous practices they had observed (*Report of the Royal Commission into Deep Sleep Therapy* 1990, p. 127). As in the case of the 'unfortunate experiment', there is room to speculate here that had nursing personnel been better prepared to recognise and respond effectively to violations of professional ethical standards, the trauma and suffering experienced by the patients at Chelmsford could have been reduced considerably, if not avoided altogether.

Not all moral calamities occurring in health care contexts are as ethically exotic as those that occurred in the 'unfortunate experiment' and the Chelmsford Private Hospital cases, however. Moral calamities can and do occur on a much more commonplace level in the health care arena. Consider, for example, the common but morally odious practice of withholding nourishing tube feeds from severe stroke patients. Wilson-Barnett (1986) cites the heart-rending case of a 66-year-old man who had suffered several strokes and as a result had been left paralysed, aphasic, depressed and suicidal. After two months of rigorous medical and nursing care, a medical decision was made to discontinue his nourishing tube feeds and to commence a three-hourly regime of restricted water. The fluid regime was not sufficient for his needs, however, and he became severely dehydrated. As his condition deteriorated, he began to pass only small quantities of offensive urine and, despite full nursing care, became malodorous and halitotic. Because of his terrible smells, few people entered his room. A senior student nurse involved in caring for him was very distressed about his discomfort, but relayed her distress only to other nurses. Her concerns were not relayed to the patient's attending physician, and she felt unable to approach him herself. (In fact, in accordance with hospital norms, students at that time were not generally encouraged to approach senior doctors.) After ten days of existing in a dehydrated, anuric, malodorous and halitotic state, the patient died. The student nurse meanwhile continued to suffer on account of what she perceived as her dismal failure to maintain her patient's dignity and to 'speak up on his behalf' (Wilson-Barnett 1986, p. 125).

Registered nurses all know that this type of scenario is common, and may occur in a ward not once but a dozen times, and in a hospital not once but a thousand times (see, for example, Lynn 1989). What may not be so well appreciated, however, is that the kind of suffering that occurs in these and similar scenarios is very often unnecessary and preventable. Had the participants in Wilson-Barnett's example been better prepared as moral negotiators and moral mediators, the simple remedy of giving more water to the stroke patient might have been quickly and simply seized upon. Instead, all involved were hopelessly paralysed by their moral ignorance and unpreparedness, and as a result both the patient and the student nurse suffered needlessly. Other registered nurses who have had experiences similar to those of the student nurse in this example have carried the guilt incurred by their experiences for years. When discussing their experiences in educational forums I have conducted, they have broken down and cried — mostly because of the relief of at least being able to discuss their experiences openly and in a non-judgmental environment.

2. Moral blindness

A second type of problem that nurses very often encounter is that of what I shall call 'moral blindness'. A morally blind nurse (or other health professional) is someone who, upon encountering a moral problem, simply does not see it as a *moral* problem. Instead, they may perceive it as either a clinical or a technical problem. Carlton (1978, p. 10) argues, on the basis of her field research, that there is a tendency by many health professionals (particularly doctors) 'to translate ethical issues into technical problems which have clinical solutions'.

Moral blindness can be crudely likened to colour-blindness. Just as a colour-blind person fails to distinguish certain colours in the world, a morally blind person fails to distinguish certain 'moral properties' in the world. Perhaps a better example can be found by appealing to a set of imageries commonly associated with Gestalt psychology and theories on the nature of perception. What I particularly have in mind here are the two drawings which are popularly presented in psychology texts to demonstrate certain perceptual phenomena, including perceptual organisation and the influence of context on the way in which an object is perceived.

The first of these drawings (figure 6.1) depicts what initially appears to be a white vase or goblet against a black background; after a more sustained glance, the drawing changes (or rather, one's

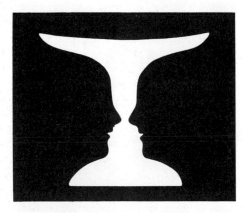

Figure 6.1 Reversible figure and background (reproduced with permission from R. L. Atkinson, R. C. Atkinson and E. R. Hilgard, *Introduction to psychology*, 8th edn, Harcourt Brace Jovanovich, New York, 1983, p. 139).

perception 'shifts') and what is perceived instead are two black facial profiles separated by a white space. Some people see the alternating vase–face images relatively quickly and easily, while others struggle to shake off what for them remains the dominant image (i.e. *either* the vase *or* the faces).

The second ambiguous drawing (figure 6.2) depicts what can be seen as either an unsophisticated-looking old woman or a very sophisticated-looking young woman. As with the vase–face drawing, some people see the alternating old woman–young woman images relatively easily, while others literally get 'stuck' with a dominant perception of *either* the young woman *or* the old woman.

Psychologists claim, however, that people's perceptions can be altered by context — in this instance, by showing photographs before the ambiguous drawings are viewed. They claim that, on an initial viewing of this drawing, 65 per cent report seeing the young woman first. If subjects are shown photographs of an old woman before seeing the drawing, however, almost all see the old woman first. The same 'reversals' can be achieved by conditioning subjects with photographs to see the young woman first (Atkinson et al. 1983, p. 147).

I am not here attempting to present an elaborate theory of moral perception but merely trying to illustrate what I believe is a common and a potentially morally dangerous phenomenon in health care contexts: that of impaired moral perception. There is, I think, some room to suggest that health professionals (including nurses) .are so dominated and conditioned by the 'clinical imagery' around

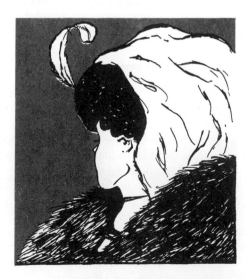

Figure 6.2 Ambiguous stimulus (reproduced with permission from R. L. Atkinson, R. C. Atkinson and E. R. Hilgard, *Introduction to psychology*, 8th edn, Harcourt Brace Jovanovich, New York, 1983, p. 139).

them that, when they do encounter a bona fide moral problem, it is very often perceived not as a *moral* problem per se, but as a *clinical* or a *technical* problem and, as such, one requiring a clinical solution, not a moral solution. Some health professionals have a healthy perception of the alternating moral–clinical images depicted by a given scenario; many, however, remain stuck with a dominant *clinical image* and just simply do not see the alternative *moral image*, which for them is less discernible. One unfortunate consequence of this, of course, is that *technically correct* decisions are made at the expense of *morally correct* decisions.

The extent to which clinical perceptions and judgments dominate over moral perceptions and judgments is well illustrated by the common hospital practice of ordering 'not for resuscitation' (NFR) on hopelessly or chronically ill patients. It is probably true to say that many doctors and nurses perceive NFR practices as involving a *clinical issue*, not a *moral issue*, and, as such, one to be rightly decided by doctors, not ethicists. The clinical–moral Gestalt problem became particularly clear to me at a nursing law and ethics conference in 1988. After presenting a paper on the nature and moral implications of NFR orders, I was approached by several registered nurses with what has now become a familiar and distressing comment: 'My God! I had never thought about it [NFR] as a *moral* issue before ... What have I done?' The issue was taken up by the media (see Miller 1988, 1989; Schumpeter 1988; Craig 1989; *Upfront* 1988); other nurses wanted to challenge or attack the view that NFR orders involve moral decisions. The Victorian State President of the Australian Medical Association, Dr Bill McCubbery, was prompted to respond to the issue, and is reported as saying that 'NFR decisions had to depend on professional judgment' (Schumpeter 1988, p. 21); the failure to mention 'moral judgment' is, I think, illuminating (see also chapter 12).

The clinical–moral Gestalt shift that has occurred in those who have been persuaded that current NFR practices constitute a fundamental moral issue has been, for me, an interesting phenomenon to observe.

Other equally compelling examples of the extent to which clinical perceptions and judgments dominate over ethical perceptions and judgments can be found in sociologist Wendy Carlton's work *'In our professional opinion ...': the primacy of clinical judgment over moral choice* (1978), in which she details a number of persuasive anecdotal case studies collected while doing field research in a university teaching hospital. One case study, which has already been briefly mentioned in chapter 2, concerns an 11-year-old Down's syndrome child who had been admitted to hospital for a hysterectomy. It will be recalled that most of the doctors and nurses involved in the case were appalled that this child was being considered for such a radical operation, yet felt that they could not go against the consulting physician's decision. Interestingly, the moral problem posed by this case was not resolved by open and honest moral debate among those involved, but by the anaesthetist declaring that because of a pre-existing heart condition the child was unfit for a general anaesthetic and surgery. As Carlton (1978, p. 37) points out, the child's heart condition conveniently 'allowed the sidestepping of ethical concerns in favor of sound clinical reasons against surgery'.

The issue of 'moral blindness' among nurses is an important and far-reaching one, and, as with the problem of moral unprepared-ness, risks the realisation of otherwise avoidable moral harms. I do not believe that this problem is insurmountable, however. Just as subjects can be 'conditioned' to see the old woman rather than the young woman in the ambiguous drawing shown in figure 6.2, so too can nurses, doctors and allied health professionals be 'con-ditioned' to see the moral dimension of an ambiguous scenario which can be perceived as involving either a moral problem or a clinical or technical problem. The critical question here, however, is: what kind of conditioning should nurses and others be given to ensure that they do experience a Gestalt clinical–moral shift in their professional perceptions?

Whatever the answer to this question, the unhappy fact remains that, unless nurses, doctors and other health professionals escape their moral blindness, they will never be in a position to either condemn or rectify morally iniquitous clinical practices, to con-demn or rectify situations entailing patients' rights violations, or indeed to condemn or rectify *any* situation entailing unethical conduct in health care settings. It hardly needs pointing out that the possible consequences of this 'moral disability' could be extemely tragic, and could result in avoidable human suffering like that which occurred in the cases of the 'unfortunate experiment' and the Chelmsford Private Hospital.

3. Moral indifference

A third type of problem which nurses may encounter is that of 'moral indifference'. Moral indifference is characterised by an un-concerned or uninterested attitude toward demands to be moral. The morally indifferent person is someone who typically refrains from expressing any desire that certain acts should or should not be done in all comparable circumstances (Hare 1981, p. 185). An example of a morally indifferent nurse would be a nurse who is both unconcerned about and uninterested in alleviating a patient's pain, or is unconcerned about or uninterested in the fact that an NFR (not for resuscitation) order or an order to perform ECT (electroconvulsive therapy) has been given on an unconsenting patient, or is unconcerned about and uninterested in any form of violation of patients' rights, for that matter. As well as this, a morally indifferent nurse would probably refrain from expressing a desire that anything should or should not be done about such situations.

The problem of moral indifference in nursing is well captured by Mila Aroskar (1986) in her illuminating article 'Are nurses' mind sets compatible with ethical practice?' Aroskar (1986, p. 72) cites the findings of a study done in the late 1970s which showed that nurses tended to defer to institutional norms 'even when patients' rights were being violated'. She also points out that, despite the United States nursing profession's formal commitment to ethical practice (as manifested, among other things, by its formal adoption of various codes and standards of practice), arguments are still widely heard among nurses that 'ethical practice is too risky and requires a certain amount of heroism on the part of nurses' (Aroskar 1986, p. 69). Although Aroskar is writing from an American point of view, I am sure all would agree that her words apply equally to many nursing care contexts outside the United States of America.

The retreat by nurses into moral indifference, while not con-donable, is understandable. The American legal cases of *Tuma v. Board of Nursing of the State of Idaho* (1979), *Warthen v. Toms River Community Memorial Hospital* (1985) and *Free v. Holy Cross Hospital* (1987) stand as sobering reminders of the kinds of difficulties nurses might find themselves in when attempting to conduct morally responsible professional practice, and the ultimate price that can be paid for taking a firm moral stand (see also Johnstone 1994, chapter 9). In the *Tuma* case, a registered nurse by the name of Jolene Lucille Tuma, a clinical teacher, had been involved in caring for a patient by the name of Grace Wahlstrom who had been suffering from leukemia for a number of years. Mrs Wahlstrom asked Tuma to discuss with her possible alternative (unorthodox) treatments to chemotherapy, which Tuma agreed to do. The patient's family, however, took exception to Tuma giving Grace Wahlstrom the information she had requested, and immediately informed the consulting physician. Upon being contacted by the patient's family, the physician asked for Tuma's name. Two weeks later, despite receiving chemotherapy, the patient died. The physician meanwhile reported Tuma's actions to the state board of nursing, and she was subsequently deregistered. The ground for her deregistration was that she had 'interfered with the physician–patient relationship', and thus was guilty of 'professional misconduct'.

Tuma took her case to the Supreme Court and appealed against the state board's decision to deregister her. Although Tuma won her case, the publicity given to it had effectively ruined her profes-sional nursing career, and she 'felt it unwise' to resume her nursing practice (King 1985, p. 162; see also Johnstone 1994, chapter 6). It is perhaps worth noting here that Tuma did not win her case on grounds of the legitimacy of the relationship she had with her patient (and of legitimately meeting her patient's expressed needs and considered wishes in that relationship), but on a technical point of law pertaining to the state nursing board's failure to make explicit just *what* constituted an 'interference with the physician–patient relationship', and, further, that interference with the physician-patient relationship constituted 'unprofessional conduct' (Johnstone 1994, chapter 6). It is also worth noting here that much non-nursing literature to date seems to have a pre-occupation with the legal and moral unacceptability of nurses interfering with the *doctor–patient* relationship, yet there is very little discussion of the moral and legal unacceptability of doctors interfering with the *nurse–patient* relationship.

In the *Warthen* case (already briefly mentioned in chapter 1) a registered nurse by the name of Corinne Warthen was dismissed after refusing to dialyse a terminally ill bilateral amputee patient. It will be recalled that Warthen cited 'moral, medical and philo-sophical objections' to performing the procedure, since it was causing the patient more harm. In the legal case that followed, the court did not accept her defence, and Warthen lost her appeal against what she argued was an 'unfair dismissal'.

Finally, in the American legal case *Free v. Holy Cross Hospital* (1987), which I have considered extensively elsewhere (Johnstone 1994), a nurse was dismissed for insubordination because she refused to evict a seriously ill and bedridden patient from hospital. (At one point the nurse was instructed to remove the patient 'even if removal required forcibly putting the patient in a wheelchair and leaving her in the park' [*Free v. Holy Cross Hospital* 1987, p. 1189].) The nurse took the case to court, arguing that her dismissal was unfair. In defence of her actions, Free argued that to evict the patient would have been:

> in violation of her ethical duty as a registered nurse not to engage in dishonourable, unethical or unprofessional conduct of a character likely to harm the public as mandated by the Illinois nursing act.
>
> (*Free v. Holy Cross Hospital* 1987, p. 1190)

The court hearing the case did not accept Free's defence, however, and she lost her fight to be reinstated.

The difficulties nurses often face when trying to deliver ethically responsible nursing care are worldwide. We all know (and, no doubt, have even personally experienced at some stage) the forces that can be brought to bear upon a nurse who takes a moral position which conflicts with established hospital norms and etiquette. The degree to which many professional nurses feel intolerably burdened in their efforts to deliver ethical nursing practice has been made clear to me by comments made at a number of nursing ethics seminars and in-service lectures I have given in Australia. For example, in two separate incidents, registered nurses openly broke down and cried in a room full of people when relating morally troubling experiences they had each personally had. In one of these incidents the registered nurse told of how she had been ordered to administer large and potentially lethal doses of narcotics to an unconscious terminally ill patient. Upon performing a thorough pain assessment of the patient in question, however, she judged the prescribed analgesia regime to be excessive, and concluded that giving the amounts ordered would almost certainly hasten the patient's death. She reasoned further that giving the prescribed analgesia regime would, in this instance, be tantamount to committing murder. The dilemma for her was that she had 'not been trained to kill people', and yet here she was being expected to do just that. When she voiced her concerns to a senior nurse administrator, she was strongly criticised and accused of being personally and professionally 'immature' — a view which the prescribing doctor also came to share. The nurse was told that, if she persisted in her objection to administering the prescribed analgesia regime, she would have to leave her job (Johnstone 1987, p. 30).

Other sobering examples of the kinds of difficulties nurses can face when taking a moral stand on a nursing matter can be found in chapter 12 in the discussion on not-for-resuscitation orders, and in chapter 13 in the discussion on conscientious objection.

It is small wonder that nurses become morally indifferent to the violations of patients' rights and other unjust practices in health care domains. The reality is that both legal and institutional constraints make it very difficult for nurses to act morally. The price paid for acting morally or for taking a moral stand can be intolerably high, as we have seen. What this signifies, however, is not that nurses should abandon the demands of morality; rather, they should seek ways in which morality's demands can be safely and effectively upheld.

4. Amoralism

A fourth type of moral problem which nurses might encounter, and which is similar to moral indifference, is that of 'amoralism', which is characterised by an absence of moral concern and a rejection of morality altogether (a position significantly different from *im-moralism*, which accepts morality, but violates its demands). An amoral person is someone who refrains from making moral judgments and who typically rejects being bound by any of morality's behavioural prescriptions and proscriptions. If an amoralist were to ask: 'Why should I be moral?', it is likely that no answer would be satisfactory. (For a helpful response to the question 'Why should I be moral?', see Nielsen 1989.)

A nurse who is an amoralist would reject any compulsion to behave morally as a professional. For example, the amoral nurse might reject that there is any moral compulsion to alleviate a patient's pain even though it was possible to do so, or not to violate a patient's rights. The amoral nurse would also probably claim that it does not make any sense even to speak of things like a patient's pain or its relief, or the violation of a patient's rights, in terms of being 'good' or 'bad'; for the amoral nurse, moral language itself has no meaning. The amoralist's position in this respect is analogous to the atheist's rejection of certain religious terms. The extreme atheist, for example, would argue against uttering the word 'God', since it refers to nothing and therefore has no meaning. Such an atheist might also claim that there is no point in engaging in a religious debate on the existence of God, since there is just nothing there to debate. To try and debate the existence of God would be like trying to debate the existence of 'a black cat in a darkened room when there isn't one!' The amoralist may argue in a similar way in relation to the issue of morality.

It can be seen that the amoralist's position is an extreme one, and one which is very difficult to sustain. (Even thieves, who may appear amoral, act on the 'moral' assumption that it is good/right to steal.) If it is encountered in health care contexts, it is likely that very little can be done, morally speaking, to deal with it. The only recourse in dealing with the amoral health professional would be to appeal to non-moral censuring mechanisms such as legal and/or professional disciplinary measures.

5. Moral complacency

A fifth type of moral problem nurses can encounter is that of 'moral complacency', defined by Unwin (1985, p. 205) as 'a general un-willingness to accept that one's moral opinions may be mistaken'. Again, we do not need to look far to find examples of moral complacency in health care contexts.

I recall being approached by a gerontology nurse specialist lamenting the 'short-sightedness' of some of her students, who were of the view that elderly people in residential care homes should be resuscitated in the event of cardiac arrest, and that the blanket NFR status given to all elderly residents upon entering a residential care home was both immoral and illegal. The nurse specialist was insistent that the students were morally wrong, and was clearly disturbed and outraged by their position.

In my response to her, I enquired concerning the discussion she had had with her students whether anyone had thought to ask the elderly residents what their preferences were — whether, in the event of cardiac arrest, *they* wished to be resuscitated or not? It should be noted that elderly people entering a residential care agency are almost invariably asked whether they wish to be cremated, and where they wish to be buried; they are not generally asked whether they wish to be resuscitated if and when they cardiac arrest. The nurse specialist became obviously agitated by my question, and exclaimed: 'Surely it is ludicrous to ask all elderly residents whether they wish to be resuscitated!' After I had expressed my disagreement and pointed out the minimal require-ments of the moral principle of autonomy, the nurse specialist retorted: 'Would you really expect us to ask each and every resident whether they wish to be resuscitated? It's ludicrous! It's silly! It's unnecessary ...' To this retort, I reminded the nurse specialist that elderly residents are already asked whether they wish to be cremated and where they wish to be buried, so what was so difficult about asking them whether they wish to be resuscitated? The nurse specialist was still unconvinced, and persisted in rejecting the view I was putting to her. She further maintained that it was right and proper that all elderly residents should be uniformly labelled NFR upon admission to a residential nursing care home. Even the thought that such a practice was tantamount to mass passive involuntary euthanasia failed to move her. The attitude of the nurse specialist in this anecdote is an example of moral complacency.

Like moral unpreparedness and moral blindness, moral com-placency is, I believe, something which can be rectified by moral education and moral consciousness raising. The objective of taking this action would be, of course, to produce in the morally complacent person the attitude that nobody can afford to be complacent in the way they ordinarily view the world — least of all the moral world. This is particularly so in instances where *other* people's moral interests are at stake. It is a grave mistake to assume that our moral opinions are 'right' *just because* they are our own opinions. As ethical professionals, our stringent moral responsibility is to *question* our taken-for-granted assumptions about the world, and not to presume their inviolability.

6.   Moral fanaticism

A sixth type of moral problem which may be encountered by nurses, and which is similar in many respects to moral compla-cency, is that of 'moral fanaticism'. The moral fanatic is someone who is thoroughly 'wedded to certain ideals' and uncritically and unreflectingly makes moral judgments according to them (Hare

1981, p. 170). Richard Hare's celebrated case of the fanatical Nazi is a good example here (Hare 1963, chapter 9). The fanatical Nazi in this case stringently clings to the ideal of a pure Aryan German race and the need to exterminate all Jews as a means of purging the German race of its impurities. The Nazi falls into the category of being a 'fanatic' when he insists that, if he discovers himself to be of Jewish descent, then he too should be exterminated along with all the rest of the Jews (Hare 1963, pp. 161–2).

Examples of moral fanaticism abound in health care contexts. The doctor who 'saves life' regardless of a patient's wishes to the contrary, or regardless of the suffering it causes, is an important example here. Morally fanatical doctors in this instance might further boost their position by claiming that it is a supremely moral one. The maintenance of absolute confidentiality, even though harm might be caused as a result, is another good example. So, too, is the example of a doctor or a nurse forcing unwanted information on a patient in the fanatical belief that all patients must be told the truth, even if the patient in question has specifically requested not to receive the information.

In the case of moral fanatics, an appeal to overriding considerations or principles of conduct would not be helpful (Hare 1981, p. 178). As with the amoralist, the problem of the moral fanatic in health care contexts is likely to have disappointing outcomes. In the final analysis, it may be that other (non-moral) mechanisms will have to be appealed to in order to resolve the moral problems caused by moral fanaticism; for example, it may be necessary to seek the adjudicating involvement of a public advocate, a court of law or a disciplinary body.

7. Moral disagreements

A seventh type of moral problem nurses will very often encounter is that involving 'moral disagreement' — concerning, for example, the selection, interpretation, application and evaluation of moral standards. Milo (1986) identifies two fundamental types of moral disagreement: internal moral disagreement and radical moral disagreement.

INTERNAL MORAL DISAGREEMENT

Three forms of internal moral disagreement can occur. The first of these involves a fundamental conflict about the force or priority of accepted moral standards. For example, two people may agree to common moral standards but disagree about what to do when these standards come into conflict. Milo (1986, p. 455) argues that the disagreement here is not necessarily attributable to 'any disagreement in factual beliefs or to bad reasoning', but to a disagreement in *attitude* (see also McNaughton 1988, pp. 17, 29).

Consider the following hypothetical example to illustrate Milo's point.

Two nurses might both accept a moral standard which generally requires truth-telling, but may disagree on when this standard should apply. Nurse A, for instance, might favour (that is, have a 'pro-attitude' towards) telling the truth to patient X about a pessimistic medical diagnosis. Nurse B, on the other hand, might not favour (i.e. might have a 'con-attitude' towards) telling the truth to patient X about this diagnosis and prefer a pro-attitude to pain avoidance (i.e. the psychological pain of learning about the diagnosis). It is not that these two nurses have different criteria of relevance, as such, but rather have *different principles of priority* (Milo 1986, p. 457).

A second type of internal disagreement centres on what are to count as acceptable exceptions and limitations to otherwise mutually agreed moral standards. As Milo explains, we generally accept that moral standards are limited by other moral standards, as well as by the competing claims of self-interest. (Morality does not usually expect us to risk our own lives or our own important moral interest in morally troubling situations.) People might agree that as a general rule we ought all to make certain modest sacrifices in terms of our own interests (a minimal requirement of justice), but may disagree 'about what constitutes a modest sacrifice' (Milo 1986, p. 459). In many respects this type of disagreement could be loosely described as a disagreement in interpretation of an accepted moral standard. Consider another example.

Two nurses might agree that patients' rights should not be violated. Nurse A might further hold that, in situations involving violations of patients' rights, a nurse should act — even if this means threatening the nurse's job security (which nurse A views as a modest sacrifice). Nurse B, on the other hand, might agree that nurses should in principle act to prevent a patient's rights from being violated, but disagree that nurses should do so if they stand to lose their jobs as a result (something which nurse B views as an unacceptable and extreme sacrifice). What these two nurses are essentially disagreeing about is not the moral standard per se (that nurses should act to prevent violations of patients' rights), but about when morally relevant considerations can be and cannot be overridden by self-interest. In disagreements like this, and where the disagreement is based on preferences rather than attitude, there may well be no happy solution, a situation which Milo calls a 'moral deadlock' (1986, p. 461).

A third and final type of internal moral disagreement centres on the selection and applicability of accepted ethical standards. This kind of disagreement has nothing to do with whether a standard can be overridden by other considerations, but concerns whether it should have been selected or appealed to in the first place.

For example, two nurses may agree that killing an innocent human being is wrong. They may disagree, however, that abortion is wrong. Nurse A, for example, might argue that, since the fetus is not a human being, abortion does not entail the killing of an innocent human being and therefore is not wrong. Appealing to a moral standard prohibiting the killing of innocent human life would then, for nurse A, be quite irrelevant. Nurse B, on the other hand, may argue that the fetus is a human being, and therefore abortion, since it entails killing an innocent human being, is absolutely morally wrong. Appealing to a moral standard prohibiting the killing of innocent human life would then, for nurse B, be supremely relevant. The disagreement between these two nurses hinges very much on a disagreement about the moral relevance of the facts on what constitutes a human being.

RADICAL MORAL DISAGREEMENT

Milo (1986) identifies two types of radical moral disagreement: the first type he calls 'partial radical moral disagreement', and the second type 'total radical moral disagreement'.

In cases of *partial radical moral disagreement*, dissenting parties might agree on some criteria of relevance but not all. For example, a nurse might argue that directly killing terminally and chronically ill patients with a lethal injection is morally wrong, whereas merely 'letting nature take its course' or 'letting patients die' is not morally wrong. Another nurse might agree that directly killing terminally and chronically ill patients is wrong, but thoroughly disagree that merely 'letting die' is less morally offensive. Here there may be no court of appeal to reconcile the distinction between direct 'killing' and merely 'letting die'. In this case, partial radical disagreement is very similar to internal moral disagreement. It may be very difficult to distinguish between the two, a point which Milo reluctantly concedes.

In cases of *total radical moral disagreement*, disputants do not agree on any criteria of relevance, and do not share any basic moral principles. For Milo (1986, p. 469), this is 'the most extreme kind of moral disagreement that one can imagine'.

An example of total radical moral disagreement would be where two theatre nurses radically disagree with each other about the moral acceptability of organ transplantations. Nurse A argues that retrieving or harvesting organs from so-called 'cadavers' is an unmitigated act of murder, since the person whose organs are being retrieved is not yet fully dead. (Nurse A, in this instance, rejects brain-death criteria as indicative of death.) Nurse A also argues that, even if the potential cadaver is restored to nothing more than a persistent vegetative state, and even if another person may die as a result of not getting a life-saving organ transplant operation, this does not justify violating the sanctity of life of the potential organ donor. The death of another person through not receiving a new organ, while 'unfortunate', cannot be helped. Such are the tragic twists of life.

Nurse B, on the other hand, argues that retrieving organs is nothing like murder since, among other things, the person is already dead. (Nurse B, in this instance, totally accepts brain-death criteria as indicative of death.) Nurse B also totally rejects a 'sanctity of life' view, arguing that it has no substance; only quality of life considerations have ethical meaning. Nurse B further argues that, even conceding the unreliability of brain-death criteria as indicative of death, retrieving the organs is still morally permissible, since the donating person can at best look forward only to a 'vegetative existence' and one devoid of any 'quality of life' (which is cruel and immoral), whereas an organ recipient could look forward to a renewed quality of life.

In the dispute between nurse A and nurse B, resolution is unlikely. As Milo points out, in total radical disagreement the disputants reach a total and irreconcilable impasse. The possibility of this situation occurring in health care contexts, is, I believe, something which needs to be taken very seriously, and which has important implications for conscientious objection claims (an issue that is given separate consideration in chapter 13 of this text).

It should be clarified here that, while moral disagreements can certainly be problematic (particularly if a person's life and well-being are hanging in the balance, and an immediate decision is needed about what should be done), these need not be taken as constituting grounds upon which morality as such should be viewed with scepticism or, worse, rejected altogether. As Stout (1988, p. 14) argues persuasively, the facts of moral disagreement 'don't *compel* us to become nihilists or skeptics, to abandon the notions of moral truth and justified moral belief'. One reason for this, he explains, is that moral disagreement is, in essence, just a kind of moral diversity or, as he calls it, 'conceptual diversity' (Stout 1988, pp. 15, 61). While moral disagreement may rightly challenge us to 'meticulously disentangle' diverse and conflicting moral points of view, it does not preclude or threaten the possibility of moral judgment per se, either within a particular culture or across many cultures (Stout 1988, p. 15).

In the previous chapter, it was argued that moral disagreement has historically been the beginning of critical moral thinking, not its end. Given this, there is room to suggest that we should be very cautious in accepting Milo's pessimistic conclusions about the irreconcilability of radical moral disagreement. Instead, we should look towards a more optimistic solution, and view such disagreements as an important and necessary opportunity for 'enriching [our] conceptions of morality through comparative inquiry' (Stout 1988, p. 70), and thereby augment our collective wisdom about what morality is, and what it really means to *be* moral in a world characterised by individual and collective (cultural) diversity. In the ultimate analysis, the solution to the problematic of moral disagreement may not be to engage in adversarial dialogue (fight/litigate), or even to negotiate a happy medium between conflicting views (compromise). Rather, the solution may be, to borrow from Edward de Bono (1985), to engage in 'triangular thinking'; to engage in moral disagreement, not as a judge or as a negotiator, but as a 'creative designer' who is able to escape the imprisonment of the positivist logic and language that is so characteristic of mainstream Western moral discourse; and to engage in moral disagreement as someone who is able ultimately to resolve the conflicts and disagreements which others have long since abandoned as hopeless and irreconcilable impasses. Such an approach, however, requires not just an ability to think about new things, but, to borrow from Catharine MacKinnon (1987, p. 9), 'a new way of thinking.'

8.   Moral dilemmas

The last type of moral problem to be considered here (and one which has been widely discussed in both nursing and bioethical literature) is that of the proverbial 'moral dilemma'. Broadly speaking, a dilemma may be defined as a situation requiring choice between what seem to be two equally desirable or undesirable alternatives; it may be crudely described as an 'awful feeling of being stuck'. A moral dilemma, however, is a little different, and can occur in one of several forms.

First, a moral dilemma can occur in the form of *logical incompatibility* between two different moral principles. For example, two different moral principles might apply equally in a given situation, and neither principle can be chosen without violating the other. Even so, a choice has to be made. Consider the case of a nurse who accepts a moral principle which demands respect for the sanctity of life, and who also accepts another moral principle which demands that persons should be spared intolerable suffering. Now, imagine this nurse in the situation of caring for a terminally ill patient who is suffering intolerable and intractable pain. In this situation, if the nurse accepts the sanctity of life principle, the administration of the large and potentially lethal doses of narcotics that might be required to relieve the patient's intolerable pain would probably be prohibited. On the other hand, if the non-maleficence principle were followed, the nurse might be required to administer the potentially lethal doses of narcotics, even though this could hasten the patient's death. In this situation, the nurse is unavoidably confronted with the profound and troubling dilemma that to uphold the sanctity of life principle could violate the non-maleficence principle, but to uphold the non-maleficence principle could violate the sanctity of life principle. The ultimate question posed for the nurse in this situation is: 'Which principle ought I to choose?'

The options open to the nurse are:

- to modify the principles in question so that they do not conflict (i.e. by adding 'riders' to them);
- to abandon one principle in favour of the other;
- to abandon both principles in favour of a third (for example, autonomy and respect for the patient's rational wishes, or compassion).

It should be noted that none of these is free of moral risk.

A second type of moral dilemma is that involving *competing moral duties*. Consider the following case. A nurse working in a specialised unit is assigned a patient with a known history of drug addiction, and is instructed to chaperone the patient when there are visitors to make sure that illicit drugs are not 'slipped in'. The nurse, however, believes that the duty to protect this patient from harm (such as might occur from receiving illicit drugs) competes with the duty to respect the patient's privacy. The question for the nurse in this scenario is: 'Which duty ought I to fulfil?'

In another case, a nurse is assigned a patient of traditional Greek background who has recently been diagnosed with meta-static cancer. The doctor has ordered that the patient not be told his diagnosis. The patient, however, keeps asking the nurse and his family for information about his diagnosis. The family knows the diagnosis, but wants the doctor to tell the patient. Here the nurse is caught between a duty to tell the truth to the patient, and a duty to respect the wishes of the family. The nurse is also bound to follow the doctor's orders (although the question of whether there is a *duty* to follow them is another matter). The question for the nurse in this scenario is, again: 'Which duty ought I to fulfil — my duty to the patient or to the family, or to the doctor, or to whom?'

Philosophical answers to questions raised by a conflict of duty are varied and controversial. In *The right and the good*, W. D. Ross (1930) argues that duties are prima facie or 'conditional' in nature. Thus, when two duties conflict, we must 'study the situation' as fully as we can until we are able to reach a 'considered opinion (it is never more) that in the circumstances one of them [the duties] is more incumbent than any other' (Ross 1930, p. 19). Once we have worked out which of the conflicting duties is the more 'incumbent' on us, we are bound to consider it our prima facie duty in that situation. Richard Hare (1981, p. 26), however, takes quite a different view. He argues that, if we find ourselves caught between what appear to be two conflicting duties, we need to look again. For it is likely that, in the case of an apparent conflict in duties, one of our so-called 'duties' is not our duty at all; we have only mistakenly thought that it was. In other words, what happens here is that one of the two apparently conflicting duties is eventually 'cancelled out', so to speak.

Williams (1973) disagrees. While he believes that one of the conflicting *oughts* has to be rejected (but only in the sense that both conflicting duties/oughts cannot be acted upon), he does not agree that this means that the duties or oughts in question do not apply equally in the situation at hand, or that one of the conflicting duties must inevitably be 'cancelled out'. To the contrary: our reasoning may assist us to deal with a conflict of duty and may assist us to find a 'best' way to act, but this does not mean that we abandon one or other of the duties in question. How do we know? Even after making a choice between two conflicting duties, we are still left with a lingering feeling of 'regret'. And it is this very feeling of regret which tells us that we have not altogether abandoned or 'cancelled out' the duty we decided could not, in that situation, be also acted upon.

In the drug addict case, we might well side with Richard Hare and unanimously agree that the nurse is mistaken in a belief that there is an overriding duty to respect the patient's privacy, and that clearly the primary duty is to prevent the patient from suffering the harms likely to be incurred by the administration of illicit drugs. But here the question arises: is it really a nurse's duty to act as a kind of police warden? What if the patient is not receiving any form of therapy for the immediate drug addiction problem, and is at risk of developing severe and life-threatening withdrawal symptoms? How is the nurse's duty to 'prevent harm' to be regarded in this instance? Does cancelling out one of the conflicting duties here relieve the moral tension created in this scenario? Or is there more to be achieved by exploring ways in which they can be reconciled with each other?

In the cancer diagnosis case, we might unanimously agree that the nurse's primary duty is to the patient, and that any apparent duty owed to the family is not a bona fide one (after all, does not the moral principle of autonomy demand respect for the patient's rational wishes in this scenario?). Placed in a cultural context, however, the scenario takes on a whole new dimension. As Kanitsaki (1988, 1989, 1993, 1994) points out, and as was considered briefly in chapter 5 of this text, families from a traditional cultural background very often play a fundamental and highly protective role in mediating the flow of information to a sick loved one. To ignore a family's request in such a situation could be to risk terrible violence to the well-being of the patient. Where this is likely, it is imperative that the nurse works closely with the family and ensures that the transfer of information to the patient is handled in a *culturally appropriate manner*. While the family may be perceived as 'interfering', in reality it may be providing an important and key link in ensuring that the patient's well-being and moral interests are fully upheld. Cancelling out one of the duties in this scenario is unlikely to relieve the moral tension generated by the patient's request for and the doctor's refusal to give the medical information on the patient's diagnosis. Had the only criterion for action been what superficially appeared to be a primary duty to the patient, the nurse may have unwittingly facilitated the flow of information in a culturally *inappropriate* and thus harmful manner. By reconciling the apparent conflict in duties, and by working closely with the family, however, the nurse is able to facilitate the flow of information to the patient in a culturally appropriate and thus less harmful manner. In this instance, by fulfilling the duty owed to the family, the nurse could also succeed in fulfilling the duty owed to the patient.

It might be objected that the examples given here do not involve difficult cases, and that the required choices are relatively easy to make. But even if we admit 'hard cases', Hare's position is somehow unsatisfactory, as is his argument that when there is an apparent conflict in duties, it is likely that one of the duties involved is not our duty at all. There is, I believe, always room to question how we can ever be really sure that a 'cancelled' duty was not our duty in the first place. The cancer diagnosis case, I think, illustrates this point well. Ross's and Williams's positions, on the other hand, remind us that matters of moral duty are never clear-cut; and, further, that we always have to be very careful in our appraisal of given situations and in the choices we make regarding to whom our moral duties are owed and what our moral duties actually are.

A third kind of moral dilemma, and one closely related to a dilemma concerning competing duties, is that entailing *competing and conflicting interests*. Here the question raised for the moral observer is: 'Whose interests ought I to uphold?'

Consider the following case. A clinical teacher on clinical placement at a residential care home was informed by a student that an elderly demented resident had been physically and verbally abused by one of the ward's permanent staff members, as witnessed by the student. The clinical teacher was temporarily undecided about what to do. It was a very serious matter — and, indeed, a very serious accusation — but it would be very difficult to prove. If the incident was not reported to the home's nursing administrator, the staff member concerned would probably continue to abuse the home's residents. If the incident was reported, there was a risk that the interests of both students and the school of nursing could be threatened. (The home's administrator might, for example, refuse to continue allowing students to be placed at the home for the purposes of gaining clinical experience.) The dilemma for the clinical teacher was whether not to report the matter and thereby protect both the students' and the school's interests in having continued clinical placements, or to report the matter fully, whatever the consequences to the school and the students, and thereby protect the residents' interests.

The teacher and the student mutually agreed that the matter was too serious to ignore and decided they would risk the consequences of reporting the incident. The exercise, as feared, proved extremely distressing and painful for both the student concerned and the clinical teacher. The accused staff member denied having abused the elderly resident, and in turn accused the student of lying and of being the one who had really committed the abuses. The opinion of the patient could not be sought, as the elderly resident concerned was demented. Fortunately, the matter was eventually resolved to everyone's satisfaction.

A fourth type of dilemma is taken from a feminist moral perspective, and is described by Gilligan (1982, 1987) in terms of being caught between attachments to people and trying to decide upon ways that will avoid 'hurting' each of these 'attached people'. Gilligan uses the example of a woman contemplating an abortion; she argues that generally a woman faced with having to make a choice in this situation 'contemplates a decision that affects both self and others and engages directly the critical moral issue of hurting' (Gilligan 1982, p. 71). Here the question to be raised in contemplating a difficult choice is: 'How can I avoid hurting the people to whom I am attached?'

It might be objected here that Gilligan's sense of 'hurt' and 'avoiding hurt' is not very different from the general moral principle of non-maleficence and its demand to avoid or prevent 'harm'. While I concede that 'hurt' is a type of harm, there is a subtle distinction between 'hurt' in the sense that I think Gilligan is using it and 'harm' in the abstract sense that philosophy uses it. It is important to draw a distinction between these two notions so as not to obscure other important distinctions which can be drawn in our moral discourse. Let us examine this point a little more fully.

The sense in which 'hurt' is being used here is not simply 'physical', but rather existential, spiritual, and even 'soulful' or 'soul-felt'. There is even room to make the radical claim that the notion of 'avoiding hurt' is not being asserted as a *principle* as such, but more as an *attitude*, and one which reminds us that we need to take very special care in our selection, interpretation and application of general moral principles in our everyday personal and professional lives. In short, it is an attitude which serves to *mediate* the use of more general moral principles. Consider, for example, the demand to 'avoid hurt' in a situation involving a patient who has yet to be told an unfavourable medical diagnosis. The demand to 'avoid hurt' reminds us that it is not enough just bluntly to *give* the patient the diagnosis (as may otherwise be required by the moral principle of autonomy), but that it must also be given in a caring, compassionate and culturally appropriate manner. Furthermore, it is not clear to me that the principle of non-maleficence fully captures the demand to be caring, compassionate and culturally appropriate in manner when performing such an unpleasant task as giving someone an unfavourable medical diagnosis. And in some instances, taken to its extreme, the principle of non-maleficence might even instruct that the diagnosis should not be given at all. 'Avoiding hurt', on the other hand, recognises that the information that needs to be given could be 'harmful' and is probably 'hurtful', but that there is a way of *lessening* if not *avoiding* this harm and hurt. To illustrate this point, consider the following case (told to me by a nursing colleague).

A young doctor walked into a patient's room, stood at the end of the bed, and in full view and hearing distance of other patients in the room, and without greeting the patient or smiling, stated abruptly: 'We've looked at your throat and the lump you have there is cancer.' Without another word, the doctor then briskly walked off. The patient had previously expressed a desire to know the diagnosis when it was available, so in many respects we could conclude that the doctor acted 'ethically' in that the patient's rational wishes had been respected and the requested information had been relayed to the patient. What is evident in this case is that the doctor had not considered ways to give the information less 'hurtfully' — or, if such ways had been considered, they were certainly not heeded. For example, the doctor might have at least greeted the patient, used a friendlier tone of voice, drawn the curtains around the patient before speaking, sat down on a chair to be at the same level as the patient, and stayed long enough to allow the patient to ask questions, which the patient stated later would have been desirable. If the doctor felt inadequate to deal with this situation, it might have been advisable to wait until a colleague or a nurse was available to help. Or, more simply, the doctor should have passed the task over to someone else who was more experienced and better prepared to deal with the situation. By using such an abrupt manner, the doctor not only failed to 'avoid hurt', but exacerbated it. To make matters worse, the diagnosis given to the patient later turned out to be incorrect. At the time of learning that in fact there was no cancer, the patient was still in a state of psychological shock. This could have been avoided had the situation been handled more compassionately and caringly, and with an attitude intent on 'lessening hurt'. Within the same week, two other patients confided in my colleague that they had had similar experiences with the same doctor.

Of course, doctors are not the only ones guilty of hurt-causing attitudes. I have seen many instances (far too many, in fact) where nurses have likewise failed to avoid or to lessen the hurt of a given situation. I recall the tragic case of a middle-aged man who was dying from advanced cancer. A close friend and members of his family were greatly distressed about his deteriorating condition, and even accused the nursing staff of 'trying to kill' their loved one by giving him morphine for his pain. On one occasion the nursing staff observed the family friend clutching his friend and pleading with him not to accept the morphine injections, telling him: 'Don't you see, they are killing you! They are killing you! You don't have to have them ...' The nursing staff tried to get the friend to leave, but he refused to go. When he became abusive, the nursing staff contacted a hospital security officer, and he was forcibly removed. There is, I believe, room to speculate about this case: had the friend's grief been properly addressed by the nursing staff, and the dynamics and benefits of effective pain management fully explained to him, both he, and the patient, the patient's family and attending nursing staff would have been spared the 'hurt' that this most unpleasant situation caused.

These two cases demonstrate that 'avoiding hurt' is not something that can be fully directed or achieved by an abstract moral principle. Rather, it requires that we draw very heavily on our past experience, intuition, feelings, and communication and interpersonal skills, as well as on a thorough and systematic analysis of the facts of the situation at hand.

Dealing with moral problems — a systematic approach

Many nurses respond to moral problems with a 'gut response'. Needless to say, this is no more appropriate than it would be to respond to *clinical problems* with a 'gut response'. Does this mean that gut feelings have no part to play in clinical or moral decision making? To the contrary. As we all know, many of our clinical findings are inspired by an intuition that 'something is not quite right with a patient', or that 'there is something wrong with the patient'. But the point is, when we have these 'clinical intuitions' we do not just leave it at that. We systematically set about to get more concrete data so as to obtain a more complete picture of what is going on. We may, for example, ask the patient how they are feeling, check the patient's vital signs, examine the patient's drug sheet and check which drugs have been administered, ask the opinions of others involved in caring for the patient, and so on. On the basis of the data collected, we then proceed to diagnose the problem, formulate objectives, plan a course of action, implement the plan of action, and evaluate the outcomes. This systematic approach (generally called the *nursing process*) is now taught to and used by nurses around the world in their clinical nursing practice.

Moral problems can be dealt with and solved in much the same way. In short, moral problems, like clinical problems, can be dealt with by a systematic decision-making process. It should be cautioned, however, that there is no *one* right way of going about solving moral problems. The following five-step process is merely one among many which might be used by nurses (see, for example, Bergman's [1973] model of ethical decision making, and Curtin and Flaherty's [1982] model for critical analysis). Nevertheless, since nurses are already familiar with the nursing process, I would suggest that the model of moral decision making I propose is one which nurses would find relatively easy to use.

A moral decision-making model

A moral problem can be approached by way of a five-step process:

1. assessing the situation;
2. diagnosing or identifying the moral problem;
3. setting moral goals and planning an appropriate moral course of action;
4. implementing the moral plan of action;
5. evaluating the moral outcomes of the action implemented.

This model may be expressed diagrammatically as shown in figure 6.3. The following is a somewhat simplistic hypothetical case study to illustrate how this model can be applied to clarify the nature of and solve a moral problem. The case involves Mrs A, a patient who has been diagnosed as having advanced cancer, but has not been told her medical diagnosis.

1. ASSESSING THE SITUATION

To make decisions with insufficient knowledge is to risk making serious errors. Making moral decisions without first obtaining the relevant information about a point of moral controversy is likewise to risk making serious errors; it is also likely to reduce the possibility of moving closer to negotiation and resolution of moral disagreement. The first step towards solving a moral problem, as with any problem, is to fully assess the problem and the factors establishing it. What the nurse first needs to do, on being alerted to the possibility that a moral problem is at hand, is to bring together all the relevant facts of the matter as well as all the relevant ethical information. Here facts and ethical information count as *relevant* if it appears that they will make a difference and will probably

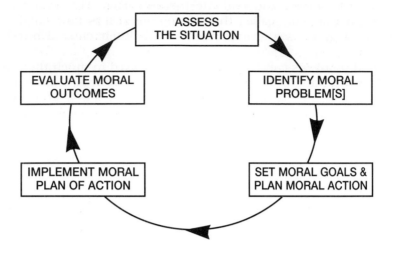

Figure 6.3 Moral decision-making model.

influence a person's ultimate choice. The information collected should include at least the following. (The hypothetical case of Mrs A is used to illustrate each point.)

1. *A detailed description of the facts of the matter.* Mrs A has recently been diagnosed with advanced cancer. The diagnosis is correct, but little can be done for her, medically speaking. Mrs A does not know that she has cancer. She has expressed a desire to know the findings of recent tests and what her medical diagnosis is; she has said there are matters in her life which are outstanding. Dr X does not have effective communication with either Mrs A or the nursing staff, and has not told Mrs A her diagnosis.

2. *A detailed description of the factors establishing the facts.* The reason Mrs A does not yet know she has cancer is that her doctor, Dr X, has ordered that she not be told her diagnosis. Dr X has given no reason for withholding this information from Mrs A. Dr X typically withholds information of this nature from his patients; Dr X has poor communication and interpersonal skills.

3. *The points of view of those who stand to be affected by any decisions made.* Mrs A repeatedly asks to be told her diagnosis, and states she does not care *who* gives it to her — she 'just wants to know'. The nurses caring for Mrs A have to give untruthful answers to her questions,

and believe this is wrong, on grounds that she has a right to be told the truth. The nurses also believe that they are bound to follow Dr X's orders. (Whether this belief is correct is another matter, and one which will also need to be subjected to moral scrutiny.) The nurses unanimously agree that Mrs A is the sort of person who will be able to cope with her diagnosis, and that she should be told what is wrong; Mrs A's children also want to know their mother's diagnosis, and furthermore, they want their mother to know what it is.

4. *Selection of a preferred ethical theory and relevant moral principles.* Preferred theories may be, for example, deontological ethical theory, utilitarian theory, feminist moral theory or transcultural moral theory. Moral principles to consider include autonomy, which demands that Mrs A's preferences should be respected; non-maleficence, which demands that otherwise avoidable harms should be prevented; beneficence, which requires that benefits should be bestowed where this can be done at minimal cost or inconvenience to self; justice, which demands that there should be an equal distribution of benefits and burdens; care, compassion and avoiding hurt, which remind the decision makers to take particular care in their approach to the patient and her family, and in applying any moral principles which have been selected.

5. *Clarification of definitions of moral principles and moral terms used.* It should be noted here that in some instances clarifying the definition of given moral terms and principles may be enough to settle a misunderstanding involving a moral problem.

6. *Prediction of possible consequences of the current position and an estimation of the probability that these consequences will occur.* Mrs A will not have time to adjust to the altered circumstances of her life. Mrs A and her family will carry an intolerable burden of anxiety at not knowing what is going on, while attending nurses will also carry an intolerable burden of having to lie to Mrs A and of not being able to fulfil their professional responsibilities to her. Mrs A will be prevented from setting in order the outstanding matters in her life before she dies, and this will have predictably undesirable consequences. On the basis of past experience, and given the nature of her tumour and its advancement, it is likely that these consequences will eventuate.

7. *Prediction of possible consequences of appealing to adjudicating moral principles, and an estimation of the probability that these consequences will occur.* The possible consequences of upholding the principle of autonomy are that Mrs A is told her diagnosis, and the family can begin to support their mother and can start the grieving process. The nurses can better support Mrs A and her family in coming to terms with the cancer diagnosis, and no longer have to feel guilty at not telling her the truth. Mrs A can begin to settle the outstanding matters of her life before she dies. On the basis of past experience, it is likely that these outcomes will be achieved; it is also likely that other predicted harms and injustices will be avoided.

8. *Availability of alternatives.* Mrs A has another consulting physician caring for her who could also tell her the diagnosis. The hospital has a patient's advocate on staff who could initiate action likely to result in the patient being told her diagnosis. The hospital has a newly established hospital ethics committee set up to deal with 'hard cases'. The hospital has access to the facilities of the public advocate, which other hospitals have successfully used in the past in similar situations, and which have resulted in the patients concerned being told their diagnoses. The charge nurse has in the past, without serious consequences, overridden Dr X's orders and told requesting patients their diagnoses.

9. *Availability of resources.* There are enough members of staff to support Mrs A in coming to terms with her diagnosis. The ward has a single room available which Mrs A can move into if she wishes and be more private with her family. Mrs A is a religious person, and the hospital chaplain is also available to comfort her.

10. *Clarification of personal values and beliefs.* The people involved in the scenario clarify personal values and beliefs, including their own selection, interpretation, weighting and application of given moral principles and their compatibility with those of other people. Dr X is using a narrowly defined principle of non-maleficence, which he interprets as requiring that Mrs A not be given the 'harm-causing' information regarding her diagnosis. The patient, her family and the attending nurses are all using a broadly defined principle of autonomy which emphasises that Mrs A's wishes must be respected and that she should be told her diagnosis even if this stands

to cause her 'harm'. (The risk of being harmed is one she is entitled to take.)

11. *Assessment of the moral competence of the ultimate decision maker and dissenting decision makers.* It should be established whether the decision makers have a least at working knowledge and understanding of the relevant moral rules and principles needed for appraising the facts of a given matter, and whether they have a sound ability to select, interpret and apply these moral rules and principles in a just and appropriate way. The decision makers should also be able to clarify:

- which features of a given situation are morally significant — i.e. Mrs A has not been told her medical diagnosis when she has explicitly requested to be told;

- which aspects of a given situation need to be morally justified — i.e. why Dr X has ordered that Mrs A not be told her diagnosis, or why Mrs A's family and attending nurses believe she should be told her diagnosis;

- where the onus of justification lies — i.e., in light of the compelling moral nature of Mrs A's rational wishes, the onus of justification for withholding the information falls squarely on Dr X;

- just what is to count as a justification — i.e. whether it is to be personal taste, habit and/or convention, or something more substantial, such as that supplied by critically reflective moral analysis;

- whose justification should be given the most weight and on what ground — i.e. the doctor's, the patient's, the family's, or the nurses'.

As with making a clinical assessment, having collected all the relevant factual and ethical information (including both subjective and objective data), and, of course, validated these, the nurse will then need to set about organising or 'clustering' the data into patterns and filling in any gaps where information appears to be lacking. On the basis of the clustered data, the nurse can then proceed to identify the specific moral problem or problems at hand.

2.   DIAGNOSING OR IDENTIFYING THE MORAL PROBLEM

Nurses need to be open-minded about the precise nature of the problem at hand when diagnosing or identifying a supposed moral problem. The possibility always exists that the nurse might in fact be mistaken, either factually (clinically or technically) or morally. As we have learned, what appears to be a 'moral problem' may not in fact be a moral problem at all, but merely a problem of poor communication, misunderstanding, misinterpretation of the facts, ignorance of legal law or institutional policy, inappropriate legal law, inadequate institutional policy, or cultural unawareness. In such instances, it is likely that the problem at hand is one to be settled by education, psychology, law or some other bureaucratic mechanism, rather than by moral reasoning. If the nurse is satisfied that the problem at hand is more than merely practical, it becomes necessary to make a more definitive 'moral diagnosis'. The possibilities, as we have learned, are numerous and can include one or a combination of the following:

- moral unpreparedness;
- moral blindness;
- moral indifference;
- amoralism;
- moral complacency;
- moral fanaticism;
- moral disagreement (e.g. internal moral disagreement, partial radical moral disagreement, and total radical moral disagreement);
- moral dilemmas (e.g. conflicting moral principles, conflicting moral duties, conflicting moral interests, conflicting personal responsibilities, and the effort to avoid hurt to those with whom one has 'attachments').

Once the nurse has made a 'moral diagnosis', the moral goals can be formulated and a moral course of action planned to achieve those moral goals.

Before continuing, it is worthwhile at this point to try and formulate a diagnosis of the moral problem in the case of Mrs A. On the surface it would appear that there are several problems at hand, including:

- moral unpreparedness (on the part of the nurses to deal with the situation at hand effectively and appropriately);
- moral fanaticism (on the part of Dr X, who is thoroughly wedded to the ideal that patients with advanced cancer should not be told their diagnosis, even when they explicitly request to know);
- moral disagreement between Dr X, Mrs A, Mrs A's family and attending nurses about the priority of the given moral principles of non-maleficence and autonomy and, further, about how each of these should be interpreted and applied.

3. SETTING MORAL GOALS AND PLANNING AN APPROPRIATE MORAL COURSE OF ACTION

Just as nursing diagnoses direct the planning of client-oriented nursing care and the setting of client-oriented health goals, so too do moral diagnoses direct the setting of moral goals and the planning of moral action. Unlike nursing diagnoses, however, the plan of action with regard to each possible moral problem is likely to be very similar. In the case of moral problems, for example, a combination of strategies will probably be required. This will involve a mixture of *moral education* (informal, formal, or both); *moral coordination* (individual or collective); *moral cooperation* (among those involved in a given scenario, as well as relevant others outside the scenario); *moral negotiation* and *moral persuasion* (again with all those involved); and, as a last resort, *mechanisms of non-moral enforcement* (particularly in instances where moral coordination, cooperation and negotiation break down). In choosing strategies, the decision maker again needs to be very mindful of the possibility of making moral errors, and needs constantly to be justifying and validating the decisions being made along the way.

In the case of Mrs A, it is likely that all those involved need to be educated about the moral dimensions of the situation. For example, Dr X needs to be made aware that his values and preferences are causing serious 'hurt' to his patient and her family, and are also forcing the nurses into an intolerable position — both morally and professionally. Mrs A and her family need to be made aware of the difficulties facing the nurses, and of why the nurses believe they cannot just go ahead and tell Mrs A her diagnosis. The nurses need to come to some understanding about whether in fact they are 'prohibited' from telling the patient her diagnosis, and, if so, to work out which alternatives are available to them to get the information to Mrs A; the nurses also need to be educated about what role they can play in terms of getting medical information to patients who request it.

The priority, as I see it, is to seek prompt communication and negotiation with Dr X — after all, he too has significant moral interests at stake, which must also be considered. If the nurse succeeds in bringing Dr X to the negotiating table, but still fails to obtain his understanding and cooperation, or if she fails to bring Dr X to the negotiating table at all, then there is no alternative but to go outside the immediate doctor–patient and doctor–nurse relationship and seek cooperation from others who can assist; for example, the charge nurse, the doctor's superior, the hospital's patient advocate, the hospital ethics committee, the public advocate, or, as a last resort, the courts. The coordinator or co-ordinators of the strategies being used must take great care to avoid 'hurting' those involved, including Dr X and, in particular, Mrs A.

Before moving on, I would suggest that the most important strategies to be used in resolving moral problems are those of *education, mediation* and *negotiation.* Often merely learning of new information or new facts about a given matter may make it possible to move closer towards negotiation and resolution of disagreement. And negotiation and reaching an agreement on a common set of principles or on the concepts and definitions of moral language may also come some way towards settling moral disagreement. Other strategies which might be employed include trying to persuade a dissenting party by using examples and counter-examples, or more simply by exposing the inadequacies and unexpected consequences of an argument being used (Beauchamp and Walters 1982, pp. 4–6). Mechanisms of enforcement (such as the law, the courts, or professional disciplinary measures) should be used only as a very last resort — for the simple reason that, once mechanisms outside moral reasoning and moral negotiation are appealed to, the matter ceases to be a problem solvable by voluntary moral means and becomes — undesirably — a problem that can now be solved only by some form of force.

4.   IMPLEMENTING THE PLAN OF MORAL ACTION

Once the nurse has formulated a plan of moral action, it is then possible to implement it. For example, the nurse may embark on a detailed educational strategy, assist in the coordination of a strategy aimed at resolving a moral problem at hand, engage in certain moral negotiations, seek cooperation with morally signifi-cant others, or, if all else fails, appeal to some outside mechanism necessary to achieve the desired moral outcomes.

In the case of Mrs A, the nurse would go ahead and seek nego-tiation with Dr X, or, if attempts to do so failed, embark on some other planned course of action aimed at ensuring that Mrs A receives the information about her diagnosis as she wishes.

In summary, what the nurse chooses to do here is to engage in the moral actions that have been chosen, or refrain from the immoral actions that have been identified and rejected.

5.   EVALUATING THE MORAL OUTCOMES OF THE
ACTION IMPLEMENTED

After implementing the planned moral course of action, the nurse should evaluate whether the projected moral goals and the desired moral outcomes have been achieved. The kinds of questions the nurse might ask here include:

- Has my action or strategy achieved the desired moral outcome? If not, why not?

- Were all the relevant facts and relevant ethical information included in the original analysis of the moral problem?

- Was the moral diagnosis correct?

- Was the moral reasoning used in identifying and planning a moral course of action faulty?

- Were the correct ethical principles selected?

- Were the selected moral principles interpreted and weighed correctly?

- Was there sufficient agreement between dissenting parties on the selection, interpretation and application of given moral principles?

- Was there sufficient agreement between dissenting parties on chosen definitions of moral terms and concepts?

It can be seen that, in attempting to answer these questions, the nurse would need to repeat the whole moral problem-solving process.

Returning one last time to the Mrs A case, the questions which would need to be asked in an effort to evaluate whether the moral plan had been successful or not would be, among others:

- Has Mrs A been told her diagnosis? If not, why not?

- If so, did Mrs A suffer, as Dr X feared she would, by receiving the diagnosis? If so, why?

- Did any other undesirable moral consequences occur as a result of implementing the moral plan of action? If so, why?

Dealing with moral problems — an experiential approach

A major problem for the nursing profession is that not all of its members have had the opportunity to study nursing ethics at a formal educational level. This has sometimes meant, as previous examples have already demonstrated, that nurses have not always been well enough prepared to detect, and respond effectively and appropriately to, moral problems arising in or as a result of the delivery of nursing care to patients.

Consideration of this problem raises at least two critical questions. First, is it always the case that nurses who lack a formal education in nursing ethics (in particular, its theoretical under-pinnings, the nature and use of a systematic approach to moral decision making, specific ethical issues in nursing practice, and so on) are incapable of ethical professional conduct when planning and implementing nursing care? Second, if not, then to what extent, if any, should nurses allow their thinking and conduct to be driven by an abstract and systematic approach to moral deliberation such as that advocated by mainstream Western moral philosophy? Let us now examine these two questions.

A calculus of experience as a guide to moral conduct

The first question to be addressed here is whether nurses who have not had the benefit of a formal education in nursing ethics, or indeed bioethics, are capable of acting morally when planning and implementing nursing care. From anecdotal evidence, the short answer to this seemingly trite question is quite obviously, yes. As the following anecdotes will show, even without a formal education on moral theory, on the nature and use of a systematic approach to moral decision making, and on specific ethical issues in nursing practice, nurses are still capable of making sound moral judgments and of acting in morally sound ways.

The ability of experienced and expert nurses to make impeccable moral judgments has become increasingly apparent to me recently while I have been exploring the issue at nursing ethics seminars and workshops. At one seminar, for example, a nurse, a bioethicist and a medical doctor (who was also a philosopher) agreed to sit on a panel and present a personal response to a real-life case scenario, which they had been given beforehand. They also agreed to receive and respond to questions from the exclusively nursing audience which had been invited to attend. As the evening progressed, many other actual case scenarios were presented by individual nurses in the audience. All the cases shared involved extremely delicate and morally complex situations. As the nurses shared their experi-ences, it became increasingly apparent to the panelists and others present that, without exception, each of the nurses involved had acted in a morally impeccable manner; despite their expressed concerns that perhaps they could have been 'more moral', careful moral analysis showed that their decisions and actions had been quite faultless.

Upon leaving the seminar venue, I asked the bioethicist whether she could explain how the nurses sharing their experiences could have got it so 'right', given that, as had been confirmed at the time, none of them had ever studied or read articles on bioethics or nursing ethics. She replied that it seemed 'beyond an immediate explanation', and that she would 'have to think about it'.

Other seminars have been equally illuminating. For example, at a seminar on ethical issues in clinical nursing practice, at which I was a principal speaker, an experienced intensive care nurse asked for advice on 'what more she could have done' in the situation which she then related as follows.

She had been involved in the care of a middle-aged woman who, after suffering a massive myocardial infarction, had been admitted (deeply unconscious) into the local intensive care unit. The woman had been intubated before admission to the unit, and was placed immediately on a respirator. A few days later the medical hopelessness of the patient's condition was confirmed, and a medical decision was made to remove the artificial life-support system that was sustaining her life.

The woman's husband, who had been present most of the time since his wife's admission, objected strongly to this decision, however, and became very aggressive towards the medical and nursing staff. He also threatened to sue the hospital. Recognising the husband's reaction as a manifestation of extreme grief, the intensive care nurse approached the woman's adult children, who were also present, and, in a private setting, discussed with them what *they* thought should or could be done to help their father deal with the situation better. The children were unanimous that what was required was 'extra time' — specifically, that the removal of the life-support system be delayed so that they could console their father and help him to see that the situation really was 'hopeless'; that, tragic as it was, nothing further could be done. Upon learning of the family's wishes, the nurse offered to act as a mediator between them and the medical staff, to herself remove the life-support from their mother, and to seek support for their wishes from the attending medical staff. This the family accepted. Over the next hour, the nurse was able to fulfil her role as 'mediator', and succeeded in obtaining full support from the medical staff involved in the case. This support included the medical staff agreeing to the nurse deciding when and how to remove the life-support system from the patient. As a result of this mediation, extra time was 'bought', and the woman's husband and children were able to come to terms with the tragic decision that had been made. The family were all able to sit with the woman as the nurse progressively turned off the artificial life-support system. Later, the husband returned to the intensive care unit and thanked the nurse for her intervention.

Upon hearing this anecdote, my initial thought was, 'How could I possibly give this nurse any advice?' It was evident to all present that the nurse had acted with extreme sensitivity, and that her actions were morally beyond reproach. As with the nurses at the seminar referred to earlier, it was later confirmed that this nurse had never read anything about or studied 'ethics'. Thus, again, the question arose: how did this nurse get it so 'right'?

It could be objected here that the nurse's actions in this case were not so remarkable, and that any experienced nurse in a comparable situation would probably have acted as this nurse did. This, however, is questionable. It will be recalled that, in the earlier discussion on moral dilemmas, a distraught visitor mourning the deteriorating condition of his friend was removed forcibly from the hospital after nursing staff called a hospital security officer to evict the man from the hospital premises. There is room to speculate here that, had the nurse in the previous example been involved in this scenario, the outcome might have been quite different. Meanwhile, we could ask: how did the nurses in the distraught visitor's case get it 'so wrong'?

There are many reasons and theories advanced by, among others, psychologists, anthropologists, sociologists, theologians and philosophers, about why some people are able to behave morally when others are not, or are able to behave more morally than others who, in the ultimate analysis, prove morally 'weak-willed'. Unfortunately, since it is not the purpose of this work to advance or elaborate a theory on moral motivation, consideration of these reasons and theories must be left for another time. Nevertheless, there is at least one nursing-specific factor that has an important bearing on the moral motivations, sensibilities and abilities of nurses, and that warrants some consideration here, and that is nurses' actual clinical practice and, more specifically, the nature of the nurse–patient relationship. (See also Yarling and McElmurry 1986; Cooper 1988, 1990, 1991; Packard and Ferrara 1988; Twomey 1989; Bishop and Scudder 1990; Benner 1991; Gaut and Leininger 1991.)

Unlike the relatively detached and decontextualised activity of academic philosophy (see chapter 3 of this text), clinical nursing practice, and the lived realities of the nurse–patient relationship, offer nurses 'hands-on' (lived) experience in detecting and recog- nising, engaging with, and responding directly to the suffering of their patients; developing the ability to make fine discretionary moral judgments about whether a patient's well-being is being violated or is at risk of being violated; building up a repertoire of possible actions that can be effectively deployed to alleviate patients' suffering in appropriate ways; and developing effective ways in which nurses' perceptions, and the morality of their judgments and actions, can be validated. Over time this lived experience can contribute to the development and refinement of nurses' perceptual apparatus (Benner 1984, 1991; de Bono 1990). This, in turn, can enable them to develop the 'background' patterns necessary to perceive correctly the moral dimensions of human suffering (Amato 1990), and to act appropriately to try and alleviate human suffering when it is encountered. In other words, nurses' vast experience as clinical practitioners can enable them to develop exquisite experience-based knowledge on what constitutes right and wrong conduct in regard to human suffering in nursing care contexts. This, in turn, can enable nurses to fine-tune their moral perceptions and moral intuitions, and concomitantly enhance their ability to make the fine discretionary moral judgments that are so often required to ensure appropriate ('right') moral behaviour during moments of human crisis, which are characterised all too frequently by intense and sometimes overwhelming feelings of fear, anxiety, loneliness, uncertainty, ambivalence, pain (at all physical, emotional, spiritual and psychic levels), hopelessness, helplessness, despair, and a deep and abiding sense of vulnerability.

It might be objected here that if *experience* is *all* that is required in order to develop moral sensibilities and moral attunement to people and their suffering, why is it that some nurses lack the ability to behave in morally acceptable ways? Why, for instance, do some experienced nurses seem blind to the suffering of their patients, or, when suffering is detected, seem quite unable to respond to it appropriately and effectively? Why are some nurses apparently indifferent to the well-being of their patients, or oblivious to the factors that may be threatening it? For example, many of the Brown Sisters of Nazi Germany (referred to in chapter 1 of this text) were 'experienced' and even 'expert' nurses, yet demonstrably immoral practitioners. Drawing on this extreme — although real — example, clearly much more than *mere experience* is required in order to develop one's moral sensibilities, and, indeed, the ability to *be* moral. The question remains: just what is required to develop these things?

The question of whether moral sensibilities ('virtue') and the ability to *be* moral can be taught is as old as Western moral philosophy itself, and, to this day, remains the subject of much controversy (a point I shall return to in the final chapter of this text). Despite the controversy, however, there does seem to be at least one factor that is crucial to a person's ability to be moral, and that is the level of personal commitment a person makes, or is prepared to make, to carefully chosen moral values (see also van Hooft 1987; Roach 1987). In the case of nursing, of particular importance is the nurse's commitment to the moral values of care and to protecting the genuine welfare (as opposed to merely upholding the rights) of people made vulnerable by their health crises. Despite a lack of empirical research to support this view, anecdotal evidence suggests strongly that critical to any nurse's ability to act morally is a personal commitment to nursing's ideal and philosophy of care, and the demand it prescribes to maximise and protect the welfare and well-being of patients who, for whatever reason, are not able to maximise and protect their own significant moral interests.

As argued elsewhere in this text, *care* has long been recognised, albeit controversially, as the moral ideal, essence and foundation of nursing. (Whether care is, in fact, any of these things is an open question, and one that has yet to be settled conclusively.) Whatever the controversies surrounding the notion of care as providing a basis and framework for moral conduct in nursing, it is anecdotally evident that it has played an important and influential role in ensuring the realisation of just outcomes in nursing care contexts. For example, it was through a guiding framework of care that the experienced intensive care nurse referred to earlier was able to perceive the reaction of her patient's distraught husband not as aggression, nor as a threat to be removed forcibly by a hospital security officer, but as an expression of profound grief and vulnerability warranting a compassionate and understanding response. This is in sharp contrast to the case discussed earlier involving a visitor, it will be recalled, whose distress at the sight of his dying friend was perceived by attending nurses not as a reaction of grief, but as an act of unprovoked aggression — a threat — to be removed quickly and forcibly, without compassion and without any understanding of the sense of despair or hopelessness the visitor was experiencing. An important lesson here is that care can not only motivate moral action, but can assist the actor to perceive correctly an instance of human suffering (this may present as little more than 'a look of suffering' on a patient's face), to decide how, if at all, to respond to the suffering that has been detected in another, and to decide when, where and by whom the suffering should be responded to.

Should nurses study ethics?

The brief attention which has been given here to speculating about the experiential factors that may have been instrumental in guiding nurses to act morally has probably raised more questions than it has answered; it has also certainly illuminated the need for extensive empirical research on the subject. Nevertheless, the examples given are quite sufficient to demonstrate that there are in existence factors and means other than abstract moral principles and moral theories which can guide nurses in their moral deliberations, and enable them to make the exquisite moral judgments that they are often required to make in the course of their everyday practice. One question that now arises is: if nurses can be moral without studying moral theories, and without developing a systematic approach to moral decision making, should educational programs and initiatives in this area be abandoned?

Do nurses really need to study ethics as it is now commonly being taught in nursing courses around the world?

The short answer to this question is that we should be very careful not to 'throw the baby out with the bath water'. While abstract moral principles and theories have their limitations, they can be extremely helpful in guiding nurses' perceptions of what constitutes right and wrong conduct — particularly in uncertain situations involving 'strangers', or patients with whom nurses have not yet had the opportunity to develop — or have been unable to develop — the level of intimacy required to achieve the degree of empathy necessary to inform and enable correct moral judgments to be made about whether the patient's well-being is being upheld or violated. Moral principles and theories can provide a quantifiable measure against which nurses can evaluate their actions in instances where they are just not sure about whether they have done or are doing the 'right' thing. Significantly, when I have asked nurses for their opinions on the value of their learning about the theoretical underpinnings of Western moral philosophy, including the nature and application of the abstract moral principles of autonomy, non-maleficence, beneficence and justice, their responses have tended to be unanimous. Firstly, the view is commonly expressed that 'it has been a relief' to learn about the four moral principles cited above, since it has provided something for them [the nurses] 'to hang their hats on'. The nurses often explain that these principles provide a useful framework in terms of which they can make sense of and, more importantly, justify their past moral actions. As a point of interest, it is not unusual for nurses to comment: 'I thought I did the right thing in such-and-such a situation, but I was never sure. Now I feel much more confident, and in a better position to justify to others why I did what I did.' Secondly, the view is commonly expressed by nurses that, upon learning of the theoretical underpinnings of Western moral thinking, they feel they can be more confident and courageous in taking the action that may be necessary to remedy moral problems that may occur at some future point in time in their places of work.

It is perhaps not surprising that nurses have responded in the way just described. With careful questioning, it soon becomes apparent that many nurses are already subscribing to the moral values and standards that have been formalised by the abstract moral principles of autonomy, non-maleficence, beneficence and justice (which, incidentally, have a firm grounding in the Judaeo-Christian values underpinning our Western culture). This I have been able to demonstrate repeatedly by the simple exercise of asking nurses whether they have ever given a wrong drug to a patient, and, if so, how they felt about it. Almost without exception, the responses have tended to be: 'I felt dreadful', 'I felt awful', 'I was devastated', and so on. When pressed to explain why they felt like this, again the responses have tended to be unanimous: 'Because I could have killed the patient', or 'Because the patient could have been harmed'. And when pressed to explain further why this mattered — that is, why did it matter to them particularly whether a patient was harmed — the nurses' responses again have tended to be unanimous: 'Because it is wrong'. At first glance, these responses might not seem very significant. But, on closer examination, what is highly significant is that the main concern of these nurses has been for the well-being of their *patients*, not themselves. Indeed, it has not been until after the above kinds of views have been expressed that, upon further prompting, the nurses concerned started to cite other, more self-interested, reasons why they were upset about their drug administration error; for example, 'I felt stupid', or 'I don't like making mistakes'; and then, finally, because they realised that their error could have resulted in some sort of disciplinary action against them if harm to the patient had occurred. From other examples and the responses to them, it has become apparent to me that nurses also subscribe to the values that have been formalised by the other moral principles of autonomy, beneficence and justice.

Although the examples given above are only anecdotal, they are nevertheless substantial enough to show that, in the ultimate analysis, nurses might not rely on experience alone or on one particular moral framework (for example, an ethic of care) for guiding their moral actions, but may in fact subscribe to a variety of frameworks (for example, an ethic of care *as well as* internalised moral principles). And they also show that, in practice, what nurses are faced with when dealing with moral problems is not a competitive struggle between a principle-orientated ethic and an ethic of care, as some have suggested, but a 'creative tension' between these two mutually enhancing guiding moral frameworks (Cooper 1991). Either way, it is evident that greater attention must now be given to exploring the critical relationship — and the creative tension — between moral reasoning, emotion and intuition, and their vital influence on guiding nurses' thinking, perceptions and values about what constitutes right and wrong conduct, and hence their overall experience as moral practitioners. And much greater attention must be given to investigating generally the experiential as well as the theoretical underpinnings of the demonstrable ability of nurses to be moral in situations where it is not always easy to decide what is the morally correct thing to do — even for accomplished moral philosophers.

Issues and recommendations

In actually planning and carrying out ethical decisions, it should be remembered that sometimes it may be difficult to take the 'morally correct' action because of various institutional and legal constraints. As has already been discussed and demonstrated in this text, nurses can suffer enormously if they take a firm moral position in relation to a clinical nursing or controversial medical matter. Life can be made 'hell' for nurses if they do not conform to the status quo, and in many instances they have no choice but to 'voluntarily' resign. Victimisation, as we well know, is often difficult to prove; a nurse may be left with a good career in shreds (see Johnstone 1994). One of the troubling things about this situation for nurses is that this reality is often perpetrated by other nurses (in particular senior clinical nurses and nurse administrators).

Despite the difficulties that nurses face when attempting to deal with moral problems, various approaches are possible to achieve a morally tolerable clinical reality. In concluding this chapter I should like to make a number of recommendations.

1. Nursing administrators must provide a clinical environment that is more conducive to open and honest debate on bioethical issues affecting nursing practice and standards of nursing care.

2. Nurse practitioners must themselves create and demand opportunities for formal discussion of the many ethical issues that derive from clinical nursing practice (see the notion of 'ethical rounds', in Davis 1982).

3. Nurses must familiarise themselves with the legal acts and statutes governing their practice.

4. Nurses must lobby for law reform in areas which are intolerable to accountable and ethically responsible nursing practice.

5. Nurses must familiarise themselves with the written policies of their employing institutions, and seek changes to those policies that are obstructive to ethically responsible and accountable nursing practice.

6. Nurses should seek membership of a professional nursing organisation and actively work towards improving the nursing profession.

7. Individual nurses must lobby their professional organisations to formulate positions on and to address the ethical issues that are found to be particularly troubling in nursing practice (for example, giving information to patients, conscientious objection claims,

unethical conduct by nursing and medical colleagues) — if nurses' professional representatives are not aware of an issue, they are powerless to effect any positive and helpful changes.

8. In extreme cases, nurses must be prepared to seek legal advice.

Moral problems are a fundamental and integral part of nursing practice, in much the same way that clinical problems are. If we do not address these moral problems, and, more importantly, address them competently, we risk a number of undesirable moral consequences, including the enforcement of morally unsound decisions and actions; a failure to prevent moral harm; the actual causing of hurt and moral harm; the creation of moral conflict; the unjust imposition of our personal values on others ('moral bullying'); and the abdication of our broader moral responsibilities ('moral buckpassing').

Caring for our patients — caring for people — is not just a task; it is itself the very moral ideal of nursing (Watson 1985, pp. 58, 63). If nurses are to uphold this ideal — and uphold it well — they must include a sound and experientially based moral point of view in their clinical nursing practice. As well as this, they must be able to function as competent moral problem solvers and decision makers, and truly make a difference in terms of promoting and protecting the welfare and genuine moral interests of all those for whom they care.

References

Amato, J. A. (1990). *Victims and values: a history and theory of suffering.* Praeger, New York.

Aroskar, M. A. (1986). Are nurses' mind sets compatible with ethical practice? In P. L. Chinn (ed.), *Ethical issues in nursing,* Aspen Systems, Rockville, Maryland, pp. 69–79.

Atkinson, R. L., Atkinson, R. C. and Hilgard, E. R. (1983). *Introduction to psychology,* 8th edn. Harcourt Brace Jovanovich, New York.

Beauchamp, T. L. and Walters L. (eds) (1982). *Contemporary issues in bioethics,* 2nd edn. Wadsworth, Belmont, California.

Benner, P. (1984). *From novice to expert: excellence and power in clinical nursing practice.* Addison-Wesley, Nursing Division, Menlo Park, California.

Benner, P. (1991). The role of experience, narrative, and community in skilled ethical comportment. *Advances in Nursing Science* 14 (2), pp. 1–21.

Bergman, R. (1973). Ethics, concepts and practice. *International Nursing Review* 20 (5), p. 140.

Bishop, A. H. and Scudder, J. R. (1990). *The practical, moral and personal sense of nursing: a phenomenological philosophy of practice.* State University of New York Press, Albany.

Bromberger, B. and Fife-Yeomans, J. (1991). *Deep Sleep: Harry Bailey and the scandal of Chelmsford.* Simon & Schuster, Sydney.

Carlton, W. (1978). 'In our professional opinion ...': the primacy of clinical judgment over moral choice. University of Notre Dame Press, Notre Dame.

Cooper, M. (1988). Covenantal relationships: grounding for the nursing ethic. Advances in Nursing Science 10 (4), pp. 48–59.

Cooper, M. (1990). Reconceptualizing nursing ethics. Scholarly Inquiry for Nursing Practice: An International Journal 4 (3), pp. 209–18.

Cooper, M. C. (1991). Principle-orientated ethics and the ethic of care: a creative tension. Advances in Nursing Science 14 (2), pp. 22–31.

Craig, O. (1989). Life or death? How doctors decide which patient gets a 'black dot'. Sun-Herald (Sydney), 12 March.

Curtin, L. and Flaherty, M. J. (1982). Nursing ethics: theories and pragmatics. Prentice Hall, Bowie, Maryland, p. 61.

Davis, A. (1982). Helping your staff address ethical dilemmas, Journal of Nursing Administration 12 (2), February, pp. 9–13.

de Bono, E. (1985). Conflicts: a better way to resolve them. Penguin Books, London.

de Bono, E. (1990). I am right — you are wrong. Penguin Books, London.

Free v. Holy Cross Hospital 505 NE 2d 1199 (III App 1 Dist 1987).

Gaut, D. and Leininger, M. M. (eds) (1991). Caring: the compassionate healer. National League for Nursing Press, New York.

Gilligan, C. (1982). In a different voice. Harvard University Press, Cambridge, Mass. (See in particular chapter 3, 'Concepts of self and morality'.)

Gilligan, C. (1987) Moral orientations and moral development. In E. F. Kittay and D. T. Meyers (eds) (1987). Women and moral theory. Rowman & Littlefield, Totowa, New Jersey, pp. 19–33.

Hare, R. M. (1963). Freedom and reason. Oxford University Press, London. (See in particular chapter 9, 'Toleration and fanaticism'.)

Hare, R. M. (1981). Moral thinking. Clarendon Press, Oxford. (See in particular chapter 10, 'Fanaticism and amoralism'.)

Johnstone, M.-J. (1987). Nursing and professional ethics. In Proceedings of the conference, 'The Role of the Nurse: Doctors' Handmaiden, Patients' Advocate or What?' Centre for Human Bioethics, Monash University, Melbourne, pp. 18–44.

Johnstone, M.-J. (1994). Nursing and the injustices of the law. W. B. Saunders/Baillière Tindall, Sydney.

Kanitsaki, O. (1988). Cancer and informed consent: a cultural perspective. Paper presented at seminar, Controversial Ethical Issues in Patients with Cancer. Heidelberg Repatriation General Hospital Melbourne, 13 October.

Kanitsaki, O. (1989). Health–illness–suffering experiences of a sample of Greek-born members of 12 Greek–Australian families living in Melbourne. Minor thesis completed in partial fulfilment of the requirements for the Degree of Master of Educational Studies, Faculty of Education, Monash University, Melbourne.

Kanitsaki, O. (1993). Transcultural human care: its challenge to and critique of professional nursing care. In D. Gaut (ed.), A global agenda for caring, National League for Nursing Press, New York, pp. 19–45.

Kanitsaki, O. (1994). Cultural and linguistic diversity. In J. Romanini and J. Daly (eds), Critical care nursing: Australian perspectives, W. B. Saunders/Baillière Tindall, Sydney.

King, P. A. (1985). Unprofessional conduct and the nursing profession: the Tuma case. Bioethics Reporter 6 (7), pp. 159–62.

Lemmon, E. J. (1987). Moral dilemmas. In C. W. Gowans (ed.), Moral dilemmas, Oxford University Press, New York, pp. 101–14.

Lynn, J. (ed.) (1989). By no extraordinary means: the choice to forgo life-sustaining food and water. Indiana University Press, Bloomington and Indianapolis.

MacKinnon, C. A. (1987). *Feminism unmodified: discourses on life and law.* Harvard University Press, Cambridge, Mass.

McNaughton, D. (1988). *Moral vision: an introduction to ethics.* Basil Blackwell, Oxford.

Miller, C. (1988). Nurses told, let sick die. *Herald* (Melbourne), 30 September, p. 3.

Miller, C. (1989). NFR system is 'dangerous'. *Australian Dr Weekly*, 20 January.

Milo, R. D. (1986). Moral deadlock. *Philosophy* 61, pp. 453–71.

Nielsen, K. (1989). *Why be moral?* Prometheus Books, Buffalo, New York.

Packard, J. S. and Ferrara, M. (1988). In search of the moral foundation of nursing. *Advances in Nursing Science* 10 (4), pp. 60–71.

Report of the Royal Commission into Deep Sleep Therapy (1990). Government Printer, Sydney.

Report of the Study of Professional Issues in Nursing (1988). Victorian State Government Printer, Melbourne.

Rice, S. (1988). *Some doctors make you sick: the scandal of medical incompetence.* Angus & Robertson, Sydney.

Roach, M. S. (1987). *The human act of caring: a blueprint for the health professions.* Canadian Hospital Association, Ottawa, Ontario.

Ross, W. D. (1930). *The right and the good.* Oxford University Press, London.

Schumpeter, P. (1988). No-rescuscitation rules are unclear: lecturer. *The Age*, 1 October, p. 21.

Stout, J. (1988). *Ethics after Babel: the languages of morals and their discontents.* Beacon Press, Boston.

Tuma v. Board of Nursing of the State of Idaho 593 P 2d 711 (1979).

Twomey, J. G. (1989). Analysis of the claim to distinct nursing ethics: normative and non-normative approaches. *Advances in Nursing Science* 11 (3), pp. 25–32.

Upfront (1988). 'Not for Resuscitation' orders leave nurses in a moral, legal and professional dilemma. 7 (4), December, pp. 6, 13.

Unwin, N. (1985). Relativism and moral complacency. *Philosophy* 60, pp. 205–14.

Van Hooft, S. (1987). Caring and professional commitment. *Australian Journal of Advanced Nursing* 4 (4), pp. 29–38.

Warthen v. Toms River Community Memorial Hospital 488 A 2d 299 (NJ Super AD 1985).

Watson, J. (1985). *Nursing: human science and human care.* Appleton-Century-Crofts, Norwalk, Connecticut.

Williams, B. (1973). Ethical consistency. In C. W. Gowans (ed.) (1987), *Moral dilemmas*, Oxford University Press, New York, pp. 115–37.

Wilson-Barnett, J. (1986). Ethical dilemmas in nursing. *Journal of Medical Ethics* 12, pp. 123–6, 135.

Yarling, R. R. and McElmurry, B. J. (1986). The moral foundation of nursing. *Advances in Nursing Science* 8 (2), pp. 63–73.

Chapter

7

Patients' rights

In July 1987, the Melbourne *Age* carried a front-page report headed 'AMA will consider secret AIDS tests', in which it was revealed that New South Wales doctors had 'been testing selected patients for AIDS without their consent or knowledge' (Conley 1987, p. 1). A little over a year later, a front-page report in the Melbourne *Herald* claimed that fifteen hundred Aborigines on Palm Island had been tested for AIDS (Miller 1988). It was alleged in this report that, while consents had been obtained for taking a 'blood test' (screening was also being carried out for diabetes and other diseases), there was doubt about the quality of these consents. A senior Aboriginal Commonwealth officer was reported as saying that the quality of the informed consent was only '50–50 at best' (Miller 1988). Equally disturbing was the report's allegation that there had been serious breaches of confidentiality regarding five Palm Islanders who had been found to be HIV-positive.

On 27 January 1985, John McEwan, an Australian water skiing champion, was left a ventilator-dependent quadriplegic after a diving accident at Echuca, Victoria. Throughout his hospitalisation, he repeatedly asked to be allowed to die. At one point he went on a hunger strike and instructed his solicitor to draw up a 'living will', which stated 'that he did not wish to be revived if and when he fell into a coma' (*Request to die* 1985, p. 2). According to media reports, this led to a psychiatrist certifying him as rationally incompetent. The psychiatrist's judgment was revoked a few days later, however, when John McEwan 'agreed to end his hunger strike and accept a course of antidepressants' (*Request to die* 1985, p. 2).

A little over a year after his accident, and despite still being ventilator-dependent, John McEwan was discharged home. The round-the-clock day care he required was given by family members and friends who had received special training in how to care for him. In the weeks following his discharge from hospital, John McEwan continued to express his wish to be allowed to die (Social Development Committee 1987, pp. 310–11). This prompted the general practitioner who was medically responsible for him to inform the senior nursing assistant that:

> John McEwan at his own request could come off the ventilator from time to time but had to be reconnected if he became distressed *even if it was against his own wishes* [italics added].

(Social Development Committee 1987, p. 312)

During one incident, while at home, John McEwan was observed to be angry at having been reconnected to the ventilator against his wishes. And in another incident shortly before his death, he talked openly with his general practitioner about 'hiring someone to blow his [John McEwan's] brains out or kill him as he felt his wish to die was being frustrated' (Social Development Committee 1987, p. 316). There was no reason to suspect that John McEwan's wishes were irrational. Before his accident he had been a committed sportsman. I have been told informally that sport was not merely an interest to him, but a fully fledged obsession. Thus, for him, the life of a helpless quadriplegic was intolerable.

At four o'clock in the morning on 3 April 1986, John McEwan was found dead by his nursing attendant. At the time of discovery he was disconnected from his ventilator.

These reports on secret AIDS testing, inadequate consent practices, breaches of confidentiality, and treating patients against their will, are just some among many examples of patients' rights violations occurring in modern health care contexts. In chapters 1, 2 and 6 of this text, several other examples of patients' rights violations have been given, and the chapters to follow will provide still more.

The issue of patients' rights

People requiring or receiving health care are not, and never have been, obliged to be the passive recipients of unnegotiated care. Yet the more we examine the realities of health care practice and the way our health care institutions and services operate, the more apparent it becomes that the rhetoric surrounding the idealism of people's rights to and in health care does not match the reality. As the bioethics, legal, professional and lay literature, and our own everyday experience, make plain, people continue to be denied equitable access to the quality and quantity of health care they need; they continue to be denied the opportunity to make informed choices about their care and treatment options; and they continue to be harmed physically, psychologically, spiritually and morally as a result of unscrupulous or at least morally questionable practices in our health care services and institutions. This is an appalling indictment, not just of 'the system', but of the health care professionals who comprise it and, more specifically, of their culpable lack of ability and moral commitment to remedy it.

It is probably true to say that, although the issue of patients' rights is widely discussed by health professionals, academics and the laity, it is nevertheless poorly understood and poorly represented — at least publicly. The media seem to treat the issue of patients' rights as little more than a curiosity — one which lends itself very well to sensational headlines and sensational drama. Bioethicists, meanwhile, tend to treat the issue of patients' rights as though it belongs to the exclusive domain of philosophical inquiry. They also seem to view the issue from the safe distance of a comfortable philosophical armchair placed conveniently behind a 'veil of ignorance'. The risk of distorting the issue from this abstract position is, I believe, very great. Health professionals (especially those in positions of power) are also guilty of distorting the issue of patients' rights. Many view it as a 'luxury' issue, in that it can be 'afforded' only if there is time, or if circumstances permit (which, from their perspective, is unlikely). Others simply view it as a non-issue, asserting that, since health care is precisely about upholding the patients' good, nothing more need be said on the matter.

Unfortunately, as a consequence of these views, the community at large is kept ignorant of the nature and purpose of the patients' rights debate and movement, or why these must be supported publicly. To complicate the issue further, there is a diversity of opinion on what rights consumers do in fact have, and whether, when, how and by whom the rights that have been identified should be protected and upheld (see, for example, Australian Consumers' Association 1988; Department of Health, Housing and Community Services 1989; Ronalds 1989; Consumers' Health Forum 1990; Health Issues Centre 1991, 1992; National Health and Medical Research Council 1990, 1991; Mental Health Consumer Outcomes Task Force 1991; Faculty of Nursing, RMIT 1992; Health Department, Victoria 1992; Longo 1992; Health Services Review Council [nd]).

Whether the media, bioethicists, health professionals or others wish to admit it or not, it is a reality that the world has a sorrowful and repugnant history of patients' rights violations. The examples given in this text barely scratch the surface of known cases worldwide involving moral abuses that patients have had to suffer — even in so-called sophisticated and well run health care institutions. Patients' rights violations have occurred, and are continuing to occur, at a scandalous level. Even the United Nations (which has formulated universal declarations on human rights, the rights of the disabled, the rights of the mentally handicapped, and children's rights) has done nothing specifically to address the problem of patients' rights violations.

In his book *Some doctors make you sick*, Stephen Rice (1988, p. 9) estimates that in Australia alone over seventy thousand patients are injured by their doctors each year (in the United States the figure is estimated to be 2.6 million). Of these seventy thousand patients, only two hundred and fifty will push their legal right to sue; and, of these, only a meagre 10 per cent will take their cases to court (largely owing to the disincentives successfully created by the powerful medical lobby and allied medical defence unions). These figures, of course, pertain only to the limited issue of patients suffering *legal* harms. The incidence of patients suffering *moral* harms, I would suggest, even on the basis of these figures, is beyond precise estimation. To give some idea of the extent to which patients' rights violations occur in Australia, consider the issue of informed consent, which is taken up in more detail later in this chapter.

As a general rule, patients admitted to hospital are required to sign what is called a 'consent form'. The signing of this form, however, does little more than provide documentary evidence that consent has been given; the question of whether the patient's consent is valid is entirely another matter (Staunton and Whyburn 1993, pp. 97–131). I shall argue in this chapter that in most cases a patient's consent to treatment is *invalid*. The implications of this claim are clearly very serious, not only in moral terms (particularly as these relate to patients' rights), but also in legal terms. Let us examine this claim further.

It is estimated that in Australia approximately 3.5 million people are admitted to hospital each year (Rice 1988, p. 9). If we consider the gross inadequacy of current consent to treatment procedures used in most Australian hospitals, it seems reasonable to hypothesise that probably most patients entering hospital do not give a truly informed and valid consent to treatment. Given this, it also seems reasonable to hypothesise that approximately 3.5 million cases of patients' rights violations occur each year in Australia (give or take the number of cases in which consent has been legally waived because of the demands of a life-threatening or emergency situation). Even if it is conceded that this hypothetical estimate is grossly exaggerated, and that at least 50 per cent of patients entering hospital give a truly informed and valid consent to treatment, the estimate of patients' rights violations would still be unacceptably high at 1.75 million (again give or take the number of cases involving legal waiver). And even if it is conceded that the unlikely figure of 75 per cent of patients entering hospital give a valid consent, we would still be left with the unacceptably high figure of 875 000 violations of patients' rights occurring in Australian hospitals each year.

These hypothetical figures do not, of course, include other more subtle instances involving the violation of patients' rights. Consider, for example, the almost infinite number of times patients are given medication without their knowing what the name of the medication is, what it is for, and what its known side effects are; or consider the numerous occasions on which patients are made 'Not For Resuscitation' (NFR) without their knowledge or consent; or consider the numerous instances in which patients who cannot read or write English are given consent-to-treatment forms to sign without any explanation whatsoever about what the form is or what the implications of signing it are. The patient is merely shown the dotted line and handed a pen! I am told that many non-English-speaking persons sign so as 'not to cause any trouble' — hardly the basis of a voluntary and informed consent.

Given other rights which patients are entitled to claim, it is likely that the 3.5 million figure already projected could be not only sustained but multiplied two, three, four, five, or even more times. This possibility is not at all far-fetched once it is considered that an individual patient's rights can be violated more than once during any *one* admission to hospital, and, further, can be violated by more than one attending health professional. Then, of course, there is the incidence of patients' rights violations occurring *outside* hospital contexts — for example, in doctors' surgeries, or even in the patient's own home when the patient is visited by a doctor, a nurse or another health professional). In the United States it is estimated that '20% of all medical negligence occurs in the doctor's surgery or during visits to the patient's home' (Rice 1988, p. 9); in Australia it is estimated that the proportion may be even higher. Translate these legal figures into moral figures, and again we are left with a scandalous statistic of patients' rights violations.

In the light of these kinds of considerations, it can be seen that it would take little to expand the number of patients' rights violations occurring in Australia to tens of millions each year. If this figure is multiplied and expanded to be universally representative, the world record of patients' rights violations would probably tally up to tens of billions each year. Even if this figure is reduced by as much as 90 per cent, the world is still left with an intolerable human rights violations scandal on its hands. And the scandal is not just that patients' rights violations have occurred, but that they are *continuing* to occur.

The issue of patients' rights has begun to receive significant attention in Australia and New Zealand over the past few years. In Australia reforms are being sought actively (and in some cases have already been achieved) in areas concerning:

- a patient's common law right to refuse orthodox medical treatment (made explicit in Victorian law by the State Government's proclamation of its controversial *Medical Treatment Act* 1988);

- review and recomposition of professional registration boards (Carter 1987);

- legislation on informed consent (an issue that has been the subject of a discussion paper produced by the now disbanded Law Reform Commission of Victoria in conjunction with the Australian Law Reform Commission, the New South Wales Law Reform Commission [1987] and the National Health and Medical Research Council [1991]);

- review of 'Not For Resuscitation' orders (Social Development Committee 1987);

- health services complaints mechanisms (already the subject of formal legislation in Victoria under its *Health Services [Conciliation and Review] Act* 1987, and the subject of formal recommendations made in the South Australian Government's 1987 report of the *Task force on patients' rights.*

New South Wales was also to pilot a 'patients' representatives scheme' but, owing to outrage by the medical lobby, this scheme appears to have been dropped [Rice 1988, pp. 110–11]). Other areas include multicultural health care (Transcultural Health Care Council, 1988; Health Department Victoria 1992); women's health (Victorian Ministerial Women's Health Working Party 1987); mental health (Mental Health Consumer Outcomes Task Force 1991); aged and residential care (Ronalds 1989; Department of Health, Housing and Community Services 1989); public advocacy; data collection and information control; and many more. As discussed in chapter 1, New Zealand has witnessed a rigorous national inquiry into allegations concerning the treatment of cervical cancer at the National Women's Hospital and into other related matters (*Report of the Cervical Cancer Inquiry* 1988). And in 1989 New South Wales saw the Chelmsford Hospital Inquiry into malpractice allegations in relation to the use of controversial psychiatric therapies and a number of patient deaths (Bromberger and Fife-Yeomans 1991).

In both Australia and New Zealand, an unprecedented number of important books pertaining to patients' rights issues were released in the late 1980s. Of particular note is the Australian Consumers' Association's book entitled *Your health rights* (1988), and the Consumers' Health Forum of Australia's report entitled *Legal recognition and protection of the rights of health consumers* (1990). Other books include Stephen Rice's *Some doctors make you sick* (1988); John Fairbanks Kerr's *Don't call a doctor* (1987), written from a layperson's perspective; Stuart Rees and Leonie Gibbons' *A brutal game: patients and the doctors' dispute* (1986); Derek Humphry and Ann Wickett's *The right to die* (1987); Sandra Coney's *The unfortunate experiment* (1988); Phillida Bunkle's *Second opinion*

(1988); Erica Bates and Susie Linder-Pelz's *Health care issues* (1987); and Judith Fordham's *Doctors' orders or patient choice?* (1988), written from a lawyer's perspective; Brian Bromberger and Janet Fife-Yeomans' *Deep Sleep: Harry Bailey and the scandal of Chelmsford* (1991); and, last but not least, Jane Gilmour's heart-rending book, *Michael: a mother's battle for the rights of her child* (1992).

For all the attention given to the issue of patients' rights, the reality in our hospitals remains grim. Few patients are informed of their rights, and even fewer are encouraged to assert them. Those who do know of and assert their rights risk being either victimised or ignored. Rice (1988) comments that the Australian legal system is 'loaded against patients' (p. 4), and that on the whole (with only one or two notable exceptions), judges are unsympathetic to patients' claims (p. 133).

While we might hope that the situation would have changed since Rice first made this observation, it appears the status quo remains unchallenged. The Consumers' Health Forum (1990) points out, for example, that the Australian legal system has not been responsive to protecting the needs of health care consumers. In its report on the *Legal Recognition and Protection of the Rights of Health Consumers*, it states:

> For some consumers the diversity of the Australian legal system has provided some benefits. Unfortunately, for the majority it has been far more effective in creating an inequitable and unresponsive legal maze. As it currently stands:
>
> - there is no comprehensive, consistent, consumer-orientated health law that recognises individual consumers' and the community's health and well-being as a fundamental objective;
>
> - there is no clear direction for consumers as to how they should act, how others should act, and what redress they have if things go wrong. Their rights depend upon which State consumers live or even whether they attend a public or private health facility; and
>
> - the interests of bureaucrats and professional groups are better reflected in existing law than the interests of consumers and the community in such matters as information, participation, accountability and openness.
>
> (Consumers' Health Forum 1990, pp. 1–2).

The medical profession also takes a very dim view of patients' rights claims. The States' medical boards appear to be more interested in complaints relating to 'advertising and publicity' than they are in complaints relating to patients' rights violations (Rice 1988; Health Call 1987). In Victoria, the State ombudsman once criticised the Victorian State medical board for its lack of 'serious public accountability' and for its dismal failure to investigate properly and to 'account for its findings on complaints made to it by health care consumers' (Ombudsman Victoria 1988, pp. 25–36).

The nursing profession's perspective

The position of the nursing profession in relation to the issue of patients' rights is also far from satisfactory. The federal Australian Nursing Federation (ANF) does not have a specific and formal position on patients' rights, and neither does the Royal College of Nursing, Australia. The Western Australian and Victorian branches of the ANF have position papers on patients' rights (see appendixes IV and V of this text). However, neither of these position papers is fully incorporated into law, and therefore they have no legal force. Legally speaking, therefore, nurses are not 'bound' by them. While such position papers carry the force of moral censure, they may not, in the ultimate analysis, be sufficient to stand up to the weight of the legal law in cases where a nurse acts to protect a patient's rights as identified in a given position statement. As Kohnke (1982, p. 124) correctly reminds us, 'when push comes to shove it is the law that carries the most weight'. We can, for example, imagine a nurse informing a patient of the moral right to seek a second medical opinion (a right stated in many patients' rights codes), only to be confronted with a defamation suit for lowering 'a doctor in respect of his [sic] professional reputation' (O'Sullivan 1983, p. 6).

The issue of patients' rights from a nursing perspective is further complicated by the problem that many registered nurses do not have the slightest idea about their profession's position on patients' rights, or, if they do have some idea, it is often a misguided or an incorrect one. In Victoria, for example, I have met many registered nurses who do not know that the ANF (Victoria Branch) has a position paper on patients' rights, and those who have known of it have not known where to obtain a copy. Further to this, I have been told informally that there are no clear guidelines outlining the ANF's position in instances where either a nurse is treated unfairly for upholding the demands of the position statement on patients' rights, or a nurse fails to uphold the statement's demands. The reason given was that the position paper 'has not been tested yet'.

The question that inevitably arises here is: if patients' rights statements are unable to be enforced ('lack teeth', as it were), what is the point of having them?

It is true that the nursing profession's position statements on patients' rights are on the whole without legal force, and in some respects (which are beyond the scope of this present text to discuss) are inadequate ethically. Nevertheless, we should not dismiss them outright. There are a number of important reasons for supporting position statements on patients' rights or, more specifically, a bill of patients' rights. There is even room to suggest that the international community urgently needs a United Nations declaration on patients' rights, and further that it would be highly appropriate for the nursing profession, worldwide, to lobby for this initiative. Whatever their faults, position statements and bills of patients' rights achieve a number of things: firstly, they help to remind people (patients, health professionals, the laity, and others) that patients do have special interests and entitlements which ought to be respected and protected. Secondly, by making patients aware of their rights, they may encourage patients to assert them and to demand respect for them. Thirdly, and perhaps more importantly, they remind all concerned that patients are not there for the convenience of health professionals (a point which some health professionals seem to forget), and further are not obliged to be passive recipients of unnegotiated care (Beauchamp and Walters 1982). Lastly, they remind attending health professionals that their relationships with patients are constrained ethically and are bound by certain correlative duties.

If nurses are to pick up the gauntlet of patients' rights, they need to be very clear, first, about what exactly patients' rights are, and second, about what can be done to ensure that a bill of patients' rights or a position statement on patients' rights achieves what it is supposed to achieve.

What are patients' rights?

To put it simply, patients' or clients' rights are merely a subcategory of human rights. Statements of patients' or clients' rights are merely statements about particular moral interests that a person might have in health care contexts and that require special protection when a person assumes the role of a patient or client. Referring to this particular set of interests in terms of 'patients' rights' or 'clients' rights' serves more the purposes of convenience and manageability than those of philosophy. For example, when the notion 'patients' rights' or 'clients' rights' is used, we know immediately what kind of context and what kind of rights claims are likely to be encountered. The notion of patients' rights or clients' rights in this instance immediately 'sets the scene', or identifies the universe of concern. In the case of human rights language, the scene that is set is much broader. Some might consider human rights language in health care contexts to be somewhat cumbersome to manage. This is not to say that it would be inappropriate to use the notion of human rights in health care contexts; quite the reverse is true. In many respects, using human rights language might be more compelling and more effective in motivating much-needed change. For example, the exclamation 'there are gross violations of *human* rights in our hospitals' may be more forceful than the exclamation 'there are gross violations of *patient* rights in our hospitals'. Human rights language tends to engender a strong feeling that the matter affects all human beings, unlike patients' rights language, which engenders a feeling that 'this is a matter which only affects patients, who after all have no real business complaining'.

The conventional term 'patient' (from the Latin *patiens*, meaning 'suffering, enduring, being patient', and the Greek *ponos*, meaning 'pain') denies autonomy and is defunct in modern nursing schools, which now favour the term 'client'. There are good reasons for abandoning it, and thus for abandoning 'patients' rights' language altogether (Johnstone 1988). It is precisely the nature of the term *patient* that tends to divert attention away from the fact that what is at issue are fundamental *human rights* violations, and not merely violations of the terms of some charitable relationship between a patient and a professional care giver. For all these concerns, I nevertheless suspect that patients' rights language is here to stay, and for this reason alone I have elected to use it in this text. It is a language that all health professionals, as well as the laity, understand, find accessible and meaningful, and use in moral discourse. Thus, for the time being at least, there is little to be gained by abandoning 'patients' rights' language in favour of 'human rights' language. However, something can be gained by making patients' rights language more meaningful and more visible from a moral point of view.

Patients' rights statements tend to include a mixture of civil rights, legal rights and moral rights (see appendixes II, IV and V). Popular examples of patients' rights include: a right to health care, a right to be informed, a right to participate in decision making concerning treatment and care, a right to give an informed consent, a right to refuse consent, a right to have access to a trained interpreter, a right to know the name and status of attending health professionals, a right to a second opinion, a right to be treated with respect, a right to confidentiality, a right to bodily integrity, the right to compensation in the case of unlawful injury, a right to the maintenance of dignity, and many others. Many of these rights statements derive from the broader moral principles of autonomy, justice, beneficence and non-maleficence, already discussed in this text. Unfortunately there is insufficient space here to discuss every type of patients' right that has been formulated at some time or another. For the purposes of this discussion, attention is given to only four broad categories of rights, under which many other narrower rights claims fall. These category claims include the rights to health care, informed consent, confidentiality and dignity (including the right to die with dignity).

1. The right to health care

The right to health care (taken here in its broadest sense, and not to be confused with *medical* care) is complex and controversial. As well as being a sensitive moral issue, it is also a highly charged political issue, as ongoing debates on health care resource allocation make plain.

Bioethicists have yet to find a happy medium between the many competing and conflicting views on the subject. Some philosophers argue that health care is something all people are equally entitled to receive, regardless of the cost. Where human life is at stake, they contend, decisions should not be constrained by economic considerations (Brody 1986); if more money is required, the solution is relatively simple: redirect society's resources (for example, away from gross expenditures on arsenals of arms and other life-threatening instruments of war). Others argue that it is implausible and impossible to provide a high standard of health care to all persons equally. At best, all that people can reasonably claim is a 'decent minimum' of health care, as measured in terms of the amount necessary to secure a minimally decent or 'tolerable' life (Fried 1982; Buchanan 1984; Engelhardt 1986, p. 336). Still others argue that there is no such thing as a right to health care. One philosopher even claims that it is *immoral* to speak of health care as a 'right' (Sade 1983), and another that the expression 'a right to health care' is nothing but a 'dangerous slogan' (Fried 1982).

Charles Fried (1982, p. 400) makes the interesting and, if taken from the perspective of medical treatment, I think correct, claim that the 'impossible dilemma posed by the promise of a right to health care' is really nothing more than a product of 'our culture's inability to face and cope with the persistent facts of illness, old age, and death'. He goes on to assert that:

Because we are little able to come to terms with the hazards which illness proposes, because the old are a burden and an embarrassment, because we pretend that death does not exist, we employ elaborate ruses to put these things out of the ambit of our ordinary lives.

(Fried 1982, p. 400)

Whether the right to health care is a bogus claim or a dangerous slogan or a cultural quirk will, however, depend very much on how the notion of 'health care' is interpreted. I suspect that many philosophers' criticisms derive from their erroneously equating 'health care' with 'medical care'. Since medical care makes up only a small proportion of overall health care, it is obviously not synonymous with health care. Once the notion of 'health care' is understood in more holistic terms, the right to such care may not seem so outrageous or fraudulent or even culturally odd as a claim. Every culture has its way of dealing with sickness, illness, pain and suffering, and of caring for the sick. Not every culture embraces Western scientific medicine as the most effective way of dealing with sickness and related illness experiences, however. And thus not every culture is posed with the dilemma of economic restrictions on resource allocation; this, I suspect, is what lies at the root of the debate about whether people have a right to health (viz medical) care. Once health care, in its more holistic sense, is seen as an important means of promoting a person's *total* (and not merely physical) well-being, it becomes increasingly difficult to deny that claims to it are valid — particularly in the light of demands imposed by the broad moral principles of beneficence, non-maleficence, justice, and even autonomy. What makes a claim to health care compelling is precisely that, once it is accepted, it has the moral power to prescribe actions to relieve the distressing symptoms caused by disease and illness, to promote human well-being (a moral end), and, indeed, to promote human life itself (also a moral end). If we deny entitlements to health care, we must also deny entitlements to a range of other interests, including those of life, happiness, and even the exercise of self-determining choices.

It is beyond the scope of this text to deal with the many arguments and counter-arguments raised in response to the question of whether people have a right to health care. What is of concern here is to clarify the *nature* of the claim to *a right to health care*, and what might be meant by such a claim.

People's entitlement to receive health care first received global recognition with the signing of the United Nations Declaration of Human Rights on 10 December 1948. Article 25 states:

> Everyone has the right to a standard of living adequate for the health and wellbeing of himself [sic] and his [sic] family, including food, clothing, housing and medical care and necessary social services, and the right to security in the event of unemployment, sickness, disability, widowhood, old age or other lack of livelihood in circumstances beyond his [sic] control.
>
> (United Nations 1978, p. 8)

It is worth noting here that the right to health care embodied by this statement extends far beyond a claim of mere *medical* care, and embraces a more holistic interpretation of health care.

Since the signing of this declaration the question of the right to health care has taken on a new meaning, and has emerged largely as a result of what people perceive to be an 'unjust or unfair state of affairs' involving present structures of health care, which are seen as diminishing and even eliminating possibilities for the enhancement of the quality of human life and for human life itself (McCullough 1983).

In speaking of the right to health care, it is important to distinguish at least three different senses in which it can be claimed: that is, the right to equal access to health care; the right to have access to appropriate care; and the right to quality of care.

The right to equal access to health care raises questions of distributive justice and of how benefits and burdens ought to be distributed. It also raises questions of whether people or institutions can be found morally negligent for failing to provide equal access to health care for persons requiring it. Responses refuting this sense of a right to health care typically centre on such arguments as: 'there is not a 'bottomless pit' of health care resources, and somebody has to do without'.

Specifically, the 'scarce resources, but unlimited wants' argument tends to be constructed as follows:

1. the demand for health care has outstripped supply;
2. this is fundamentally because health care resources are limited;
3. different people have different health needs, and different views on how existing resources should be used to meet these needs;
4. it is true that existing health care resources can be used in alternative ways;
5. nevertheless, health care resources are limited, so it is not possible to satisfy everybody's needs and wants (Johnstone 1990, p. 3; see also Council for Science and Society 1982; Fuchs 1983, p. 4).

The ultimate conclusion drawn from these premises — the 'bottom line', so to speak — is that, inevitably, choices will have to be made. In particular, borrowing from Sheehan and Wells (1985, p. 59), choices will have to be made about:

1. the conditions for which scarce resources should be made available; and
2. the priority with which given conditions should be treated.

It remains an open question, however, whether we have to accept the premises of this 'scarce resources, but unlimited wants' argument, and, further, whether we have to accept its apparent 'inevitable' conclusions. As I have argued elsewhere (Johnstone

1990), it is far from clear that we do have to accept them —
particularly when the politics of health care resource allocation is
considered fully, including the vested and powerful interests that
the whole health care economics debate is serving. Further, it is
also open to serious question whether we are obliged to accept that
economic principles ought to supplant morality as the ultimate
test of conduct, as an economic rationalisation approach to health
care dictates. Human life is not something that can be reduced,
like an object, to mere economic worth, and as moral beings we
ought to resist attempts to do so; if we do not resist, we risk seeing
'worthless' human beings denied the health care entitlements they
would otherwise be entitled morally to receive.

The arguments of economic rationalism are less than convincing
when considered in relation to the demands of morality. On a more
practical level, they are also less than convincing when considered
in the light of the wastages that occur in scientific health care
contexts (particularly hospitals) and the misallocation of health
care resources generally. Consider, for example, the once routine
usage in many hospitals of the seemingly inexpensive oxygen
humidifier used on patients receiving oxygen by nasal cannula.
Research done in the United States has shown that humidifying
oxygen administered by nasal cannula has no therapeutic value
and unnecessarily adds to hospital costs and expenditure
(Campbell et al. 1988). Despite these research findings, many
hospitals continued to advocate the routine use of humidification
on patients receiving nasal oxygen. It is not insignificant that, in
the United States alone, the manufacture of bubblejet humidifiers
was an 18-million-dollar industry (Campbell et al. 1988, p. 293).

The cost-effectiveness of medical technology is already a subject
of much controversy, both in Australia and overseas. Bates and
Linder-Pelz (1987), for example, argue that since the 1980s it has
become increasingly evident that damages inflicted by some
medical technology by far outweigh many of the expected benefits,
a problem which they see as being largely attributable to the lack of
adequate evaluation of technology before its widespread acceptance
(p. 124). Mulley (1984) also raises questions about the
appropriateness of the high costs incurred by running technology-
dependent intensive care units, given that the effectiveness of
intensive care units is as yet unproven. Suspicion also surrounds
the cost-effectiveness of highly priced diagnostic machinery. Rice
(1988), for example, cites a research study conducted over a six-
year period at Westmead Hospital, Sydney, in which the cases of
218 women who had attended the hospital for mammography were
examined. The researchers discovered that in 95 (44 per cent) of
these cases, the mammogram failed to detect an existing tumour
(Walker and Langlands 1986, pp. 185–7; Rice 1988, p. 15).

Similar claims about the apparent unreliability of mammograms have also been made by medical authors. Mendelsohn (1982, pp. 109–10), for example, cites a screening program conducted over a three-year period between 1973 and 1976. Of the 1800 cases of cancer detected, 48 were found to be cases of mistaken diagnosis, and of these 37 had resulted in the needless removal of breasts. Mendelsohn (1982, pp. 110–11) argues further that routine mammography for women under fifty years of age is actually 'potentially dangerous' to health, and can, ironically, predispose to iatrogenic breast cancer later in life. Following numerous studies, and warnings to a United States congressional subcommittee, routine mammography in women under the age of fifty years was finally abandoned by the National Cancer Institute (NCI) and the American Cancer Society (ACS) (Mendelsohn 1982, p. 110).

Other medical authors have claimed that, in 5 per cent to 69 per cent of cases, mammography can yield false negative results, leading to failure to diagnose cancerous conditions (Inlander et al. 1988, p. 106):

> In one study of 48 'negative' mammograms of women who later turned out to have breast cancer, one-third had cancers that were clearly visible on the X-rays, but had been overlooked or misread by the X-ray personnel or physicians.
>
> (Inlander et al. 1988, p. 106)

These and other examples raise serious questions about the wisdom of spending vast amounts of money on equipment that cannot be relied upon to give accurate results.

The issue of medical technology aside, the cost-effectiveness of medical treatment itself is also open to dispute. Kerr (1987), for example, makes the controversial claim that 75 per cent of patients who see a doctor 'receive no benefit whatsoever from medical treatment' (p. 10). He also cites the findings of a Melbourne study revealed by the comments of Dr J. L. Frew, Chairman of the Victorian State Committee of the Royal Australasian College of Physicians, during an address at an annual meeting of the Australian Association of the Ethical Pharmaceutical Industry, which indicate that 10 per cent to 15 per cent of patients admitted to hospital are suffering from iatrogenic illness; i.e., illness caused by previous medical treatment (Kerr 1987, p. 8). Commenting on the issue of how many people are in fact made worse by medical treatment, Kerr further states:

> Unremarkably enough, no precise figures are available on this subject. The information which medical practitioners are required to furnish to the Department of Health does not include an item such as 'The number of patients whom I made worse last month'.
>
> (Kerr 1987, p. 9)

It can be seen that the issue of resource allocation goes far beyond the simple question of merely how to allocate dollars and cents. It involves much broader questions of how to measure quality of life, efficacy of health care and medical treatment, and quality of care, and of how to calculate cost-effectiveness, as well as complex socio-cultural questions pertaining to power, politics, elitism and greed (Johnstone 1990; see also David Lindorff's controversial and provocative text *Marketplace medicine: the rise of the for-profit hospital chains* [1992]).

Unless nurses address these other broader questions — both academically and professionally — they will never be in a position to offer a convincing account of why *care* (whatever form this may take) needs to be better recognised as an intrinsic part of health care generally, and why it must be more appropriately funded. Someone has to take a strong stand on the need to recognise and to fund *care* better, and there is considerable scope to argue that it would be very appropriate for the nursing profession to do so. That the nursing profession is not doing so is clearly evident in its lack of public support in relation to at least two critical issues: care of the elderly, and lay care of AIDS sufferers. On both these issues nurses (both individually and collectively) have been conspicuously silent.

One particular case that warrants mention here is that involving David Zuber, a lay carer. David was seeking a carer's pension so that he could care for his live-in companion, who was suffering from the advanced stages of AIDS and had been diagnosed as only having six to eight weeks to live. As a point of interest, David first learnt that his friend had AIDS when 'he overheard nurses chatting in a hospital lift' (Birnbauer 1987a). David's application for a carer's benefit was rejected by the Department of Social Security without explanation. A spokesperson for the Minister for Social Security eventually confirmed that 'under the Social Security Act, heterosexuals in de facto relationships were eligible for the carer's pension, but homosexuals were not' (Birnbauer 1987a). In an editorial comment about the case in *The Age* (12 February 1987, p. 13), the then Minister for Social Security, Mr Howe, was reported as saying 'if homosexual partners caring for AIDS sufferers became eligible for the pension it might be difficult to exclude "aunts and uncles and second cousins and next-door neighbours and so on"'. The Social Security Appeals Tribunal later recommended that 'the Federal Government pay the carer's pension to David for looking after his homosexual partner' (Birnbauer 1987c). The pension being sought at the time amounted to $106.20 per week (given his friend's six-to-eight week prognosis, the total sum needed would ultimately have been less than $1000); the Health Department of Victoria meanwhile estimated that caring for an AIDS patient in hospital at that, time would have cost on average about $150 000

(Birnbauer 1987b). Mr Adam Carr, president of the Victorian AIDS Council, also pointed out that of the predicted $8.6 million cost for AIDS care in Victoria, over $2 million would be offset by the Council's two hundred volunteers, who were providing free counselling and care to AIDS sufferers twenty-four hours a day (McIntosh 1987).

The case of David and his dying companion is interesting and provocative from the point of view of supporting the role of lay carers in our community, something which the nursing profession endorses (Kitson 1987). Holistic nursing philosophy endorses the involvement of 'significant others' and of the ill person being surrounded by and cared for by those whom she or he wishes to be near; these may well include uncles and aunts, next-door neighbours or friends. Furthermore, holistic nursing philosophy also endorses the validity and role of alternative health modalities outside immediate scientific health care institutions, including those provided by lay and folk carers in a person's *own home* (a notion also fully endorsed by the modern hospice movement). Yet, throughout the publicity about David's case, the nursing profession was conspicuously silent; not one official word supported David, nor the role of the lay carer, nor the need to support lay carers generally. The publicity given to David's case is unusual. Individuals (mostly women) care for the ill and infirm every day without one cent of recompense, or without receiving media attention. Nevertheless, it provided an important opportunity for the nursing profession publicly to support the issue of *care*. Sadly, it neglected to take this opportunity. This analysis can of course also be made in relation to care of the elderly, the disabled, and others. The nursing profession has a moral obligation to lobby effectively for the community as a whole, and the individuals who comprise it, to have better access to holistic health care, and not merely to scientific medical care.

The right to have access to appropriate care is a second sense in which a right to health care can be claimed. This sense raises important questions concerning the cultural relativity or ethno-specificity of care and its ability to accommodate people's personal preferences, health beliefs, health values and health practices. Failing to provide health care in an appropriate manner can have disastrous consequences (clinically, legally and morally). For example, Kanitsaki (1983; 1988a) offers a thought-provoking case study concerning an elderly woman of Greek origin who had been admitted to hospital for the treatment of a chronic leg ulcer, with a view to amputation. In this case, the woman's doctor and attending nursing staff viewed amputation as being the 'treatment of choice', whereas the elderly woman viewed this treatment option as being both personally abhorrent and culturally taboo; she would rather die than have the amputation. Fortunately, thanks to a sympathetic charge nurse who had a cultural understanding of the woman's plight, alternative remedies were tried and the woman's leg eventually healed.

Many other examples can be given here. The holistic health movement has posed all sorts of new dilemmas for the scientific health professional, particularly in instances where patients prefer to try scientifically 'unproven' vitamin or herbal remedies, meditation, and other therapeutic agents for serious diseases, rather than risk the known and unpleasant side effects of more orthodox medical treatments. To some extent this type of problem has been overcome by health professionals combining orthodox and unorthodox treatments (for example, performing surgery as well as administering vitamin and herbal therapies, or administering orthodox drugs as well as performing spinal manipulation, acupuncture and acupressure, facilitating meditation, and the like) — something which once would have been unheard of in the domains of scientific Western medicine (see also Moyers 1993; Dossey 1991; Chopra 1989).

Another aspect of 'appropriate care' entails patients having access to people (lay, folk and professional) of their own choosing. It also includes patients' entitlements to seek a second medical opinion, to refuse a recommended medical therapy or folk therapy, to choose an alternative health therapy, to be surrounded by family and friends, to have unrestricted visiting rights, and to decline to be 'ordered' to do anything they do not wish to do (including getting out of bed, having a shower every day, and taking prescribed medication). As the Australian Consumers' Association (1988, p. 16) correctly points out, patients do not need a doctor's or nurse's 'permission' (to be distinguished here from *advice*) for anything!

If nurses are to respond to this sense of a right to health care, they need to gain knowledge and understanding of their patients' health beliefs and health practices and to negotiate ways in which these can be accommodated and met appropriately.

A right to quality of care is a third and final sense in which the right to health care can be claimed. This sense raises questions concerning the accountability, responsibility and competency of health professionals and health care providers, and about the standard of care that is actually delivered. Not only are practical and technical skills at issue here, but also attitudinal factors such as a health care provider's attitude towards patients as human beings with needs and interests, who are entitled to participate in decision making concerning their care. A claim to receive quality care also raises questions concerning what should be done in the case of the 'impaired professional' (Somerville 1986) — someone who functions below an otherwise acceptable professional standard.

Quality health care as a right is an ambiguous and complex notion. Nevertheless, an attempt must be made to understand and use it in a meaningful way. Among the best measures of such terms as 'quality care' or 'substandard care' are past experience and quality assurance formulae. Until anything better can replace these, the commonsense notion of quality of care has to be relied upon. The task for the nursing profession is to ensure that health care delivery never falls to a level that compromises patient safety and well-being; nurses in many parts of the world have already demonstrated their willingness to take strike action when patient safety is compromised by substandard conditions and resources.

It can be seen that all three senses of the right to health care pose a significant challenge to the nursing profession. As far as the right to equal access is concerned, nurses have much to contribute. Nurses know very well the areas in which access to health care has effectively been denied people, and why (for example, lack of appropriate resource allocation, inappropriate structuring of health care delivery, obstructive institutional policies and legal laws, language and cultural barriers). Despite their knowledge and experience in relation to these matters, however, nurses are more often than not excluded from participating in important policy making and resource allocation initiatives in the health care arena. Nurses are not usually consulted on how and where the health dollar should be spent or on how health care services should be structured and could be improved.

As a point of interest, nurses comprise 70 per cent of health care workers. Yet they have next to no say in the management of the health industry or the health care arena as a whole. The moral as well as professional implications of this situation are serious. What is particularly of concern is that the exclusion of nurses from top-level decision making and policy formation effectively prevents them from fulfilling their broader moral responsibilities towards the community at large in terms of ensuring its access to appropriate and quality health care services. The lesson to be gleaned from this observation is clear: nurses must directly participate in high-level decision making concerning health care matters, an imperative already well argued for by Paul Gross (1985). If nurses fail to influence policy and decision making, the prospects for patients' rights, not to mention the nursing profession's ability to promote and protect these, will remain pessimistic.

The right to health care, in the senses pertaining to both appropriate health care and quality health care, also poses significant challenges to the nursing profession, in terms not only of its own standards, but also of those applied in health care contexts generally. If the nursing profession is to succeed in providing appropriate nursing care (a subcategory of health care), it needs to pay careful and continuous attention to developing its curricula and to ensuring that its members are educationally prepared to meet and to respond to the needs of society, and in particular the needs of the culturally and individually diverse people comprising it. As well as this, the nursing profession must pay careful attention to developing reliable mechanisms for guiding its members in their attempts to deliver safe, therapeutically effective, culturally appropriate and morally accountable care, and for censuring those of its members who fail to do so.

Nurses, individually and collectively, have a moral responsibility to respond to the serious threats mounting against a person's right to health care; they must therefore develop a well organised and effective lobby to champion a more balanced approach to resource allocation and a more balanced approach to the structuring of health care facilities generally. Nurses also have a moral responsibility to inform the community at large of its entitlements to, in and against health care, and to educate it that the 'technologically big' is not necessarily the 'health care best'.

2. Informed consent

Traditionally, doctors have assumed ultimate decision-making authority in health care contexts. The notion of 'doctor knows best' has been, and in many instances continues to be, widely accepted by the lay community. Unfortunately, as numerous anecdotal case studies show, doctors have not always used their authority wisely, much less to the benefit of their patients' interests. In some instances (as happened in the John McEwan case cited at the beginning of this chapter), doctors have made and implemented decisions against their patients' expressed and considered wishes.

The role and authority of the doctor as ultimate decision maker is, however, being increasingly questioned by the laity, academics, consumer rights groups, other health professionals and governments. In King et al. (1988), the conceptual underpinnings of physician authority are critically examined and successfully challenged. The unanimous conclusion of all twelve contributors to this volume is that it is no longer appropriate or necessary for doctors to be 'the captain of the ship', a metaphor borrowed from American legal law and used to describe the doctor as being in charge of 'the clinic, the operating theatre and the health care team'.

Of all the patients' rights which may be claimed and which impose correlative duties on attending health professionals (including doctors), none threatens the power and authority of doctors more than the patient's right to give informed consent to medical treatment. This probably helps to explain why some doctors tend to oppose the introduction of a reasonable *patient* standard model of consent in Australia in favour of the current reasonable *doctor* standard model of consent. For example, a past president of the Victorian branch of the Australian Medical Association (AMA) is reported as saying that informed consent is 'an ideal that can be very rarely achieved' (Schauble and Willox 1987, p. 19).

Change is on the horizon, whether or not the medical profession finds proper informed consent procedures plausible or desirable. Consumer interest groups, women's health groups and patients' rights groups are all pushing for reforms in the area of informed consent, a demand which shows no sign of abating. As already mentioned, the Law Reform Commissions of Australia, Victoria (now disbanded), and New South Wales jointly produced a discussion paper on informed consent to medical treatment, in which current procedures are critically examined and recommendations made for reforms (1987).

More recently, the National Health and Medical Research Council (1991) released a preliminary paper entitled *General guidelines for medical practitioners on providing information to patients.* Undoubtedly, however, one of the most significant challenges to the status quo has been the High Court of Australia's ruling in November 1992 that 'doctors have a duty to provide patients with information about the possible risks and side effects of a proposed treatment' (*Healthsharing Women* 1933, p. 1; Kingston 1992, p. 3; Wallace 1992). Significantly, as *Healthsharing Women* notes:

> the judgement supersedes previous rulings that have allowed some doctors to successfully defend charges of negligence on the grounds that their failure to provide such information was in accordance with a practice accepted as proper by a responsible body of doctors.
>
> (*Healthsharing Women* 1993, p. 1)

However, Wallace (1992) contends that the decision still has not challenged the *reasonable doctor standard*, and hence that the status quo, in essence, has been preserved.

Whether the informed consent debate will succeed in achieving the urgently needed reforms being sought will depend very much on the public support it receives and on how seriously the nursing profession takes up the issue. In my view, the nursing profession has been conspicuously silent on the issue of informed consent, and, despite the obvious and serious professional as well as moral implications of current consent to treatment practices, has not done all that it could do to support reforms in this area. If nurses are to make a meaningful contribution to the informed consent debate — one of the most important bioethical issues facing Australia and New Zealand — they need to be clear about just what exactly the nature and function of informed consent is, and, further, why it is of concern to nurses. Let us consider these two points further.

WHAT IS INFORMED CONSENT?

The doctrine of informed consent, although having a profound ethical dimension, is essentially a legal doctrine developed partially out of recognition of the patient's right to self-determination and partially out of the doctor's duty to give the patient 'sufficient information about proposed treatment so as to provide him or her with the opportunity of making an "informed" or "rational" choice as to whether to undergo the treatment' (Robertson 1981, p. 102).

In distinguishing the differences between a legal and a moral approach to informed consent, Faden and Beauchamp (1986) explain that the legal law's approach to informed consent 'springs from pragmatic theory', which focuses more on a doctor's duty to disclose information to patients and not to injure them. By contrast, moral philosophy's approach to informed consent 'springs from a principle of respect for autonomy that focuses on the patient or subject, who has a right to make an autonomous choice' (Faden and Beauchamp 1986, p. 4).

Whether such a clear-cut distinction can be drawn between a legal and a moral approach to informed consent is a matter of some controversy, however. The moral demand to respect autonomy is clearly the prime motivator of the doctor's duty to disclose information, and the moral principle of non-maleficence the prime motivator of the doctor's duty not to injure or harm patients. It seems that, while the moral and legal approaches to informed consent can be loosely distinguished, they are nevertheless inextricably linked. It is this linkage which highlights the other important functions, besides the promotion of patient autonomy, that the application of the doctrine of informed consent also serves, namely those of protecting patients, avoiding fraud and duress (i.e., as occurs when information is not disclosed), of encouraging self-scrutiny by health professionals, of promoting 'rational' and systematic moral decision making, and of involving the public 'in promoting autonomy as a general social value and in controlling biomedical research' (Capron 1974).

The need to revise current consent to treatment procedures in Australia is long overdue. Despite popular medical opinion to the contrary, current consent procedures are inadequate and are open to abuse. Nurses witness consent abuses in hospital contexts almost every day, and are sometimes unwitting (sometimes witting) accomplices to these abuses. For example, I have been told of several instances in which nurses have been 'ordered' by an operating surgeon to obtain the written consent of a patient who has already been given a pre-medication and who is drowsy and awaiting transfer to the operating theatre. In each instance, the fact that consent given under the influence of sedating or narcotic drugs is legally invalid seems to have been largely ignored by the surgeons in question. In one case, the gynaecologist 'ordered' a registered nurse to obtain the signature of a non-English-speaking and already pre-medicated woman on whom he was about to perform a dilatation and curettage (D&C) of the uterus. However, there was some suggestion that the gynaecologist also intended to sterilise this woman, and the nurse involved in the case was deeply concerned that the matter of surgical sterilisation had not been properly discussed with the woman. Further, the patient was in no state to give a valid consent, since she was very drowsy from the effects of her pre-medication. As well, no interpreter was immediately available to transmit to the woman the information she needed in order to give an informed consent. On the basis of her assessment of the situation the registered nurse refused to comply with the gynaecologist's order. Upon hearing her refusal the gynaecologist became abusive and was overheard to yell at her. Fortunately, other nurses on the ward came to her defence and supported her decision not to seek the woman's signature. Needless to say, the woman did not go to theatre that day.

The Victorian organisation Health Call (1987) cites an even more alarming case, which is worth quoting at length here, since it is very similar to the case just discussed and serves to show that this kind of case is by no means unique.

> Four weeks prior to giving birth a 26-year-old woman, pregnant with her fourth child, attended an antenatal appointment with her Medical Specialist.
>
> The physician initiated a discussion about sterilization during which the woman made it quite clear to him she had no wish to undergo sterilization.
>
> On admission to hospital for a caesarian section the woman was approached by nursing staff and asked to sign a form consenting to sterilization and the caesarian section. The woman again made a clear verbal statement refusing sterilization.
>
> After undergoing the caesarian section the woman was informed by the Medical Specialist that a tubal ligation had been performed. The woman asked the doctor why he had performed the procedure despite her consent not having been given. He replied: 'In my medical opinion you should not have any more children'.
>
> (Health Call 1987, p. 5)

These two cases are in no way isolated examples. Kanitsaki (1992), for example, cites the case of a 66-year-old Greek woman

('Mrs G') who had been admitted to hospital for elective surgery to treat a kidney disorder. As in the previous cases, informed constent was not obtained. Describing the circumstances surrounding the failure to obtain an informed consent from this woman, Kanitsaki writes:

> The morning of Mrs G's operation arrived, and it was observed by the nurse who was to prepare her for theatre, that Mrs G's consent form was not signed. The nurse reported this to the charge nurse who rang the relevant doctor to come and obtain Mrs G's signature on the consent form. The surgical registrar arrived, and in an irritable tone asked 'why this was not done the day before'. The nurse remarked that Mrs G only spoke a few words of English, and would need an interpreter to explain to her what she was signing and why. The doctor replied 'I know. But I have no time to wait. It will be alright.' He then proceeded to instruct Mrs G how to sign the consent form. Mrs G sat up in bed, however, and looking puzzled, uttered 'Me no understand. Me no understand'. The doctor then proceeded to pick up Mrs G's hand, placed a pen into it, and by holding and directing her hand, made a cross on the consent form. Once this was achieved, the doctor gently touched Mrs G's hand and said 'Good. Good.' He then left the ward.

> (Kanitsaki 1992, pp. 2–3)

While women feature large in allegations of consent abuses, they are of course not the only ones to fall victim to unscrupulous consent-to-treatment practices and related patients' rights violations. In one extraordinary case, which occurred in 1986, a 35-year-old man had been admitted to a major city hospital for a surgical fusion of his cervical spine. He was a self-employed carpenter, who had worked hard to build up his small business. Worried about the risks associated with the procedure for which he had been admitted, the man asked an attending junior registered nurse what the risks were of being left a quadriplegic following a cervical fusion. In response to this question, the nurse informed the patient that he really needed to discuss the matter with his doctor, and that she would contact him to come and answer any questions. The patient at this point informed the nurse that his brother was a doctor and had advised him to ask the operating surgeon a number of questions pertaining to the procedure, including the question just ventured about the risk of quadriplegia.

A short time later the ward's junior medical resident came to see the patient to answer his questions. The patient was not, however, satisfied to discuss the matter with the junior resident, and asked to see the consulting surgeon. Three days later the surgeon walked briskly into the patient's room and, without greeting him by name, asked in a stern tone of voice: 'What is all this nonsense going on?' The patient calmly replied that he had been informed by his medical brother that there was a significant risk of being left a quadriplegic following surgery to the cervical spine and that he simply wanted some reassurance that the risk was minimal. The surgeon replied curtly 'it's not worth worrying about' and further that the procedure was 'perfectly safe'. The patient then asked the surgeon whether he would be doing the operation *personally*. To this the surgeon replied, again in a curt tone of voice, 'you will be operated on by *whoever* is available — probably my registrar'. This is not an uncommon occurrence in Australian hospitals, and in fact the consent forms signed by patients generally carry explicit wording to the effect: 'I understand that an assurance has not been given that the operation will be performed by a particular surgeon' (see figure 7.1).

The man became very concerned about receiving this piece of information, and insisted that, as he had been admitted under the surgeon Mr X, surely he had a right to be treated by Mr X, and surely Mr X had an obligation to treat him? To this the surgeon replied: 'As a Medicare patient, the answer is no. You are only entitled to be treated by whoever is available.' The surgeon then went on to inform the patient that either he accept that the registrar would be performing the operation, or else he was free to discharge himself.

Despite the severe neurological symptoms he was experiencing in his arm (including a loss of function and muscle wasting) the patient discharged himself. The matter was reported to the nursing supervisor who just shrugged, raised her eyebrows, and stated: 'there is nothing we can do...' None of the nurses involved in this case felt they could intervene on the patient's behalf. Their main reason was that they feared the wrath of the surgeon, who had a reputation for being 'abusive and difficult'.

Strong objections may issue forth against the examples given here. A typical response may be: 'Of course the actions of the doctors in these examples deserve universal condemnation. But these are, after all, "one off" examples . . .' I would suggest that any number of experienced nurses could show that the examples given here are not 'one off'. Critics might also begin their inquiries with ex-patients, such as the 948 unconsenting women and the unconsenting parents of the 2200 newborn baby girls involved in the National Women's Hospital 'unfortunate experiment' in New Zealand, or the unknown number of unconsenting women patients used as teaching objects when under general anaesthetic (Bone 1987). It would not take long to build up a very strong case against popular medical opinion on the matter of informed consent to treatment.

CONSENT FOR OPERATION AND ANAESTHETICS

I, ...of ....

....hereby consent to

undergo

the submission of my (child)(ward) .... to undergo

the operation of...

the nature and purpose of which have been explained to me by

Dr/Mr ....

I also consent to such further or alternative operative measures as may be found appropriate during the course of the above-mentioned operation, and to the administration of general, local or other anaesthetics for any of these purposes.

No assurance has been given to me that the operation will be performed by any particular practitioner.

Date ....Signed ....
                                                        *Patient/Parent/Guardian

I confirm that I have explained the nature and purpose of this operation to the *patient/parent/guardian.

Date ....Signed ....
                                                        *Medical/Dental Practitioner

*Delete as appropriate

Figure 7.1 Typical consent form for operation and anaesthetics procedure (from J. Fordham, *Doctor's orders or patient choice,* Leo Cussen Institute, Melbourne, 1988, p. 68).

One reason why consent practices in Australia and New Zealand are less than desirable is the model they are based on. Unlike the United States and Canada, which use a *reasonable patient standard* model of consent (emphasising trespass and battery), Australia and New Zealand use a *reasonable doctor standard* model (emphasising negligence and malpractice). Understanding the difference between these two models is important to any debate on informed consent, and I will briefly outline them here. (For a more detailed discussion on the legal aspects of informed consent to medical treatment, see Andrews 1985; Faden and Beauchamp 1986; Law Reform Commission of Victoria et al. 1987; Wallace 1991; Staunton and Whyburn 1993.)

In the *reasonable doctor standard* model of consent, a consensus of reasonable and established medical opinion provides the 'objective' measure. On the basis of this model, a doctor has the duty to use reasonable skill and may *withhold* information if, in the doctor's opinion, its disclosure would be injurious to the patient. If patients are successfully to sue for damages on account of a failure to disclose information relevant to the consent process, they have to show, first, that the doctor failed to provide information and advice to a patient that accords with the 'practice existing in the medical profession' (Law Reform Commission of Victoria et al. 1987, p. 8), and, second, that injury was suffered as a (causally) *direct result* of this negligence. In establishing whether the doctor did in fact use 'reasonable skill', the law would appeal to the *reasonable doctor standard* and would ask what most or many reasonable and competent doctors in a given particular branch of medicine would do and say in such circumstances; that is, what would be considered 'accepted medical practice' in this situation? If there were conflict, the answer to this question would be sought from an expert medical witness, or witnesses, who would testify what they, as reasonable and competent doctors in a particular branch of medicine, would probably do or say in the circumstances under question. For example, the question of whether a doctor should have disclosed to a patient a 0.1–0.2 per cent risk of quadriplegia in cases involving cervical spinal surgery would ultimately be decided on the basis of whether *other* reasonable and competent doctors in the field usually disclose this information. If it could be established that other reasonable doctors do not disclose to their patients a 0.1–0.2 per cent risk of quadriplegia in cases involving cervical spinal surgery, it is likely that a doctor who failed to disclose such information to a patient would *not* be found negligent or causally responsible for the patient's injuries in the case of a material risk manifesting itself (such as quadriplegia).

In the *reasonable patient standard* model, on the other hand, the standard is set 'by reference to hypothetical behaviour of adult, competent people in the sorts of situations which are presented to courts and other tribunals for decision' (Law Reform Commission of Victoria et al. 1987, p. 8). On the basis of this model, a doctor has the duty to *disclose* to the patient all the information necessary to making an intelligent and 'rational' choice (including information pertaining to small material risks). For example, consider the hypothetical case of a patient who has suffered the complication of quadriplegia following a cervical spinal fusion. Consider further that the patient claims that, had information been given about the associated risk of quadriplegia, the operation would never have been consented to in the first place. The famous *Sidaway* case provides a good and thought-provoking example of this kind of situation (Law Reform Commission of Victoria et al. 1987, pp. 3–4, 37–9; Andrews 1985, p. 14). In the hypothetical case, the question of whether a doctor should have disclosed to the patient a 0.1–0.2

per cent risk of quadriplegia in cases involving cervical spinal surgery would ultimately be decided on the basis of whether:

1. the information that was withheld was critical to the patient's making an intelligent choice;

2. the information would have caused the patient to make a different choice had she or he been informed of the associated risks before giving consent; and

3. the patient's desire to know of the given associated material risks was consistent with the desires of a hypothetical reasonable and competent adult.

If it could be established, in this instance, that the patient would not have consented to the procedure, and that the patient's declining to give consent would have been consistent with what a hypothetical reasonable and competent adult would do in a similar situation, then the patient's original consent would be vitiated and the doctor would be found guilty of trespass and battery.

Both models depend on the further consideration of a patient's rational or legal *competence* — a matter that, rightly or wrongly, the courts ultimately decide (the question of patient competency will be considered later in this discussion).

The issue facing us is whether we should totally abandon the reasonable doctor standard model in favour of the reasonable patient standard model, or whether we should opt for some middle ground between the two. There is some suggestion that this middle position has already been opted for in one or two Australian court cases (Russell 1987, p. 18); however, further legal opinion would be necessary to explore the issue in more depth.

Whatever the legal considerations and arguments for or against these models, from a moral point of view (and, indeed, a pragmatic point of view) neither is free of difficulties. It takes little imagination to see how the reasonable doctor standard can be unreliable. As books, articles, anecdotal case studies and media commentaries make plain, doctors are on the whole loath to testify against their colleagues. A Sydney developmental physician and advocate, Dr Cary Ooi, has even alleged that many of the so-called 'expert witnesses' provided by the Medical Defence Union of the United Kingdom (whose Australasian Secretariat is based in Sydney) give false and fraudulent testimonies in a bid to support colleagues brought before the courts for negligence or malpractice claims. In his unpublished paper 'Paediatrics — a new version', Dr Ooi argues that medical fraud occurs on an international scale and 'there is evidence that it is committed quite often without shame or effective sanction' (p. 1). He has also commented elsewhere that in one court case 'the evidence of a UK trained general nurse and midwife was completely ignored by the learned judge, and the false medical testimony of a paediatrician-defendant was accepted without thought that it was served by self-interest' (personal communication, 1988). The implication of this situation for the nursing profession is self-evident, and supports the view that judges/the courts have little regard for a nursing perspective on professional, clinical or moral matters (see in particular Johnstone 1994). Commenting on Australia's medical defence unions, Stephen Rice (1988) writes:

> the medical defence unions operating in Australia claim they do not object to their members testifying against colleagues. But they stress to members in newsletters: — 'Avoid unnecessary criticism of the work or conduct of other practitioners.'
>
> (Rice 1988, p. 124)

Rice also cites the experience of a Sydney solicitor (and former legal secretary of the Australian Medical Association) who, when addressing a medico-legal seminar organised by the AMA, was unable to find *one* doctor in the audience who was prepared to give evidence against another doctor at a court hearing. Rice comments further: 'Even with his impeccable contacts in the medical community, he [the solicitor] has discovered it is not easy to find willing witnesses' (p. 124).

The reasonable patient standard, however, can also be un-reliable. For example, who is to say what is to count as a 'reasonable' patient, hypothetical or otherwise? Are we really expected to believe and accept that an abstract 'hypothetical reasonable and competent adult' — divorced from any cultural, social, historical, spiritual context of living — is able to represent reliably and truthfully what an actual person whose 'reason-ableness' is at issue would ultimately desire? What one patient might consider *reasonable*, another might equally reject; and vice versa. The case of Jehovah's Witnesses and their well recognised refusal to accept life-saving blood transfusions is a point in question. It is not difficult to imagine a 'reasonable patient' of the Jehovah's Witness faith refusing a blood transfusion against an overwhelming body of opinion that such a refusal was 'unreason-able' and even 'crazy'. In the case of culturally different persons, as in the Kanitsaki (1983) example of the elderly Greek woman who refused amputation of her leg, it is not difficult to imagine a 'reasonable patient' of a traditional and non-scientific cultural background refusing scientific medical treatments against an overwhelming body of opinion that such a refusal would be 'unreasonable' and even 'odd'.

In dealing with these and other difficulties, as well as with other more general objections which may be raised against the doctrine of informed consent, it is important not to lose sight of the underlying moral principles justifying informed consent and what their application (as interpreted through the informed consent doctrine) is supposed to achieve. The principles of particular importance here include those of:

- *autonomy* — demands respect for patients as autonomous choosers and justifies allowing them the option of accepting risk;
- *non-maleficence* — demands the protection of patients from battery and other harms that may result from inadequate or inappropriate disclosure;
- *care* — demands that patients be approached carefully and sensitively for their consent;
- *utility* — demands the maximisation of patients' preferences; and
- *justice* — demands fairness and the equal distribution of benefits and burdens.

It should be noted that autonomy is *a* value underlying the doctrine of informed consent but not *the* value, nor an *absolute* value. As Faden and Beauchamp (1986, p. 18) point out, at best autonomy is only a prima facie value, and to regard it as having overriding value would be both historically and culturally 'odd'. This is not to say that autonomy does not have a significant place in a moral approach to informed consent. It merely means that it does not have a sole place, and can be justly restricted by other competing moral principles, such as those already mentioned.

Having now reviewed the moral principles governing the doctrine of informed consent, and having also examined the function of informed consent, let us proceed critically to examine the constituents and nature of informed consent.

THE ELEMENTS OF AN INFORMED AND VALID CONSENT

It is generally recognised within moral philosophy that disclosure, comprehension, voluntariness, competence and consent form the analytical components of the concept of informed consent (Faden and Beauchamp 1986, p. 274).

Morally speaking, for a consent to be regarded as informed, it must satisfy a number of criteria, including those relating to the *informational* aspect of the consent and those relating to the *giving of consent* itself. Beauchamp and Childress (1989, pp. 74–119) argue that for consent to be informed: there must be a *disclosure* of all the relevant information (including both benefits and risks); the patient must fully *understand* (comprehend) *both* the information which has been given *and* the implications of giving consent; the consent must be voluntarily given (i.e., the patient must be free of coercion or manipulation); and, lastly, the patient must be competent to consent (i.e., be both 'rational' and prudent). Faden and Beauchamp (1986) argue along similar lines, but recommend what they believe are less 'overdemanding' and more plausible criteria, notably:

> (1) a patient or subject must agree to an intervention based on an *understanding* of (usually disclosed) relevant *information*, (2) consent must not be controlled by influences that would engineer the outcome, and (3) the consent must involve the intentional giving of *permission* for an intervention.
>
> (Faden and Beauchamp 1986, p. 54)

It needs to be noted that patients frequently do not realise that in giving consent they are not merely acknowledging the receipt of information concerning a recommended medical treatment or procedure, but are also actually *giving permission* to an attending health professional to go ahead and perform the treatment or procedure in question.

Faden and Beauchamp's theory of informed consent is probably one of the most comprehensive and convincing to date, and one which, although written from the cultural perspective of the United States, deserves to be given serious attention by those furthering the informed consent debate in Australia, New Zealand and other common law countries. As well as advancing their ethical theory, these authors also make a number of useful practical suggestions on how informed consent practices could be made more 'workable'. It should be noted that their comments on the need for consent seekers to improve their communication and interpersonal skills and the need to create a better 'climate' for seeking consent have often been made by nurses. This is another example of knowledge already accepted by nurses now being legitimised by others outside nursing. It is frustrating to think that the medical profession and other academic groups deny that nurses ever had knowledge on this subject in the first place.

It should be noted that the doctrine of informed consent has been the subject of much controversy, most notably amongst health professionals. Popular objections include:

- obtaining an informed consent is unacceptably time-consuming;
- when patients are told the information they need to know, they forget it;

- most patients do not want to know all the details of the risks and benefits associated with a recommended medical treatment or procedure, and forcing information on them would be just as paternalistic as withholding it;

- most patients would not understand the information required to make an informed choice;

- giving information to patients can be harmful (for example, they might refuse a life-saving procedure or drug because of a negligible risk);

- informed consent is impractical and thus unworkable.

Despite their popularity, however, these and similar objections are difficult to sustain in the face of research findings, anecdotes and professional experience. For example, it is well recognised that people in stressful and unfamiliar situations are vulnerable both to information overload and short-term memory loss (Faden and Beauchamp 1986, pp. 324–5; Robinson and Merav 1983). The stress of being admitted to hospital; of coping with feelings of pain, fear and anxiety; of being separated from the familiarity of one's home, family and friends; the general disruption of one's life, not to mention the effort required to adapt to a new (hospital) environment characterised by strange smells, sights, noises, tastes, routines, faces, procedures and sensations — all contribute, predictably, to lessening an individual's capacity to pay attention to and to recall information that has been disclosed. It is small wonder that patients forget. Information overload and short-term memory impairment in turn compromise the individual's actual understanding of information received.

To complicate matters, health professionals seeking consent or giving information do not always manage their encounters with patients very well (see, in particular, the example given in chapter 6. Some use a hurried, uninterested and sometimes positively intimidating approach when seeking a patient's consent. (Significantly, this has been the subject of formal complaint to the Victorian Health Services Commissioner [*Victorian Health Services Commissioner Annual Report 1991*]; see also Spitzer 1988). When seeking consent from a patient, health professionals too often give little attention to controlling their tone of voice, choosing a suitable time and place to approach the patient, ensuring privacy, using the appropriate body language and facial expressions, choosing the right words, avoiding complicated jargon, sitting at the patient's level, and so on. I can recall many instances in my career of doctors standing at the end of the bed looking down on the patient lying in bed when offering an explanation of an impending procedure. No doubt the doctors in question regarded their towering position as being perfectly 'natural', and probably even now would consider nothing wrong with it. What some doctors do not seem to realise, however, is that standing above a patient in that manner can be very intimidating and can serve more to hinder the communication process than to enhance it. In such situations, patients may find it extremely difficult to ask the questions they really want to ask. Of course, many doctors do sit down, do face the patient at a mutually agreeable level, and are unafraid to touch their patients in a gesture of reassurance and care; unfortunately some others still do not follow their colleagues' example.

When dealing with non-English-speaking patients, these problems are considerably worse. For example, health professionals may shout unnecessarily (a problem which also sometimes occurs when they are dealing with blind or physically handicapped people who nevertheless have perfect hearing), or they may use inappropriate body language and facial expressions, use the wrong intonations in speech, or use terms which cannot be readily interpreted into the patient's spoken language.

As far as patients who do not want to know the details of an impending medical procedure are concerned, there are few who seem to fit into this category. In some instances patients have declined information (on the basis of personal and cultural health beliefs and practices), but even then only certain select pieces of information have been declined; in these instances, patients have not voiced a blanket and unconditional rejection of all relevant information. In many instances, what has superficially appeared to be a 'refusal' was in fact more a demand that the information be given in a culturally appropriate manner (Kanitsaki 1988b). If, however, patients do make an informed refusal to receive certain relevant pieces of information, and on reflection are not open to changing their minds about receiving the information in question, then to give this information to the patients would certainly count as a paternalistic act, as Vandeveer (1980) and Kanitsaki (1988b) have already contended elsewhere.

The objection that patients would not be able to understand the information necessary in order to make an intelligent and informed choice is also difficult to sustain. It is sometimes difficult to avoid the impression that the claim that a patient cannot understand is more an assumption than a matter of sound deliberation and determination. Buchanan (1978, p. 386), for example, argues that to assume a patient would not understand given information is to make a 'dubious and extremely broad psychological generalisation', which, of course, ordinary doctors and nurses are not particularly qualified to make. Faden and Beauchamp (1986) also argue that most patients are able to understand the information given to them, and, what is more, that a patient's level of understanding can be ascertained and measured.

Even if patients do not fully understand the information given, this does not always imply that it is the fault of the patient. A patient's inability to understand is probably attributable just as much to a doctor's or a nurse's inappropriate behaviour and communication as it is to a patient's cognitive inability (Roth et al. 1983, p. 176). The onus then is on consent seekers to improve their approach to patients, and to presume a patient's *ability* to understand information rather than an inability to understand. On this point Muyskens argues:

> as in a court of law in which one's innocence is presumed until proven otherwise, the client's ability to comprehend and understand what is going on and to be able to make judgments based on the data must be presumed until firm evidence establishes the contrary.

> (Muyskens 1982, p. 119)

Just as there is no compelling evidence to suggest that patients would not understand information disclosed to them about a proposed medical procedure, there is no compelling evidence to suggest that patients would be unduly injured or harmed by disclosures. Bok (1980), for example, cites studies which show that very few patients withdraw their consent when informed of material risks or other so-called 'harmful' pieces of information concerning a proposed medical procedure. She further contends that in fact 'it is what patients do not know but vaguely suspect that causes them corrosive worry' (Bok 1980, p. 234).

Buchanan (1978) is even more scathing in his criticism of the 'information causing harm' objection, arguing that it reeks of nothing more than wide and unfounded 'psychiatric generalisations', which, again, ordinary doctors and nurses are simply not qualified to make. He argues further that even qualified psychiatric specialists would probably find it very difficult to judge correctly whether a patient would be significantly harmed by disclosure.

The 'information causing harm' objection, of course, also ignores the moral point that, even if a patient refused to undergo a recommended medical procedure on the basis of information received about certain material risks, this is, after all, something which any competent patient is morally entitled to do — whatever the risks involved and regardless of what others might think of their refusal. At best, all attending health professionals can morally do is *non-coercively* to persuade patients about the known benefits of undergoing a given medical procedure; but they are not entitled to interfere with the patient's choice if such persuasion fails (Faden and Beauchamp 1986).

Even if critics concede that these objections cannot be sustained, the objection still remains that informed consent procedures are impractical because they are unrealistically and unacceptably time-consuming. It is quite true that obtaining a voluntary consent (i.e., one free of coercive or manipulative influences) and a truly informed consent from a patient will take more time than the type of consent that is likely to be obtained in an 'assembly line' approach. But, then, so it should take more time! People are at issue here, not hamburgers or car parts or toasters. Health professionals *should* take more time (and as much as is required) to interact and communicate with their patients in a way that facilitates making informed choices and realising morally acceptable outcomes. If health professionals really do care about the well-being of their patients, there can be no excuse whatsoever for denying patients the time needed to deal with an anxiety, to answer a worrisome question, or to be reassured. Patients must have sufficient time to make an adequate decision and must have sufficient time to contemplate viable and real alternatives; anything less will result in information overload and will undermine their ability to make voluntary and informed choices (Faden and Beauchamp 1986, p. 326).

The so-called problem of 'time constraint' may be only a pseudo-problem. In some respects it may even be an *excuse* — to avoid respecting patients as autonomous choosers; to restrict and constrain the role of patients in decision making concerning their own care; to avoid the intrusion of patient authority into physician authority — in short, an excuse to maintain the status quo and to avoid doing what is morally just.

In a culture so heavily dominated and constrained by considerations of 'time', it is very easy to accept 'time constraint' as a valid excuse for abrogating one's moral responsibilities. This, however, is not acceptable morally. There are ways around the difficulties posed by time constraints, and these must always be fully explored. In the case of the informed consent, the one possible solution is to involve others in the business of information transfer to and sharing with patients.

While it is obviously and properly the responsibility of treating doctors to obtain informed consents to treatment required from the patients they are treating, there is neverthless considerable room to suggest that a collaborative approach to meeting patients' information needs would contribute substantially to maximising the patients' moral interests. Rightly or wrongly, nurses already play a major although unacknowledged role in meeting patients' information needs. This situation has arisen for many reasons, including the reality that treating doctors sometimes fail to meet the information needs of their patients — even when specifically requested to do so, either by patients themselves, or by nurses, or even by other doctors. In situations like this, an attending nurse is often the only immediately available person patients have to turn to in order to obtain the information they want. Indeed, nurses are very often the ones whom patients ask directly about what to expect of a given or pending medical procedure or treatment. (The experience of Ann Oakley, the internationally reputed English medical sociologist, considered in the final chapter of this book, is a case in point.) In such instances, nurses can find themselves in a very difficult situation — particularly if an attending doctor will not respond appropriately to a patient's request for information, as happened in the case of the man scheduled for spinal surgery, given earlier, and in Ann Oakley's case to be cited later. The nurses' dilemma is compounded by the fact that they know they can contibute a great deal to allaying patient anxiety related to knowledge deficits concerning proposed and rendered medical care and treatment options, but do not have the legitimated authority to undertake this role. Thus, if and when they are giving information to patients about medical treatments, nurses know they are 'taking a risk', since this could be construed as 'interfering with the physician–patient relationship' — as, indeed, happened in the *Tuma* case, cited earlier in this text (see also Johnstone 1994).

Recent studies have also shown that nurses can greatly assist patients in coming to understand their illness experience and physician directives given during medical consultations (Uyer 1986). One study also shows that the task of giving information to patients and satisfying patients' information needs is '*impossible* [emphasis added] without systematic collaboration between medical and nursing staff' (Engstrom 1986). It is clear that this is a matter which requires much greater attention than it has been given up until now.

A second obvious strategy which could be used to help resolve the time constraint problem is to restructure the time frame itself during which consents are usually sought. In elective admissions, consents are usually sought on the day before or evening before (or, as we have seen, even the minute before!) a scheduled medical or surgical procedure. The moral disadvantages of this are obvious. As Faden and Beauchamp ask:

> who would want, on the eve of surgery after having disrupted one's life, gathered one's courage, and entered the hospital, to change one's mind? And thus who would want to pay attention to information that challenges the wisdom of the decision?
>
> (Faden and Beauchamp 1986, p. 325)

The 'night before' time frame is hardly conducive to patients exercising voluntary and informed consent. One possible solution here would be to give patients all the 'usual' information during a pre-admission clinic a week or so before the procedure. In this way, patients would have time to go home, contemplate the information received, discuss it with family and friends, formulate any further questions they would like to ask, or even change their minds and decline the recommended therapy or procedure if they so desired. If patients were allowed time to reflect on the information given to them, not only would their consents to treatment be of better quality, but so too would their decisions to enter hospital.

The time factor involved in obtaining consent is crucial to the realisation of morally just outcomes. If sufficient time is not allocated for the purposes of gaining a patient's consent, a very real risk exists that the voluntary and informed nature of the consent will be seriously compromised, thus having the domino effect of violating underlying moral principles such as autonomy, non-maleficence, beneficence, justice, care and utility. In other words, a complete moral collapse of the situation could occur. In emergency or life-threatening situations, of course, it is not always possible to seek an informed consent and it could be hazardous to try and do so. The law recognises that in emergency or life-threatening situations consent can be 'waived'; morality likewise recognises situations in which consent can be justly waived.

The challenge to doctors and nurses and other health professionals is to restructure their thinking on informed consent, and to view it as something which 'should help overcome the inclination that many people have to yield compliantly to proposals from powerful authority figures' (Faden and Beauchamp 1986, p. 372). Faden and Beauchamp (1986, p. 305) argue that the questions that all health professionals and policy and law makers should be asking are not what patients should be told or even who should tell them, but 'What can professionals do to facilitate obtaining informed consents based on substantial understanding?', or 'How can professionals enable patients and subjects to make informed autonomous choices?'.

If informed consent procedures are to work and to achieve their desired ends, a number of other practical considerations need to be attended to. First, consent forms must be made available in the patient's own language. Where this cannot be done, the patient must be given access to a *trained health interpreter*. To illustrate the need, although over 25 per cent of Victoria's population are from non-English-speaking backgrounds, in 1988 fewer than twenty-nine full-time health interpreters were employed by the Victorian Central Health Interpreters Service. I was told by a coordinator from the Interpreters Service that, while interpreters have completed a general interpreters course, they have not been specially trained as health or medical interpreters. She further commented that the supply of health interpreters at the time was grossly inadequate to meet the demand of non-English-speaking patients. As an example, it was reported to me by a colleague that when she sought from the Central Health Interpreters Service the services of an Arabic-speaking interpreter (the patient was due to go to theatre the next day), she was informed that there was a six-week waiting list. Currently, the situation is in fact worse than it was a few years ago. The economic rationalisation of interpreter services in hospitals has in some instances seen a return to the situation of the 1950s, during which a lack of appropriate interpreting services risked the health and lives of immigrants who could not speak English (Johnstone 1991).

It is often the practice to ask cleaners or orderlies or kitchen hands who speak languages other than English to interpret for a non-English-speaking patient (see also Stone 1991, p. 4). This practice is, however, wholly undesirable. First, orderlies and cleaners and kitchen hands are not trained as interpreters and thus may seriously misinterpret the information being relayed, or may give their own assessment of and interpretation of a question being asked. For example, Olga Kanitsaki describes a case in-volving a Greek-speaking patient. In this case, a cleaner called in to interpret for the doctor exclaimed to the patient, in Greek, 'Well, if you only have a headache why don't you take an aspirin? What did you come into hospital for? Why are you bothering the doctor?' (personal communication).

Another problem here, and one often overlooked by health professionals, is that orderlies and cleaners and kitchen hands do not have a professional relationship with the patient; thus, involving them as interpreters is tantamount to breaching confid-entiality. Who is to know whether these 'informal' interpreters will keep confidential the information disclosed? Since they are not bound by any professional code of ethics, they may not fully appreciate their moral responsibilities not to disclose the confidential information they have become privy to while acting as interpreters.

A second practical consideration is that patients' consent must be continuously *re-evaluated* so as to check whether their original consent still holds. This is particularly crucial in situations involving 'Not For Resuscitation' orders or refusal to consent to given life-saving therapies. In some instances, the terms of patients' original consent may need to be modified. It has been asserted informally by those working in the area that the term 'informed consent' should be abandoned in favour of the term 'informed decision-making'. The rationale given is that the notion of *informed consent* has an air of finality about it — that is, once consent has been obtained, that is the end of the process. With the notion of *informed decision making*, however, the connotations are quite different. In contrast, it has an air of 'open-endedness' about it —

of a process that is *ongoing*. Given this, it is thought, the notion of informed decision making, unlike the notion of informed consent, seems to invite the continuous re-evaluation of any decisions made about care and treatment options. This change in thinking, however, has yet to be reflected fully in literature on the subject.

A third consideration is that patients must be informed of their entitlement to *refuse* a recommended medical or nursing procedure, and the opportunity to refuse must always be present without prejudice to the patients. Fourth, patients must be kept up to date on the relevant details pertaining to their cases. Details which are not readily understood should be explained (in understandable language), and reinforced through planned patient health education programs (something that nurses are educationally prepared to undertake).

Lastly, health professionals need to remind themselves constantly that many factors can deter patients from exercising informed and voluntary choices, including, but not limited to, fear of victimisation. For example, patients may fear that if they refuse to give consent to some aspect of the proposed procedure they may be victimised by being denied other forms of treatment or by being verbally and emotionally abused. Other factors include feelings of guilt where patients might feel, for example, that somehow they ought to give consent for the sake of their families (see Roberts, 1987); fear of unknown outcomes, as happened in the cervical spinal fusion case cited earlier; frank disagreement and value conflict, where patients might refuse simply because they do not agree with a given recommended medical therapy and would prefer to try an alternative health modality; pain or grief states which can cloud patients' prudence; 'rational incompetence', and an associated inability to exercise self-determining choices; and incompetent or impaired health professionals, who may, for instance, be poor communicators, have poor interpersonal skills, be rushed or hurried, or lack the relevant information to give to the patient.

Before concluding this discussion one further issue remains to be addressed — the problem of the so-called 'rationally incompetent' patient. This is an issue of particular concern to those working in psychiatric institutions and residential care homes.

THE PROBLEM OF RATIONAL COMPETENCY

The issue of competency is controversial and complicated. There is no substantial agreement on the characteristics of a 'competent person' or on how 'competency' should be measured. To complicate this matter further, there is also no substantial agreement on what constitutes *rationality* (as already discussed in previous chapters).

Roth et al. (1983) argue that the concept of competency is not merely a psychiatric or medical concept, as some might assume, but is also fundamentally social and legal. They warn, however, that there is no magical definition of competency, and that the problems posed by so-called 'incompetent' persons are very often problems of personal prejudices and social biases, or of other difficulties associated with trying to find the 'right' words.

The critical issue in developing tests of competency is how to strike a happy balance between serving a rationally incompetent person's autonomy and also serving that person's health care, nursing care and medical treatment needs. Also of critical concern is finding a competency test which is comprehensive enough to deal with diverse situations, which can be applied reliably, and which is mutually acceptable to health care professionals, lawyers, judges, and the community at large.

Roth et al. suggest that competency tests proposed in the literature basically fall into five categories:

1. evidencing a choice;
2. 'reasonable' outcome of choice;
3. choice based on 'rational' reasons;
4. ability to understand;
5. actual understanding.

(Roth et al. 1983, p. 173*)

The test of *evidencing a choice* is as it sounds, and is concerned only with whether a patient's choice is 'evident'; that is, whether it is *present or absent*. For example, a fully comatose patient would be unable to evidence a choice, unlike a semi-comatose patient or a brain-injured person, who could evidence a choice by opening and shutting their eyes or by squeezing someone's hand to indicate 'yes' or 'no'. The *quality* of the patient's choice in this instance is quite irrelevant. One problem with this test, however, is whether, say, the blinking of a patient's eyes can be relied upon as evidencing a choice; in a life and death situation one would need to be very sure that a patient's so-called 'evidencing a choice' is more than just a reflex.

The test of *reasonable outcome of a choice* is again as it sounds, and focuses on the *outcome* of a given choice, as opposed to the mere presence or absence of a choice. The objective test here is

---

* From L. H. Roth, A. Meisel and C. W. Lidz, Tests of competency to consent to treatment, *American Journal of Psychiatry* 134 (4), 1977, pp. 279–84. Copyright © 1977, The American Psychiatric Association. Reprinted by permission.

similar to that employed in law, and involves asking the question: 'What would a reasonable person in like circumstances consider to be a reasonable outcome?' The reliability of this measure is, of course, open to serious question — as previously objected, what one person might accept as reasonable another might equally reject.

The test of *choice based on rational reasons* is a little more difficult to apply. Basically, it asks whether a given choice is the product of 'mental illness' or whether it is the product of prudent and critically reflective deliberation. A number of objections can be raised here. For example, contrary to popular medical opinion, there is nothing to suggest that a person's decision to suicide is always the product of mental disease or depression. A patient could without contradiction 'rationally' choose to suicide as a means of escaping an intolerable life characterised by suffering intractable and intolerable pain. Alternatively, a depressed and so-called 'irrational' person might refuse a particular psychiatric treatment, such as psychotropic drugs, electroconvulsive therapy, or psycho-surgery, out of a very 'rational' and well-founded fear of what undesirable effects these treatments might ultimately have.

The test of *ability to understand*, on the other hand, asks whether the patient is able to comprehend the risks, benefits and alternatives to a proposed medical procedure, as well as the implications of giving consent. Here objections can be raised con-cerning just how sophisticated a patient's understanding needs to be. The problem also may arise of patients perceiving a risk as a benefit. Roth et al. (1983, p. 175), for example, cite the case of a 49-year-old woman psychiatric patient who was informed that there was a one in three thousand chance of dying from ECT. When told of this risk she replied, happily: 'I hope I am the one!'

The fifth and final competency test is that of *actual under-standing*. This test asks how well the patient has actually understood information which has been disclosed. This can be established by asking patients probing questions and inviting them to reiterate the information they have received. On the basis of educated skill and past experience, the health professional is usually able to ascertain the level at which the patient has understood the information received and what data gaps or misunderstandings remain.

Whatever the patients' competency to decide and quality of their autonomous choice may be, any duty of respect owed would still ultimately depend on the demands of other competing moral principles, as already discussed. Thus what may appear to be a dilemma involving whether to respect a patient's autonomy may not in fact be a dilemma at all. For example, if an elderly demented patient keeps wandering aimlessly from his bed, and is at risk of falling and fracturing his hip, overriding considerations do exist which would justify interfering with the choice to wander. If, after careful analysis of all available alternatives, the only way to stop this elderly patient from sustaining a fractured hip is to restrain him, it may well be that the use of a comfortable restraining device is the morally compelling option in this case. If, however, the elderly person is not at risk of falling and sustaining a fractured hip, and his wandering is merely an 'inconvenience' to staff, the solution might be better found in securing door locks so as to prevent the patient from wandering out onto the street where there is a very real risk of injury — say, of being hit by a car. This solution is already employed in a number of residential care homes which have installed combination locks on all their doors; only those residents who know the combination of the locks on the doors can freely come and go. Either way, entitlements and corresponding duties in the case of 'rational incompetence' must ultimately be determined by critical reflection and not, as tends to happen, by misguided or unfounded assumption.

It should be noted that competency is a key issue not just in psychiatric nursing, but in any health care context where judgments of competency are critical to deciding: (1) whether a patient can or should decide and/or be permitted to decide for her or himself; and (2) the point at which another or others will need to or should decide for the patient — that is, become what Buchanan and Brock (1989) term *surrogate decision makers*. The question remains, however, of how these things can be decided in a morally sound and just way. This question becomes even more problematic when it is considered that patients deemed 'rationally incompetent' can still be quite capable of making self-interested choices, and, further, that the choices they make — even if 'irrational' — are not always harmful.

Commenting on the moral standards which should be met when deciding whether to respect or override the expressed preferences of a patient deemed 'incompetent', Buchanan and Brock (1989) argue that it is important to be clear about what statements of competence refer to. They argue, for instance, that statements of competence usually refer to a person's competence to *do something* (in this instance, to *choose and make decisions*); by this view, competence is, therefore, 'choice and decision-relative'. Given this, determining competence in the psychiatric context fundamentally involves determining a person's ability to make particular choices and decisions under particular conditions (Buchanan and Brock 1989, pp. 311–65).

An important problem in psychiatric contexts is that severe mental illness can significantly affect the capacities needed for competent decision making (for instance, understanding, reasoning, and applying values), and hence the ability generally of severely mentally ill persons to make sound decisions about their own well-being — including the need for care and treatment (Buchanan and Brock 1989). For example, as Buchanan and Brock comment:

> a person may persist in a fixed delusional belief that proferred medications are poison or are being used to control his or her mind. Such delusions or fixed false beliefs obviously may also impair a person's capacity to reason about whether hospitalization and treatment will on balance serve his or her well-being. Severe mental illness can also affect and seriously distort a person's underlying and enduring aims and values, his or her conception of his or her own good, that one must use in evaluating hospitalization and treatment for an illness.
>
> (Buchanan and Brock 1989, p. 318)

It is precisely in situations such as these that attending health care professionals need a reliable framework within which to decide how best to act — notably: (1) whether to respect a patient's preferences even though the patient is deemed 'incompetent', or (2) whether to override patients' preferences in the interests of protecting or upholding what has been deemed by *others* to be in the patient's overall 'best interests'. Just what such a framework would — or indeed should — look like, is, however, a matter of some controversy. Neverthless, as Buchanan and Brock's substantive work *Deciding for others: the ethics of surrogate decision making* (1989) has shown, it is possible to devise at least a prima facie working framework to guide professional ethical decision making in this sensitive, complex and problematic area. Specifically, Buchanan and Brock (1989) suggest that the whole issue hinges on:

1. setting and applying accurately standards of competency to choose and decide; and

2. achieving a balance between (i) protecting and promoting the patients' well-being (human welfare), (ii) protecting and promoting the patients' entitlement to and interest in exercising self-determining choices, and (iii) protecting others who could be harmed by patients exercising harm-causing choices.

In regard to setting and applying accurately standards of competency to choose and decide, Buchanan and Brock suggest that, among other things, ethical professional decision making in this problematic area should be guided by the following considerations:

No single standard of competence is adequate for all decisions. The standard depends in large part on the risk involved, and varies along a range from low/minimal to high/maximal. The more serious the expected harm to the patient from acting on a choice, the higher should be the standard of decision-making capacity, and the greater should be the certainty that the standard is satisfied.

(Buchanan and Brock 1989, p. 85)

In other words, the extent to which an attending health care professional is bound morally to respect the choices of a person deemed 'rationally incompetent' depends primarily on the severity of the risks involved to the patient if her or his choices are permitted. The higher and more severe the risks involved, the higher and more rigorous should be the standards for determining the patient's decision-making capacity, and the more certain attending health care professionals should be that the patient has met these standards. This framework is expressed diagrammatically in figure 7.2.

For example, if a patient with severe mental illness chooses to refuse hospitalisation, the extent to which an attending health professional is obliged morally to respect this choice will depend on how severe the risks to the patient of not being hospitalised are — for instance, whether a failure to hospitalise the patient will result in her or him suiciding, or will result only in her or him being left in a state of moderate, although not life-threatening, depression. In the case of suicide risk, the grounds for not honouring a patient's choices do seem at least prima facie stronger than possible grounds for overriding the choices of a patient who is only moderately depressed. (Whether or not the risk of suicide does provide strong grounds for overriding a patient's choices to refuse hospitalisation and treatment is another question, however, and one which is considered separately in chapter 11 of this text.)

While Buchanan and Brock's (1989) framework appears hopeful, it is not free of difficulties. For instance, there remains the problem of how to determine what is a harm, what is a low/minimal and high/maximal risk of harm, and who properly should decide these things — the answers to which involve complex value judgments. Consider, for example, the following case:

An involuntary psychiatric patient refuses to take the psychotropic medication he has been prescribed. (For a helpful discussion on this problematic issue, see Feather 1985.) In defence of his refusal, the patient argues 'reasonably' that the adverse side-effects of the drugs he is being expected to take are intolerable, and that he would prefer the pain of his mental illness to the intolerable side-effects of the drugs that have been prescribed to treat his mental illness. Staff on the ward in which he is an involuntary patient are divided about what they should do. The more

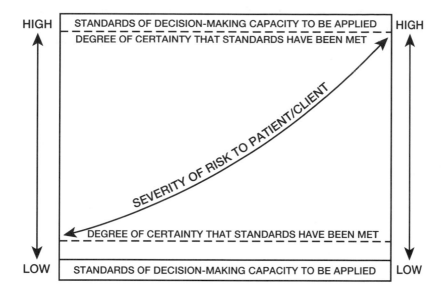

Figure 7.2 Assessing risks and permitting choices of patients deemed 'rationally incompetent'.

experienced staff in this case insist that the patient should be given his medication forcibly by intramuscular injection. They argue in defence of this decision that the patient's condition is deteriorating rapidly, and that if he does not receive the medication prescribed he will 'spiral down into a psychiatric crisis' (in other words a total exacerbation of his condition), which would be even more intolerable and harmful than the unpleasant side-effects he has been experiencing as a result of taking the psychotropic drugs in question. They make the additional value judgment that it would be 'better' for the patient if his psychiatric condition was prevented from deteriorating, and that their decision to administer his prescribed medication forcibly against his will is justified on these grounds.

The less experienced staff on the ward disagree with this reasoning, however, and argue that, even though the patient's psychiatric condition is deteriorating, and this is a preventable harm, the patient is nevertheless able to make an informed choice about this and therefore his wishes should be respected. In defence of their position, they argue that the patient's complaints are justified — the adverse side-effects of his psychotropic drugs have indeed been 'awful', and are commonly experienced by other patients as well; and that he has experienced a decline in his psychiatric condition before, and hence knows what to expect. Further, they argue, if he is given the medication against his will, an even greater harm will follow: specifically, he will trust the nursing staff even less than he does already, and will be even less willing to comply with his oral medication orders than he is now.

In this case, the more experienced staff outnumbered the less experienced staff, and the patient was held down and forcibly given an intramuscular injection of the medication he had refused. Later, after recovering from this incident, the patient was, as predicted by the less experienced nursing staff, grossly mistrustful of the nursing staff on the ward, and even less willing to comply with his oral medication orders. His requests for different and less drugs, and more counselling, went unheeded.

This case scenario demonstrates the difficulties that can be encountered when accepting/rejecting a patient's ability to choose and decide care and treatment options, and deciding when and how to override a patient's preferences. Not only is there the problem of how to determine accurately what a harm is and how a given harm should be weighted morally when evaluating whether a patient's choices should be respected or overridden; there is the additional problem that attending health care professionals may disagree radically among themselves about how these things should be determined — to a point that may even cause rather than prevent harm to the patient, as happened in this case. What else then should health care professionals do?

One response is to insist on the development of reliable (research-based) criteria for deciding these sorts of problematic issues. The need to do this becomes even more acute when the problem of determining and weighting harms is considered in relation to the broader demand to achieve a balance between protecting and promoting the patient's well-being, protecting and promoting the patient's autonomy, and protecting others who could be harmed if a mentally ill person is left free to exercise harm-causing choices (as happened in the *Tarasoff* case, to be considered later in this chapter.

Just what these criteria should be, however, and how they should be applied, is an extremely complex matter, and one that requires much greater attention than it is possible to give here. Nevertheless, Buchanan and Brock (1989) provide an important starting point by identifying the following three factors which should be (and are already being) taken into consideration when deciding whether to override a mentally ill person's choices, namely (1) whether the person is a danger to her or himself; (2) whether the person is in need of care and treatment; and (3) whether the person is a danger to others. In regard to the consideration of being a danger to self, Buchanan and Brock (1989, pp. 317–31) correctly argue that what are needed are stringent criteria of what constitutes a danger to self; in the case of the need for care and treatment, that what are needed are stringent criteria for ascertaining deterioration and distress; and in the case of harm to others, that what are needed are stringent criteria of what constitutes a danger to others. And while applying the criteria developed may inevitably result in a health care professional assuming the essentially paternalistic role of being a surrogate decision maker for a given patient, this need not be problematic provided the model of surrogate decision making used is patient centred — that is, committed to upholding the patient's interests and concerns in so far as these can be ascertained (something which was not done in the case given above).

A patient-centred model of surrogate decision making, in this instance, would have as its rationale *preventing harm to patients*, and would embrace an ethical framework which is structured 'for deciding *for* patients for *their benefit*' (Buchanan and Brock 1989, pp. 327, 331). This is in contrast with a non-patient or 'other'-centred decision making model, which would have as its rationale *preventing harm to others*, and which embraces an ethical framework 'for deciding *about* others for *others' benefits* (Buchanan and Brock 1989, pp. 327, 331). It should be noted, however, that these two models are not necessarily mutually exclusive and indeed could, in some instances, be mutually supporting (a man contemplating a violent suicide involving others is not only a danger to himself but to the innocent others he plans to 'take with him'). Just which model or models are appropriate, and under what circumstances they should be used, will, however, depend ultimately on the people involved (and the relationships between them), the moral interests at stake, the context in which these moral interests are at stake, the resources available (human and otherwise) to protect and promote the moral interests that are at risk of being harmed, and, finally, the accurate prediction of possibilities and probabilities in regard to the achievement of desirable and acceptable moral outcomes. This, in turn, will depend on the ability, experience and moral integrity of the decision makers, and the degree of commitment they have: (1) to ensuring the realisation of morally just outcomes, and (2) to protecting and promoting the well-being and moral interests of those made vulnerable not just by their mental illnesses, but by the inability of their care-givers to respond to the manifestation of their illnesses in morally sensitive, humane, therapeutically effective and culturally appropriate ways.

INFORMED CONSENT AND NURSES

The discussion given here on informed consent is less than complete; much more can be said on the matter. Nevertheless, in the light of what has been discussed it is quite evident that nurses have much to contribute to the informed consent debate. Further, it is evident that nurses also need to pay much greater attention to the doctrine of informed consent and its moral implications for nurses — not least the duties it imposes on nurses to obtain patients' informed consent to *nursing* care and procedures. It is perhaps important to emphasise that, although the doctrine of informed consent has traditionally been discussed primarily in regard to medical treatment and care, the underlying moral values, moral principles and moral requirements of this doctrine apply equally to other kinds of health care practices and procedures, including nursing care and procedures — the point being, of course, that nurses are no less exempt than are any other health care professionals from the moral standards governing consent procedures, including the demands to: (1) disclose all relevant information necessary for making an informed choice about proposed nursing cares and procedures; (2) ensure that the patient understands the information received and the implications of giving consent; (3) ensure that the consent is given voluntarily (that is, that nurses do not coerce or manipulate the patient into giving consent); and (4) ensure that the patient has the capacity to make an informed choice, and, if not, that any surrogate decision making on the patient's behalf is in accordance with rigorous moral standards.

The nursing profession can obviously do much more than it has done up until now to challenge the status quo in regard to the informed consent issue. Specifically, the nursing profession could develop a systematic program to confront the many issues raised by the informed consent debate, and to develop ways in which these issues could be addressed constructively. For instance, nurses could:

1. work closely with other groups (including health consumer groups) to ensure that the informed consent debate is kept firmly on the public agenda;

2. organise a nursing action lobby group to push for positive changes to current consent practices which do not protect or promote patients' interests and entitlements in regard to making informed choices about proposed medical and psychiatric treatments and nursing cares;

3. work for the development of sound, reliable and flexible institutional health care policies that are responsive to meeting the information needs of patients, and that can be appealed to in order to adjudicate troubling situations in which patients' information needs are not being met by an attending health care professional; and

4. work to secure the legal, moral and professional freedoms necessary to encourage patients to ask questions about proposed medical and psychiatric treatments, nursing cares and other health care procedures, and to ensure that patients receive the information they need in appropriate ways so they can make informed and intelligent choices.

By working to achieve these and like changes, the nursing profession will not only demonstrate its commitment to promoting and protecting the entitlements of patients to make informed choices about their care and treatment options, but also its commitment to upholding the view that patients are not — and never have been — obliged to be the passive recipients of un-negotiated care.

3.   Confidentiality

The principle of confidentiality has long been recognised as an important guide to action in health professional–client relationships. This principle is recognised in law as well as in ethics. In so far as the law is concerned, Wallace (1991) explains:

> It is unlawful for any person to disclose any information relating to patients, except with their consent, when required by law, or to lessen a serious threat to the life and health of the individual.

> (Wallace 1991, p. 146)

The moral position on confidentiality is very similar to the legal position, as will now be shown.

The International Council of Nurses (ICN) *Code for Nurses* (1973) states: 'the nurse holds in confidence personal information and uses judgment in sharing this information' (see appendix I). By contrast, the *International Code of Medical Ethics* (1983) states: 'A physician shall preserve absolute confidentiality on all he [sic] knows about his [sic] patient even after the patient has died' (p. 6).

The principle of confidentiality (traditionally upheld by a variety of professional groups, including priests, doctors and lawyers, and more recently nurses and other allied health workers) demands roughly that information gained in a professional–client relationship must be kept secret, even when its disclosure might serve a greater public good. Both real and hypothetical cases, however, have exposed the inappropriateness and moral un-acceptability of holding confidentiality as being an *absolute* principle (i.e., it may not be overridden under any circumstances). It will be noted that confidentiality is held to be absolute by the *International Code of Medical Ethics*, but, interestingly, not by the

ICN *Code for Nurses* — something which immediately raises the prospect of moral disagreement between these two professional groups and the possibility of significant moral conflict.

In cases where innocent victims stand to be significantly harmed by a failure to disclose, the demand to breach confidentiality becomes morally compelling. This was the view taken in the United States legal case *Tarasoff v. Regents of the University of California* (1974), the subject of Dennis Daley's (1983) thought-provoking article 'Tarasoff and the psychotherapist's duty to warn'. The case involved a university student, Prosenjit Poddar, who had met and fallen in love with a young woman, Tatiana Tarasoff. Unfortunately, Tarasoff did not share Poddar's feelings, and told him so. Consequently, Poddar became very depressed and sought psychiatric help on a voluntary out-patient basis at the Cowell Memorial Hospital at the University. During a consultation with his psychologist, Dr Lawrence Moore, Poddar revealed that he seriously intended to kill Tarasoff. After receiving this information the psychologist wrote to the campus police and informed them that Poddar was 'at this point a danger to the welfare of other people and himself', also pointing out that Poddar had been threatening to kill an unnamed girl who he felt had 'betrayed him' and had 'violated his honour' (Daley 1983, p. 243). The psychologist then went on to ask the police for assistance in detaining Poddar for psychiatric assessment. Daley writes that the campus police detained Poddar 'but released him when he appeared rational and promised to stay away from Tarasoff (p. 235).

Following this, Poddar's psychologist was directed by a superior to take no further action and to destroy his client's records (a practice which is sometimes followed by psychologists and psychiatrists in order to ensure confidentiality). Two months later, as he had threatened to his psychologist, Poddar carried out his intention and killed Tarasoff with a butcher's knife.

Daley (1983) notes that neither the girl nor her parents were warned of Poddar's threat. It seems that none of the psychotherapists involved considered it part of their professional morality to warn the victim. Even the California Supreme Court acknowledged recognition of the general rule that 'there is ordinarily no duty to control the conduct of another or to warn those endangered by such conduct' (Daley 1983, p. 235). However, the Supreme Court also recognised certain exceptions to the general rule, and its final decision in the *Tarasoff* case imposed a new duty to warn upon doctors and psychiatrists. The psychiatric profession 'reacted with alarm' to the California Supreme Court's ruling, claiming that it would 'cripple the use of psychotherapy by destroying the confidentiality vital to the psychiatrist–patient relationship' (Daley 1983, p. 234).

The *Tarasoff* case raises interesting and thought-provoking questions about the nature and force of the principle of confidentiality and the extent to which health professionals are really bound by it.

In general the demand to keep secret information disclosed in a professional–client relationship is thought to derive from the broader moral principles of autonomy, non-maleficence, justice and the obligation to keep one's promises. In the case of autonomy, it is held that individuals are entitled to choose who should have access to information about themselves, as well as what information should be disclosed, if any. Non-maleficence, on the other hand, demands that people are entitled to be protected from the harms that might flow from disclosure (which, as we know, can be both considerable and intolerable). And justice demands that a person disclosing information deserves to be treated fairly. Promise keeping, simply put, demands that 'added respect is due for that which one has promised to keep secret' (Bok 1980, p. 149), although it is generally recognised that a promise to do morally evil things is either not binding at all or 'deficient in its binding power' (Freedman 1978, p. 12).

In health care contexts, the supremacy of the principle of confidentiality is thought to be particularly justified on grounds that it is crucial to preserving the fiduciary (trust) nature of the doctor–patient relationship, and any other health professional–patient/client relationship, for that matter (Beauchamp and Childress 1989, p. 4). If patients/clients can trust their attending health professionals to keep secret certain information disclosed in the professional relationship, it is thought that patients/clients will be more likely to reveal information crucial for making a correct assessment/diagnosis, and thus a correct prescription of care and treatment.

Understandably, if it were common practice to breach confidentiality, patients/clients would probably lose their trust and confidence in their attending health care professionals, and would probably 'refrain from divulging critical information to them' (Beauchamp and Childress 1989, p. 4). Worse, they might not seek professional help at all — something which might have the undesirable consequence of individuals, groups and indeed the community at large, suffering a health status inferior to that which might otherwise be enjoyed. This argument is particularly persuasive when considered in relation to the world's current AIDS crisis.

The question remains, however, of whether the principle of confidentiality really is as binding as professionals seem to think it is. Where does it come from? As Bok (1980, p. 154) correctly asks: 'Was it ever meant to stretch so far as to require lying?' and 'Why is it so binding that it can protect those who have no right to impose their incompetence, their disease, their malevolence on ignorant and innocent victims?'.

In answering these questions, it is important to understand the nature of the principle of confidentiality. One reason why I think it has been so problematic and has caused so many controversies in health professional practice is that people mistakenly view it as an absolute principle — that is, one which cannot be overridden under any circumstance, as the *International Code of Medical Ethics* seems to demand. If we examine its parent principles, that is, the broader moral principles from which it has been derived, we can soon see that this absolutist view is quite mistaken.

CONFIDENTIALITY AS A PRIMA FACIE PRINCIPLE

On close analysis it can be seen that, at best, the principle of confidentiality is, and can only ever be, a prima facie principle. Confidentiality has a special link to a person's *right to privacy*, which may be loosely defined as the right to 'have control over information about ourselves' or 'control over who can sense us' (Parker 1974; McCloskey 1980; Thomson 1975). This in turn is connected with the principle of autonomy, which demands that people should be respected as autonomous choosers, and have the right to act on their choices provided these do not seriously impinge on the moral interests of others. Given this, it seems reasonable to hold that, where the maintenance of confidentiality results in the moral interests of others being violated, the principle can and must be overridden. This conclusion is also partially supported by the principles of non-maleficence and justice. Thus, in instances where keeping a confidence or a secret has the unhappy consequence of causing or failing to prevent an otherwise avoidable harm, and/or indeed results in an unequal distribution of harms over benefits, there is a very strong case supporting disclosure of the information being kept secret.

When subjected to the scrutiny of broader moral principles, it can be seen, first, that there are serious limits to the duty of secrecy and of maintaining confidentiality. Second, it is clear that, while in some instances the norm of confidentiality might justifiably extend to include lying, this does not hold unconditionally in all cases. (Given a consequentialist analysis, lying can only ever be justified on the grounds that it is necessary to prevent an otherwise avoidable harm from occurring, and that there is no other alternative action which can be taken to prevent the foreseen harm in question.) Third, it can be seen, given the competing demands of the moral principles of non-maleficence, justice and care, that the principle of confidentiality can never be used morally to protect those who would impose their incompetence, their diseases and their malevolence on to innocent and ignorant victims.

Unfortunately, the moral principle of confidentiality has sometimes been (ab)used to prevent the disclosure of unscrupulous practices. A poignant example of this can be found in the Chelmsford case referred to in chapter 6. Of particular relevance to this discussion is the point that, after the '60 Minutes' program in 1977, when some advice was sought by medical authorities on how to deal with the Chelmsford case, the principle of confidentiality was used to impose a duty of silence on the matter, or at least to delay its exposure. When, for example, an eminent professor of psychiatry at Cambridge University was approached about the matter, he advised:

> The inhumanity and cruelty to which the patients appear to have been subjected is quite unique in my experience, and the Scientologists and other organisations will have obtained ammunition for decades to come. There is therefore a pressing need for maintaining strict confidentiality at this stage until one can set these unique barbarities in the context of contemporary practice in psychiatry in a carefully prepared statement that comes from colleges and other bodies concerned.

> (Sir Martin Roth, cited in Bromberger and Fife-Yeomans 1991, p. 143)

This appeal to the principle of confidentiality should, however, be seen for what it is: an abuse of moral principles and the perversion of morality, not the reverse. Indeed, this stands as an example of how conventional ethical principles of conduct can be (ab)used to maintain and reinforce the status quo rather than to challenge it. And when the more parochial interpretations and applications of the principle of confidentiality are considered, what emerges is not a profound respect for professional ethical principles, but rather what Bok (1980) describes as 'primeval tribal emotions: the loyalty to self, kin, clansmen, guild members as against . . . the unrelated, the outsiders, the barbarians' (p. 149). Bok (1980, p. 149) concludes that the principle of confidentiality thus serves little more than the drive for 'self-preservation' and 'collective survival in an hostile environment'.

It is not being argued here that the principle of confidentiality ought not to be respected. On the contrary: confidentiality is an important moral requirement of any health care professional–patient/client relationship, and one that is crucial to ensuring the protection of a patient's/client's well-being and moral interests. Indiscriminate breaches of confidentiality can have morally undesirable and catastrophic consequences for patients/clients. For example, careless breaches of confidentiality concerning persons who are HIV positive can result — and have resulted — in people being dismissed from their jobs, being evicted from their rented accommodation, and being subjected generally to a wide range of negative discrimination and abuse. Similarly, careless breaches of confidentiality concerning a person's mental health status (including mild depression and grieving states) can also result — and have resulted — in harmful consequences, including those persons losing their jobs or having their career prospects hampered. It is crucial, therefore, that every effort is made to ensure that information disclosed in the professional–client relationship is kept secret. This is not to say, however, that there is not a need for the principle of confidentiality to be interpreted better and applied more justly than it has been in the past. Points of clarification which need particularly to be addressed are summarised as follows:

1. confidentiality is at best only a prima facie principle, not an absolute one, and thus is one which may be overridden by stronger moral considerations;

2. confidentiality should not be upheld in instances where doing so would result in otherwise avoidable harms occurring to innocent others; and

3. while patients/clients as a general rule have an entitlement to have certain information about themselves kept secret, the entitlement is forfeited where it stands seriously to impinge on the moral interests of innocent others.

If these points of clarification are accepted, it must also be accepted that patients (or anybody else, for that matter) might not always be entitled to have certain information about themselves kept secret; and that disclosure, in some instances, might even be an overriding moral duty, particularly in cases where non-disclosure entails the probability of innocent others suffering unnecessary and avoidable harms. This second demand is also enshrined in legal law, which requires health professionals to report certain infectious diseases (commonly referred to as 'notifiable diseases'), suspected cases of child abuse, and other activities 'which [are] potentially or actually dangerous to the health of others' (Wallace 1991, p. 303).

Whatever the situation at hand, nurses' decisions to keep secret or to disclose certain information gained in a professional–client or other type of relationship (for example, an employee–employer relationship) must always be based firmly on sound ethical principles and sound moral decision-making procedures. Nurses also need to remember that arbitrary disclosure is just as morally capricious as arbitrary non-disclosure, and may have just as many devastating consequences. As in any morally troubling situation, dilemmas posed by a controversial application of the principle of confidentiality must be resolved in a way which ensures the realisation of morally just outcomes.

4. Dignity and dying with dignity

The last patients' right to be considered in this chapter is that of *the right to the maintenance of dignity*, and, in particular, *the right to die with dignity.*

The terms dignity and dying with dignity have gained popular usage in contemporary debates concerning the invasive and sometimes encroaching nature of technological scientific medical care. They have also featured as key words in debates concerning the moral rights and wrongs of euthanasia. Yet, while the terms 'dignity' and 'dying with dignity' have been and are freely used, there is room seriously to question whether those who use them have a clear understanding of what exactly they mean.

Another concern is that these terms have come to be used in a rather clichéd sense, and thus could have the undesirable con sequence of a blanket definition of dignity being applied uncritically in all situations, regardless of their ethically significant differences, and in a way which could result in a serious distraction from (rather than a focus on) the moral issues at stake. For example, some speak of the removal of a life-support system, or the withdrawal of some other orthodox medical therapies, as tanta-mount to 'letting a person die with dignity' (Social Development Committee, Victoria 1986, 1987). What such views dangerously presume, however, is that the terms 'dignity' and 'dying with dignity' in these contexts have a clear-cut, commonsense meaning and use, and, furthermore, implicitly justify the acts or omissions in relation to which they have been expressed.

Two central questions invariably arise here. How should the notions 'dignity' and 'dying with dignity' be defined? What might be the implications of given definitions of these terms for nursing practice?

CAN DIGNITY BE DEFINED?

The word dignity comes from the Latin *dignitas*, meaning 'merit', and *dignus*, meaning 'worthy'. Needless to say, there are as many definitions of 'dignity' as there are dictionaries. *Collins English dictionary*, for example, defines dignity as:

> [1]. a formal, stately, or grave bearing ... [2]. the state or quality of being worthy of honour ... [3]. relative importance; rank ... [4]. sense of self importance ...

According to the *Oxford English dictionary*, dignity is:

> [1]. the quality of being worthy or honourable; worthiness, worth, nobleness, excellence . . . [2]. Honourable or high estate, position, or estimation . . . [4]. Nobility or befitting elevation of aspect, manner, or style . . .

Webster's dictionary says dignity is:

> [1]: the quality or state of being worthy: intrinsic worth: EXCELLENCE . . .

> [2]: the quality or state of being honoured or esteemed: degree of esteem . . .

> [5]: formal reserve of manner, appearance, behaviour, or language: behaviour that accords with self-respect or with regard for the seriousness of occasion or purpose . . .

Interestingly, the unabridged international edition of *Webster's dictionary* also gives consideration of the word 'decent' (i.e., of the mind and character) as a definition of dignity. It is perhaps worth noting here that the term 'decent' comes from the Latin *decens*, meaning 'suitable', and from *decere*, meaning 'to be fitting'.

Significantly, the question of dignity has also been a topic of philosophical debate. For example, in 1651 the English philosopher Thomas Hobbes defined it as:

> (T)he publique worth of a man [sic], which is the Value set on him [sic] by the Common-Wealth . . . And this Value of him [sic] by the commonwealth, is understood, by offices of Command, Judicature, public Employment; or by Names and Titles, introduced for distinction of such Value.
>
> (Hobbes 1968 edn, p. 152)

Later philosophers, however, rejected this 'social worth' view and sought to define dignity in more sophisticated moral terms. The German philosopher Immanuel Kant, for instance, defines dignity in quite different terms as 'an intrinsic, unconditioned, incomparable worth or worthiness' (1972 edn, p. 35). Rejecting the 'market value' or 'social worth' interpretations of dignity, he goes on to assert that:

> Morality or virtue — and humanity so far as it is capable of morality — alone has dignity. In this respect it cannot be compared with things that have economic value (a market price) or even with things that have an aesthetic value (a fancy price).

The incomparable worth of a good man [sic] springs from his [sic] being a [moral] law making member in a kingdom of ends.

(Kant 1972 edn, p. 35)

More recent definitions and interpretations have tended to capture the essence of Kant's views. One modern philosopher, for example, argues that dignity is akin to 'justified happiness' (a happiness which is 'interpenetrated with a sense of meaning, reason, and worth') and the attainment of 'just goals', that is, morally valuable ends (Swenson, 1981). The behaviourist B. F. Skinner (1973, pp. 48–62) sees dignity and what he calls the 'struggle for dignity' as having many features in common with freedom and the 'struggle for freedom'.

Some of the most revealing and instructive definitions of dignity and dying with dignity might, however, come from a group of students from the Phillip Institute of Technology (now the Royal Melbourne Institute of Technology), first-year Diploma of Applied Science (Nursing) in Victoria. Comments were sought from the students after their clinical placement at a residential care home for the elderly. The results are summarised as follows:

- 'dying with dignity is dying the way you want to die';
- 'dignity is a feeling of pride . . . of feeling good about yourself';
- 'dignity and dying with dignity is maintaining self-value, self-respect, and self-image . . .';
- 'I don't know, but I think, as it is used today, it all boils down to having to look good for other people';
- 'dignity is having pride without shame';
- 'dignity and dying with dignity is being happy with oneself, and what one has achieved in life';
- 'dying with dignity is having no pain, no fear. Feeling valued, and having your opinions valued. Yes. That's it! It involves having control and being valued';
- 'dying with dignity is putting yourself above whatever is going on around you';
- 'dignity is concerned with self-respect, and how this is related to society — your social worth';
- 'dignity is being accepting of one's self, and of what's to come . . . the problem is, however, that a lot of people base their self-worth on what other people think of them.'

As the last student voiced her comments, another student interjected with frustration, exclaiming: 'Oh! How can you die with dignity if you have no say about it?'

In considering all these definitions, it soon becomes apparent that the notions 'dignity', and 'dying with dignity', essentially defy precise definition. What this inevitably warns, of course, is that nurses — and indeed health care professionals generally — must never take the notion of dignity (and its usage) for granted. They must also be cautious in treating these terms as if they had clear-cut, commonsense interpretations. What one person might consider 'dignity', another person might equally reject — and this has important implications for nursing care delivery in particular, and health care management generally.

How, then, should dignity be defined? And what might be the implications of a given definition for nursing practice?

IMPLICATIONS FOR NURSES

Despite the variety of definitions and interpretations of the notions dignity and dying with dignity, there are a number of common elements. In summary, these include:

1. that persons have intrinsic moral worth, and thus ought to be treated as ends in themselves, and not as mere means to the ends of others;

2. that persons should be respected as autonomous choosers, and thus as beings capable of exercising self-determining choice;

3. that persons should be facilitated and supported in the course of exercising their autonomous choices;

4. that persons should be facilitated and supported in their attempts to maintain their self-respect and self-esteem.

Whatever nurses or allied health workers take dignity and/or dying with dignity to mean, it is important that they do not unfairly impose their interpretations on their patients. It is a moral imperative of the first order that patients' preferences are respected, even if others do not agree with these. This means that, where possible, and where it is culturally appropriate, patients are morally entitled to participate in decision making concerning their care, and are morally entitled to give a fully informed consent to the use and withdrawal of recommended medical or other therapies. If patients are not able to participate in decision making concerning their care and treatment, every effort must be made to establish what their considered preferences might be. Either way, in the final analysis, what is to count as dignity and dying with dignity must be decided from the patients' (or their advocates') point of view, not that of the health professionals.

Given this, nurses should not be asking 'What is dignity?' or 'What does it mean to die with dignity?'; rather, they should be asking: 'What is dignity for *this* or *that* person?' and 'What is dying with dignity *for them*?' If nurses want valid answers to these questions, they need to ask these questions in the first place.

The challenge to nursing is not just to allow patients the right to the maintenance of dignity, but actually to find out what the patient considers as being dignity and/or a dignified death, and ensuring that this is permitted and upheld on terms of what the patient wants, and not on what the *nurse thinks* the patient wants.

Issues and recommendations

To understand the nature and purpose of patients' rights claims is one thing; to protect these rights is quite another.

On 1 May 1986, Health Call, an independent health complaints telephone service set up under the auspices of the Health Issues Centre, was opened in Melbourne. In its first year of operation, Health Call received 1735 calls and recorded 2617 complaints. Of these, 500 'general enquiries' were referred to appropriate services (Health Call, 1987). In its 27 months of operation, Health Call recorded a total of 5052 calls. Of these, 3317 were complaints, 1531 were enquiries, 158 were follow-up calls, and 46 were general calls (Health Call, 1988, p. 3).

Just over two years after being set up as a pilot scheme with funding from the Victorian State Government, Health Call was closed. This was partly due to the passage of the *Health Services (Conciliation and Review) Act* 1987 (Vic.) and the establishment of the Office of the Health Services Commissioner under the Act, together with the appointment of a health services commissioner. The closure was also partly due to a lack of funds (Health Issues Centre 1988, p. 3).

The passage of health services complaints legislation and the establishment of the Office of the Health Services Commissioner represents a milestone achievement for the patients' rights movement. The Office of the Health Services Commissioner now provides consumers with a statutory authority through which health complaints can be made, investigated and conciliated.

In the first nine months of office, the health services commissioner received nearly 1867 inquiries, of which 954 were viewed as actual complaints. Out of the 135 cases already formally investigated by the commissioner, only eleven have been found to be of 'no merit' (Burchill, 1989, p. 1). The Australian Medical Association's response has been that the number of complaints received by the commissioner 'do not mean anything' (Burchill

1989, p. 6). There have been no media reports of either the Australian Nursing Federation or the Royal College of Nursing, Australia (RCNA) responding to these figures. Neither have there been any media reports of responses from other allied health professional groups. During the seven days immediately following the initial report of these inquiry and complaint figures, no further comments or letters to the editor on the matter were printed in *The Age*.

Despite the obvious importance to health consumers of the Victorian Health Services Act, it had a sunset clause, and was due to expire just three years after the date of its commencement. Fortunately, a review of this sunset provision has seen the retention of the health services commissioner. In 1991, the number of complaints registered under the Act totalled 2063 — a rise of 33 per cent over 1990 (during which 1547 complaints were registered), and a substantial rise over 1988, during which 876 complaints were registered under the Act (*Victorian Health Services Commissioner Annual Report 1991*, p. 9).

Significantly, the history of Victoria's health complaints units is not unique. The New South Wales Complaints Unit, established in 1984, has also had a troubled history. When it was set up it had no statutory existence and hence had an uncertain future. As Stephen Rice (1988, p. 156) put it, the New South Wales Complaints Unit was essentially left to hang precariously in the balance of 'political whim', because it had no statutory existence and hence was vulnerable to being 'dismembered or dismantled by the government without reference to Parliament'.

On 16 September 1992, a Health Care Complaints Bill was tabled in the New South Wales Parliament by the Minister for Health, Ron Phillips. The Bill, however, became the subject of 'bitter debate, division among community organisations, and attacks from some professional organisations, 'owing to a lack of community consultation and the Bill's potential 'to limit access to the complaints system rather than enhance and strengthen it' (Petrie 1993, p. 23).

The New South Wales Department of Health has since responded to the many criticisms of the Bill, and fears that it might disappear into a legislative 'black hole' have been allayed. At the time of writing, the Bill had been revised and was due to be re-tabled in Parliament. It is reported that the Bill has a 'positive future', but that:

> Community groups are holding fire in the hope that the outcome will be a positive one, but determined to fight on if necessary to ensure the strongest possible legislation to protect the interests of health care consumers in New South Wales.

(Petrie 1993, p. 24)

The fragility and vulnerability of past and existing health complaints units afford little optimism for the future of patients' rights. The examples just given of the Victorian Health Call, the *Victorian Health Services (Review and Conciliation) Act*, and the New South Wales Complaints Unit, all sternly warn of the need for vigilance by the laity, professionals and politicians. When considering the extraordinary lengths that the powerful medical lobby appears to have gone to in order to block initiatives in the area of health complaints, it is difficult to avoid asking what the medical lobby might have to hide and what it is so concerned about, particularly if the professional practice of its members is beyond reproach. Why is the medical lobby apparently so intent on dismissing or trivialising the issue of patients' rights and the comments of anyone trying to further the patients' rights debate? (See, for example, Cunningham 1987.)

There is room for grave concern about the Australian Medical Association's and other medical professional groups' repeated attempts in the media to trivialise or dismiss the significance of health complaints statistics and their failure to reflect health complaints trends in their reports — an observation shared by Health Call (1987, p. 2) and the Victorian Ombudsman (1988, pp. 25–36). There is further room for concern about the apparent lack of response to health complaints figures from other health professional groups, particularly the nursing profession (which is by no means exempt from complaints being made against its members), and not least consumer interest groups. One question which must be raised here is: Is this apparent lack of reported response from other health professional and consumer interest groups because they have genuinely not responded, or is it because newspaper reporters do not seek their comments, or, if they do, because newspaper editors decline to publish them?

Whatever the answers to these questions, the direction the nursing profession needs to take in relation to the patients' rights and health complaints issues is clear: it must lobby, and it must lobby hard. In particular it must lobby for:

1. the formulation and global recognition of a comprehensive list of principles, together with a set of interpretive statements, which can be appealed to for both identifying patients' rights and guiding their protection (in short, a universal declaration of patients' rights);

2. the establishment and maintenance of accessible, just, reliable and enforceable health complaints mechanisms;

3. the improvement of health professional education programs aimed at preparing health professionals better

to recognise and respond appropriately to patients' rights claims;

4. the introduction of broadly based community information programs aimed at better informing its community members of their rights to, in and against health care; and

5. the staging of regular state, national and international multidisciplinary and transcultural symposiums on patients' rights, with a commitment by all concerned (including health care professional groups and governments) to act upon these symposiums' findings.

If such aims can be achieved, the prospect for patients' rights will be considerably brighter than is suggested by present social, political and legal indicators.

———————

Section 4, 'Dignity and dying with dignity', is revised from M.-J. Johnstone, 'Dying with dignity', New Zealand Nursing Journal *81(12), 1989, pp. 34, 37.*

———————

References

Andrews, K. (1985). Informed consent: adrift on a trans-Atlantic crossing. *Lawyer* 3 (6), August, pp. 12–16 (published by Victorian Young Lawyers).

Australian Consumers' Association (1988). *Your health rights.* Australasian Publishing Company and Australian Consumers' Association, Sydney.

Bates, E. and Linder-Pelz, S. (1987). *Health care issues.* Allen & Unwin, Sydney.

Beauchamp, T. L. and Childress, J. F. (1989). *Principles of biomedical ethics,* 3rd edn. Oxford University Press, New York.

Beauchamp, T. L. and Walters, L. (1982). *Contemporary issues in bioethics,* 2nd edn. Wadsworth, Belmont, California.

Birnbauer, B. (1987a). Pension refusal adds to pain of AIDS tragedy. *The Age,* 6 February, p. 1.

Birnbauer, B. (1987b). Pension promised for AIDS partners: adviser. *The Age,* 7 February, p. 3.

Birnbauer, B. (1987c). Appeals tribunal recommends carer's pension for AIDS victim's partner. *The Age,* 13 March, p. 3.

Bok, S. (1980). *Lying: moral choice in public and private life.* Quartet Books, London.

Bone, P. (1987). Pelvic check 'by patient's consent' only. *The Age,* 18 September, p. 5.

Brody, B. (1986). Should there be a distinctively Jewish medical ethics? *Isaac Frank Memorial Lecture,* Kennedy Institute of Ethics, Georgetown University, Washington DC, ICC Auditorium, 2 June.

Bromberger, B. and Fife-Yeomans, J. (1991). *Deep Sleep: Harry Bailey and the scandal of Chelmsford.* Simon & Schuster, Sydney.

Buchanan, A. (1978). Medical paternalism. *Philosophy and Public Affairs* 7 (4), pp. 370–90.

Buchanan, A. (1984). The right to a decent minimum of health care. *Philosophy and Public Affairs* 13 (1), Winter, pp. 55–78.

Buchanan, A. E. and Brock, D. W. (1989). *Deciding for others: the ethics of surrogate decision making.* Cambridge University Press, Cambridge.

Bunkle, P. (1988). *Second opinion.* Oxford University Press. Auckland.

Burchill, T. (1989). 194 patients' complaints investigated. *The Age,* 6 January, pp. 1, 6.

Campbell, E. J., Baker, M. D. and Crites-Silver, P. (1988). Subjective effects of humidification of oxygen for delivery by nasal cannula: a prospective study. *Chest* 93 (2), February, pp. 289–93.

Capron, A. (1974). Informed consent in catastrophic disease and treatment. *University of Pennsylvania Law Review* 123, December, pp. 364–76 (cited in T. L. Beauchamp and J. F. Childress [1983], *Principles of biomedical ethics,* 2nd edn, Oxford University Press, New York, pp. 67, 102).

Carter, M. (1987). *Review of registration for health practitioners: interim report,* Health Department Victoria, Melbourne.

Chopra, D. (1989). *Quantum healing: exploring the frontiers of mind/body medicine.* Bantam Books, New York.

Coney, S. (1988). *The unfortunate experiment.* Penguin Books, Auckland.

Conley, J. (1987). AMA will consider secret AIDS tests. *The Age,* 4 July, p. 1.

Consumers' Health Forum (1990). *Legal recognition and protection of the rights of health consumers.* Consumers' Health Forum of Australia, Curtin, ACT.

Council for Science and Society (1982). *Expensive medical techniques.* Calvert's Press, London.

Cunningham Dax, Dr E. (1987). Health complaints take staff away from care. Letter to the Editor, *The Age,* 14 November, p. 12.

Daley, D. W. (1983). Tarasoff and the psychotherapist's duty to warn. In S. Gorovitz, R. Macklin, A. L. Jameton, J. M. O'Connor and A. Sherwin (eds), *Moral problems in medicine,* 2nd edn, Prentice Hall, Englewood Cliffs, New Jersey, pp. 234–46.

Department of Health, Housing and Community Services (1989). *A guide to residents' rights in nursing homes and hostels.* AGPS, Canberra.

Dossey, L. (1991). *Meaning and medicine: a doctor's tales of breakthrough and healing.* Bantam Books, New York.

Engelhardt, H. T. (1986). *The foundations of bioethics.* Oxford University Press, New York.

Engstrom, B. (1986). Communication and decision-making in a study of multidisciplinary team conference with the registered nurse as conference chairman. *International Journal of Nursing Studies* 23 (4), pp. 299–314.

Faculty of Nursing, RMIT (1992). *Proceedings of the Conference 'Meeting the Challenge of Patients' Rights — Issues for the 1990s',* RMIT Faculty of Nursing, Nursing Law and Ethics 4th Victorian State Conference, held 20 November, Dallas Brooks Hall, Melbourne. Royal Melbourne Institute of Technology, Faculty of Nursing, Melbourne.

Faden, R. R. and Beauchamp, T. L. (1986). *A history and theory of informed consent.* Oxford University Press, New York.

Feather, R. B. (1985). The institutionalised mental health patient's right to refuse psychotropic medication. *Perspectives in Psychiatric Care* 23 (2), pp. 45–68.

Fordham, J. (1988). *Doctors' orders or patient choice?* Leo Cussen Institute, Melbourne.

Freedman, B. (1978). A meta-ethics for professional morality. *Ethics* 89, pp. 1–19.

Fried, C. (1982). Equality and rights in medical care. In Beauchamp and Walters 1992, pp. 395–401.

Fuchs, V. R. (1983). *Who shall live? Health, economics and social choice.* Basic Books, New York.

Gilmour, J. (1992). *Michael: a mother's battle for the rights of her child.* Little Hills Press, Sydney.

Gross, P. F. (1985). Nursing care in the 1980s and beyond: the challenge to be relevant, ethical and accepted. *Australian Nurses Journal* 15 (1) July, pp. 46–8.

Health Call (1987). *Health complaints advisory link line annual report, 1 May, 1986–30 April, 1987.* Health Call, Melbourne.

Health Call (1988). *Health Call annual report 1988.* Health Issues Centre, Melbourne.

Health Department, Victoria (1992). *Working with people from non-English speaking backgrounds: guidelines for health agencies.* Health Department Victoria, Melbourne.

Health Issues Centre (1988). *Health Issues Centre annual report 1988.* Health Issues Centre, Melbourne.

Health Issues Centre (1991). *Our better health: getting it together.* Health Issues Centre, Melbourne.

Health Issues Centre (1992). *Casemix: quality and consumers.* Health Issues Centre, Melbourne.

Health Services (Conciliation and Review) Act 1987, no 25, Government Printer, Melbourne.

Health Services Review Council (nd). *Patient access to medical records, a discussion paper.* Health Services Review Council, Health Services Commission, Melbourne.

Healthsharing Women (1993). Doctors must disclose all information. 3 (3), December 1992–January 1993, pp. 1–2.

Hobbes, T. (1968 edn). *Leviathan* (reprinted from 1651 edition with notes by C. B. Macpherson). Penguin Books, Harmondsworth, Middlesex.

Humphry, D. and Wickett, A. (1987). *The right to die.* Collins, Sydney.

Inlander, C. B., Levin, L. S. and Weiner, E. (1988). *Medicine on trial: the appalling story of ineptitude, malfeasance, neglect, and arrogance.* Prentice Hall, New York.

International Code of Medical Ethics (1983). In Amnesty International, *Ethical codes and declarations relevant to the health professions,* Amnesty International, London, 1985.

International Council of Nurses, Code for Nurses (1973). International Council of Nurses, Geneva, Switzerland.

Johnstone, M.-J. (1988). Ethical issues in planning rehabilitation in patients with advanced cancer. Paper presented at seminar, 'Rehabilitation in Patients with Advanced Cancer — a Contradiction in Terms?' College of Nursing, Australia, in conjunction with Victoria Association of Hospice Care Programs, Melbourne, 17 October.

Johnstone, M.-J. (1990). Bioethics and the health care economics debate: a nursing perspective. Paper presented at the NSW Nurses' Association's 45th Annual Conference/Professional Seminar Day, Bioethical Considerations and Opportunity Cost, Sydney. Reprinted in full in M.-J. Johnstone (1992 edn), *Module 601E. Ethics and Nursing — Book of Readings.* Distance Education Division of Royal College of Nursing Australia, Melbourne, Reading 2.1.

Johnstone, M.-J. (1991). Government's rationalisation of language services spells disaster for NESB patients. *Transcultural Health Care Council Newsletter,* March–April, pp. 1–4.

Johnstone, M.-J. (1994). *Nursing and the injustices of the law.* W. B. Saunders/Baillière Tindall, Sydney.

Kanitsaki, O. (1983). Acculturation — a new dimension in nursing. *Australian Nurses Journal* 13 (5), November, pp. 42–5, 53.

Kanitsaki, O. (1988a). Transcultural nursing: challenge to change. *Australian Journal of Advanced Nursing* 5 (3), March–May, pp. 4–11.

Kanatsaki, O. (1988b). Cancer and informed consent: a cultural perspective. Paper presented at seminar, Controversial Ethical Issues in Patients with Cancer, Heidelberg Repatriation General Hospital, Melbourne, 13 October.

Kanitsaki, O. (1992). Meeting the challenge of patients' rights: a transcultural perspective. *Proceedings of the conference 'Meeting the Challenge of Patient's Rights — Issues for the 1990s', RMIT Faculty of Nursing, Nursing Law and Ethics, 4th Victorian State Conference*, held 20 November, Dallas Brooks Hall, Melbourne Institute of Technology, Faculty of Nursing, Melbourne.

Kant, I. (1972 edn). *The moral law* (translated by H. J. Paton). Hutchinson University Press, London.

Kerr, J. Fairbanks (1987). *Don't call a doctor.* Veritas, Bullsbrook, Western Australia.

King, N. M., Churchill, L. R. and Cross, A. W. (1988). *The physician as captain of the ship.* D. Reidel, Dordrecht.

Kingston, M. (1992). Onus on doctors to disclose risks. *The Age*, 20 November, p. 3.

Kitson, A. L. (1987). A comparative analysis of lay-caring and professional (nursing) care relationships. *International Journal of Nursing Studies* 24 (2), pp. 155–65.

Kohnke, M. F. (1982). *Advocacy: risk and reality.* C. V. Mosby, St Louis.

Law Reform Commission of Victoria, Australian Law Reform Commission, and New South Wales Law Reform Commission (1987). Informed consent to medical treatment, discussion paper no 7. Law Reform Commission of Victoria, Melbourne.

Lindorff, D. (1992). *Marketplace medicine: the rise of the for-profit hospital chains.* Bantam Books, New York.

Longo, E. (1992). Bid for health rights charter. *The Age*, 15 December, p. 6.

McCloskey, H. J. (1980). Privacy and the right to privacy. *Philosophy 55*, pp. 17–38.

McCullough, L. B. (1983). The right to health care. In S. Gorovitz, R. Macklin, A. L. Jameton, J. M. O'Connor and A. Sherwin (eds), *Moral problems in medicine*, 2nd edn, Prentice Hall, Englewood Cliffs, New Jersey, pp. 536–44.

McIntosh, P. (1987). Volunteers offset cost of care, says AIDS Council. *The Age*, 24 April, p. 6.

Medical Treatment Act 1988. no 41, Government Printer, Melbourne.

Mendelsohn, R. S. (1982). *Male practice: how doctors manipulate women.* Contemporary Books, Chicago.

Mental Health Consumer Outcomes Task Force (1991). *Mental health statement of rights and responsibilities.* AGPS, Canberra.

Miller, C. (1988). 1500 Aboriginals tested for AIDS — 5 positive. *The Herald* (Melbourne), 31 August, pp. 1, 2.

Moyers, B. (1993). *Healing and the mind.* Doubleday, New York.

Mulley, A. G. (1984). The triage decision. In S. J. Reiser and M. Anbar (eds), *The machine at the bedside*, Cambridge University Press, Cambridge, pp. 221–6.

Muyskens, J. L. (1982). *Moral problems in nursing: a philosophical investigation.* Rowman & Littlefield, Totowa, New Jersey.

National Health and Medical Research Council (1990). *Discussion paper on ethics and resource allocation in health care.* AGPS, Canberra.

National Health and Medical Research Council Working Party on General
Guidelines on Informed Decisions about Medical Interventions (1991).
*General guidelines for medical practitioners on providing information to
patients. Preliminary discussion paper.* AGPS, Canberra.
Ombudsman Victoria (1988). *15th Annual Report*, 30 June 1988. Government
Printer, Melbourne.
O'Sullivan, J. (1983). *Law for nurses*, 3rd edn. The Law Book Company,
Sydney.
Parker, R. (1974). A definition of privacy. *Rutgers Law Review* 27 (2),
pp. 275–96.
Petrie, C. (1993). Down but not out for health complaints system in New South
Wales. *Health Issues*, March, pp. 23–4.
Rees, S. J. and Gibbons, L. (1986). *A brutal game: patients and the doctors'
dispute.* Angus & Robertson, North Ryde, NSW.
Report of the Cervical Cancer Inquiry (1988). Prepared by the Committee of
Inquiry into Allegations Concerning the Treatment of Cervical Cancer at
National Women's Hospital and Other Related Matters. Government
Printing Office, Auckland, New Zealand.
Request to die (1985). *Bioethics News* 5 (1), October.
Rice, S. (1988). *Some doctors make you sick.* Angus & Robertson, Sydney.
Roberts, M. (1987). The nurse as an advocate between patient and family.
*Proceedings of the conference, 'The Role of the Nurse: Doctors' Handmaiden,
Patients' Advocate or What?* Centre for Human Bioethics, Monash
University, 16 November, pp. 98–111.
Robertson, G. (1981). Informed consent to medical treatment. *The Law
Quarterly Review* 97, January, pp. 102–26.
Robinson, G. and Merav, A. (1983). Informed consent: recall by patients tested
postoperatively. In S. Gorovitz, R. Macklin, A. L. Jameton, J. M. O'Connor
and A. Sherwin (eds), *Moral problems in medicine*, 2nd edn, Prentice Hall,
Englewood Cliffs, New Jersey, pp. 182–6.
Ronalds, C. (1989). *Residents' rights in nursing homes and hostels: final report.*
AGPS, Canberra.
Roth, L. H., Meisel, A. and Lidz, C. W. (1983). Tests of competency to consent
to treatment. In S. Gorovitz, R. Macklin, A. L. Jameton, J. M. O'Connor and
A. Sherwin (eds), *Moral problems in medicine*, 2nd edn, Prentice Hall,
Englewood Cliffs, New Jersey, pp. 172–9 (reprinted from *American Journal
of Psychiatry* 134 (4), pp. 279–84).
Royal Australian Nursing Federation (Vic.) (1987). Position paper: patients' bill
of rights. In Royal Australian Nursing Federation, *Ethics in perspective*, vol.
1, RANF, Melbourne, pp. 123–6.
Royal Australian Nursing Federation (WA) (1987). Position paper: patients' bill
of rights. In Royal Australian Nursing Federation, *Ethics in perspective*, vol.
1, RANF, Melbourne, pp. 119–22.
Russell, H. (1987). What you don't know can hurt. *Health Issues*, 11,
September, pp. 17–19.
Sade, R. M. (1983). From 'Medical care as a right: a refutation'. In S. Gorovitz,
R. Macklin, A. L. Jameton, J. M. O'Connor and A. Sherwin (eds), *Moral
problems in medicine*, 2nd edn, Prentice Hall, Englewood Cliffs, New Jersey,
pp. 532–5.
Schauble, J. and Willox, I. (1987). Government reviews law on consent to
medical treatment. *The Age*, 21 August, p. 19.
Sheehan, M. and Wells, D. (1985). The allocation of medical resources. In C. L.
Buchanan and E. W. Prior (eds), *Medical care and markets: conflicts
between efficiency and justice*, George Allen & Unwin, Sydney, pp. 55–69.
Skinner, B. F. (1973). *Beyond freedom and dignity.* Penguin Books,
Harmondsworth, Middlesex, England.

Social Development Committee (Vic.) (1986). *First report on inquiry into options for dying with dignity.* March, Government Printer, Melbourne.

Social Development Committee (Vic.) (1987). *Inquiry into options for dying with dignity: second and final report.* April, Government Printer, Melbourne.

Somerville, M. (1986). Rights to, in and against medical treatment. *Bioethics News* 5 (3), April, pp. 5–17.

Spitzer, R. B. (1988). Meeting consumer expectations. *Nursing Administration Quarterly* 12 (3), pp. 31–9.

Staunton, P. and Whyburn, B. (1993). *Nursing and the law*, 3rd edn., W. B. Saunders/Baillière Tindall, Sydney.

Stone, D. (1991). Hospitals forced to use cleaners as interpreters. *The Sunday Age*, 10 February, p. 4.

Swenson, D. F. (1981). The dignity of human life. In E. D. Klemke (ed.), *The meaning of life*, Oxford University Press, New York, pp. 20–30.

Task Force on Patients' Rights: First Report (1987). South Australian Health Commission, Adelaide.

The Age (1987). A case for compassion. Editorial, 12 February, p. 13.

Thomson, J. J. (1975). The right to privacy. *Philosophy and Public Affairs* 4 (4), Summer, pp. 295–314.

Transcultural Health Care Council Inc. (Vic.) (1988). *3rd Annual Report, 1987–1988.* Transcultural Health Care Council, Melbourne.

United Nations (1978). *The International Bill of Human Rights*, United Nations, New York.

Uyer, G. (1986). Effect of nursing approach in understanding of physicians' directions, by mothers of sick children in an out-patient clinic. *International Journal of Nursing Studies* 23 (1), pp. 79–85.

Vandeveer, D. (1980). The contractual argument for withholding medical information. *Philosophy and Public Affairs* 9 (2), pp. 198–205.

Victorian Health Services Commissioner Annual Report 1991. Flash Print, Melbourne.

Victorian Ministerial Women's Health Working Party Report (1987). *Why women's health? Victorian women respond.* Government Printer, Melbourne.

Walker, Q. J. and Langlands, A. O. (1986). The misuse of mammography in the management of breast cancer. *Medical Journal of Australia* 145, 1 September, pp. 185–7.

Wallace, M. (1991). *Health care and the law: a guide for nurses.* The Law Book Company, North Ryde.

Wallace, M. (1992). Meeting the challenge of patients' rights: a legal perspective. *Proceedings of the conference 'Meeting the Challenge of Patients' Rights — Issues for the 1990s'*, RMIT Faculty of Nursing, Nursing Law and Ethics, 4th Victorian State Conference, held 20 November, Dallas Brooks Hall, Melbourne, Royal Melbourne Institute of Technology, Faculty of Nursing, Melbourne.

Chapter

8

The question of
nurse–patient advocacy

ONE OF THE MOST COMPLEX QUESTIONS to confront nurse theorists and
practitioners over recent years has been the question of patient
advocacy, and the extent — if any — to which nurses should
assume the role of patients' advocate. The need to address the
advocacy question has become somewhat pressing in the light of
increasing and ongoing developments of and reliance on scientific
medical technology, and the impact these have had on patients'
rights generally.

During the twentieth century, particularly since the 1960s, the
Western world has witnessed spectacular advances in the development and use of medical technologies, which have come to represent an awesome optimism (sometimes false, sometimes not) for
therapeutic success. These technologies include new drugs, new
and sophisticated machinery, perfected palliative and curative
medical and surgical procedures, and the establishment and
development of 'new organisations and support systems for the
purposes of delivering technological medical therapies and cares'
(Bates and Lapsley 1985, p. 1). The flood of medical technology has,
for some, also come to represent a welcome escape from the many
troubling dilemmas all too often posed by the uncertainties of
disease and illness (Bursztajn et al. 1984, p. 183). Whether medical
technology does, in fact, offer such an escape is another question
entirely.

Despite its apparent successes, medical technology has received
enormous criticism. Its methods have been criticised on the
grounds of its dehumanising impact and its seeming disregard for
human dignity. Its efficacy has been challenged on the grounds
that it has caused widespread iatrogenesis and, equally disturbing,
has not been properly evaluated (Bates and Lapsley 1985; Bates
and Linder-Pelz 1987; McKinlay 1984; Mendelsohn 1979; Kingston
1992). In short, rather than promoting human values, rights and

interests, medical technology has, according to its critics, seriously undermined these.

Proponents of medical technology have responded to these criticisms by arguing that, far from undermining human values, medical technology merely requires 'that human values be exercised or pursued more intelligently', and, it might be added, more responsibly (Mitcham and Grote 1978, p. 1642). Thus, it is not technology in itself that has erred, but rather those who have used it.

In discussing medical technology it is important that its effects and impact on human values and human well-being are kept in proper perspective. For example, while it is true that many people have suffered at the hands of medical technology, it is equally true that many people have benefited from it. The relief obtained from taking a simple aspirin, the grief spared by the prevention of diseases through effective immunisation, and the control of some disease processes through effective scientific diagnoses and treatment all stand as specific instances. What this point wisely instructs is that a careful distinction needs to be made between technology *as such* (i.e. technology viewed as an *object*), and technology's *use* (i.e. as *knowledge, process* or *volition*), together with the *conditions* under which it is actually used (Mitcham and Grote 1978, p. 1638). Making this distinction will, in turn, help to clarify that it is not the mere existence of medical technology that carries the potential for creating profound moral conflict, but rather its unjustified discriminate and/or indiscriminate uses (and non-uses) that do so.

The problem of moral conflict involving the use (or non-use) of medical technology becomes particularly acute in situations where, for example:

1. it has not been used or has been withdrawn when patients (or their advocates) have wished it to be used;

2. it has been used when the patients (or their advocates) have not wished it to be used;

3. it has been used, but not in a way that patients (or their advocates) have expected or intended it to be used — for example, it may have been more painful or more inconvenient than expected, or, more seriously, it may not have had the therapeutic effect or outcome that patients (or their advocates) hoped to receive.

In other words, medical technology becomes morally troubling when its use or non-use does not accord with the recipient's (the patient's) considered preferences and health goals, or does not achieve a morally desirable outcome. And it is here that serious questions arise concerning patients' rights and interests, and the mechanisms which might be usefully employed for either upholding or enforcing these.

The notion of nurse–patient advocacy

Rightly troubled by the threat that an uncritical or unjust use of medical technology poses to patients' rights and interests, and by the many instances in which patients' interests and well-being have been seriously compromised by its controversial uses and non-uses, the nursing profession has sought to explore and develop a number of ways in which it can be more effective in promoting the interests and well-being of patients in health care domains. One of the nursing profession's responses has been to argue that the nurse has a legitimate and unique role to play as a *patient's advocate*. This is particularly so in situations where the patient is being denied the opportunity to exercise truly self-determined choices.

Defending the notion of nurse–patient advocacy has involved at least four important philosophical activities, most notably:

1. formulating, establishing and developing acceptable criteria for determining just *what is* a patient's advocate;

2. arguing for and defending the *need* for a true patient's advocate in health care contexts;

3. debating and defending a hypothesis that nurses are in a *unique* position and are the ones *best suited* to act as patients' advocates;

4. clarifying the *conditions* and *circumstances* under which nurses acting as patients' advocates ought to fulfil their role.

Nursing literature to date strongly supports the notion of the nurse rightly assuming and fulfilling the role of a patient's advocate. Some authors even go so far as to suggest, controversially, that advocacy forms the very philosophical basis of nursing and, not least, the nurse–patient relationship (Curtin 1986; Gadow 1980). Others suggest that advocacy should be taught as a discrete subject in nursing courses — even at the expense of more structured courses in applied ethics (Kohnke 1982).

Despite its superficial attractiveness and popular acceptance among nurses (it has become almost a universal catchword among nurses in the Western world, and has been legitimised in several nursing codes of ethics), the notion of nurse–patient advocacy is vulnerable to philosophical criticism. Its main weakness is that, as it stands, it is plagued by a number of serious theoretical flaws, partly because little or poor attention has been given to establishing sound philosophical bases for both the *concept* of advocacy and the *role* which depends on it. The validity and moral force of advocacy has been, in a somewhat question-begging fashion, merely assumed rather than critically determined. In an attempt to support their views, nurse theorists have tended to rely on colourful rhetoric rather than sound philosophical argument. As a result, they have largely failed to defend convincingly the four important philosophical activities mentioned. Nurse theorists, in defending the need for advocacy, have tended to ignore the possibility of employing other more reliable mechanisms for ensuring that the significant moral interests of patients are maximised in health care contexts. Second, as to whether nurses really are in a unique position to act as patients' advocates, arguments tend to reject the notion that *others*, for example, a patient's spouse or family, or other attending health care professionals, might likewise have a role to play as a patient's advocate. Third, there is, for example, always room to question whether nurses are morally and professionally bound to assume and fulfil the role of advocate. With regard to the question of whether nurses are the ones *best suited* for the role of advocate, it will be recalled that, in the New Zealand Cervical Cancer Inquiry, the Commissioner ruled that, while nurses 'most appropriately should be the advocate for the patient', they generally felt too 'intimidated' by medical staff, and for this reason could not be relied upon to be effective patient advocates (Bickley 1988). Lastly, nurse theorists have failed to show convincingly that patients do in fact *want* nurses to act as their advocates. I can think of many examples where patients would most certainly not want attending nurses to act as advocates on their behalf, and where attending nurses would have been incapable of acting as advocates. This has been particularly evident in cases involving culturally different persons whose health beliefs and practices have been quite at odds with those of the attending nurses, and the nature of which nurses have failed abysmally to understand (see also Kanitsaki 1983, 1988a, 1993; Johnstone and Kanitsaki 1991).

One important point to be gleaned from these four concerns is that while advocacy may be a worthy notion, and one warranting serious attention by the nursing profession, it should not be accepted uncritically in its present form. If it is to be accepted, careful attention should first be given to its philosophical basis and content — else we risk falling prey to a corrupting metaphor or, equally bad, building an empire on an empty and meaningless neologism.

In the remainder of this chapter, an attempt is made to answer the questions: what is the substantive nature of nurse–patient advocacy; how should the notion of nurse–patient advocacy be structured (i.e. how should it be constituted and what should its philosophical content be); and, finally, what can be done to ensure that nurse–patient advocacy fulfils its task of protecting and upholding important human values and interests in health care domains?

What is advocacy?

In critically examining the nature of advocacy, it is instructive to first give some consideration to both its historical and conventional usage in the English language.

The word 'advocate' has been in use since the early 1300s. It comes from the Latin *advocatus* and the old French *avocat*, meaning 'one summoned or "called to" another, especially one called in to aid one's cause in a court of justice'. *The Oxford English dictionary* defines 'advocate' as:

> [1] One whose profession it is to plead the cause of anyone in a court of justice ... [2] One who pleads, intercedes, or speaks for, or in behalf of, another; a pleader, intercessor, defender ... [3] One who defends, maintains, publicly recommends, or raises his [sic] voice in behalf of a proposal or tenet ... [4] The secular defender or 'patron' of a church or religious house.

Advocacy is defined as:

> [1] The function of an advocate; the work of advocating; pleading for or supporting ... [2] Advocation ...

'Advocation' is defined by the *Oxford English dictionary* as:

> [1] A calling of people to council; a summoning or convocation; [2] The calling of an action before itself by a superior [e.g. Papal] court; [3] The act of calling to one's aid; an appeal (for aid or defence); [4] The function of an ADVOCATE (1, 2) or pleader; pleading, advocacy, advocateship; [5] ... the function or office of a patron; guardianship, protection or patronage of a church, or benefice; right of presentation to a living.

As a point of interest, the now obsolete term 'advocatess', meaning a 'female advocate' derives from the medieval Latin *advocatissa*, 'patroness of a benefice' (*Oxford English dictionary* 1961).

Modern usage of the terms advocate and advocacy tends typically to refer to a courtroom situation where an agent, usually a lawyer, pleads the cause of another. (Note that in the Scottish city of Aberdeen, the term advocate is used as a local title for a solicitor.) While the legal sense of the term advocacy is the one most popularly used, it is not the only sense or context in which it can be meaningfully employed. Nothing suggests that lawyers have, or should have, a monopoly on the term's usage (as some would perhaps contend), which helps to collapse the popular objection sometimes raised in the advocacy debate that advocacy is rightly and solely the domain of lawyers (or even physicians), and thus something which nurses (or any other health care professionals, for that matter) have no business or legitimacy in pursuing.

Given that others besides lawyers and physicians can have a valid role to play in 'pleading the cause of another' (in this instance, patients) the question remains of what particular sense or senses of advocacy nurses should adopt (if any) in their attempts to uphold important human values and interests in health care contexts. It is also important to assess whether a non-legal sense of the term would necessarily offer nurses the tool they are seeking in order to explain and strengthen the philosophical basis of the nurse–patient relationship.

In seeking possible answers to these questions, attention will be given to three popular nursing views on advocacy and the role of the nurse as a patient's advocate. Before considering these, it should be noted that there are many other views on patient advocacy, some of which not only contradict but also seriously compete with each other. Unfortunately, there is not space here to consider all these. Thus, for the purposes of this discussion, consideration is given to the views of only three influential writers: Leah Curtin (1986), Sally Gadow (1980) and Mary Kohnke (1982). The views of each of these authors are critically examined separately and then collectively in an attempt to explore more fully the philosophical notion of patient advocacy, as well as some of the implications of holding that notion as unique to nursing philosophy.

Leah Curtin and the notion of 'human advocacy'

In her celebrated essay 'The nurse as advocate: a philosophical foundation for nursing', Leah Curtin (1986, p. 12) argues that '[t]he end or purpose of nursing is the welfare of other human beings', and further that '[t]his end is not a scientific end, but rather a moral end'. The moral nature of nursing, she suggests, is derived from the involvement of nurses with other human beings (in this instance patients), the actual relationship they (nurses) have with those human beings (patients), and the promotion in that relationship of what is mutually seen (by both the nurse and the patient) as good — notably, health.

Recognising a need to protect the 'humanity of the sufferer' when it is threatened by the effects of illness, Curtin rejects both the patients' rights and legal concepts of advocacy, proposing instead a new concept of advocacy, which she calls 'human advocacy' (p. 14). Human advocacy, she argues, is fully derived from the *common* humanity, *common* needs and *common* human rights that nurses and patients share. And it is this very 'commonality' in humanity which gives rise to the need for advocacy, and which stands to compel nurses to accept human advocacy as the very foundation of the nurse–patient relationship. (Whether this 'commonality' between nurse and patient is as substantive as Curtin suggests, and whether it does, in fact, have the moral force to oblige nurses to accept human advocacy as the basis of the nurse–patient relationship, is, however, another issue altogether; it is likely that cultural anthropology and moral philosophy would both yield quite a different analysis to that suggested by Curtin.) That nurses are uniquely qualified as human advocates is explained by Curtin as being precisely because nurses attend patients for 'sustained periods of time' and provide patients with 'intimate details of physical and emotional care', and thus have the opportunity to gain knowledge and experience of patients as unique human beings. By experiencing patients as unique human beings, Curtin argues, nurses are particularly qualified to act uniquely as human advocates.

What is the proper role of the human advocate? For Curtin, it is simply to 'create an atmosphere that is open to and supportive of the individual's decision making' (p. 19). By doing this, Curtin suggests, nurses will be performing their 'greatest service' to patients and their families. She concludes that human advocacy is not only simple but, controversially, 'as natural as living and dying' (Curtin 1986, p. 19). Curtin's notion of human advocacy is an interesting one, which will undoubtedly find appeal among those who are opposed to a positivistic approach to moral conduct and support a more relational ethic of care. Nevertheless, at least three important objections to it can be raised.

The first is her troubling insistence on drawing a firm distinction between human rights and patients' rights. What this distinction fails to recognise, however, as clarified in chapter 7 of this text, is that patients' rights are merely a subcategory of human rights, and that nothing can really be gained by drawing a firm distinction between them. While this observation might not collapse her thesis, it certainly raises some serious questions about its reliability and usefulness.

A second troubling concern is Curtin's insistence that nurses are in a *unique* position to act as patients' advocates. Just why nurses are uniquely placed — as opposed to other health care professionals, or other lay persons, for that matter — to experience patients as unique human beings, or to act as human advocates, Curtin does not convincingly show. Her reasoning plainly ignores the reality that no single nurse (except in some very exceptional circumstances) spends a total 24-hour period with a patient. And even within a shift of eight, ten or twelve hours, it is doubtful that a nurse spends the time with a patient that is necessary for gaining an 'intimate knowledge' of the patient, much less a unique or 'holistic' view (as time and motion studies already suggest). Even in ordinary life, two people can live together for years and still not know all there is to know about each other — including the kinds of choices each would be likely to make in a health crisis. Given this, there is something absurd and naive in suggesting that nurses, *as* nurses, are in a unique position to come to know the patient intimately as a unique human being. It is certainly doubtful that the nurse is in any better position than anybody else in terms of knowing a patient intimately enough to assume the role of that patient's advocate.

A third and final concern relates to Curtin's provocative and highly controversial claim that human advocacy is 'as natural as living and dying'. Leaving aside the philosophical difficulties of how the notion 'natural' should be interpreted, given the extraordinary demands that may be placed on an advocate, and the skills required to fulfil such a role competently and effectively, there is every indication, as Kohnke's work shows, that advocacy is very much an *acquired* role, demanding learned skills, not just a *natural* role, as Curtin asserts.

Gadow and the notion of existential advocacy

A second respected and influential author on the subject of advocacy is Sally Gadow. In her widely acclaimed article 'Existential advocacy: philosophical foundation of nursing', Gadow (1983), like Curtin, argues that advocacy is the 'philosophical foundation and ideal of nursing' (p. 42). Like Curtin, she also contends that advocacy determines the actual form that the nurse–patient relationship should take. Rejecting both the concept of advocacy as implied in patients' rights movements (what she calls 'consumer advocacy') and the concept of advocacy *in extremis* as upheld by paternalism, Gadow further argues that nurses should not masquerade as a 'bill of rights brochure', but rather should engage themselves in actively assisting individuals 'to authentically exercise their freedom of self-determination' (p. 45). Implicit in Gadow's view here is the notion that, unless individuals (patients) exercise their freedom of self-determination (for her, the most fundamental and valuable of human rights), their integrity (their wholeness) as persons will be seriously and unjustly compromised. With regard to the role of the existential advocate, Gadow makes it quite clear that this:

> is not based on an assumption about what individuals *should want* to do, nor does it consist in protecting individuals' *right* to

do what they want. It is the effort to help persons *become clear about what they want* to do, by helping them discern and clarify their values in the situation, and on the basis of that self-examination, to reach decisions which express their reaffirmed, perhaps recreated, complex of values. Only in this way, when the valuing self is engaged and expressed in its entirety, can a person's decision be actually *self*-determined instead of being a decision which merely is not determined by others.

(Gadow 1983, p. 46)

Gadow's thesis does contain some persuasive arguments, and the notion of assisting individuals 'to authentically exercise their freedom of self-determination' does have some merit, but only in so far as *authenticity* holds as a condition of autonomy (see Faden and Beauchamp 1986, pp. 262–8). Nevertheless, her thesis is vulnerable to criticism. First, Gadow does not adequately show why, if at all, the supposed right to self-determination is (if, indeed, it is) *the* most valuable and important human right. As discussed elsewhere in this text, morally compelling instances sometimes rightly require that a person's autonomous wishes be overridden. Furthermore, as also discussed in this text, there is something profoundly historically and culturally odd in holding autonomy as being *the* most important value (Faden and Beauchamp 1986, p. 18). Second, Gadow does not convincingly show how a *human rights* claim to self-determination differs significantly from a *patients' rights* claim to self-determination. I suspect that, like Curtin, she has not understood that patients' rights are merely a subcategory of human rights, and therefore share common properties with human rights.

A third criticism is that Gadow fails to show convincingly just what is to count as 'authentically exercising one's freedom of self-determination'. The notion of authenticity used by Gadow here seems to rely on its somewhat existential sense, of being '*one's own*' (as in 'one's own' values, beliefs, motivations, choices, actions). This sense, however, is so inherently vague, and open to such a multitude of interpretations, that its worth as a component in any advocacy doctrine is at best dubious, and at worst unhelpful. One obvious question which arises here is: can nurses be relied upon to assist fully a patient to exercise truly authentic choices? For example, nurses might set about assisting patients to make an authentic and *self-determined* choice. What nurses fail to realise, however, is that during the process of helping patients 'to become clear about what they want to do, by helping them discern and clarify their values in the situation' and so on, they might inadvertently exert manipulative or coercive influences over those patients, and so inadvertently influence the patients' choice. This, in turn, raises the additional question of whether it is necessarily wrong to benevolently 'manipulate' or 'coerce' another's choice — particularly if the choices that person is making are potentially harmful (an issue which is considered more fully in chapter 11 on suicide).

Then, of course, a further problem is posed by cultural difference. Not only might nurses be quite unable to assist culturally different patients to exercise an authentic choice, but they might set about doing it in a culturally inappropriate and thus harmful manner. (The risk of this happening is particularly high in situations where nurses do not know or understand the intricate cultural prescriptions and proscriptions governing patients.) For example, a nurse's chosen method of supporting and assisting (advocacy) might be quite foreign and even unacceptable to the culturally different patient, as Kanitsaki's (1993, 1994) discussion on what she calls the 'Family Cultural Advocacy Communication Model' makes plain. (See also the discussion on transcultural ethics in chapter 5 of this text.) The nurse might have feelings of being genuinely concerned and of caring about a patient, but, as Kanitsaki repeatedly emphasises in her work, these are not always reliable guides towards ensuring the cultural appropriateness of professional behaviour. Consider, for example, the patient who belongs to a traditional cultural group and who values collective decision making within the group above so-called 'individual' decision making (Kanitsaki, 1988b; see also Johnstone and Kanitsaki 1991). In such cases, it would be quite inappropriate for a nurse to set about assisting that patient to exercise an 'authentic' (which in non-traditional cultures almost always means *individual*) decision. For such a patient, a choice would be 'authentic' if, and only if, it derived from shared values and beliefs, and the *collective* thinking and decision-making processes of the *collective family group* (Kanitsaki, 1988b, 1993, 1994).

There is undoubtedly room for caution in holding that an individual (in this instance, a patient) could, especially in an institutional health care context, ever exercise a truly 'authentic choice' — irrespective of the information received for the purposes of, and the assistance given in, making such a choice. Assistance and information, by their very nature, stand to significantly influence choice, and it is doubtful that in health care contexts they could ever be given *impartially*. In other words, the whole notion of 'authenticity' in patient decision making needs to be seriously questioned. As argued elsewhere, the very selection of 'relevant' information or the 'helpful' recommendation of a 'treatment of choice' or a 'preferred drug', or the like, all import value judgments (Johnstone 1988; Fisher 1988; Veatch 1987).

There are other difficulties in the case of patients whose prudence and capacity to make critically reflective choices have been clouded by, for example, pain, grief, fear, anxiety and drug administration. In such cases, all the support and assistance in the world would probably contribute little to patients' exercising an *authentic* choice — at least in the 'one's own' sense. Gadow's thesis does little to rescue nurses faced with dilemmas of determining whether patients' choices are, in the final analysis, *authentic*, or what to do when patients exercise choices which, while autonomous, are not their 'own', so to speak — such as when patients are unduly influenced by pain, grief, anxiety and the like. It is evident that Gadow's notion of authenticity needs to be much more sophisticated if it is to be helpful to the formulation of a substantive theory of advocacy. Faden and Beauchamp's (1986, pp. 262–8) thesis of authenticity being 'reflective non-repudiation' (i.e. of personally held values, beliefs, motivations, and the like) offers some promise here.

Lastly, Gadow's thesis is vulnerable to the objection that what is of ultimate concern in this debate is not so much that individuals exercise authentic choices (this is only a part, though an important one, of overall moral endeavours), but that in exercising their choices individuals achieve morally desirable outcomes — the measure of which, incidentally, is a matter for *morality* to decide, not *advocacy*, as is shown in the following pages.

Kohnke and the notion of advocacy as informing and supporting the patient

The last influential author to be considered here is Mary Kohnke. In her popular text *Advocacy: risk and reality*, Kohnke (1982) argues that, unlike the lawyer advocate, who 'actually presents the client's case and either pleads for justice or defends the client from accusations' (p. 2), the role of the nurse advocate is simply to *inform* and *support* patients in whatever decision they make.

Informing, in this instance, is interpreted as supplying patients with the information they need in order to make informed decisions. Kohnke (1982, pp. 13–38) warns, however, that, before engaging in this activity, nurses must first decide whether they want to be advocates; whether they want clients to have the previously undisclosed information; whether they understand what it will mean personally to go through with the disclosure; and, lastly, whether they have the most up-to-date and relevant information to give to the patient (bearing in mind the ever-present legal as well as moral dangers of giving incorrect information, and of causing harm by disclosing information).

Supporting, on the other hand, consists of two roles, notably an *action* role and a *non-action* role (Kohnke 1982, pp. 26–7). The *action role* is described by Kohnke as being comprised of two functions: first, of *assuring* patients that they have both the *right* and the *responsibility* to make their own self-determining choices;

and, second, of *reassuring* patients that they do not have to 'give in to pressure from others to change [their] decisions if [they] do not choose to' (Kohnke 1982, pp. 26–7). The *non-action* role, on the other hand, demands that the advocate refrains 'from subtly undermining a patient's decision' — especially if it is a decision with which the advocate does not agree (Kohnke 1982, p. 27). Here Kohnke warns that the advocate must take great care not to move out of the 'advocacy role' into what she terms the 'rescuing role' — viz, of 'fighting patients' battles for them'. This, she suggests, would be not only inappropriate but also outright hazardous, unless the advocate had a legitimate authority base upon which to interfere with the actions of those others who are otherwise obstructing a patient's self-determining choices.

Kohnke's thesis rests on a number of controversial claims, which I will summarise. The first claim is that individuals have an absolute right to self-determination. The second claim is that ethics and professional codes are inadequate to protect this right. As a point of clarification, it should be noted that in her discussion Kohnke treats *ethics* and *codes of ethics* as synonymous. As clarified in chapter 2 of this text, however, these two notions are quite separate, and care should be taken to distinguish the two (see also Johnstone 1987). The third claim is that ethics and advocacy, while 'related', are clearly different. For Kohnke, the distinction is drawn on the basis that *ethics* speaks to the 'rescuer in us' — that is, urges us to rescue patients by making decisions for them and 'accepting the responsibility for [those] decisions' (p. 30) — whereas *advocacy* is simply 'the *process* of informing people so that they can make decisions and then supporting them in their decisions' (p. 75). Fourth, Kohnke claims that professional codes (and, as seems to be implied, ethics) are merely 'one aspect of the larger knowledge base of advocacy and the role of the advocate' (p. 3). Fifth, the claim is made that ethics does not *teach* the role of advocacy (p. 3). And, lastly, it is claimed that advocacy has the outstanding merit of acting as 'a bridge between ethics and law' — something which ensures that the legal requirements to inform a client *and* the moral requirements to honour a person's right to self-determination are both met (p. 89). This last claim is not only seriously misleading, however, but dangerous, since it ignores the important relationship that ethics has with law and the important role it plays in scrutinising morally bad laws and instructing their reform (see also the discussion on legal law in chapter 2 of this text); it also ignores the compelling force that morality exerts as an action guide in both health care domains and the 'ordinary world' .

Unlike Curtin and Gadow, Kohnke implicitly rejects the notion of advocacy being *natural*. Rather, as her book in itself stands to suggest, advocacy is very much a learned skill and, furthermore, very much involves an acquired (not a natural) role. Kohnke's work clarifies that, if nurses are to be effective patients' advocates, they must satisfy at least two important conditions: they must first have a number of important and necessary 'advocacy qualities'; and they must also have a very sound knowledge base. Thus advocates must, minimally, be informed; have access to relevant information; be able to determine available choices and probable consequences of those choices; be able to make decisions and assume responsibility for their outcomes; have the ability to communicate; be culturally sensitive; and have a broad knowledge base about people generally, about society (its values, norms and practices) and, not least, about social order (including legal laws governing professional practice) (Kohnke 1982, pp. 3–11).

Kohnke also goes to considerable lengths to point out that the role of the advocate is far from glamorous and in reality entails a number of serious hazards and risks, all of which need to be fully contemplated by nurses before they decide to assume the role of patients' advocate. These risks include: misinforming the patient; using an inappropriate method or approach when informing a patient; losing their job, or at least having their career prospects hampered (particularly if an advocacy action stands to violate certain institutional norms or even legal law); and the risk of the processes of sound and just decision making and patient support being totally disrupted by, for example, racism, ethnocentrism, ageism and sexism, or personal prejudice and bias, to name some, which may prevail and impinge on the advocate–patient relationship.

Kohnke's comprehensive approach to the issue of advocacy is commendable, most notably on account of its practical approach. Unfortunately, like those of other authors, her thesis is not entirely free of difficulties, and is vulnerable to at least three serious objections. First, in insisting on a firm distinction being drawn between ethics and advocacy, and in rejecting ethics as a significant contributor and force in assisting patients to exercise truly autonomous choices, Kohnke's entire notion of patient advocacy stands to be substantially weakened, and risks collapse as a coherent and compelling theory (as is shown shortly).

Second, her thesis is troubled by an internal logical contradiction and inconsistency. On closer analysis, for instance, it soon becomes evident that Kohnke, like Curtin and Gadow before her, has committed the logical error of holding that advocacy *both involves and does not involve* upholding patients' rights. As already discussed, Kohnke argues that the notion of advocacy she is advancing is *quite distinct from a patients' rights sense of the term.* And yet, despite this claim, her entire thesis rests precisely on a patients' rights claim — notably on the supposed *right to self-determination in health care contexts.*

Third, it is difficult to see how Kohnke's theory of advocacy differs significantly from a substantive moral theory of informed consent and the behaviours such a theory motivates in attending health professionals. It will be recalled from our discussion of patients' rights that the overriding moral imperative of any substantive theory of informed consent is to ensure that patients give voluntary (i.e. free of coercive or manipulative influences) and truly informed (i.e. based on relevant factual as well as ethical information) consents to medical treatment, nursing care and other health cares. It will also be recalled that, at best, all health professionals can do in decision-making situations is 'reflectively persuade' a patient about the benefits of a recommended therapy; they can never use coercion or manipulation — something which is wholly compatible with Kohnke's advocacy theory.

A critical examination of advocacy

Given the views of Curtin, Gadow and Kohnke, the question remains of whether advocacy does provide the philosophical basis of nursing, and whether it does stand as a coherent and comprehensive theory of the nurse–patient relationship. In attempting to answer this question, consideration will be given to critically examining a number of points which the views of these three authors have in common.

To start with, the very sense in which the term 'advocacy' may be meaningfully used needs to be examined. While it is true that the term/concept of advocacy can be meaningfully defined and used in a non-legal sense (as dictionary definitions make plain), it is far from clear that the new 'nursing-specific sense' formulated by the theorists discussed here is in any way meaningful if considered independently of a patients' rights sense of the term. Consider the following.

In defining advocacy, the theorists have gone to considerable lengths to reject the connotation of *consumerist* or *patients'* rights. Curtin argues, for example, that it is *human* rights which are at issue in the advocacy debate, not *patients'* rights. Gadow and Kohnke argue along similar lines. What this view fails to understand, however, to re-emphasise an earlier point, is that patients' rights are merely a subcategory of human rights, and as such share common features with human rights. In particular, they share the common feature of imposing corresponding duties onto others (i.e. either not to interfere with another's preferences, or to act positively to bestow benefits on that other). Thus, to distinguish between them would be to advance a logically inconsistent and contradictory position, and to risk the collapse of any theory which might be based on that distinction. Related to this is the additional point that, regardless of the status of patients' rights in relation to human rights, the nurse–patient relationship, as correctly pointed out by Curtin, is by its very nature a moral relationship, and thus imposes on nurses certain corresponding moral duties. Nurses are morally bound to fulfil the corresponding duties imposed upon them whether they desire to fulfil these duties or not. On this point, Kohnke's assertion that nurses *must first decide* whether they 'want' to be advocates, or 'want' the client to have certain information, and so on, should be viewed with suspicion, since if something is a moral duty of nurses then they *ought* morally to do it — regardless of any personal desires to the contrary. (In this instance *personal desires* are to be distinguished from *significant moral interests* which a duty-bound individual might otherwise have, and which might validly compete with a given moral duty, as the discussion on moral problems in chapter 5 helps to explain.)

A second troubling concern here is the implicit view (in Kohnke's case, the explicit view) that advocacy is distinct from, and perhaps even superior to, ethics. Kohnke (1982) makes the additional radical claim that ethics is inadequate since it is profession, time and culture relative, and since it does not teach advocacy (p. 3).

What is troubling about this view, however, is that it erroneously presumes that advocacy is *not* profession, time and culture relative — a claim which is extraordinary. As pointed out earlier, the very term advocate is recorded as having been in use only since the 1300s. Further to this, by all accounts, the notion of advocacy as first advanced by lawyers, and as now being advanced by nurse theorists, is every bit a product of 'professional culture'; furthermore, in the case of the nursing profession, had it not been for the multitude of problems generated by the dominance of 'medical culture', it is likely that patient advocacy discourse would never have found currency in nursing philosophy in the first place. Advocacy, then, is no less profession, time and culture relative than is ethics — and, even then, it is open to dispute whether ethics, in the Western philosophical sense, while admittedly culturally and historically relative, is as 'profession relative' as Kohnke claims. Ethics is here apparently confused with the more *parochial* forms of 'professional ethics', which, as already discussed in the preceding chapters of this text, are not generally regarded in moral philosophy as supplying reliable action guides.

Another troubling concern about the way advocacy has been defined by these authors is that it ignores the fundamental overriding nature of ethics, and its role in guiding conduct and overriding the self-interested preferences of attending health care professionals in practical contexts. It also ignores (against Kohnke's claim) the compelling force that a critically reflective moral schema has in terms of directing and indeed instructing or 'teaching' autonomous moral agents how best to respond and act in morally significant human relationships (in this instance, the nurse–patient relationship). In short, the new nursing-specific sense of advocacy, as advanced by nurse theorists, fails to capture the essence of moral commitment and obligation. Further, it fails to show why supporting patients' attempts to make self-determined choices is the only moral interest that advocates should aim to protect. (For example, there is room to argue that advocates should aim to protect patients from suffering unnecessary harm — even if this means, in defiance of Kohnke, 'fighting patients' battles for them' (1982, p. 27). And, while it claims to be a device for protecting certain interests a patient might have (most notably of being informed and supported when attempting to make self-determined choices), it also fails to show convincingly that this, in fact, is its *real* intention, and, further, that it is an effective mechanism for achieving those outcomes.

On this note, it seems pertinent at this point to raise the questions of what really is the ultimate purpose of formulating a unique concept of advocacy and what its practical application is supposed to achieve.

There are at least two possible answers here: either advocacy aims to achieve a *metaphor of power* for nurses (and one which might be useful as a political bargaining chip for furthering the interests of the nursing profession [Winslow 1984; Clay 1987, pp. 38–54; Bandman and Bandman 1985]); or it aims to provide a *reliable mechanism for upholding and protecting a patient's considered preferences* and/or *perceived best interests*.

If we accept the first answer, we are left in the morally uncomfortable position of engaging in a kind of 'moral bartering' — using the issue of patients' rights and interests as a kind of 'moral capital' for buying, or as a means for furthering, the nursing profession's ends. If this is the case, it seems that nurses have fallen prey to a corrupting metaphor and to being mischievously led along the path of moral error. If we accept the latter answer, however, we are left in an equally untenable position. For if advocacy is, after all, a mechanism for upholding and protecting patients' considered preferences (as the theorists discussed contend), then it is not clear that any meaningful distinction can be drawn between advocacy per se, and a sound critically reflective morality which demands, among other things, that it 'maximise a person's considered preferences,' or 'respect that person as a self-determining chooser,' or the like. In short, unless the concept of advocacy itself can be shown to have a sound philosophical basis (and to carry the force of an overriding moral command), it may be that it is, in the final analysis, nothing more than an empty and meaningless neologism.

This discussion so far demonstrates that, unless advocacy is clearly articulated as a substantive moral concept (and one which carries an overriding morally prescriptive force), it will never provide a sound philosophical basis for the nurse–patient relationship, or any other health professional–patient relationship for that matter. Furthermore, while advocacy remains morally void, so to speak, it will always remain open to nurses to ask: 'Why should I be an advocate?' or 'Why should I inform or support this patient or that patient'? — questions which only a substantive *moral* theory can answer, not a theory of advocacy per se. Even if advocacy is clearly articulated as a moral concept, it still may not escape criticism, and may yet collapse under the objection that, from a moral point of view, at least, it is, quite simply, redundant. For example, if questions pertaining to its purpose can be answered only by appealing to the concepts and language of morality — and the prevailing forces of sound, critically reflective moral principles (such as autonomy, justice, beneficence and non-maleficence) — it would seem that we are committed to accepting (against advocacy's proponents) that it is not advocacy that is at the seat of moral initiative and a morally appropriate attitude in the nurse–patient relationship, but rather a substantive and critically reflective morality. This point finds further support when it is recognised that nurses' duty to respect patients' interests in exercising self-determined choices derives *not* from their role as advocates per se, but from the ultimate moral values and standards that govern the nurse–patient relationship and that come into play from the very moment of its inception. Thus, given that contemporary notions of advocacy are neither morally articulate nor morally compelling, it seems reasonable to conclude that the philosophical basis of the nurse–patient relationship is not advocacy but a sound and critically reflective ethic.

A third and final objection to be considered here is in response to the claim that nurses are in a *unique* position to act as patients' advocates. What such a view presumes is that nurses not only have the skills required to be effective advocates, but are also in a position of authority to be so. It also seems to presume, as briefly mentioned earlier, that others who have a morally significant relationship with the patient (such as the patient's family or close friends or other allied health workers) do not have any advocacy-type responsibilities or duties toward the patient. Given the broader demands of a sound professional ethic, it is highly questionable to assert that others do not have any discrete or independent responsibilities towards the patient they are caring for. If advocacy is, contrary to the objections raised here, a reliable mechanism for protecting patients' interests (in particular, in exercising autonomous and authentic choices), then surely this is a role which *everybody* who has a morally significant relationship with a given patient ought to fulfil — not just an attending nurse, or nurses in general. Given this, any claim by nurses to the effect that they *alone* have a unique role to play as patients' advocate deserves to be viewed with suspicion, not moral optimism, and should be challenged as incorrect and misleading.

Where, then, does this leave the concept and role of advocacy? Does advocacy have the power to achieve what it has supposedly been designed and promoted to achieve — notably, to assist individuals in exercising self-determined choices when in the role of a patient? More specifically, is advocacy really adequate to deal with the many other moral problems and crises that arise in health care contexts (such as those considered throughout this text), and that result in the violation of patients' rights or significant moral interests?

It is significant that patient advocacy as such finds no special consideration in contemporary bioethical literature, save for the issue of public advocacy in relation to the question of social justice and upholding the public good. Instead, discussion has tended to focus on patients' rights or interests, and on ways in which these might be protected or maximised. While nurses might well choose either to agree or disagree with this omission, they cannot afford to ignore it (see also Bernal 1992).

If advocacy is to be advanced as a credible theory, nurse theorists must turn their attention to developing sound philosophical arguments for its defence, and must not rely on mere metaphor or rhetoric. One possible solution here might be found in articulating advocacy as a coherent and comprehensive *moral* theory; that is, as a *subcategory of moral duty* rather than as a distinct and separate concept or theory in its own right. In developing the concept or theory of advocacy, nurses must also seriously consider the real moral issues at stake in relation to the difficulties experienced by individuals in their attempts to ensure that their significant moral interests are protected and promoted. There is surely far more to be gained by encouraging and engaging in honest, open and accessible debate about violations of patients' rights — i.e. human rights — in health care settings, than by advancing spurious and unhelpful philosophically flawed metaphors.

Issues and recommendations

Fulfilling one's duty may be extremely difficult, even for the morally best of us. This does not mean, however, that the demands of patients' rights and interests should be abandoned or discarded into the 'too-hard basket'. On the contrary, it simply means that helpful strategies aimed at better protecting patients' interests and well-being should be pursued more rigorously. As discussed elsewhere in this text, there are a number of helpful strategies which nurses and allied health professionals alike can employ. In summary, these include:

- educationally preparing *all* health professionals to respond better to their moral obligations to promote and protect patients' significant moral interests in health care contexts (education in this instance should not only include discrete, and relevant, courses in applied bioethics, but also in law, cultural anthropology, systematic decision making, interpersonal skills, communication skills, and the like);

- lobbying for law reform (particularly in areas which are intolerable to morally responsible nursing practice);

- pursuing excellence rather than mere competence in professional nursing practice;

- establishing reliable policies and guidelines for dealing with morally troubling situations in the health care environment;

- encouraging personal commitment by nurses to work actively towards improving the nursing profession as a whole, and recognising the collective responsibility that all nurses share in upholding the individual's, the group's and the community's good.

By implementing these and similar strategies, the nursing profession may well achieve its goals in terms of promoting patients' interests, and thus may ultimately succeed, to borrow from Curtin, in performing its greatest service to patients and their families, not to mention to the community as a whole.

———————————

An earlier version of this chapter was presented at the Mater Misericordiae Hospital's Expo Conference, 'Nursing and Technology', Brisbane, 2 September 1988. The paper has been revised for publication in this text.

———————————

References

Bandman, E. L. and Bandman, B. (1985). *Nursing ethics in the life span.* Appleton-Century-Crofts, Norwalk, Connecticut.

Bates, E. and Lapsley, H. (1985). *The health machine: the impact of medical technology.* Penguin Books. Ringwood, Victoria.

Bates, E. and Linder-Pelz, S. (1987). *Health care issues.* Allen & Unwin, Sydney.

Bernal, E. W. (1992). The nurse as patient advocate. *Hastings Center Report* 22 (4), pp. 18–23.

Bickley, J. (1988). What the cervical cancer inquiry report means for nurses. *New Zealand Nursing Journal* 81 (9), pp. 14–15.

Bursztajn, H. J., Hamm, R. M. and Gutheil, T. G. (1984). The technological target: involving the patient in clinical choices. In S. T. Reiser and M. Anbar (eds), *The machine at the bedside*, Cambridge University Press, Cambridge, pp. 177–92.

Clay, T. (1987). *Nurses: power and politics*. Heinemann Nursing, London.

Curtin, L. L. (1986). The nurse as advocate: a philosophical foundation for nursing. In P. L. Chinn (ed.) (1986), *Ethical issues in nursing*, Aspen Systems, Rockville, Maryland, pp. 11–20.

Faden, R. R. and Beauchamp, T. L. (1986). *A history and theory of informed consent*. Oxford University Press, New York.

Fisher, S. (1988). *In the patient's best interest: women and the politics of medical decisions*. Rutgers University Press, New Brunswick, New Jersey.

Gadow, S. (1983). Existential advocacy: philosophical foundation of nursing. In C. P. Murphy and H. Hunter (eds), *Ethical problems in the nurse–patient relationship*, Allyn & Bacon, Boston, pp. 40–58.

Johnstone, M.-J. (1987). Nursing and professional ethics. *Proceedings of the conference, 'The Role of the Nurse: Doctors' Handmaiden, Patients' Advocate or What?* Centre for Human Bioethics, Monash University, Melbourne, 16 November, pp. 18–44.

Johnstone, M.-J. (1988). Quality versus quantity of life: who should decide? *Australian Journal of Advanced Nursing* 6 (1), September–November, pp. 30–7.

Johnstone, M.-J. and Kanitsaki, O. (1991). Some moral implications of cultural and linguistic diversity in health care. *Bioethics News* 10 (2), pp. 22–32.

Kanitsaki, O. (1983). Acculturation — a new dimension in nursing. *Australian Nurses Journal* 13 (5), November, pp. 42–5, 53.

Kanitsaki, O. (1988a). Transcultural nursing: challenge to change. *Australian Journal of Advanced Nursing* 5 (3), March–May, pp. 4–11.

Kanitsaki, O. (1988b). Cancer and informed consent: a cultural perspective. Paper presented at seminar on Controversial Ethical Issues in Patients with Cancer, Heidelberg Repatriation General Hospital, 13 October, Melbourne.

Kanitsaki, O. (1989). Transcultural nursing. *Peter MacCallum Cancer Institute Annual Lecture* (presentation), 14 March 1989, Peter MacCallum Cancer Institute, Melbourne.

Kanitsaki O. (1993). Transcultural human care: its challenge to and critique of professional nursing care. In D. Gaut (ed.), *A global agenda for caring*, National League for Nursing Press, New York, pp. 19–45.

Kanitsaki, O. (1994). Cultural and linguistic diversity. In J. Romanini and J. Daly, *Critical care nursing: Australian perspectives*, W. B. Saunders/Baillière Tindall, Sydney, pp. 94–125.

Kingston, M. (1992). Prescriptions blamed for 900 deaths a year. *The Age*, 15 July, p. 1.

Kohnke, M. F. (1982). *Advocacy: risk and reality*. C. V. Mosby, St Louis.

McKinlay, J. B. (ed.) (1984). *Issues in the political economy of health care*. Tavistock Publications, New York.

Mendelsohn, R. S. (1979). *Confessions of a medical heretic*. Warner Books, New York.

Mitcham, C. and Grote, J. (1978). Technology. In W. T. Reich (ed.), *Encyclopedia of bioethics*, The Free Press, New York, pp. 1638–43.

Winslow, G. R. (1984). From loyalty to advocacy: a new metaphor for nursing. *Hastings Center Report* 14 (3), June, pp. 32–40.

Chapter

9

Matters of life and death: I

Abortion

THERE ARE NO ETHICAL ISSUES quite so emotionally charged as those involving matters of life and death. Television news media continue to depict anti-abortionists being dragged, kicking and screaming, from their protest positions outside lawful abortion clinics, and current affairs programs across the nation's radio and television networks compete with each other to bring into our living rooms the personal tragedies of strangers who are suffering painful and life-threatening diseases and seeking the option of active voluntary euthanasia. Punctuating these dramatic sequences are emotionally charged advertisements, sponsored by the Australian Kidney Foundation, inviting people to 'donate a life' (an invitation which, as we shall see later, can be interpreted in more ways than one). Sitting inconspicuously on the sidelines of these issues are politicians, not game to be seen taking a position one way or another for fear of political repercussions. Those politicians who do take a firm stand risk experiencing the negative consequences of doing so.

Nurses are no less affected by and no less involved in life and death matters than other health professionals or other members of the community. Yet their involvement, experiences and views are almost always ignored. This has been particularly so in relation to the controversial issues of abortion, euthanasia, suicide, Not For Resuscitation (NFR) orders, and organ transplantation. Although they are directly and actively involved in the care of patients at the centre of abortion, euthanasia, suicide, NFR, and organ transplantation decisions, nurses are expected not to question, not to have a view, not to complain, not to dissent, and in some instances not even to care or have feelings about the matters at hand. The cost of this attitude has been high. Because nurses' views and experiences have not been considered and responded to appropriately, they have had to bear intolerable and disproportionate moral as well as legal burdens, and have suffered enormously on both a personal and professional level as a result.

On a personal level, nurses have had to assist with and perform acts to which they have been opposed conscientiously; of those who have had the courage to take a stand, many have lost their jobs, or have had their career prospects seriously hampered, as examples already considered in this text have shown. In one notable case, nurses conscientiously opposed to abortion also experienced the indignity of being labelled as suffering from an acute *psychiatric disorder* (Char and McDermott 1972). On a professional level, standards of nursing care have been eroded and violated, reducing further the power and esteem of the nursing profession as a whole. So successful has been this erosion of professional morale in contexts involving matters of life and death, and the ethical issues arising from them, that many nurses feel quite unable to speak out. This is evident from the appalling lack of attention given to bioethical issues in the *Australian Nurses Journal* and the *New Zealand Nursing Journal* — both major Australasian nursing journals. It is significant, I think, that neither of these journals features regular columns on ethical issues in nursing practice. The *Australian Nurses Journal* has for years had a regular column addressing legal issues in nursing practice ('The nurse and the law'), but, as we know, legal law is quite distinct from moral law and the discipline of ethics, and the discussions given in this column have been quite inadequate in terms of addressing the many *ethical issues arising in*, and the *ethical aspects of*, clinical nursing practice.

In this and the following three chapters, an attempt is made to address six critical life and death issues — abortion, euthanasia, suicide, the quality of life question, 'not for resuscitation' (NFR) orders, and organ harvesting and transplantation — and to show how each has serious implications for nurse practitioners. It is hoped that, by addressing these issues, nurses will be able to take a strong and informed position on the need to effect positive structural change in the health care arena and to develop better policies and legislation governing health care and related practices.

Abortion — raising the issues

In January 1988, Canada shredded its 19-year-old abortion law. An article in the *Leader Post* signed 'The Canadian Press' (1988) reported that everyone was scrambling to gauge what this legislative reform would mean — 'particularly [to] *politicians* and *doctors* [italics added]'. It went on to report:

> Most authorities agree the ruling will not mean abortion on demand — at least not immediately and not ever in the sense that *doctors have the right to refuse* to perform the procedure [italics added].

(Canadian Press 1988)

In the 1200-word article reporting on this reform, not once is the term 'nurse' mentioned, nor is any thought given to the impact that the new liberal abortion laws might have on nurse practitioners generally. The Canadian Medical Association is reported as having 'advised its 45 000 members to honour the law until lawyers have studied the ruling', but no mention is made of any response from the Canadian Nurses Association. Pro-abortionist and anti-abortionist groups are widely quoted, as are eminent theologians and legal authorities — but no nurses.

In the United Kingdom, midwives have long been expected to participate actively in abortion work, and until the later 1980s this included supervising the abortion of fetuses of 24–28 weeks' gestation. As a result of the 28-week limit (permitted by abortion laws), abortions were resulting in viable births. In 1985, one midwife is reported have have confirmed that her unit had 'one [live] baby born under 28 weeks every three weeks' (*Nursing Times*, 24 July 1985, p. 5). Another midwife confirmed that viable births resulting from abortions were posing serious problems, not least that of forcing midwives and medical staff to 'decide how to dispose of live babies' (*Nursing Times*, 24 July 1985, p. 5). This intolerable situation prompted the question of whether nurses should be asked to participate in abortions of fetuses that might be capable of independent existence (Holmes 1988, p. 19). The problem was partially 'resolved' by the legislative reforms restricting the time limit for 'social' abortions to 18 weeks — where fetal viability is low (*Nursing Times*, 17 February 1988, p. 8).

The issue of abortion has, on the whole, proved to be both a complex and an unhappy one from a nursing perspective. In the past, nurses have been systematically discriminated against and have lost their jobs for refusing to participate in abortion procedures (Thompson and Thompson 1981, p. 84; Muyskens 1982, p. 59; Davis and Aroskar 1983, p. 129). Some states in the United States of America have since enacted legislation aimed at protecting individuals who conscientiously refuse to participate in abortion work by making it a felony for employers to dismiss employees (such as nurses) on grounds of conscientious objection (Davis and Aroskar 1983, p. 129). In the United Kingdom, abortion laws now permit nurses, by way of a 'conscience clause', conscientiously to refuse, in non-emergency situations, to participate in abortion work (Tschudin 1986; Rumbold 1986). In Australia, the banning of religious discrimination in public hospitals ensures that *believers*, at least, are not placed in 'situations of moral dilemma' (Broekhuijse 1988). The situation for *non-believers* is not clear, although most nurses I have spoken to have indicated that, on the whole, conscientious objection in cases involving abortion is reasonably well accepted in Australian hospitals, despite not being supported legally.

Despite these protective provisions and this general tolerance, however, nurses still suffer unfair discrimination, stereotyping and harassment if they have a moral objection to participating in abortion work. The International Council of Nurses (ICN) (1977), for example, cites the case of a midwifery student who had 'problems on ethical grounds' in assisting with abortion and sterilisation procedures. When the student approached the teaching hospital's director of nursing to discuss the matter, she was asked by the director of nursing why she had 'bothered' to come to the hospital to do her midwifery training at all. The student unsuccessfully tried to explain that, for her, midwifery did not entail assisting with abortions or sterilisations. Commenting on her eventual decision to withdraw from the midwifery course, the student wrote: 'Rather than continue in these sad circumstances I packed my bags and returned home the next day. I was a disappointed midwifery student but happy that I had taken the correct action' (International Council of Nurses 1977, p. 13).

In February 1988, a similar case occurred in Australia. The case involved a registered nurse and midwife who was allegedly refused employment at a large New South Wales rural hospital because she was conscientiously opposed to participating in abortion and sterilisation work (Broekhuijse 1988). The nurse had apparently been offered a position at the hospital concerned, and had written back accepting the offer. In her letter of acceptance, however, she pointed out that she was conscientiously opposed to abortion and sterilisation procedures, and that if she was asked to participate in such procedures she would exercise her right to refuse. To this, the director of nursing is reported to have replied: 'It would be quite impractical for you to be excluded from any involvement in the care of these patients' (Broekhuijse 1988, p. 13).

After several more letters had passed between the nurse and the director of nursing, and after the nurse had declined the offer of an alternative position, the original offer of employment was withdrawn. Interestingly, a New South Wales Health Department document is reported as stating that: 'In the case of junior *medical staff* [italics added] reasonable steps must be taken to reorganise work so as not to place individuals in situations of moral dilemma'

(Broekhuijse 1988). Whether this provision also applies to *nursing staff* is a point in question.

One of the most extraordinary examples of negative attitudes toward nurses who are opposed conscientiously to abortion is to be found in a 1972 article published in the *American Journal of Psychiatry*. The article in question, written by two psychiatrists, Walter Char and John McDermott, also provides a classic example of 'an ethical issue being translated into a technical problem which has a clinical solution'. As well as this, it vindicates feminist criticism of abstract objectivity, and of Western moral philosophy's arbitrary rejection of the emotions. Since this article provides such an important and compelling example of so many things, I make no apology for discussing and quoting from it at length.

On 11 March 1970, Hawaii became the first of the United States of America to liberalise its abortion laws, paving the way for abortion to be available virtually on demand. Psychiatrists applauded the reformed legislation, since it meant that society no longer required them 'to conjure up psychiatric reasons to justify abortion' (Char and McDermott 1972, p. 952). Within a month of the passage of the new abortion bill, however, many nurses began conscientiously to refuse to participate in abortion work, and some threatened resignation. This led to a chief of staff of a major hospital contacting the consulting psychiatrists, Walter Char and John McDermott, and requesting them to help 'deal with the acute psychological reactions of many of their nurses who were so upset by their abortion work' (some were in fact assisting with up to ten abortions a day) (Char and McDermott 1972, p. 952). Soon after, a second hospital also sought the assistance of these two psychiatrists. Char and McDermott (1972) later dubbed the crisis an 'acute *psychiatric* problem [italics added]' and one which 'no-one foresaw' would occur as a result of Hawaii legalising abortion.

It is perhaps not surprising that the psychiatrists in this case should perceive the nurses' *moral distress* as a *psychiatric problem*. Nevertheless, their overall analysis of the nurses' reaction deserves to be described as misguided and wrong.

Significantly, Char and McDermott 'found' that all of the nurses 'suffered from strong emotional reactions to their abortion work and welcomed the opportunity to talk about them' (p. 953). In support of this finding, they write:

> The nurses' strong reactions were a surprise to even some of them since many of them, including some of the Catholic nurses, appreciated the problem of unwanted pregnancies and had approved of the new abortion law before it went into operation. But once the nurses became *personally, intimately, and constantly involved* with abortions, their *intellectual* and *professional objective* attitudes favoring legalized abortions were

replaced by deeply *personal emotional reactions* so strong that many of them were *even* questioning the wisdom of the new law [italics added].

(Char and McDermott 1972, p. 953)*

Char and McDermott further stated that all the nurses showed symptoms of anxiety and depression:

They [the nurses] complained about being tired and being unhappy about their work; they cried *too easily* and got angry *too quickly*; they had difficulty sleeping and had bad dreams; during the day they found themselves preoccupied with disturbing thoughts about their abortion work; and they were *overly sensitive* when their friends teased them about working in a 'slaughter house'. One nurse *even* worried about what her mother [. . .] would think of her if she found out that she was working in an 'abortion mill' [italics added].

(Char and McDermott 1972, p. 9 53)*

The psychiatrists concluded that the nurses' 'symptomatology' fell into the category of 'a transient reactive disorder'. They pointed out, however, that only one nurse appeared to have a more 'severe psychiatric disability', manifested by her going about 'compulsively blessing dead fetuses' (a problem which they judged was caused by a pre-existing 'deep-seated emotional difficulty').

One of the disturbing features about this psychiatric assessment is that it assumes that the nurses' reaction to their abortion work was abnormal, and even pathological. Also disturbing is its overt disdain for emotion as a professional behaviour guide, and its rejection of the validity of being personally and intimately involved in one's work. The psychiatrists' labelling of the nurses' reactions as being over-sensitive is also disturbing: it would be interesting to know just what standard they used to measure this 'oversensitivity'. What is particularly noteworthy, however, is the case of the nurse 'compulsively blessing dead fetuses'. This nurse's cultural and religious background is not given. Placed in the context of strong cultural and religious beliefs, her actions might not seem so obviously the manifestation of psychiatric illness. As we saw in chapter 2, in the case of the young Maori woman who spontaneously aborted her twenty-week fetus, practices of 'compulsively blessing' dead or dying fetuses can have a perfectly reasonable explanation.

---

* From W. F. Char and J. F. McDermott (1972), Abortions and acute identity crisis in nurses, *American Journal of Psychiatry* 128 (8), pp. 952–7. © 1972, The American Psychiatric Association. Reprinted by permission.

Char and McDermott also 'found' that many of the nurses 'over-identified with the aborted fetus'. This, they reasoned, largely came about because in the wards fetuses of twelve to twenty weeks were mostly aborted. Abortions in these cases were procured by injecting saline into the uterus, causing labour and the subsequent expulsion of the fetus twelve to twenty-four hours later. Nurses working with patients having this type of abortion found it most disturbing 'to hold a well-formed aborted fetus with movement and with its eyes "still alive"' (Char and McDermott 1972, p. 953). Nurses involved in abortions procured by the dilation and curettage method were also deeply disturbed by seeing 'formed fetal parts such as hair and bits of limbs being sucked out or scraped out'. The psychiatrists concluded that this distress was quite unnecessary, and was largely the product of nurses 'over-identifying' with the fetus and projecting 'into the protoplasmic masses real, live, grown-up individuals' (p. 953). The psychiatrists also concluded that the nurses who over-identified the most with the aborted fetuses were themselves adopted, or had adopted children, or had had difficulty conceiving.

The leap in logic taken by Char and McDermott in making their assessments must not go unchallenged. Holding a little fetus, feeling it move, hearing it trying to 'cry' (something which usually only happens with older fetuses, those of around twenty weeks' gestation or more), seeing it trying to open its eyes (again, usually with the older fetuses), smelling its death, and the like, are not trivial experiences; nor are they particularly pleasant ones. The psychiatrists' report on nurses' comments do not in fact suggest that the nurses perceived the fetuses as 'grown-up individuals'; live, yes, but not 'grown up'. What they saw was a tiny and uniquely human form of life made vulnerable by medical intervention. This sight — as any delicate sight has the power to do — caused in the nurses feelings of emotion in exactly the same way that nurses observing the removal of 'beating hearts' from cadavers experience strong feelings of emotion. This feeling of emotion is hardly startling, and is in this case a highly questionable basis for making a sound psychiatric diagnosis. Yet a diagnosis was made, and the process effectively medicalised the nurses' emotions — something which all caring, sensitive and feeling people should view with concern.

A third diagnosis formulated by Char and McDermott was that 'the nurses felt hostile toward most of the abortion patients' (1972, pp. 953–4). This, they suggested, was largely influenced by the nurses 'own sexual problems', as well as the by nurses' difficulty in identifying positively with the abortion patients.

The 'catch-22' should be obvious here: on the one hand the nurses were accused of *over-identifying* with the aborted fetuses, and on the other of *under-identifying* with the aborting/aborted mothers. These nurses were thus firmly placed in a 'no-win' situation. It is doubtful whether any degree of identification with the aborting mothers would lessen the emotion provoked by the sight of a tiny moving fetus. Further, the assessment that the nurses' problems stemmed from their own sexual difficulties seems hardly a suggestion to be taken seriously. For instance, it is not difficult to imagine a nurse who has no sexual problems whatsoever still being overwhelmingly distressed by the sights likely to be witnessed during abortion work (including the sights of distressed and grieving mothers, as in cases involving therapeutic abortions of planned pregnancies).

Char and McDermott make one further controversial assessment of the nurses, notably that they 'suffered from an acute identity crisis regarding their nursing role and function' (pp. 954–5). This, the psychiatrists reasoned, occurred predominantly as a result of role conflict: on the one hand nurses were trained to save life; now they were being asked to assist in terminating life. This role conflict was exacerbated by the fact that the nurses, unlike doctors (including junior residents), did not have the option of refusing. The reasons given for nurses not having this option were solely practical ones, that is, 'whether she [sic] was in the operating room or on the floor, the nurse *had* [italics added] to cover whatever case came on her [sic] service' (p. 954). Further to this, the nurses claimed that 'many of the physicians were not as readily available to help in the care of abortion patients as with other patients' (p. 954) — a problem which still persists and in some cases is even legitimated by law (see in particular *Royal College of Nursing v. DHSS* (CA) [1981] AC 800; Rea 1981).

The psychiatrists' diagnosis of identity crisis and role conflict is, in my view, simplistic and open to serious question. The judgment of 'role conflict' in this instance erroneously presumes that the nurse is torn between two bona fide roles. If it can be shown, however, that one of the roles is not in fact a bona fide nursing role, the psychiatrists' diagnosis of role conflict and related identity crisis is immediately without basis. In this instance, it is open to serious question whether *assisting with an actual abortion procedure* (to be distinguished here from *caring for women who have had or are about to have an abortion*) is a bona fide nursing role. Nurses may well be able to fulfil a *practical role* in assisting with an actual abortion procedure, but this in no way implies that the role is a bona fide *professional nursing one*. This argument becomes persuasive when we consider the very concept and definition of nursing itself. *Nursing* is typically defined in terms of *caring* and *fulfilling a caring role* (see, for example, Watson 1985; Benner and Wrubel 1989). It is difficult to see, on the basis of this definition, how handing over a set of surgical instruments to a doctor performing an abortion, and/or counting a set of swabs after the procedure has been completed, is the fulfilment of a caring (viz nursing) role. If, for example, we analyse the tasks performed by assisting nurses during a surgical abortion procedure, we soon see that their role quickly reduces to being little more than *technical assistance* — nothing more, nothing less — and, what is more, of a kind that does not particularly draw upon *nursing* skills. While nurses may well use their learned skills during the pre-operative and post-operative/recovery stages, it is open to serious question whether they do so in an operating theatre situation. Against Char and McDermott, then, I would suggest that, at least in the case of surgical abortions performed in the operating theatre, it is not the nurse's role to assist. Even if it is conceded that nurses do have a role in assisting with abortion procedures, this still does not rescue Char and McDermott's diagnosis. For what the Hawaiian nurses were clearly suffering from in this case was not *role conflict* but fully fledged *moral conflict*, complete with all the psychological and moral distress associated with it.

Char and McDermott's solution to the abortion crisis came in the form of psychiatric therapy, notably abreaction, the use of psychiatrists as positive therapeutic figures, assisting nurses to establish a more positive identification with their patients, helping the nurse to 'regain objectivity' about abortions, and calling for the role, philosophy and ethics of nursing and medicine guiding abortion practices to be redefined.

The psychiatrists both felt they had been successful in resolving the crisis. They felt that they had been particularly effective in helping to 'bridge the gap that was separating the nurses from administrators and the medical staff and brought the hospital "family" closer together again' (p. 955). They also felt they had been successful in helping the nurses regain their 'objectivity', and to see 'again that what is aborted is a protoplasmic mass and not a real, live, grown-up individual' (p. 956). Char and McDermott conceded, however, that where nurses continue to 'react poorly' they should be transferred to another type of duty.

The treatment of this moral issue as a psychiatric problem to be solved by a clinical solution has parallels to the 'doubling' described by Robert Jay Lifton (1986) in his analysis of the Nazi doctors and their psychology of evil. What is disturbing about this case, however, is that the psychiatrists in question had the power to 'condition' a group of others (nurses) to 'double' — to see abortion not as a moral issue but as *good medicine*, and to see the fetus not as a *human form* but as a *protoplasmic mass*. It should be of some concern that psychiatrists have the legitimated authority to function in this way (see also Wikler and Barondess 1993).

It could be argued against the use of this example that the article was after all written a generation ago, and thus is somewhat outdated for the purposes of discussing present-day issues. Significantly, however, the attitudes expressed in Char and McDermott's article are still current. On the basis of informal comments received from nurses involved in organ retrieval work, autopsies and abortion work, or who work with patients who refuse care or for whom decisions have been made to withhold or withdraw medical treatment, I have good reason to believe that these attitudes are far from outdated, and remain relevant to present-day concerns. I have been told, for instance, that psychiatrists are playing an increasing role in 'debriefing' nurses in situations where patients have refused care and treatment, but where these patients' wishes have been overridden on the basis of recommendations made by a consulting psychiatrist.

In one notable case (occurring as recently as 1988), for example, a severely debilitated patient expressed a wish to be allowed to die. When her wishes were refused, she proceeded to decline offers of food and fluids. A consulting psychiatrist was called in, and subsequently declared the patient 'rationally incompetent'. Nursing staff who were distressed by the fact that this woman's wishes were not being respected (and they had no reason to believe that her wishes were not rational) were later 'counselled' by the psychiatrist, and assisted to regain their 'objectivity' about the 'medical facts' of the case. When it became evident that the nursing staff could not cope with the woman being force-fed against her will, she was discharged by the hospital into the care of her husband.

All the cases given here succeed in raising a number of important questions.

1. What is abortion, and is it morally wrong?
2. If abortion is morally wrong, can nurses be decently expected to assist with abortion procedures and/or care for women who have had them?
3. If abortion is not morally wrong, are nurses really entitled conscientiously to refuse to assist with abortion procedures and/or care for women who have had them?
4. Either way, to what extent, if any, should the nursing profession publicly support social policy formulation on the abortion issue?

It is to answering these questions that this discussion now turns.

What is abortion?

As with any moral debate, it is important first to clarify the terms of reference being used. Not surprisingly, abortion is defined differently by those who do support it and those who do not. This is interesting and significant, in that it again raises questions concerning the supposed value neutrality of so-called 'objective' moral definitions and concepts, and the extent to which these can be ethically loaded.

In its 1985 report, *Human embryo experimentation in Australia*, the Senate Select Committee on the Human Embryo Experimentation Bill defines 'abortion' as a 'spontaneous or induced termination of pregnancy' (p. xix), and 'miscarriage' as the 'the spontaneous loss of an early pregnancy at any stage before the twentieth week after conception' (p. xxi). Pro-abortionists use similar language when discussing abortion, tending typically to define it in terms such as 'terminating pregnancy' or 'ridding the products of unwanted conception'. The language in this instance is 'objective' and focuses attention away from the emotional aspect of the issue. It also seems to imply the conclusion that abortion is morally permissible. Anti-abortionists, by contrast, tend typically to define abortion in such terms as 'artificially causing the miscarriage of an unborn child', or of 'killing an innocent human being' (Fisher and Buckingham 1985). The language used in these and similar definitions is 'emotive', and focuses attention on the emotional aspect of abortion. It also seems to imply the conclusion that abortion is morally wrong.

In the light of the ongoing radical disagreement between pro- and anti-abortionist groups, it is unlikely that a consensus on the definition of abortion will ever be achieved. This serves as a timely warning that it is unlikely that the abortion debate itself will ever be resolved to everybody's satisfaction. The question of whether abortion is *moral* (to be distinguished here from it being *legal*) is, however, not one to be answered by a popular vote on what is to count as an acceptable definition. Rather, it is something which can only be decided by rigorous moral analysis.

Is abortion morally permissible?

Abortion has an interesting history. Anthropological studies suggest that abortion has been widely practised across cultures and throughout human history, and probably dates back even to prehistoric times (Thomas 1986, p. 77). Abortion techniques have been described in early Chinese, Egyptian and Greek texts, and continue to be widely practised in non-industrialised societies and other Third World countries. Muslim traditions permit abortion, so long as it is procured while 'the embryo is unformed in human shape' (Thomas 1986, p. 79). Japan did not introduce anti-abortion laws until the Meiji Restoration (1869–1912).

Contrary to what many Christian fundamentalists believe, opposition to abortion is not justified by appealing to either the Bible — it simply 'does not discuss it' (Badham 1987), to church traditions or to Christian reasoning. The early religious fathers, including St Augustine, St Jerome and St Thomas Aquinas, did not believe that the embryo was a human being from the moment of conception, and 'all insisted that early abortion could not be classed as homicide' (Badham 1987, p. 11). They also drew a firm distinction between early and late abortions. As far as the personhood of the fetus is concerned, this too 'has virtually no significant support' in the Christian tradition until the teachings of Pope Pius IX (1846–78). And in the Hebrew version of Exodus 21, accidental abortion is seen as an offence (and one punishable by death) 'only if the woman dies' (Thomas 1986, p. 78).

Where then has contemporary anti-abortion sentiment arisen from? There is much to suggest that it is largely the product of Catholic dogma dating back to the 1854 proclamation of the *Dogma of the Immaculate Conception* and the subsequent series of papal decrees (for example, in 1884, 1889, and 1908), 'which forbade direct termination of a pregnancy even in circumstances where, as in ectopic pregnancies, the result of non-intervention was the certain death of both mother and child' (Badham 1987, p. 12). Given this, it is difficult to avoid the impression that the ongoing abortion debate is as much a matter of disagreement of religious dogma as it is of moral values.

Abortion is usually viewed as both a moral and a legal problem. In this instance, morality and legal law have vitally interdependent roles to play in ensuring the realisation of just outcomes. Common questions which both law and morality attempt to answer include: who, if anyone, ought to be permitted to have an abortion? under what circumstances or conditions might abortion be allowed?

Generally speaking, there are roughly three positions that can be taken on abortion: a conservative position, a moderate position and a liberal position.

The conservative position

According to the conservative position (see, for example, Brody 1982; Noonan, 1983), abortion is an absolute moral wrong, and thus something which should never be permitted under any circumstances — not even in self-defence, such as cases where a continued pregnancy would almost certainly result in the mother's death. A common concern among conservative anti-abortionists is that, if abortion is permitted, then respect for the sanctity of human life will be diminished, making it easier for human life to be taken in other circumstances. Arguments typically raised against abortion here are almost always based on the sanctity-of-life doctrine. One example of the kind of reasoning which might be employed to argue against abortion is as follows:

It is wrong to kill innocent human beings; fetuses are innocent human beings; therefore it is wrong to kill fetuses.

(Warren 1973, p. 53)

Or, to use another example:

Human beings have a natural right to life; fetuses are human beings; therefore fetuses have a right to life and killing them is wrong.

Whether human beings do in fact have a natural right to life, and whether fetuses are in fact human beings, are matters of philosophical controversy.

The moderate position

According to the moderate position (see, for example, Werner 1979; Bolton 1983) abortion is only a prima facie moral wrong, and thus prohibitions against it may be overridden by stronger moral considerations. Werner (1979), for example, argues that abortion is permissible provided that it is procured during pre-sentience (i.e. before the fetus has the capacity to feel). Since a pre-sentient fetus cannot feel, it cannot be meaningfully harmed or benefited. Thus, as with other non-sentient or pre-sentient entities, it makes no sense to say a fetus has rights, much less a right to life. In the case of post-sentience, Werner argues that abortion may still be justified on carefully defined grounds, namely: *self-defence* (for example, where the life or health of the mother would be at risk if the pregnancy was allowed to continue); or *unavoidability* (for example, where abortion cannot be avoided, such as in the case of ectopic pregnancy or accidental injury). Abortions performed on lesser grounds are, according to Werner, unjustified.

Bolton (1983) takes a slightly different line of reasoning. She argues that, since fetuses are not undisputed persons, they do not have the same rights not to be killed as do actual undisputed persons. Thus, in the case of life-threatening pregnancy, at least, a woman's right to life overrides that of the fetus. Bolton (1983) also argues, controversially, that if women are not permitted to have abortions, the community might find itself deprived of the beneficial contributions that a woman freed of the burdens of child rearing would otherwise be free to make (p. 335). She concedes, however, that there are also cases 'in which others stand to benefit from the pregnant woman's bearing a child' (Bolton 1983, p. 337), and that this too might contribute to the community's benefit. The bottom line of Bolton's position is that abortion is morally permitted in some situations, and might even be 'morally required' in others, and it is not morally permitted in some other types of situations.

Either way, the facts of the matter need to be carefully assessed and analysed before an abortion decision is made.

Another popular argument raised in defence of abortion under a moderate's banner is that a woman is under no moral obligation to bring a pregnancy to term, particularly in instances where the pregnancy has been forced upon her (as in the case of rape), or where the pregnancy has not resulted from a voluntary and informed choice (as in cases involving the intellectually impaired, the ignorant and uneducated, or, quite simply, contraceptive failure). In her celebrated article 'A defence of abortion', Judith Jarvis Thomson (1971) contends, for example, that even if it is conceded, for the sake of argument, that a fetus is a person, this still does not place an obligation on a woman to carry it to full term. Her reasoning is simply that morality does not generally require individuals to make large sacrifices to keep another alive. Thus, if pregnancy requires a woman to make a large sacrifice — and one which she is not willing to make — it is morally permissible for her to terminate the pregnancy.

It could, of course, be objected that the kinds of sacrifices a woman might ultimately be required to make by giving birth could be avoided by her allowing the unwanted child to be adopted. And, indeed, many view the *adoption option* as a respectable way out of the abortion dilemma — even in cases involving severely disabled fetuses or severely disabled newborns (see, for example, Rothenberg 1987). Thomson, however, rejects the adoption option, arguing that it can be utterly devastating on relinquishing mothers — a claim which finds considerable support in research studies on the subject (see in particular Howe et al. 1992; Lancaster 1983; Harper 1983; Winkler and van Keppel 1983). It can also be utterly devastating on adopted children, who may grow up 'wondering who they are' and spending a lifetime searching for their unknown biological parents (Health and Community Services 1992). In some countries, babies born out of wedlock (especially 'rape babies') can face a life of shame and rejection (see in particular Doder 1993, p. 8). 'Rape babies' can even be prevented by law from being adopted. In Bosnia, for example, it is reported that the government has prohibited adoption of the children of rape victims, in the hope that their natural mothers will one day accept them (Williams 1993, p.48). The American feminist Barbara Ehrenreich (1985) also strongly rejects the adoption option, and her views on the matter are worth quoting at length here. She writes:

> Anyone who thinks for a moment about a woman's role in reproductive biology could never blithely recommend 'adoption, not abortion' because women have to go through something unknown to foetuses [sic] or men, and that is pregnancy. We are

talking about a nine-month bout of symptoms of varying severity, often including nausea, skin discoloration, extreme bloating and swelling, insomnia, narcolepsy, hair loss, varicose veins, haemorrhoids, indigestion and irreversible weight gain, and culminating in a physiological crisis, which is occasionally fatal and almost always excruciatingly painful.

If men were equally at risk for this condition — if they knew that their bellies might swell as if they were suffering from terminal cirrhosis, that they would have to go for nearly a year without a stiff drink, a cigarette or even an aspirin, that they would be subject to fainting spells and unable to fight their way on to public transport — then I am sure that pregnancy would be classified as a sexually transmitted disease and abortion would be no more controversial than emergency appendectomies.

(Ehrenreich 1985, p. 7)

Ehrenreich's conclusion, among other things, reminds us that, placed in its complete historical, cultural, social and political context, the issue of abortion would probably be viewed in quite a different light.

The liberal position

The third stance on abortion, the liberal position (see in particular Tooley 1972; Warren 1973; Thomson 1971), holds that abortion is morally permissible on demand. Michael Tooley (1972) argues, for example, that since fetuses are not persons, they cannot meaningfully claim a right to life. He points out that the notion 'person', in this instance, is a purely moral concept, and that the unfortunate tendency by some to use it as if it were synonymous with the notions of 'human being' and 'human life' is grossly misleading. Warren (1973) argues along similar lines. She contends that a fetus is not a *human being* and to claim that it is only begs the question. She points out that it is one thing to use *human* to refer 'exclusively to members of the species *Homo sapiens*', but quite another to use it in the sense of being 'a full-fledged member of the moral community' (p. 53). In other words, it is one thing to be human in the *genetic* sense, but it is quite another to be human in the *moral* sense. These two senses are quite distinct, and care must be taken to distinguish between them. She concludes:

In the absence of any argument showing that whatever is genetically human is also morally human . . . nothing more than genetic humanity can be demonstrated by the presence of the genetic human code.

(Warren 1973, p. 53*)

---

* Copyright © 1973, *The Monist*, La Salle, Il 61301. All quotations from this work are reprinted by permission.

The consequence of this is unavoidable. It has yet to be demonstrated that the genetic humanity of fetuses alone qualifies them to have fully fledged membership of the moral community.

Judith Jarvis Thomson (1971) also argues that a fetus is not a person. She contends that it is nothing more than a 'newly implanted clump of cells'. In defence of this claim, she argues that a fetus is 'no more a person than an acorn is an oak tree'. The analogy can be extended further to show that, just as stepping on an acorn is significantly different from cutting down an oak tree, so too is aborting a fetus significantly different from killing an actual person.

The conclusion of these and similar views is that, once it is admitted that a fetus is nothing more than a clump of genetically human cells (or a 'protoplasmic mass', as it was called by the psychiatrists cited earlier), the abortion issue is immediately rendered a non-issue. It would make no more sense to speak of the right of a fetus to life than it would be to speak of some other piece of genetically human tissue's right to life, say, a strand of human hair or a piece of human toenail (both of which are genetically human).

A 1987 Saulwick poll conducted by *The Age* suggested that 66 per cent of Australians approved of abortion in some circumstances, and another 19 per cent approved of abortion generally. Only a minority of 14 per cent disapproved entirely (Stephens 1987, p. 5). On the basis of our discussion so far, these findings may be diagrammed as shown in figure 9.1.

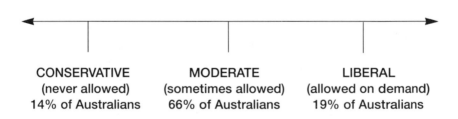

CONSERVATIVE	MODERATE	LIBERAL
(never allowed)	(sometimes allowed)	(allowed on demand)
14% of Australians	66% of Australians	19% of Australians

Figure 9.1 Australian attitudes to abortion.

Fetal and maternal rights

It can been seen that the abortion issue turns on two key points: (1) the moral status of the fetus; and (2) the moral rights of pregnant women to control their bodies and their lives. To recap, anti-abortionists argue that the human fetus is a human being, and therefore has a right to life. Pro-abortionists, however, reject this view, arguing that, while a human fetus is genetically human, this in no way implies that it is morally a human being with a full set of rights claims. Pro-abortionists argue further that fetuses are also not *persons*; the moral criteria of *personhood*, they contend, are quite different from the criteria of *fetalhood*. Let us consider this claim further.

Warren (1973) argues, controversially, that, for an entity to be a person, it must satisfy a number of criteria, namely:

1. consciousness (of objects and events external and/or internal to the being), and in particular the capacity to feel pain;

2. reasoning (the developed capacity to solve new and relatively complex problems);

3. self-motivated activity (activity which is relatively independent of either genetic or direct external control);

4. the capacity to communicate, by whatever means, messages of an indefinite variety of types, that is, not just with an indefinite number of possible contents, but on indefinitely many possible topics;

5. the presence of self-concepts, and self-awareness, either individual or racial, or both.

(Warren 1973, p. 55)

Warren admits that there are numerous difficulties involved in formulating and applying precise criteria of personhood. Even so, it can be done. Commenting on the criteria she has formulated, Warren argues that an entity does not need to have all five attributes described, and that it is possible that attributes given in criteria 1 and 2 alone are sufficient for personhood, and might even qualify as necessary criteria for personhood. Given these criteria, all that needs to be claimed to demonstrate that an entity (including a fetus) is not a person is that any entity which fails to satisfy all of the five criteria listed is not a person. She concludes that if opponents of abortion deny the appropriateness of the criteria she has identified, she knows of no other arguments which would convince them. She writes: 'We would probably have to admit that our conceptual schemes were indeed irreconcilably different, and that our dispute could not be settled objectively' (p. 56).

Michael Tooley (1972), like Warren, also interprets 'person' in rationalistic terms. He argues that in order for something to be a person it must have a serious moral right to life. And in order to have a serious moral right to life, it must possess 'the concept of self as a continuing subject of experience and other mental states, and believe that it is itself such a continuing entity' (Tooley 1972, p. 44). Since fetuses do not satisfy this basic 'self-consciousness requirement', as Tooley calls it, they are not persons — they do not have a serious moral right to life, and therefore to kill them is not wrong.

For some, the personhood argument does little to settle the abortion question. For example, it might be claimed that, even if it is true that a fetus is not a person, it nevertheless has the potential to become one, and therefore it has rights (see also Warren 1977). Thus abortion is still wrong on grounds of the potentiality of the fetus (Glover 1977, p. 122). Or, to borrow from Warren's analogy cited earlier: even though an acorn is not an oak tree, it nevertheless has the potential to become one; therefore crushing an acorn is tantamount to chopping down an oak tree.

There are a number of obvious difficulties with this view. First, the argument tends to presume that what is potential will in fact become actual. In the case of zygotes, however, this is quite improbable. As Engelhardt points out, only '40%–50% of zygotes survive to be persons (i.e. adult, competent human beings)' (1986, p. 111). It might then be better, suggests Engelhardt, to speak of human zygotes as being only '0.4 probable persons'.

Second, the argument strongly suggests that it is not the fetus per se that is valued, but rather *what it will become* (Glover 1977, p. 122). It is difficult to interpret just what kind of moral demand this creates. As Glover points out:

> It is hard to see how this potential argument can come to any more than saying that abortion is wrong because a person who would have existed in the future will not exist if an abortion is performed.
>
> (Glover 1977, p. 122)

If we take the potentiality argument to its logical extreme, we are committed to accepting, absurdly, that contraception, the wasteful ejaculation of sperm, menstruation and celibacy are also morally wrong, since these too will result in future persons being prevented from existing (Warren 1977, p. 277).

The main unresolved question, however, is: can a *potential* person be meaningfully said to have *actual* rights and, if so, can these rights meaningfully override the existing rights of actual persons? Or, to put this another way, can a fetus (a potential person) have actual rights and, if so, can these meaningfully override the existing rights of its mother (an actual person)? The crux of the dilemma posed here is whether the more immediate and actual rights of the pregnant woman should be recognised before the more remote and potential needs of the fetus, or vice versa.

One answer is that, given our understanding of the nature of moral rights and correlative duties, there is something logically and linguistically odd in ascribing rights to fetuses (non-persons), particularly during the pre-sentient stage. If we were to accept that non-sentient fetuses have moral rights, we would be committed, absurdly, to accepting that all sorts of other non-sentient things have moral rights — including human toenails, strands of hair, or pieces of skin. For argument's sake, however, let us accept that the fetus does have moral rights and, further, that these can meaningfully conflict with the mother's moral rights. The question which arises here is which fetal/maternal rights are likely to conflict?

The most obvious is the fetus' and the mother's common claim to a right to life. This is particularly so in cases where the mother's life would almost certainly be lost if the pregnancy were allowed to continue. In such situations it seems reasonable to claim that the mother's right to life must at least be as strong as the fetus' right to life. And, further, since both stand to die unless the pregnancy is terminated, then surely it is better, morally speaking, that only one life is lost instead of two? It is difficult to see how anyone could reasonably and conscientiously choose an outcome which would see both the mother and the fetus die. Furthermore, as has already been discussed elsewhere in this text, morality does not generally require us to make large personal sacrifices on behalf of another, and thus it would be morally incorrect to suggest that the mother has a duty to sacrifice her life in defence of the fetus. In the case of life-threatening pregnancies, then, it seems reasonable to conclude that the pregnant woman's right to life has the weightier claim.

A second set of rights which may conflict is the mother's *right to have control over her body and life's circumstances* versus the fetus' *right to life*. It might be claimed, for example, that a woman's right to choose her lifestyle, career, economic circumstances, standard of health, and similar, override any claims the fetus might have to be 'kept alive'. The mother may then withdraw her 'life support' even if this means the fetus will die in the process (an unfortunate, but nevertheless unavoidable, consequence). Against this, however, it might still be claimed that the inconveniences and other psychological, physical or social ills caused by an unwanted pregnancy are still not enough to justify killing the fetus and violating its right to life (Brody 1982; Noonan 1983). The demand not to kill the fetus becomes even more persuasive when it is considered that there are alternatives available for helping to prevent or alleviate the ills of unwanted pregnancies, such as child welfare and other social security benefits, adoption, counselling, medication, or, as some have suggested controversially, even extracting the fetus and placing it in a surrogate or an artificial uterus (Glover 1977, p. 135). (It should be noted that this latter suggestion is not as far-fetched as it seems. Work is already being carried out overseas on 'maintaining uteri extracted from women outside of a woman's body', and implanting embryos into these wombs [Rowland 1992, pp. 288–9]. Aborted fetuses have been 'kept alive for up to forty-eight hours' in these research projects [Rowland 1992, p. 289].) In cases where alternatives are available, it seems difficult to sustain a claim that the mother's rights ought to be given overriding consideration over those of the fetus.

A third set of rights which might conflict is the mother's *right to health* (and to a quality of life) versus the fetus' *right to life.* In this instance, the mother's health and quality of life are threatened not by her pregnancy but by a progressive debilitating disease, such as Alzheimer's, Parkinson's or diabetes. The mother might, for example, contemplate getting pregnant for the sole purpose of growing tissue which can be harvested and transplanted into her brain or pancreas in an attempt to restore her health. The issue of fetal tissue transplantation is already the subject of intensive debate (see in particular Mandel 1985; The foetal brain cell debate, 1988, p. 10; Griffiths 1988; Gillam 1989; Engelhardt 1989). Although governments are striving hard to prevent this type of scenario from occurring, it is not difficult to imagine cases of women getting pregnant and having abortions for the sole purpose of supplying fetal tissue for transplantation — if not for themselves, for other people. It is rumoured that poor women are already being given financial incentives to supply fetal tissue, in much the same way as the poor are being encouraged to sell their kidneys. (See also the discussion on organ transplantation in chapter 12.) Meanwhile, there are already documented cases of women getting pregnant and giving birth for the sole purpose of providing life-saving tissue (such as bone marrow) for transplantation into a newly born's sibling (see Gibbs 1990; Morrow 1991). In the light of this, it is difficult to imagine that women will not become — and are not already becoming — pregnant and undergoing 'altruistic abortions' in order to supply fetal tissue for therapeutic transplantations for a loved one, a needy stranger, or, indeed, themselves.

A fourth set of rights which may conflict, and one which is beginning to be given increasing publicity, involves not only the competing claims of a fetus and its mother, but also those of the father (see also Leo 1993, p. 59). Media reports suggest that around the world there is an increasing trend of fathers undertaking legal action in an attempt to stop their (ex)wives and (ex)girlfriends from having abortions (PA 1987; Lowther 1988; AFP 1989; Beyer 1989). In 1987, for example, a 23-year-old father is reported to have taken court action in an English court of appeal to try and stop his 21-year-old girlfriend, an Oxford University student, from having an abortion (PA 1987, p. 6). The court is reported to have rejected the father's appeal — significantly, not on the grounds of the woman's right to choose, but on the grounds that the fetus was:

> so underdeveloped that, if separated from its mother, it would be unable to breathe either naturally or through a ventilator, was not capable of being 'born alive'.
>
> (PA 1987, p. 8)

Upon learning of the court's decision, the 21-year-old Oxford University student is reported to have taken the position that:

> It is her decision what she does now, but it is a point of principle that she is now able to control her own body.
>
> (PA 1987, p. 8)

The 23-year-old man responsible for her pregnancy is reported to have been 'disappointed and very surprised at the result' (PA 1987, p. 8).

A year later, a similar case occurred in the United States of America. It involved a 24-year-old man who is reported to have 'lost a lower-court appeal for the right to force his estranged [19-year-old] wife to have their baby' (Lowther 1988, p. 8). The court is reported to have ruled against the father, on the grounds that the abortion concerned only the estranged wife (Lowther 1988, p. 8). Rejecting the court's decision, the man decided to 'fight to seek a legal precedent' in favour of fathers — even though his estranged wife had gone ahead and had an abortion after the court's findings. In explaining his decision to take further legal action, the man is reported to have said:

> I was willing to take full responsibility and raise the baby and take care of it; there's nothing for me to do now but let the wounds heal. Maybe the next guy will have it easier.
>
> (Lowther 1988, p. 8)

Critics of his stance, and advocates of a woman's right to choose, argued, however, that 'it is nothing short of involuntary servitude to order a woman to carry a child she does not want' (Lowther 1988, p. 8). Against this, an Indiana lawyer argued in support of the man's actions that what they were asking the court to do was merely:

> to find that there should be a balancing of the interests of the father against those of the mother on a case-by-case basis.
>
> (Lowther 1988, p. 8)

In 1989, one year later again, a similar case was reported in Canada. This time it involved a 25-year-old man who took court action to stop his 21-year-old ex-girlfriend from having an abortion (Beyer 1989). The case took a dramatic twist, however, when, with considerable embarrassment, the woman's lawyer announced, before the court case had concluded and all arguments completed, that his client, 'worried that it might be too late for an abortion even if she won the case, had decided not to wait' (Beyer 1989). Commenting on the case, Beyer writes:

> Defying a lower-court injunction, she had gone ahead with the operation. The Court was stunned. But it went on nonetheless to rule unaminously that the injunction barring the abortion was invalid. The Court thus seemed to be ending a recent spate of injunctions against abortion sought by angry ex-boyfriends.
>
> (Beyer 1989, p. 60)

Not surprisingly, this upsurge in paternal interest has met with little sympathy from women who historically have been left alone with the burden and hardships of child-rearing after the fathers of their children have long abandoned them. Further, some even worry that, if the paternity rights debate is allowed to progress to its logical extreme, it could pave the way for even rapists to prevent their victims from having abortions, and to press for access rights after the baby has been born. It has also been suggested that recognition of paternal rights may see the courts inviting rapists 'to be present at the birth' (Rogers 1992).

Women's history (or rather *her*story) is, however, unlikely to settle the debate on paternity rights. Given the tenuous relationship women historically have had with the law, it is possible that men may well eventually succeed in obtaining the legal remedies they seek in regard to protecting their paternity, viz 'property rights over the fetus' (Petchesky 1986, p. 328). It is also possible that they will win their patriarchal fight against 'female-controlled' abortion and the rights of women to control their own bodies and lives (Chesler 1991, pp. 241–5). Just what the ultimate outcome of the 'mothers' rights versus fathers' rights' debate will be, however, remains an open question, and to a very large extent probably will not depend on the genuine moral rights of individuals, or even on substantive ethical arguments. Rather, the outcome will probably depend on the power of the courts — and, more specifically, the men who preside over them — and the extent to which they wish to ensure the 'continual subordination of women to men through the exploitation of pregnancy' (Tribe, cited in Graycar and Morgan 1990 p. 209; see also Luker 1984; Petchesky 1986; Eisenstein 1988; Keown 1988; Messer and May 1988; Rhode 1989; Graycar and Morgan 1990; Chesler 1987; Smart 1992).

Issues and recommendations

The abortion issue is enormous and complex; it is also extremely political, as some other spectacular overseas incidents have shown. For example, in 1990, Belgium was thrown into a constitutional crisis after King Baudouin, Belgium's reigning monarch, stepped down from his throne temporarily 'because his conscience would not let him sign a law legalising abortion' (Reuter 1990a, p. 7). As a result, the government had to take over the King's powers and pass the abortion law. It is reported that once the abortion law was passed the King's inability to reign ceased, and he resumed his position on the throne (Reuter 1990a, p. 7).

In the same year, it was reported that disagreement over abortion law threatened to 'derail a treaty on German unity' (Reuter 1990b, p. 7). The disagreement was primarily over whether 'West German women may take advantage of East Germany's liberal abortion laws after unification' (Reuter 1990b, p. 7).

More recently, in 1992, Ireland (where abortion is illegal) witnessed political uproar and large public demonstrations after the High Court banned a 14-year-old rape victim from travelling to Britain for an abortion (the girl had been raped repeatedly by a friend's father over a one-year period) (Barrett 1992c, 1992d). It was reported that many European constitutional lawyers considered the ban a breach of the Treaty of Rome, which brought the European Community (EC) into being thirty-six years ago, and, among other things, 'permitted the right to free movement within the EC' (Barrett 1992c). The situation reached crisis point when it was evident that the ban threatened the European Community's Maastricht Treaty on European political union, which Irish voters were due to vote on a few months later (*Independent* 1992, p. 6; Barrett 1992a, 1992b, 1992f).

The case is reported to have aroused the concerns of a number of influential groups, including Irish legislators and lawyers and members of human rights and women's groups, and to have raised serious questions about how far the state and its officials should interfere in the fundamental rights of its citizens (*Independent, New York Times* 1992, p. 9). The travelling ban was eventually lifted by the Supreme Court in Dublin, and the girl was able to travel to Britain for an abortion (*Independent* 1992 p. 6). Later in the year, two Dublin counselling clinics appealed successfully to the European Court of Human Rights against the Irish Government's prohibition on women gaining access to information about abortion services overseas (Barrett 1992e, p. 8). The judges who heard the case are reported to have decided that the Irish Government was 'violating fundamental human rights by preventing women from gaining access to information about having abortions abroad' (Barrett 1992e, p. 8). The counselling clinics were also reported to have been awarded costs and damages of more than $400 000 (Barrett 1992e, p. 8).

Abortion was also a major issue in the American presidential election of 1992, with the then presidential contenders Bill Clinton and Ross Perot both trying 'to lure pro-choice voters to their side' (Barrett, L. I. 1992, p. 54). During the campaign, the Bush camp (whose law reforms saw the loss of civil rights protection for United States abortion clinics [Baltimore *Sun* 1993] and the banning of abortion counselling at federally funded clinics [Toner 1993]) admitted publicly that anything raising the profile of the abortion issue was 'a problem for us' (Barrett, L. I. 1992, p. 54). Initially, the Clinton camp also wanted to avoid too much attention being paid to the abortion issue. It was reported that basically 'he wanted to avoid the appearance of catering to "special interests", including feminists' (Barrett, L. I. 1992, p. 55).

The abortion debate in the United States took a dramatic and historic turn in 1993, when an anti-abortion protester shot and killed a doctor during a pro-life demonstration outside a lawful abortion clinic (Rohter 1993, p. 7). Abortion rights groups took the shooting of the doctor as a 'symbol of the increasing harassment' of health workers involved in abortion work, which has seen abortion clinics increasingly vandalised and destroyed by arsonists. In one case, a clinic was even firebombed and razed (Rohter 1993, p. 7).

The politics of abortion in the United States is taking another turn, however, as President Clinton moves to 'reverse a decade of Republican edicts on abortion and other issues, including a repeal on the ban on abortion counselling at federally funded clinics' (Toner 1993, p. 6). The Clinton administration is also reported to be planning a repeal of the 1977 *Hyde Amendment* (see Eisenstein 1988, p. 188), which effectively:

> barred Medicaid federal funding for poor women to obtain abortions, even when pregnancies arise from incest and rape or when they are deemed medically necessary.
>
> (Cornwell 1933, p. 8)

Despite severe criticism of these plans by proponents of anti-abortion legislation, the White House is reported to be 'determined to fulfil a promise made repeatedly by Mr Clinton during the campaign' (Cornwell 1993, p. 8).

Closer to home, Australia has also experienced the politicisation of abortion, with a small number of politicians attempting, unsuccessfully, to introduce legislation aimed at restricting abortion services for women. In 1988, for example, the Reverend Fred Nile, a New South Wales independent MP, attempted unsuccessfully to introduce his *Unborn Child Protection Bill*, which could have seen doctors performing abortions jailed for up to fourteen years and fined $100 000 (Ansell 1988, p. 21). The Reverend Nile was reported to have said that the Bill would allow abortion only if the mother's life was in danger, and that 'no exceptions would be made for any threat to the mental health of the mother' (Ansell 1988, p. 21). The medical director of the Family Planning Association of New South Wales is reported at the time to have condemned the Bill on the grounds that it would 'not stop women having abortions — it would just drive them underground' (Ansell 1988, p. 21).

Alistair Webster (a Liberal politician in New South Wales) has also made several attempts over the years to introduce legislation aimed at eliminating Medicare rebates for abortion services. An attempt in 1990 was condemned by the Women's Electoral Lobby, who reminded politicians supporting the move that 'no legislation has ever prevented desperate women from terminating unwanted pregnancies' (Schnookal 1990, p. 2). Further, as one ALP member responded during parliamentary debate on the matter:

> Medicare benefits do not cause abortion. It will not go away if we remove the benefit, just as unemployed people will not disappear if we remove the unemployment benefit [. . .] The best way to reduce abortion numbers is better sex education, family planning and support for pregnant women — from their partners and from the government.
>
> (Dr Ric Charlesworth, cited by Wainer 1990, p. 8)

At a broader international level, however, perhaps one of the most controversial examples of an attack on abortion comes from the Pope. In February 1993, the Pope is reported to have told Bosnian women pregnant as a result of wartime rape that 'they should not seek abortions, but give birth to the children' (*Bioethics News* 1993, p. 3). It is estimated that between twenty thousand and seventy thousand women have been raped — the majority of violated women being Muslims (Corlett 1993, p. 4). It is reported that the Pope addressed the women in a letter as follows:

> 'Do not abort. Your children are not responsible for the ignoble violence you have undergone.' He asked the women to 'accept the enemy' into them, and make him the 'flesh of their own flesh'.
>
> (*Bioethics News* 1993, p. 3)

The Pope's comments have since been the subject of much criticism by Muslims and Catholic theologians alike. One outspoken German Catholic theologian (a woman) is reported to have said that the Pope 'had no right to get involved in matters of which he can have no understanding' and that 'no bachelor [. . .] could decide on matters such as these. A decision can be made only by those who have been raped' (*Bioethics News* 1993, p. 3).

There remains much more to be said on the politics of and the moral controversies surrounding abortion than there is space here to do. For example, we have yet to address the problems of: restrictive abortion laws and the real suffering these stand to cause women who find themselves trapped by an unwanted pregnancy; sex-selected abortions (see in particular Mary Anne Warren's [1985] challenging text *Gendercide: the implications of sex selection*); the risk to women having abortions from the terrible side-effects that abortion procedures can have (see also Fisher and Buckingham 1985, p. 60); the dilemmas arising in cases of pregnancies that result from rape, and in cases of deformed fetuses, whether the deformity is slight or severe (for example, there is anecdotal evidence that pregnancies are being aborted even in cases where a fetus is not severely deformed — for instance, has one leg slightly shorter than the other); or the dilemmas arising in cases of pregnant women who engage in health injurious behaviours such as cigarette smoking, illicit drug taking, alcoholism, and the like, despite knowing that these behaviours could be injurious to the health of their unborn children. Another problem is that of determining the point at which a fetus actually becomes a person — for example, is it at conception/syngamy, upon achieving viability, or at birth? (See also Buckle and Dawson 1988; Warren 1988; Glover 1977, pp. 123–6.) We have also yet to examine the so-called 'slippery slope' arguments which reason that, if abortion is permitted, our moral characters and expectations will seriously decline; that is, if we allow abortion today, we will allow infanticide tomorrow and the next day we will allow euthanasia of other 'useless' persons. Regrettably, consideration of these and similar problems must be left for another time.

Although falling far short of a complete examination of the abortion issue, the discussion should clarify the nature of the abortion debate and its implications for nurses. It has been shown that abortion is a highly complex and controversial issue, and one which is unlikely to be satisfactorily resolved. This means that nurses will invariably encounter moral disagreement in abortion contexts — many of which may not be able to be reconciled. The discussion has also warned the nursing profession that it cannot afford to be complacent or indecisive about taking a formal position on policy formulation in relation to abortion practices and procedures and the questions of social justice these raise (see also Bandman and Bandman 1985, p. 136). While nurse leaders and administrators remain indecisive or complacent about reaching a just position on the subject, nurse practitioners will continue to suffer intolerable moral, personal, professional and legal burdens on account of their conscientious opposition to abortion. This in turn could have the unhappy consequence of nursing standards of care being eroded, which could place intolerable and unnecessary burdens on women requiring nursing care before, during and after an abortion procedure. An important question raised by this prospect is: to what extent, if at all, should a nurse's conscientious objection to a given abortion procedure be permitted if, in permitting it, the life, health or well-being of the woman seeking the abortion is compromised or violated? It may be that nurses' conscientious objections in such instances should not be permitted, and, if that is the case, the onus falls on nurses not to work in areas where their conscientious objections to morally controversial (although not unequivocally immoral) procedures cannot be accommodated. Since the issue of conscientious objection is important in its own right, it is considered separately in chapter 13 of this text.

Perhaps most importantly, this discussion demonstrates the need for the abortion issue to be opened up for formal and informed discussion within the ranks of the nursing profession. It can never be assumed that nurses have had a trouble-free path to conscience-free participation in abortion work. If we do not know what experiences nurses have had in this area, we will never be in a position to champion a substantive nursing perspective on the moral permissibility of abortion, much less on the extent to which nurses can be reasonably expected — against their moral conscience — to assist with abortion work. In formulating policies on the abortion issue, however, the nursing profession must be careful not to lose sight of its moral commitment to respecting women's personal choices (no matter how disagreeable these might appear to be). Individual nurse practitioners, meanwhile, must take great care not to fall into the moralising trap of imposing their personal values on others — in this instance, women who have decided, for whatever moral reason, to abort a pregnancy which, if carried to full term, promises intolerable consequences.

References

AFP (1989). Toronto Court has rethink to allow women's abortion. *Australian*, 13 July, p. 8.

Ansell, K. (1988). Nile's abortion bill would jail doctors. *The Age*, 28 June, p. 21.

Badham, P. (1987). Christian belief and the ethics of in vitro fertilization and abortion. *Bioethics News* 6 (2), January, pp. 7–18.

Baltimore Sun (1993). US abortion clinics lose civil rights protection. *The Age*, 15 January, p. 6.

Bandman, E. L. and Bandman B. (1985). *Nursing ethics* in the life span. Appleton-Century-Crofts, Norwalk, Connecticut.

Barrett, G. (1992a). Ireland abortion law poll likely. *The Age*, 20 February, p. 9.

Barrett, G. (1992b). Abortion ruling is threat to EC treaty. *The Age*,
21 February, p. 8.

Barrett, G. (1992c). Parents of girl in abortion row to appeal against ban.
The Age, 22 February, p. 7.

Barrett, G. (1992d). Pressure for change in Irish abortion ban. *The Age*,
24 February, p. 8.

Barrett, G. (1992e). Court rules against Ireland on abortion. *The Age*,
31 October, p. 8.

Barrett, G. (1992f). Election, abortion vote in Ireland. *The Age*, 26 November,
p. 7.

Barrett, L. I. (1992). Abortion: the issue Bush hopes will go away. *Time*
magazine, 13 July, pp. 54–5.

Benner, P. and Wrubel, J. (1989). *The primacy of caring*. Addison-Wesley,
Menlo Park, California.

Beyer, L. (1989). The globalization of the abortion debate. *Time* magazine,
21 August, pp. 60–1.

Bioethics News (1993). Pope: rape victims should not have abortions.
12 (3), April, p. 3.

Bolton, M. Brandt (1983). Responsible women and abortion decisions.
In S. Gorovitz, R. Macklin, A. Jameton, J. O'Connor and S. Sherwin (eds),
Moral problems in medicine, 2nd edn, Prentice Hall, Englewood Cliffs, New
Jersey, pp. 330–8.

Brody, B. (1982). The morality of abortion. In T. L. Beauchamp and L. Walters,
Contemporary issues in bioethics, 2nd edn, Wadsworth, Belmont, California,
pp. 240–50.

Broekhuijse, P. (1988). Nurse loses job over abortion. *Sunday Telegraph*,
21 February, p. 13.

Buckle, S. and Dawson, K. (1988). Individuals and syngamy. *Bioethics News*
7 (3), April, pp. 15–30.

Canadian Press (1988). Abortion ruling: What does it mean? *Leader Post*,
29 January, p. 1.

Char, W. F. and McDermott, J. F. (1972). Abortions and acute identity crisis in
nurses. *American Journal of Psychiatry* 128 (8), pp. 952–7.

Chesler, P. (1987). *Mothers on trial: the battle for children and custody*.
Harcourt Brace Jovanovich, New York.

Corlett, D. (1993). Former Yugoslavia. *Victorian Foundation for Survivors of
Torture Newsletter*, Spring, p. 4.

Cornwell, R. (1993). US plans to reverse abortion, labor laws. *The Age*, 2 April,
p. 8.

Davis, A. and Aroskar, M. (1983). *Ethical dilemmas and nursing practice*,
2nd edn. Appleton-Century-Crofts, Norwalk, Connecticut.

Doder, D. (1993). Balkans rape babies face life of shame, rejection. *The Age*,
5 July, p. 8.

Ehrenreich, B. (1985). After two abortions, a clear choice and few regrets.
The Age 'Saturday Extra', 23 March, p. 7.

Eisenstein, Z. R. (1988). *The female body and the law*. University of California
Press, Berkeley.

Engelhardt, H. Tristram Jr (1986). *The foundations of bioethics*. Oxford
University Press, Oxford.

Engelhardt, H. Tristram Jr (ed.) (1989). *Journal of Medicine and Philosophy*
14 (1). Special edition: *Harvesting cells, tisssues, and organs from fetuses
and anencephalic newborns*.

Fisher, A. and Buckingham, J. (1985). *Abortion in Australia*. Dove
Communications, Melbourne.

Gibbs, N. (1990). The gift of life — or else. *Time* Magazine, 10 September, p. 49.

Gillam, L. (ed.) (1989). *Proceedings of the Conference: The Fetus as Tissue Donor: Use or Abuse?* Centre for Human Bioethics, Monash University, Melbourne.

Glover, J. (1977). *Causing deaths and saving lives.* Penguin Books, Harmondsworth, Middlesex.

Graycar, R. and Morgan, J. (1990). *The hidden gender of law.* Federation Press, Sydney.

Griffiths, L. (1988). Foetal transplants spark controversy. *Australian Dr Weekly,* 20 May.

Harper, P. (1983). Lost, but still alive — the natural parents' need to know. In *Proceedings of the Conference: Adoption and AID: Access to Information?* Centre for Human Bioethics, Monash University, Melbourne, 2 November, pp. 29–38.

Health and Community Services (1992). *Adoption: myth and reality. The Adoption Information Service in Victoria.* Health and Community Services Promotions and Media Unit, Melbourne.

Holmes, P. (1988). Over the limit? *Nursing Times* 20 (84), p. 19.

Howe, D., Sawbridge, P. and Hinings, D. (1992). *Half a million women: mothers who lose their children by adoption.* Penguin, London.

Independent (1992). Jubilation in Ireland as abortion ban lifted. *The Age* 28 February, p. 6.

Independent, New York Times (1992). Abortion trip ban on rape victim, 14. *The Age,* 19 February, p. 9.

International Council of Nurses (1977). *The nurse's dilemma.* International Council of Nurses, Florence Nightingale International Foundation, Geneva, Switzerland.

Keown, J. (1988). *Abortion, doctors and the law.* Cambridge University Press, Cambridge.

Lancaster, K. (1983). Secrecy in adoption: a historical perspective'. In *Proceedings of the Conference: Adoption and AID: Access to Information?* Centre for Human Bioethics, Monash University, Melbourne, 2 November, pp. 21–8.

Leo, J. (1983). Sharing the pain of abortion. *Time* Magazine, 26 September, p. 59.

Lifton, R. J. (1986). *The Nazi doctors: a study of the psychology of evil.* Macmillan, London.

Lowther, W. (1988). Father seeks right to stop wife's abortion. *The Age,* 26 August, p. 8.

Luker, K. (1984). *Abortion and the politics of motherhood.* University of California Press, Berkeley.

Mandel, T. E. (1985). The use of immature pancreas as a source of tissue for transplantation in diabetes. *Bioethics News* 5 (1), October, pp. 14–22.

Messer, E. and May, K. E. (1988). *Back rooms: an oral history of the illegal abortion era.* Simon & Schuster, New York.

Morrow, L. (1991). When one body can save another. *Time Magazine,* 17 June, pp. 46–50.

Muyskens, J. L. (1982). *Moral problems in nursing: a philosophical investigation.* Rowman & Littlefield, Totowa, New Jersey.

Noonan, J. T. (1983). From 'An almost absolute value in history'. In S. Gorovitz, R. Macklin, A. Jameton, J. O'Connor and S. Sherwin (eds), *Moral problems in medicine,* 2nd edn, Prentice Hall, Englewood Cliffs, New Jersey, pp. 303–8.

Nursing Times (1985). Midwives demand 24-week time limit for abortions. 81 (30), 24 July, p. 5.

Nursing Times (1988). Nurses in abortion row. 84 (7), 17 February, p. 8.

PA (1987). Law Lords reject father's plea to stop abortion. *The Age,* 26 February, p. 8.

Petchesky, R. P. (1986). *Abortion and women's choice: the state. sexuality, and reproductive freedom.* Verso (imprint of New Left Books), London.

Rea, K. (1981). Legal semantics. *Nursing Times* 77 (9), p. 351.

Reuter (1990a). Belgian king steps down over legalising abortion. *The Age,* 5 April, p. 7.

Reuter (1990b). Abortion issue threatens German treaty. *The Age,* 31 August, p. 7.

Rhode, D. L. (1989). *Justice and gender: sex discrimination and the law.* Harvard University Press, Cambridge, Mass.

Rogers, J. (1992). Rights for rapists. *The Age,* 'Access Age', 19 February, p. 12.

Rohter, L. (1993). Anti-abortion protester kills doctor. *The Age,* 12 March, p. 7.

Rothenberg, L. S. (1987). An ethicist urges offering all options in disability cases. *Kennedy Institute of Ethics Newsletter* 1 (8), February/March, pp. 1–2.

Rowland, R. (1992). *Living laboratories: women and reproductive technologies.* Pan Macmillan, Sydney.

Royal College of Nursing v. DHSS (CA) [1981] AC 800.

Rumbold, G. (1986). *Ethics in nursing practice.* Baillière Tindall, London.

Senate Select Committee on the Human Embryo Experimentation Bill 1985 (1986). *Human embryo experimentation in Australia.* Australian Government Publishing Service, Canberra.

Schnookal, R. (1990). Re-introduction of the Bill to abolish Medicare funding of abortion announced. *Alive and WEL* (official newsletter of the Women's Electoral Lobby), October, p. 2.

Smart, C. (ed.) (1992). *Regulating womanhood: historical essays on marriage, motherhood and sexuality.* Routledge, London and New York.

Stephens, P. (1987). Tolerance of abortion is much wider now. *The Age,* 7 December, p. 5.

The foetal brain cell debate (1988). *Bioethics News* 7 (4), July, pp. 10–11.

Thomas, S. (1986). *Genetic risk.* Penguin Books, Harmondsworth, Middlesex.

Thompson, J. B. and Thompson, H. O. (1981). *Ethics in nursing.* Macmillan, New York.

Thomson, J. J. (1971). A defense of abortion. *Philosophy and Public Affairs* 1 (1), pp. 47–66.

Toner, R. (1993). President in move to reverse policy on abortion. *The Age,* 25 January, p. 6.

Tooley, M. (1972). Abortion and infanticide. *Philosophy and Public Affairs* 2 (1), Fall, pp. 37–65.

Tribe, L. (1985). *Constitutional choices.* Harvard University Press, Cambridge, Mass.

Tschudin, V. (1986). *Ethics in nursing: the caring relationship.* William Heinemann Medical Books, London.

Wainer, J. (1990). Abortion funding abolition Bill. *Alive and WEL* (official newsletter of the Women's Electoral Lobby), February, p. 8.

Warren, M. A. (1973). On the moral and legal status of abortion. *The Monist* 57 (1), January, pp. 43–61.

Warren, M. A. (1977). Do potential people have moral rights? *Canadian Journal of Philosophy* 7 (2), June, pp. 275–89.

Warren, M. A. (1985). *Gendercide: the implications of sex selection.* Rowman & Allanheld, Totowa, New Jersey.

Warren, M. A. (1988). The moral significance of birth. *Bioethics News* 7 (2), January, pp. 32–44.

Watson, J. (1985). *Nursing: human science and human care.* Appleton-Century-Crofts, Norwalk, Connecticut.

Werner, R. (1979). Abortion: the ontological and moral status of the unborn. In R. A. Wasserstrom (ed.), *Today's moral problems*, 2nd edn, Macmillan, New York, pp. 51–74.

Wikler, D. and Barondess, J. (1993). Bioethics and anti-bioethics in light of Nazi medicine: what must we remember? *Kennedy Institute of Ethics Journal* 3 (1), pp. 39–55.

Williams, C. (1993). Children of rape in Bosnia trapped by new policy. *The Age*, 26 July, p. 8.

Winkler, R. and van Keppel, M. (1983). The long term adjustment of the relinquishing mothers in adoption: a research summary. Reprinted as an appendix in *Proceedings of the Conference: Adoption and AID: Access to Information?* Centre for Human Bioethics, Monash University, Melbourne, 2 November, pp. 39–40.

Chapter

10

Matters of life and death: II

Euthanasia

In 1990, JANET ADKINS, A VICTIM of Alzheimer's disease, died after pushing a red button on a suicide machine — or 'mercitron', as it has been called — designed by a retired pathologist, Dr Jack Kervorkian, whom she had approached for assistance to die (Gibbs 1990, 1993). Adkins, who is reported to have 'feared an excruciating future', soon came to be viewed as a 'symbol of all those patients who confront a horrible disease and vow to maintain some dignity in death' (Gibbs 1990, p. 70). Dr Kervorkian, meanwhile, found himself in the forefront of the pro-euthanasia debate and, as *Time* magazine put it:

> a standard-bearer for all those who fail to see a moral difference between unplugging a respirator and plugging in a poison machine.

> (Gibbs 1990, p. 70)

Despite being dubbed 'Dr Death', and 'the devil that doctors deserve' (because of the alleged deceitful, insensitive and neglectful way they often treated dying patients), Dr Kervorkian is continuing his crusade for the legalisation of euthanasia/assisted suicide, or, as he calls it, 'medicide' (Gibbs 1993, p. 52).

The assisted suicide of Janet Adkins has received — and continues to receive — international media attention, and remains the subject of much controversy. Central to the controversy is the fundamental question of whether a doctor should intentionally and actively assist a patient to die, and, if so, by what means. These same questions can, of course, also be asked of nurses — and that they have not been asked of nurses is curious, particularly when it is considered that nurses play a fundamental role in caring for and promoting the dignity of patients who are incurably ill, suffering intolerably and dying; that these questions *should* be asked of nurses will become self-evident in this chapter.

Before continuing this discussion, it should be noted that, while euthanasia is certainly an important life and death moral issue for nurses, it is not the only one deserving attention by them at this time. Another equally — if not more important — ethical issue in this area is that which I shall refer to as *unassisted suicide*. Indeed, anecdotal evidence suggests that, in several respects, the ethical aspects of unassisted suicide are in more urgent need of being addressed than are the ethical aspects of assisted suicide/ euthanasia. This became apparent to me recently when I was canvassing the experiences of students in relation to these two important issues. Specifically, I asked students (in classes ranging in size from sixty to three hundred) the following two questions.

1. How many of you have known, been involved in the care of, or have known others who have been involved in the care of, someone who has explicitly requested assistance to die — viz euthanasia?

2. How many of you have known, been involved in the care of, or have known of others who have been involved in the care of, someone who has independently attempted suicide or succeeded in suiciding?

The responses to these two questions have been both unexpected and disconcerting. In one class of about three hundred pre-registration students, for example, only ten students indicated their personal knowledge of a person's explicit request for euthanasia. This was in sharp contrast to the 290 students or so who went on to indicate their involvement, or the involvement of someone known to them, in the care of a person who had independently attempted suicide or succeeded in suiciding. This response was replicated in two additional classes of approximately three hundred students. This disparity is not so great in smaller classes of post-registration students who have worked or who are working in areas where requests for assistance to die may be more prevalent (for example, intensive care units, spinal units, renal dialysis units, cancer care units, and so on), but the students indicating their personal knowledge of someone who has independently attempted suicide or succeeded in suiciding still outnumber significantly those students indicating their personal knowledge of someone requesting euthanasia. While it is acknowledged that nothing conclusive can be drawn from these informal observations, the observations of these responses of over a thousand students nevertheless suggest the possibility that unassisted suicide is a more pressing ethical issue for nurses than is euthanasia/assisted suicide. It is conceded that there are a number of difficulties associated with trying to distinguish clearly the philosophically and morally significant differences between euthanasia and unassisted suicide. Nevertheless, I hope this and the following chapter will demonstrate that euthanasia and unassisted suicide do give rise to different ethical issues for nurses, and thus warrant separate discussion.

In this and the following chapter, attention focuses on two key questions.

1. What is the nature and what are the moral implications of euthanasia and unassisted suicide?

2. Why, if at all, are these two life and death ethical issues of significance and importance to members of the nursing profession?

Euthanasia and its significance for nurses

Next to abortion, euthanasia is probably one of the most controversial bioethical issues to confront the modern Western world. And, like the abortion issue, it is unlikely to be resolved to everybody's satisfaction.

Euthanasia and the so-called 'right to die' are not new issues for nurses. In Australia, one of the first articles addressing the subject was published as early as 1912 in the *Australasian Nurses Journal*. Reprinted from the *British Medical Journal*, the article contains concerns and viewpoints which remain current — including the agonising question of whether euthanasia should be legalised. Citing an 1873 essay on the subject, the article contends that 'a modified *hari kari* should be made lawful in England' (and, one presumes, her colonies, including Australia), and, quoting the essay's author, that:

> on the whole it cannot be doubted that the benefits resulting from a change in the law would be simply enormous.
>
> (Lionel Tollemache, cited in the *Australasian Nurses Journal*, 16 September 1912, p. 304)

While euthanasia may not be a new issue for nurses, it has nevertheless become a more substantive and intense one. Evidence of this can be found in the increasing attention being given to the experiences of nurses in regard to euthanasia in both the professional and lay press. In 1987, for example, the English nursing periodical *Nursing Times* carried a provocative report on the fate of four Dutch nurses who had been arrested in Amsterdam after it was alleged they had practised euthanasia on three hopelessly ill patients. The report concluded that, if the nurses were found guilty of killing the patients, they could face prison sentences of up to twenty years (*Nursing Times*, 25 March 1987, p. 8). More recently, it has been alleged that:

> British nurses are often involved in euthanasia; but that due to the illegality of euthanasia practices, it is difficult to assess the exact extent of the problem — particularly in a culture which prescribes that nurses should not 'tell on colleagues'.
>
> (Turton 1992, pp. 92–3)

And in Australia, a controversial survey of Victorian nurses conducted by Kuhse and Singer (1992) (already referred in chapter 1 of this text) found that the majority of those surveyed supported euthanasia, with 566 nurses (66 per cent of those who responded) indicating that if the law was changed they would be prepared to practise euthanasia. This survey compared favourably with an earlier study of the views of doctors in Victoria, in which 60 per cent of doctors responding indicated their support for active euthanasia (Kuhse and Singer 1988).

The legal status of euthanasia

At present, euthanasia is illegal, and anyone who wilfully assists a person to die would be viewed by the courts as having committed the criminal offence of homicide (Wallace 1991, p. 265, ss. 14–65). Despite this, euthanasia is practised almost every day in Australian, New Zealand and other overseas hospitals. Acts of euthanasia usually escape public attention, however. One reason for this is, as a former Victorian Law Reform Commissioner, Mr David Neal, was reported as explaining: 'There [is] a general attitude by both hospitals and the law agencies — such as the police and the Department of Public Prosecutions — of "letting sleeping dogs lie"' (Burchill 1989b, p. 4). Others suggest that, because 'the subject is so emotive and so difficult to discuss, it remains silent' (Hawley 1983).

Over the past decade, public opinion in Australia has consistently favoured voluntary euthanasia (Radic 1982; Humphries 1983; Kuhse and Singer 1988, p. 626; *Australian Dr Weekly*, 10 August 1990, p. 19; Kuhse 1991, pp. xii–xiii); and the State governments are trying to effect positive law reforms aimed at better protecting a person's right to 'die with dignity' — despite being 'wary' of the Right to Life movement (*The Age*, 1983; Scott 1991). The articulate pro-euthanasia lobby in Australia is also gaining increasing support, encouraged in its activities by the successes of its Dutch counterpart. According to the Royal Dutch Medical Association, in

1986 there were five thousand to six thousand cases of voluntary euthanasia each year in Holland (reported in British Medical Association 1986). In 1990, the overall incidence of euthanasia was estimated by formal sources to be between four thousand and six thousand cases annually (dc Wachter 1992, p. 24). However, others. contend that the overall incidence of euthanasia is, in reality, unknown and, if informal sources are to be relied upon, could range from between two thousand and twenty thousand cases a year (ten Have and Welie 1992; de Wachter 1992; Keown 1992). In Holland, under certain clearly defined conditions, euthanasia is not viewed by the courts as a punishable offence (Vervoorn 1987; Browne 1990, p. 11; Keown 1992; Kuhse 1993; Hirschler 1993). Although euthanasia is still technically illegal, a new law passed in February 1993 clarified and affirmed the strict conditions under which it (euthanasia) is permitted. The passage of this new law is reported as 'giving the Netherlands the world's most lenient policy on mercy killing' (Hirschler 1993, p. 7). For all this, however, the courts and the powerful medical lobby in Australia remain unmoved; for example, in the much publicised 1986 Queen Victoria Hospital case (the first of its kind in Australia), involving the selective non-treatment of a severely handicapped ten-day-old infant with spina bifida, Mr Justice Vincent of the Supreme Court is reported to have told the court that:

> no parent, no doctor, no court has any power to determine that the life of any child, however disabled the child may be, will be deliberately taken from them. The law does not permit decisions to be made concerning the quality of life nor any assessment of the value of any human being.
>
> (*The Age*, 1986b)

This case received public attention after the infant's grand-parents sought a court order to have the baby treated against the wishes of its parents.

In another case, involving a 28-year-old terminally ill leukemia patient who had been resuscitated against his will after he attempted suicide, Mr Justice Fullagar of the Victorian Supreme Court is reported as saying:

> There is, in the present circumstances, no legal right to die. It is not for me to say whether this is a good or happy, or bad and unhappy state of affairs.
>
> (Burchill 1989a)

This case received public attention after the patient's wife, Mrs Talila Kinney, sought a Supreme Court injunction to stop attending doctors at St Vincent's Hospital treating her husband. In trying to resuscitate Mr Kinney after he had taken a drug overdose, doctors caused substantial bleeding while trying to insert an oropharyngeal gastric washout tube. He was subsequently intubated for maintenance on a ventilator and given successive blood transfusions to sustain his life. Mrs Kinney is reported to have told the court that 'her husband wanted to die because he had a terminal disease' (Burchill 1989a). Mr Justice Fullagar took the view, however, that:

> The prevention of medical treatment amounts to carrying into execution the attempted suicide of the person concerned. To grant the injunction would be to assist the person in his suicide.
>
> (Burchill 1989a)

Despite the court's ruling, Mr Kinney was removed from his artificial life-support system, since he was found to be 'brain dead'.

Although these and other cases have received prominent media attention, the Australian Medical Association (AMA) and other independent medical authorities have consistently opposed the legalisation of euthanasia. For example, in 1983, the then secretary of the Victorian Branch of the AMA, Dr Bill Ryall, was quoted as saying that 'legislation was not necessary and could result in more confusion than it was worth' (Birnbauer 1983). In 1986 the then President of the AMA and Past President of the Victorian AMA, Dr John Mathew, was also reported to be opposed to the legalisation of euthanasia. He was quoted as saying that 'legislation in favour of active euthanasia is undesirable', and that he believed 'most doctors did not want the responsibility of actively terminating life' (Cossar 1986). Dr Nell Muirden, of the Peter MacCallum Cancer Institute, is reported to have argued that euthanasia should not be legalised because there are too many risks and dangers associated with it — not least the danger of it being abused by 'unscrupulous relatives' (Athersmith 1986).

More recently, Dr Muirden (1993) has reaffirmed her view, arguing controversially that:

> Sick and elderly patients are very vulnerable, and they could be under subtle pressure from relatives to request euthanasia, as we now sometimes see them gently coerced in other areas affecting their care.
>
> If euthanasia were an option, it would add to the distress and guilt of those who wondered whether they were too great a burden on others. At present they are protected by euthanasia being illegal, and I think it would be a tremendous stress if this protection were removed. *By allowing some people the right to choose, you would force on everyone the obligation to make a choice.*
>
> (Muirden 1993, p. 14).

It is probably true that most doctors do not 'want the responsibility' of terminating life; this is already evident from their consistent failure to assume responsibility for the euthanasia-type decisions they make every day in health care settings. Anecdotal evidence fully supports the claim that, while doctors are more than willing to make euthanasia-type *decisions*, they are not so willing actually to carry them out, preferring attending nurses to do so. This is certainly true in at least four types of cases.

The first type of case typically involves a medical decision to withhold nourishment and fluids from a chronically or terminally ill patient with the intention of hastening that patient's death. (An example of this has already been given in chapter 6.) In such cases, *a doctor prescribes* (often by verbal order only) the withholding of nourishment and fluids, but it is almost always the patient's *attending nurses who do the actual withholding.* The second type of case typically involves a medical decision not to resuscitate a patient. As in the previous case, *a doctor prescribes* 'Not For Resuscitation' or 'Do Not Resuscitate' (NFR/DNR) for a patient, but again it is the patient's *attending nurses who tend to do the refraining* in the case of cardiac arrest. (This issue is discussed at length in chapter 12.) A third type of case involves the administration of unnecessarily large and potentially lethal doses of narcotics or sedatives to patients with and without organic pain syndromes. (An example of this has been given in chapter 6 of this text.) Here, a doctor prescribes a heavy narcotic or sedative regime, but again it is left to the nurses actually to administer the drugs prescribed. The last type of case involves the removal of life-support systems from so-called 'brain-dead' patients. Here, a doctor orders the removal or 'switching-off' of a respirator/ventilator supporting a patient's life, but again it may be left to the nurse to actually 'switch off' the machine (a practice which was first disclosed publicly in the United Kingdom as early as 1969 [*Nursing Times*, 12 June 1969, p. 739]). While it might be objected that this type of case is unusual (I know personally of at least one medical director of an intensive care unit who always takes full responsibility for switching off a ventilator and who will not, under any circumstances, allow nurses to do it), anecdotal evidence suggests that there is an increasing trend towards nurses being left with this ultimate task. One nurse commented to me informally that if the task was left to doctors, they would just 'walk in and switch it [the machine] off, then walk out . . .'. Nurses, on the other hand, are in an 'ideal position' to remove life supports, since they can withdraw them at their own pace and 'according to the needs of the patient's family'. The nurse was quick to point out, however, that any nurse who did not wish to be involved in the removal of a life-support system was not compelled to be involved and could 'opt out'.

Public debate over the past few years has contributed enormously to a much greater awareness by health professionals as well as the lay community about the nature of euthanasia, the moral and legal problems associated with it, and the extent to which it is already being practised in our hospitals. In some instances, the community and its policy makers have been brave enough to respond to public concerns by initiating long overdue law and social policy reforms which have clarified a person's common law right to refuse orthodox medical treatment. In South Australia, for example, the *Natural Death Act* (1983) provides for a patient who is terminally ill to refuse 'extraordinary measures' to prolong life; in Victoria, the *Medical Treatment Act* (1988) clarifies and protects a person's existing common law right to refuse (any) unwanted orthodox medical treatment (excluding palliative care); and, in 1993, the New South Wales Health Department launched its *Dying with dignity: interim guidelines*, which aim to 'give precedence to the wishes of patients and their families, and acknowledge that artificially prolonging life is sometimes inappropriate' (New South Wales Health Department, 5 May 1993). More recently, the former Federal Health Minister, Senator Richardson, was reported as indicating publicly that 'he will push to introduce laws to protect doctors who practise mercy killing' (Middleton 1994, p. 3).

Despite these reforms, however, and despite public support from politicians, the status quo remains largely unchanged. Doctors still retain the ultimate authority to decide what is in a patient's 'best interests' (which tends to be interpreted in medical/clinical rather than moral terms), and retain the legitimated authority to override a patient's wishes if they deem it 'necessary'. Another relatively unknown problem is that legislation designed to protect or clarify patients' common law rights to refuse orthodox medical treatment is not always used in situations where it would be entirely appropriate to do so; for example, anecdotal evidence suggests that, in Victoria, the *Medical Treatment Act* (1988) is, in fact, under-used for reasons for which are yet to be investigated formally.

Equally troubling is the problem that the situation for nurses has not improved. The presence and role of nurses in caring for hopelessly ill and dying patients continues to be marginalised and ignored in policy and law reforms, making it increasingly difficult for nurses to avoid being placed in morally intolerable situations on account of having to uphold the life and death decisions made by doctors whose legal authority to decide is not easily challenged. A good example of this can be found in the New South Wales Health Department's *Dying with dignity* guidelines mentioned above. The guidelines ignored totally the fundamental role nurses play in caring for people who have life-threatening illnesses, and, indeed, the fundamental role nurses play in promoting the dignity of patients who are ill and dying. While doctors, the clergy and social workers are mentioned in the guidelines, nurses are not. In fact, nowhere in the document is the word 'nurse' used. This is another example of the marginalisation of, and the failure to recognise, not just the moral problems experienced by nurses in this area, but also the important work that nurses do when caring for people who are ill and dying — which, as the American ethicist George Annas points out, is often 'when there is nothing more medicine can offer' (cited by Gibbs 1993, p. 50).

The nursing perspective on euthanasia is further complicated by the fact that the nursing profession itself does not have a formal position on euthanasia. While the Federal Australian Nursing Federation (1987) has a substantive position statement on 'Assuring quality care for those who are dying' (see appendix VI of this text), this position statement does not express a view on euthanasia as such. Whatever the reason for the nursing profession not having a formal position on euthanasia, it is becoming increasingly evident that nurses cannot avoid the issue and its implications for nursing practice. As Pat Turton (1992) points out:

> Nurses often suffer great stress in the long time before death occurs through non-intervention which they may feel adds unnecessary suffering to the family, and possibly the patient. It can also be argued that the decision to seek aid-in-dying is as much a patient's right as any other part of their care — for instance, refusing antibiotics.
>
> There are no easy solutions, but [. . .] total rejection of euthanasia in all its complex aspects is surely no longer tenable for the nurse in the clinical setting.
>
> (Turton 1992, p. 94)

Turton (1992, p. 94) concludes that 'it is not only desirable, but vital that the nursing profession take part in open debate on the subject.' Although she writes from the cultural context of the United Kingdom, Turton's views hold equally for nurses in other countries. There is little doubt that the nursing profession must confront the realities of its members' involvement in euthanasia practices, and must refuse to continue to accept responsibility for the decisions doctors make but do not carry out — and in some cases plainly refuse to carry out. If nurses are to take an informed position on the euthanasia question, however, they need to have a sound understanding of its moral nature and its implications for nursing practice. It is to addressing these two concerns that this discussion now turns.

What is euthanasia?

The term euthanasia comes via New Latin from Greek *eu* (meaning 'easy', 'happy' or 'good') and *thanatos* (meaning 'death'); it is translated literally as 'good death' or 'happy death'. Contrary to popular opinion, the Greeks did not use the term euthanasia (or equivalents) to imply either 'a means or method of causing or hastening death' (Carrick 1985, p. 127). Rather, it was used in a broader and somewhat metaphorical sense 'to describe the *spiritual state* of the dying person at the impending approach of death' (Carrick 1985, p. 127). Historical evidence also suggests that euthanasia, as we understand it today, was in fact prohibited in ancient medical circles (Carrick 1985, p. 81). Plato, for one, even went so far as to suggest that physicians who attempt to poison another 'must be punished by death', whereas the lay person who attempted such a thing should only be fined — indicating that physicians were regarded as having the greater burden of responsibility to refrain from causing death (Carrick 1985, p. 83). Carrick comments that 'if someone's life was terminated without his (sic) consent, normally this was prima facie a case of homicide' (p. 128).

Contemporary English definitions of euthanasia vary. The *Oxford English dictionary*, for example, defines it as 'the action of inducing a quiet and easy death', and the *Collins English dictionary* as 'the act of killing someone painlessly, especially to relieve suffering from an incurable illness'. *Webster's dictionary*, similarly, defines euthanasia as 'an act or practice of painlessly putting to death people suffering from incurable conditions or disease'.

Whether euthanasia *is* any of these things, however, is a matter of some controversy. For example, we can imagine a case of 'inducing a quiet and easy death' which is a case not of euthanasia but of cold-blooded murder. I could, for example, slip a calming and sleep-inducing sedative into my fit grandmother's nightcap, and the moment she starts blissfully sleeping in her armchair administer to her a lethal dose of intravenous morphine. My sole intention might be nothing more than to secure her premature death so that I may receive the large inheritance I know she has left me in her will. There is something about this example which, to borrow from Beauchamp and Davidson (1979, p. 295) 'omits all the subtle aspects of our notion of euthanasia'. Likewise, we can imagine cases involving patients with incurable diseases or conditions who would nevertheless not be candidates for euthanasia. Diabetes, for example, is an incurable disease, and colour blindness an incurable condition. Yet, we would not, I think, regard either of these incurable states as grounds for euthanasia.

The notion of 'painlessly' inducing death is also unhelpful. We can, for example, imagine a *painless means* of causing death (for example, injecting a lethal substance through the side arm of an intravenous line, or removing someone from a life-support system or withholding food and fluids) but where the *death itself* is nevertheless painful and/or distressing (for example, where a patient is acutely aware of the sensations of suffocation after being taken off a respirator or after being given a large dose of narcotics, or is aware of both hunger and thirst sensations when food and fluids have been withheld). Just because the *means* of death was 'painfree', it does not always follow that the *death itself* was a 'good death'.

All three dictionary definitions are also inadequate in that they say nothing about the kinds of reasons which should be considered for killing another person, leaving it wide open for motivations of self-interest to be admitted (Beauchamp and Davidson 1979, p. 295). The questions remain: how should euthanasia be defined? how can we be sure that a given act is an act of euthanasia rather than some other kind of act, such as murder or unassisted suicide?

Beauchamp and Davidson (1979) argue that for an act to be an instance of euthanasia, it must satisfy at least five conditions.

1. *Intentionality.* Death must be intended and not be merely accidental, and further must be intended by at least one other human being.

2. *Suffering and evidence of suffering.* Here suffering may be in the form of conscious pain, mental anguish, and/or serious self-burdensomeness (as may occur in cases of high quadriplegia, or tetraplegia, or the like). This interpretation of suffering fully upholds the view that ending a person's pain is not always tantamount to ending that person's suffering (see also Cassell 1982; Kuhse 1982; Hill, 1992; Starck and McGovern 1992). In assessing a person's level of suffering, every effort must be made to gain 'sufficient current evidence' (Beauchamp and Davidson 1979, p. 301); in this instance, it is simply not enough to rely on mere guesswork or on supposition based on ignorance.

3. *Reasons for death and the means of death.* Beauchamp and Davidson contend that death-causing acts must be motivated by beneficence or other humanitarian considerations (such as the demand to end suffering). Killing acts which are not motivated by these things are not acts of euthanasia, but murder. Further to this, any means of death chosen must also be of a nature that does not cause more suffering than is already being experienced (Beauchamp and Davidson 1979, p. 302).

4. *Painlessness.* This condition is related to the previous one and demands, quite simply, that any death act

performed must be as painless and as merciful as possible. Beauchamp and Davidson (1979. p. 303) explain that if the means of bringing about death causes more suffering than if that particular means was not used, then the individual will be effectively deprived of a 'good death'.

5. *Non-fetal humanity.* Beauchamp and Davidson (1979, p. 303) contend that if this simple qualification is not included then we would not be able to distinguish acts of abortion from acts of euthanasia.

Beauchamp and Davidson maintain that the five conditions they have formulated supply a 'nonprescriptive definition' of euthanasia, and thus one which avoids dictating a particular moral conclusion. Whether they have totally succeeded, however, is another matter. The definition still seems ethically loaded, and therefore carries prescriptive properties. Nevertheless, the five conditions given supply an important step towards the formulation of a substantive concept and definition of euthanasia, and one which can be meaningfully applied in the euthanasia debate.

Types of euthanasia

Bioethics literature typically distinguishes between voluntary and involuntary euthanasia, and active and passive euthanasia. In the case of *voluntary euthanasia*, the patient voluntarily and freely chooses death, and may even ask for assistance to die (hence the notion of 'assisted suicide'). For example, doctors or nurses may be asked by patients to administer a lethal injection to hasten their death. By contrast, in the case of *involuntary euthanasia,* death-causing actions are carried out without the patient's consent, and may even be imposed against the patient's wishes or desires. There is some suggestion that a further distinction should be drawn here between 'involuntary' euthanasia and 'non-voluntary' euthanasia. McGuire (1987), for example, suggests that the term 'involuntary' implies an action which is carried out against the wishes of the patient, unlike 'non-voluntary' which simply implies that there is *no* voluntariness — in the sense that the patient is not capable of either denying or giving consent (as in the case of the permanently comatose or brain-injured patient). In the case of the permanently comatose, McGuire contends, euthanasia would be 'neither voluntary nor involuntary, but is simply non-voluntary'.

Active euthanasia, meanwhile, typically involves a deliberate act (or commission) which results in the patient's death. The deliberate act of administering a lethal injection or a lethal dose of pills is an example of active euthanasia. This type of euthanasia is sometimes referred to as positive euthanasia. *Passive euthanasia*, on the other hand, involves a deliberate omission or the withholding of certain life-supporting cares and treatments. Withholding antibiotics, nutrition and fluids, mechanical life supports, or other life-supporting measures from terminally or chronically ill patients are examples of *passive euthanasia*. This type of euthanasia is sometimes referred to as negative euthanasia (Glaser 1975).

These two distinctions generate four types of euthanasia: voluntary passive euthanasia; voluntary active euthanasia; involuntary passive euthanasia; and involuntary active euthanasia (Beauchamp and Perlin 1978, p. 219). This can be expressed diagrammatically, as shown in figure 10.1.

	PASSIVE	ACTIVE
VOLUNTARY	Voluntary passive euthanasia	Voluntary active euthanasia
INVOLUNTARY	Involuntary passive euthanasia	Involuntary active euthanasia

Figure 10.1 Four categories of euthanasia.

Is euthanasia morally justified?

Like other controversial bioethical issues, euthanasia has both its proponents and opponents. Attitudes towards it range from liberal and moderate acceptance to absolutist conservative prohibition. Opinion polls suggest that on the whole the public favours voluntary euthanasia.

A 1986 Morgan Gallup Poll showed, for example, that 74.2 per cent of people surveyed favoured voluntary euthanasia, while only 18.3 per cent opposed it; 7.5 per cent were undecided (Social Development Committee 1987, p. 134). In 1990, a Morgan Gallup Poll showed that little had changed, with over 70 per cent of those surveyed still supporting euthanasia. These figures show a marked increase over the past thirty years; the first Morgan survey on the subject, taken in 1962, indicated that only 54 per cent of those surveyed supported euthanasia (*Australian Dr Weekly*, 10 August 1990, p. 9).

Arguments in support of euthanasia

Those who support euthanasia typically argue that it is morally evil to allow people to suffer unnecessarily. As one author writes:

the most horrible thing in the world for us, living and sentient beings, is inexorable suffering, pain without any possible compensation when it has reached this degree of intensity; and one must be barbarous, or stupid, or both at once, not to use the sure and easy means now at our disposal to bring it to an end.

(Reiser 1975, p. 28)

Popular arguments in support of euthanasia (and, in particular, in support of legalising it) fall roughly under four main categories:

1. arguments from individual autonomy and the right to choose;

2. arguments from the loss of dignity and the right to the maintenance of dignity;

3. arguments from the reduction of suffering;

4. arguments from justice and the demand to be treated fairly.

(adapted from Beauchamp and Perlin 1978, p. 217)

A fifth more recent and controversial category of argument raised in support of euthanasia is that, in some instances, patients have a 'duty to die' (Beloff 1992, pp. 52–6).

1. Arguments from individual autonomy and the right to choose. We generally accept that people have a right to choose. And, as we have already seen in chapter 3, the moral principle of autonomy demands that we respect other people's choices, even if we consider them to be mistaken or foolish. The only grounds upon which a person's autonomous choices can be justly interfered with is if they stand to impinge seriously on the significant moral interests of others. Proponents of voluntary euthanasia argue that the right to choose includes the right to choose death (abbreviated as 'the right to die'). Given the right to die, this means that others (including the state) should not interfere with a person's decision to die, and in some instances may even entail a positive duty to assist a person to die — as in cases where a person desires death but is physically unable to end his or her own life (Johnstone 1988). Voluntary euthanasia is thought to be justified here on grounds of autonomy and the demand to respect a person's autonomous wishes.

2. Arguments from the loss of dignity and the right to the maintenance of dignity. Related to the demand to respect a person's autonomous choices is the further demand to respect and maintain a person's dignity. Advances in medical technology have increased medicine's capacity to prolong a person's life. Its methods, however, are not always humane, and can seriously erode a person's self-concept, character, sense of self-worth and self-esteem, and the like. As Beauchamp and Perlin (1978) point out, some patients 'are not only subjected to intense and abiding pain, they are often aware of their own deterioration, as well as of the burden they have become to others' (p. 217). They conclude that under these conditions 'it seems uncivilised and incompassionate' not to allow patients to choose their own death. Euthanasia in some pain states as well as in some chronic disease states may well be the most dignified option.

3. Arguments from reduction of suffering. Suffering is generally regarded as morally unacceptable and, as we have already seen in chapter 3, morality demands that, where possible, persons should be spared or prevented from suffering unnecessarily. In cases where patients' suffering is intense, protracted, unendurable and intractable, it seems cruel to deny them the choice of death as a means of release from their suffering. Euthanasia in these kinds of cases is said to be justified on grounds of 'prevention of cruelty' or 'mercy' (Beauchamp and Perlin 1978, p. 217). It is also thought to be justified on the grounds that people have the indisputable right to judge their suffering as unbearable, and the concomitant right to request euthanasia to end their unbearable suffering (see, for example, Admiraal 1991, p. 11). This, in turn, is grounded in the fact that, despite the achievements of modern medicine, doctors still cannot relieve all suffering (Admiraal 1991, p. 16).

4. Arguments from justice and the demand to be treated fairly. It is argued that everybody is entitled to be treated fairly and to share equally the benefits and burdens of life. To deny patients the option of being spared intolerable and intractable suffering is to treat them unfairly, and to make them carry a burden which others do not have to carry. Furthermore, to deny patients the right to die (that is, in a manner and time of their choosing) is to impose unfairly on them the values of others. Only patients, or those intimately involved with them (for example, family and friends), can judge what is in their own best interests. For others to deny patients the right to choose death is therefore to violate unfairly these patients' autonomy, dignity, and entitlement to be spared the harms that will flow from suffering intolerable and intractable pain. Where euthanasia is the only thing that can end patients' intolerable and intractable pain, it stands as a morally just alternative.

5. Arguments from altruism and the 'duty to die'. It is argued that in certain circumstances (such as in the case of old age, chronic illness, or when medical treatment is futile) it may be a person's duty to volunteer for euthanasia (Kilner 1990; Beloff 1992; Schwartz 1993). Beloff, for example, apparently finds it quite plausible that:

> the mere thought of becoming a burden to others, not to mention a drain upon society, would suffice to make [some] choose voluntary euthanasia as the only honourable course of action still open to them.
>
> (Beloff 1992, p. 53)

In situations where a person's primary care-givers are burdened to the point where they cannot live their lives fully and are themselves beginning to suffer as a result of their burden of care, euthanasia, argues Beloff, is not only permissible, but required and deserving of moral praise. Beloff explains that this is because:

> If there *is* a duty to die it is one that arises from our basic human predicament, the fact that we are dependent on others, and it is a duty we owe to those we cherish.
>
> (Beloff 1992, p. 54)

Arguments against euthanasia — three approaches

Not surprisingly, those who are against euthanasia are not moved by these kinds of arguments. The anti-euthanasia response typically entails three main approaches: to assert a number of counter-claims and counter-arguments against the views put forward in support of euthanasia; to assert a number of distinctive arguments against euthanasia; and to reject altogether the notion of passive euthanasia (killing by omission) on the grounds that there is a morally significant difference between directly killing a person and merely letting a person die (referred to in the bioethics literature as the 'killing/letting die distinction').

COUNTER-ARGUMENTS TO VIEWS SUPPORTING EUTHANASIA

1. Autonomy and the right to choose death. While the moral principle of autonomy is well established in Western moral thinking, it nevertheless has limits. Whether 'autonomy' was ever meant to stretch so far as to impose a moral duty on a doctor or a nurse to comply with a patient's request for euthanasia — to intentionally and actively assist that patient to die — is an open question. If complying with a patient's request for euthanasia has the foreseeable consequence of harming or affecting pre-judicially the significant moral interests of others (for example, the doctor[s] or nurse[s] receiving the request, or the patient's family and friends), there is considerable scope for arguing that the doctor(s) and nurse(s) in question have no duty to perform euthanasia, no matter how autonomous the patient's request for it. Further, given the complex nature of the morality of euthanasia, it is rather simplistic to hold that euthanasia can be justified on the grounds of patient autonomy *alone* without consideration being given to other important moral values and principles which might also have a significant bearing on a patient's choosing active or passive euthanasia, and on a doctor's, a nurse's, a family member's or a friend's providing it.

2. Dignity and the right to die with dignity. Dignity and dying with dignity does not necessarily entail choosing death over the artificial prolongation of life. The demand to respect and maintain a person's dignity might equally entail respect for a person's autonomous wish that 'everything possible be done' to prolong or sustain her or his life — and to sustain a sense of hope that is fundamental to living that life meaningfully, even though (and when) dying. Here, it is important to understand that the ethical controversies surrounding the care of dying patients are not just about management at a technological, medical or institutional level. As Campbell (1992, p. 255) points out, they should also be seen 'as a sign of a deeper crisis of meaning in our culture', and as an indication of how impoverished our society has become in 'assessing the significance of suffering, dying and death as part of a whole human life'. Given this, as Campbell goes on to explain:

> The emergence of the individual asserting inviolable rights to self-determination becomes intelligible in this void as a way to create meaning through a freely-chosen style of life and an authentic manner of death.
>
> (Campbell 1992, p. 255)

One way to respond to this crisis of meaning is to 'provide compassionate presence to the sufferer', not to 'end the suffering by killing the sufferer' (Campbell 1992, pp. 269, 276). Another is to deny altogether the philosophical bases for a 'right to die' (see, for example, Kass 1993).

3. Suffering and the demand to end it. Suffering is not just a medical problem; it is also an existential problem involving profound questions concerning the meaning and purpose of human life and destiny (Campbell 1992; Starck and McGovern 1992; Amato 1990; Klemke 1981). To 'end suffering by killing the sufferer' is, to borrow from Campbell (1992, p. 276), to misunderstand 'both suffering and ourselves in a way that threatens [infinitely] our moral integrity'.

4. Justice and the demand to be treated fairly. To deny patients the right to *choose treatment* — including the artificial prolongation of 'hopeless life' — is as unjust as to deny patients the right to choose death. Denying patients' requests for 'everything possible to be done', where this conforms with their notions of dignity, meaning, value and quality of life, is to impose unfairly on them the values of others. As in the case *for* euthanasia, only patients (or those close to them) can judge what is in their best interests, and they must be permitted to make these judgments.

5. Altruism and the 'duty to die'. In some circumstances, people may have a 'duty to live' in order to spare the pain of their grieving loved ones, who desire their ill loved one to live 'as long as possible'. Being dependent on others is not necessarily being a burden on them (see, for example, Kanitsaki 1993, 1994). Even if dependency does become burdensome — either for the dependent person or her or his carers — it is not clear how, if at all, this gives rise to a so-called 'duty to die'. At best, it may only substantiate 'our basic human predicament' that:

> the very experience of illness, and more fundamentally the process of aging that inevitably culminates in death, not only reveals our shared vulnerability and dependency, but also that we are all subject to some kind of ultimate powers beyond our control. Through our knowledge and technology we may aspire to a mastery of nature and the immortality of the gods, but we continually receive reminders of our dependency and finitude. From this it follows that any control we assert over our dying is already limited, and that dependency and dignity are not mutually exclusive.
>
> (Campbell 1992, p. 270)

At worst, to embrace a 'duty to die' may be to embrace an all-pervasive sense of pessimism and hopelessness which would blind people to understanding that 'the lives of even the terminally ill are precious and matter, right up to the last second of breath' (Mirin, reported by Gibbs 1993, p. 53). And it may risk blinding people to the fundamental insight which has been articulated so well by the late French philosopher and feminist, Simone de Beauvoir (1964, 1987 edn, p. 92), that, while all people must die, death is still an accident, and that, even if people know this, and consent to it, death remains 'an unjustifiable violation' (de Beauvoir 1964, 1987 edn, p. 92). By this view, therefore, to embrace a duty to die emerges as an embracement of the unjustifiable violation of human life and all that it stands for. It also risks the perversion of morality — and of its ultimate aim, notably, how best to *live* the 'good life'. Finally, if currency is given to the notion of people having a 'duty to die', this might have the undesirable effect, as argued earlier, of adding 'to the distress and guilt of those who wondered whether they were too great a burden on others' (Muirden 1993, p. 14).

SPECIFIC ARGUMENTS AGAINST EUTHANASIA

Specific arguments commonly raised against euthanasia (and the need to legalise it) include:

1. arguments from the sanctity-of-life doctrine;
2. arguments from misdiagnosis and possible recovery;
3. arguments from the risk of abuse;
4. arguments from non-necessity;
5. arguments from discrimination;
6. arguments from irrational or mistaken or imprudent choice;
7. the 'slippery slope' argument.

1. Arguments from the sanctity-of-life doctrine. A popular argument raised against euthanasia draws heavily on the sanctity-of-life doctrine and contends that, since life is sacred and inviolable, *nothing* (not even intolerable and intractable suffering) can justify taking it. Sanctity-of-life arguments against euthanasia run something like this:

1. human life is sacred, and taking it is wrong;
2. euthanasia is an instance of taking human life; therefore
3. euthanasia is wrong.

Whether human life is sacred, and whether taking it is always wrong is, however, a matter of philosophical controversy. For an enlightening discussion on the sanctity-of-life doctrine, I recommend Helga Kuhse's controversial book *The sanctity-of-life doctrine in medicine: a critique* (1987).

2. Arguments from misdiagnosis and possible recovery. An argument often used against euthanasia is that which speaks to the risk of misdiagnosis and the possibility of recovery. Doctors themselves argue that they are fallible and can make mistakes (see in particular the comments of Dr John Mathew, President of the Victorian Branch of the Australian Medical Association [AMA], reported in *The Age*, 4 August 1986a, p. 5). Furthermore, patients can sometimes recover spontaneously (see, for example, Chopra 1989; Dossey 1991), or a new cure might be found. (For example, it was reported recently that scientists have shown that the 'human spinal cord may have the capacity to reconnect and regenerate, and that treatment for spinal injuries may be tested on humans within a couple of years' [Ewing 1994, p. 1]. If a cure for spinal injuries were found, quadriplegics, for example, might not request assistance to die as they are now doing.) What is of concern about the euthanasia option is that once euthanasia is performed it cannot be reversed. Once done, it is done. The risk of error is unacceptable, and overrides any other considerations which might favour euthanasia in a particular case (see also Kamisar 1978; Muirden 1993).

3. Arguments from the risk of abuse. The possibility of euthanasia being abused is an argument frequently raised against euthanasia. For example, as already mentioned earlier in this chapter, Dr Nell Muirden, of the Peter MacCallum Cancer Institute in Melbourne, has emphasised the danger of euthanasia being abused by unscrupulous relatives (Athersmith 1986; Muirden 1993). Further to this, Dr John Mathew is reportedly concerned about legislation giving one group the power to terminate life. The fear that 'the giving of power to terminate life to any one group can easily be misused' is, according to the AMA, by no means 'trivial' (*The Age*, 4 August 1986, p. 5).

For the anti-euthanasiasts, the risk of abuse is unacceptable and militates against the moral permissibility of euthanasia.

4. Arguments from non-necessity. Another type of argument which seems to be emerging in public debate is that it is simply 'not necessary' to legislate or to support euthanasia. The reason commonly offered (mostly by conservative doctors) is that 'the medical profession has been successful over the years in allowing patients to die with dignity' (see in particular Dr Ken Sleeman's reported comments in Harari and Clarke, 1987). Since patients are 'dying well' or are having 'good deaths' anyway, why take the matter any further?

5. Arguments from discrimination. Also gaining increasing popularity is the objection that euthanasia entails blatant discrimination, notably by treating some lives as less worthy than others. Margaret Tighe, president of the Victorian Right to Life, for example, repeatedly argues that euthanasia is detrimental to terminally ill, sick and incompetent people. She maintains that euthanasia 'reinforces the concept that there are some lives not worthy to be lived' (Maslen 1986; Harari 1987). By this view, just as any other act of discrimination is morally offensive, so too is euthanasia.

6. Arguments from irrational, mistaken or imprudent choice. It is sometimes argued that any person requesting euthanasia is not really exercising a rational or prudent choice, and that, for this reason, among others, an individual's request for euthanasia should not be taken seriously. One of the staunchest supporters of this view is the Vatican. In its 1980 *Declaration on euthanasia*, it states:

> The pleas of gravely ill people who sometimes ask for death are not to be understood as implying a true desire for euthanasia; in fact it is almost always a case of an anguished plea for help and love.
>
> (Vatican 1980, p. 7)

(Whether a death wish is always the product of irrational or imprudent choice is however a matter of philosophical controversy.)

7. 'Slippery slope' arguments. Also popular in the anti-euthanasia debate, as it is in the anti-abortion debate, is the 'slippery slope' contention. It will be recalled that the slippery slope argument holds that we risk a decline in our moral standards once we permit the taking of human life. For example, if we permit abortion today, we will permit infanticide the next day, and euthanasia the next. In the case of euthanasia, a slippery slope argument might run as follows: once we allow euthanasia for consenting persons, we will permit euthanasia for unconsenting and non-consenting persons, such as infants, the intellectually impaired and the severely brain-injured. Once we compromise the standards for protecting human life, we compromise all other standards pertaining to human life and well-being. Euthanasia, then, should never be justified.

The arguments for and against euthanasia given here are not the only arguments raised in bioethics literature, but they are nevertheless common, and nurses need to become familiar with them. It should be pointed out that none of these arguments is uncontroversial, and that much more remains to be said about them than there is space here to do. Nevertheless, the discussion so far succeeds in supplying a starting point from which nurses can begin to address the question of the moral permissibility of euthanasia.

The killing/letting die distinction

Another response to the euthanasia debate is to argue that there is a morally significant difference between 'killing' and merely 'letting die'. Opponents of euthanasia claim that so-called *passive euthanasia* is merely 'letting die'; it is not euthanasia at all, and is therefore morally permissible. Let us explore this argument further.

It is sometimes argued that where medical treatment is relatively 'expensive, unusual, difficult, painful or dangerous' (sometimes referred to as 'extraordinary' treatment), no moral obligation exists to use it in order to prolong a person's life (Glover 1977, pp. 195–6; Vatican 1980, pp. 10–11). Furthermore, where a given life-prolonging treatment is unduly 'burdensome' to the patient, or even costly, it may, in conscience, be withdrawn (Vatican 1980, pp. 10–11). Even though the withdrawal of life-restoring or life-prolonging therapy may causally result in a patient's death, this need not be regarded as an intentional termination of a life, and therefore an act of passive euthanasia, but rather as merely 'letting nature take its course'. To put this another way, it is merely 'letting die', not direct and intentional killing. Withholding or withdrawing life-saving or life-prolonging treatment is therefore not, strictly speaking, euthanasia.

Bonnie Steinbock (1983) argues that withdrawing or withholding life-prolonging treatment should not be viewed as the intentional termination of life, but as 'the avoidance of painful and pointless treatment' (p. 293). Where decisions are made to withdraw treatments, these are really decisions about 'the most appropriate treatment for a given patient', not about killing that patient. She further contends that if a case of ceasing treatment is to hold as a case of euthanasia, it must first be shown that a particular treatment has been withdrawn with the *intention of causing death.* Where this cannot be shown, a claim of killing simply does not hold.

There are cases in which a doctor is simply 'not at liberty', argues Steinbock, to continue treatment — such as where a competent patient has explicitly refused a recommended life-saving therapy. In such cases it seems odd to hold the doctor culpable for failing to provide treatment or for causing the patient's death. Similarly, in cases involving hopelessly ill patients, where 'nothing more can be done', it seems implausible to hold that the discontinuation of a given treatment directly *caused* a patient's ultimate death (Steinbock 1983, p. 294). Here it is *disease* which has provided the causal link to a patient's death, not some act or omission on the part of a doctor or a nurse.

The ultimate conclusion of Steinbock's argument is that the discontinuation of life-prolonging treatment cannot be considered the intentional killing of another — viz an act of euthanasia. At best, it is merely 'allowing nature to take its course' or allowing the 'natural flow of events to continue'.

The case for 'letting die' fails to consider, however, that deliberately *not acting* in life-threatening situations is itself a kind of *act* (see also Weinryb 1980). In this respect, a conscious decision to withdraw or withhold life-saving therapy still amounts to a 'deliberate inducement of death' (Trammell 1978). As Fletcher (1973) points out:

> It is naive and superficial to suppose that because we don't 'do anything positively' to hasten a patient's death we have thereby avoided complicity in his [sic] death. Not doing anything is doing something; it is a decision to act every bit as much as deciding for any other deed.

> (Fletcher 1973, p. 675)

By this view, it can be seen that withdrawing or withholding life-saving treatment still involves deliberate choice, just as positively administering treatment does, and as such still has 'a place among events' (Green 1980, p. 204). In this respect discontinuing or withholding life-saving treatment may overwhelmingly hold as at least one way of intentional killing.

The view that withholding or withdrawing life-saving treatment is tantamount to intentional killing becomes even more compelling when considering the very nature of medical/health care contexts, which generally have the facilities to restore and/or prolong life. As Gruzalski (1981) points out, failing to treat in a medical setting is one way of killing *precisely because* in such settings there are the means to prolong life; where these means are not used, then a *failure to treat* can be differentiated from *disease* as a causal factor in a patient's death. A good example of this is the celebrated Clarence Herbert case (cited in Veatch and Fry 1987, p. 175). Mr Herbert, a 55-year-old security guard, suffered a respiratory arrest following an uneventful closure of an ileostomy. He was subsequently intubated and transferred to intensive care for treatment. There was, however, some controversy about whether Mr Herbert should be maintained on a ventilator. Nevertheless, the decision was made to discontinue his respiratory support. Although unconscious, Mr Herbert continued to breathe spontaneously and his vital signs stabilised. Despite this stabilisation, a second decision was made to withdraw all intravenous and nasogastric fluids, and to transfer Mr Herbert from the intensive care unit to a room in the hospital's surgical unit. Six days after his respiratory arrest, Mr Herbert died. An autopsy listed 'anoxia and dehydration as two of the causes of death' (Veatch and Fry 1987, p. 175). Here then is one case in which a failure to treat (namely the withdrawal of respiratory support and hydration) contributed causally to a patient's death; in this case a *failure to treat* was clearly distinguishable from mere *disease*.

The killing/letting die distinction is vulnerable to criticism on other grounds as well. Tooley (1980), for example, argues that there is no morally significant difference between *intentionally* killing and *intentionally* letting die, and that it is therefore just as wrong to 'intentionally refrain from interfering with a causal process as it is to initiate it' (p. 58). One of the consequences of this view is that, if there is no significant distinction between intentional killing and intentional letting die, it is probably the case that there is also no real distinction between active and passive euthanasia, since, like killing and letting die, these share the same intention — that of bringing about or hastening a patient's death. This, suggests Tooley, forces us to conclude that either euthanasia is somehow justified and therefore not morally wrong, or that we are morally confused or insincere in our thinking about it being wrong.

Arguing along similar lines, James Rachels (1975) contends that not only is there no distinction between killing and letting die, but that letting die 'has no defence' (p. 496), particularly where the period of letting die entails a period of prolonged and intolerable suffering. Cases involving the withdrawal or withholding of fluids and nourishment from severely disabled newborns and severe stroke patients are examples of this (Battin 1983). Rachels further argues (p. 495) that where letting die is allowed for so-called 'humane reasons', it amounts to much the same thing as killing; that is, the *cessation of treatment* amounts to *intentionally terminating another's life*. Consider, for example, the common practice of withholding nourishing fluids from severely disabled newborns. As a result of this practice, the severely disabled newborn almost always dies (mostly as a result of dehydration and starvation). The decision to withhold fluids from a severely disabled infant is usually considered a 'humane' course of action, since if the infant were to live it could only look forward to a burdensome life. In these kinds of cases, withholding fluids from a severely disabled newborn amounts to exactly the same thing as administering lethal injections to it, since both acts have the same intention (and outcome) — that is, of hastening the newborn's death and thereby preventing it from living or having to live a burdensome life.

If we accept these views, against the proponents of the killing/letting die distinction, we are also committed to accepting that there is no morally significant difference between withholding nourishment and fluids and administering a lethal injection. This is particularly so in cases where both have as their intention the hastening of a patient's death, the ending of a patient's suffering, and where both ultimately stand as a causal link to the patient's death when it actually occurs. If we accept this, we are further committed to accepting that in the ultimate analysis there is no intrinsic difference between active and passive euthanasia.

Intentional killing versus alleviating pain

At this point some comment needs to be made on the issue of narcotic administration to chronically and terminally ill patients. Is this, in some cases, tantamount to killing patients? I have spoken to many nurses who feel that their actions in administering prescribed narcotic analgesia to some patients have been tantamount to 'murder'. The question which arises here is: is the administration of narcotics in some cases the same as intentional killing? If so, is this always morally wrong?

It must be remembered, first, that many cases of medically prescribed narcotic administration are *not* cases of intentional killing, and in fact may prolong life. It is also likely that some cases fall somewhere between prolonging life and intentional killing. Third, it is probably true that some cases of medically prescribed narcotic administration are cases of intentional killing. Let us refer to these three kinds of cases respectively as analgesia without death; analgesia with unintentional death; and analgesia with intentional death.

Analgesia without death. There are some pain states which can only be relieved by the administration of narcotic agents. An effective narcotic regime — even when entailing enormous doses — can, however, control pain without necessarily 'doping' or debilitating the patient. Indeed, many patients receiving large doses of narcotics remain alert, pain-free and as active as their disease will allow. Muirden (1993), for example, cites the case of a 55-year-old man who had cancer and who, at one stage of his illness, was receiving up to 3600 milligrams of morphine by injection (the usual dose is about 10 milligrams every four hours, a total of just 60 milligrams a day). She writes: 'He did not die of an overdose, and did not remain in a drowsy or drugged state' (Muirden 1993, p. 18). In such cases the administration of narcotics is clearly nowhere near tantamount to intentional killing. In fact, it may be quite the reverse. As pain specialists are quick to point out, the correct prescription of narcotic agents (for example, morphine) is more likely to prolong patients' lives than shorten them, because patients are 'able to rest, sleep, eat more and take a renewed interest in life' (Twycross and Lack 1984, p. 183; Muirden 1993).

Analgesia with unintended death. There are other pain states which can only be relieved by the administration of narcotic analgesia. However, unlike the previous type of case, these pain states require the administration of narcotics at a level which may compromise patients' alertness and physical ability, and may even render them semi-comatose. In these types of cases, death is almost always hastened, even if not directly intended. Fortunately, these types of cases are not the norm, although they do occur frequently enough to be of concern to nurse practitioners.

Analgesia with intentional death. In another type of case, ill or debilitated patients do not have an organic pain state, or have only trivial pain states, but are nevertheless prescribed potentially lethal narcotic regimes. Pat Turton (1987, 1992), for example, cites the case of an elderly stroke patient who was prescribed what one nurse considered an 'unnecessary and dangerous' dose of morphine. The nurse's views were shared by the hospital pharmacy. When the nurse questioned the drug order, however, she was asked by the prescribing doctor, 'Is this your first ward?' the implication being that the nurse was naive. Turton comments that the drug was given by another nurse and the woman died within hours. Similar cases occur every day in residential care homes and in some general hospital wards. In other cases, analgesia is given to seriously ill patients who have neuropathogenic pain states which conventional medicine is unable to alleviate. The drug regime given is clearly intended to hasten death, although this intention may be 'disguised' in some way — for example, by stating a rationale to 'alleviate pain', even though it is known that the pain cannot be alleviated. It is difficult to avoid the impression that in all these cases the administration of a given narcotic regime is tantamount to intentional killing or the intentional shortening of life.

Given these three situations, the question remains: is the administration of potentially lethal doses of narcotics always morally wrong?

The case of *analgesia without death* is morally uncontroversial. Here narcotic regimes enhance not only patients' well-being but also patients' lives. Since no moral standards are compromised, the administration of enormous doses of narcotics in this instance is morally permissible.

The case of *analgesia with unintentional death*, however, is not so morally clear-cut. Although a patient may well be spared intolerable suffering by the administration of large and potentially lethal doses of narcotics, this cannot be achieved without compromising the patient's sanctity of life. For some nurses, the conflict between the demand to alleviate a patient's pain and the demand to respect and preserve a patient's life is the most troublesome of all. When caught in such a conflict, these nurses generally find the preservation-of-life principle too compelling to override and, rightly or wrongly, opt for withholding the analgesia. As a point of interest, Donovan et al. (1987), in researching the use of analgesia, found that some nurses administer only one-fourth of prescribed analgesia to their patients, although these patients have significant pain. (The widespread undertreatment of pain is also reported by Hill [1992, p. 76].) Donovan et al. do not identify conscientious objection as a possible variable influencing this incredible degree of negligence, but it cannot be altogether dismissed. While 'opting out' might alleviate the nurse's conscience, it does little to alleviate the patient's pain. Thus we are still left with a moral problem on our hands.

Catholic theologians have long recognised the dilemma posed by intolerable pain and the use of potentially lethal doses of narcotics as a means of suppressing pain. Interestingly, although the Vatican totally prohibits euthanasia, it nevertheless permits the use of narcotics as a means of alleviating pain — and, furthermore, permits dosages which might suppress a patient's level of consciousness and even shorten a patient's life (Vatican 1980, p. 9). There are, however, clearly defined conditions which must be met. First, there must be no other means of alleviating the patient's pain; in other words, potentially lethal doses of narcotics must never be prescribed except as a last resort. (This condition has interesting implications for the use of narcotics in cases involving severely disabled newborns and the chronically ill who are given narcotics as a means of suppressing hunger pains.) Second, the intention of using narcotics must be only to *alleviate pain*, not to cause death.

The first condition, that of last resort, is consistent with the general principles governing effective and safe pain management and, as it stands, is relatively uncontroversial. The second condition, however, that of intentionality, takes its force from the controversial 'doctrine of double effect', and thus is vulnerable to the same criticisms as is the doctrine itself.

The doctrine of double effect was developed by Catholic theologians. It states, roughly, that it is always wrong to do a bad act for the sake of good consequences, but that it is sometimes permissible to do a good act even knowing it might have some bad consequences. To illustrate this doctrine, consider the case of a patient suffering intolerable and intractable pain. In this case, ending the patient's life would also result in ending the patient's intolerable and intractable pain. While ending the patient's *pain* would be a 'good thing', ending the patient's *life* would not. Indeed, given the sanctity-of-life doctrine, deliberately ending an innocent patient's life would be a morally evil thing to do. Thus, we could say here, it would always be wrong to end an innocent patient's life (a bad act) in order to alleviate that patient's pain (a good consequence).

Given the 'good' of alleviating pain, however, we are morally permitted to give the patient analgesia — even though this might have the foreseeable and unfortunate consequence of shortening the patient's life. This is permitted since, even though the act of narcotic administration is associated with the foreseen possibility of hastening death, ending the patient's life is not the conscious intention behind the act. In short, the decision and action of giving the narcotics was not done with 'murder in your heart', to borrow from Cattanach (1985). To express the doctrine of double effect another way, we could say: it is always wrong to end patients' lives for the sake of alleviating their pain, but it is sometimes permissible to give potentially lethal doses of narcotics to alleviate pain, even though this might result in the patient's death — *as long as the patient's death is not the intended outcome.*

The doctrine of double effect has been the subject of much philosophical criticism, most notably on account of its over-reliance on what is called the foreseeability/intentionality distinction. This distinction holds roughly that foreseeing that a bad consequence will occur as a result of a given act is not the same thing as intending that bad consequence. For example, foreseeing that a patient will die as a result of being given large doses of narcotics is not the same thing as intending to end that patient's life; therefore the person who administers the narcotic is not morally culpable.

Critics reject this, however, and argue that the distinction drawn here is misleading. They contend that foreseeing a bad consequence of an action is exactly the same as intending it, since the agent knows that a bad consequence is pending but deliberately refrains from preventing it. To some extent, this position is also upheld in legal law. As Kuhse (1984) points out, the law presumes: 'everyone must be taken to intend that which is the natural consequence of his [sic] actions' (p. 26).

Given these criticisms, then, it seems that we cannot rely on the distinction between merely alleviating a patient's pain and intentionally ending a patient's life. Although it might perhaps be psychologically more tolerable to admit this distinction, it is not morally tolerable to do so. Where does this leave us?

The position is clear: nurses must all pursue a path of rigorous moral analysis of their actions. Acts involving narcotic prescription and administration must satisfy the ultimate standards not only of medicine and nursing, but also of morality.

First and foremost, narcotic administration must accord with patients' considered preferences. This means that every effort must be made to establish what patients' preferences are, and to what extent patients are prepared to tolerate or not tolerate pain. Nurses must be open to the possibility, for example, of some patients preferring to suffer a certain degree of pain rather than compromise their mental alertness and physical ability. While a nurse might not agree with this kind of decision, it is nevertheless the patient's prerogative to make it.

Second, pain management must itself be guided by the moral principles of beneficence, non-maleficence, justice, and the moral virtues of compassion and care.

Lastly, those involved in the administration of narcotics must be free conscientiously to refuse to administer drug regimes which they judge to be morally controversial or unacceptable.

Like analgesia with unintentional death, *analgesia with intentional death* is morally controversial. It should also be pointed out that it is illegal and would be viewed by the courts as homicide. This is an issue which requires open and honest intellectual debate, as the entire debate on active euthanasia makes plain.

Implications for nurses of narcotic administration

Narcotic administration will always remain a controversial issue for some nurses. Nevertheless it is not insurmountable. In most cases, a sound knowledge of the principles of pain management, proper pain assessment, and correct drug administration will help to reduce the likelihood of moral dilemmas occurring. In other cases, a clear articulation of relevant moral standards and values will help to reduce and/or resolve many of the moral problems associated with pain management and drug administration. Either way, the position nurses are morally obliged to take is clear: the patients are always the nurses' primary concern. If nurses have good reason to believe that a patient's safety, dignity, autonomy and well-being will be compromised by a given drug order or regime, then they must question it. This is not only a moral requirement, but also a legal requirement. It is far better to question a narcotic order and be wrong than not to question a narcotic order and be wrong — with the former, what is at stake may be only a little self-pride; with the latter, the stake may be a patient's life.

'Nursing care only' orders

Some nurses will no doubt find this analysis of euthanasia and its conclusions disturbing. It can be seen that many of the so-called 'routine' omissions of certain cares and treatments in hospital contexts are tantamount to acts of euthanasia. Even more troubling is that many patients are not given the opportunity to give an informed consent to the withholding or withdrawal of certain life-supporting or life-prolonging measures. What this invariably means is that it is involuntary and non-voluntary euthanasia which is being widely practised in our hospitals. Furthermore, nurses have for years been unwitting accomplices to these practices. It is small wonder that some doctors, as we have seen, publicly insist that legislative changes favouring euthanasia are 'not needed', on the grounds that the *medical profession* has been 'successful' in allowing patients to die with dignity. It hardly needs pointing out, however, that, if the medical profession has indeed been 'successful' in allowing patients to die (whether with or without dignity), it is often in the context of ordering nurses to perform acts of euthanasia on its behalf. These acts have essentially gone uncensured by law enforcement agencies, not so much because of a 'let sleeping dogs lie' attitude, but because the medical profession has rather cleverly succeeded in upholding an almost universal euphemism for prescribing passive and in some instances active euthanasia — namely, the proverbial 'medical order' 'Nursing Care Only'. This claim becomes compelling when it is considered that sometimes what doctors in fact order is not *nursing care,* but rather the *withdrawal* of nursing care. To illustrate this point, consider the widely discussed Dr Leonard Arthur case (Kuhse 1984), and the Danville case (Robertson 1981).

The Dr Leonard Arthur case

On 1 July 1980, in a small English city, a Down's syndrome infant named John Pearson died in the arms of a nurse. The case would have escaped public attention had it not been for a member of staff reporting the circumstances of the case to Life, an anti-abortion organisation. On the basis of the information obtained by Life, John Pearson's attending physician, Dr Leonard Arthur, was charged with murder. The charge was based on the prosecution's claims that:

1. Dr Arthur had ordered the administration of the drug DF118 with the intention of bringing about the baby's death;
2. the fact that Dr Arthur had ordered 'nursing care only' showed that he had intended the infant to die.

(Kuhse 1984, p. 22)

Dr Arthur's 'nursing care only' order in this instance directed the feeding of *water only* to the infant, and the administration of the drug DF118 '*at the discretion of the nurse in charge* [italics added] but not more than every four hours' (Kuhse and Singer 1985, p. 2). Since John Pearson had no organic pain syndrome as such, it would seem that the DF118 was prescribed for the purposes of sedating him and suppressing his hunger sensations.

However we look at this case, it is clear that what Dr Arthur ordered was *not* nursing care, or, if it was, it was highly negligent nursing care. For example, feeding water only to an infant who is perfectly able to take and tolerate a full and nourishing fluid regime falls far short of reasonable and acceptable standards of nursing care, as does the administration of a narcotic to an infant who does not have a commonly recognised organic pain syndrome. Let us explore this claim further.

Nurses are formally educated to assess individuals' fundamental health needs, to diagnose needs deficits (viz health problems), and to plan nursing interventions aimed at helping people to meet their own health needs. Nurses are also formally educated to evaluate the outcomes of their nursing interventions and to modify their plans of care if an individual's health needs and health goals have, for some reason, not been met. Among the ten or so basic health needs which nurses are taught to assess are nutrition (including hydration), comfort (including being pain-free), and safety (including being kept free of injuries which might be caused by the over-prescription or inappropriate prescription of certain drugs). The formal education given to nurses in this area provides the minimal legal standard of reasonable and acceptable nursing care. Any nurse who fails to assess and diagnose correctly a person's health problems and plan nursing interventions to help meet the health needs of a patient is practising below a reasonable and acceptable standard of nursing care, and is thus practising negligently. The line between failing to meet the nutrition, comfort and safety health needs of a severely disabled newborn and professional negligence is, then, a very thin one.

Even if hunger is conceded as a genuine pain syndrome, this still does not justify the administration of large doses of narcotics or sedatives, nor does it rescue nurses administering these from culpability. There are at least two reasons for this. First, it is not normal practice to administer large doses of narcotics or sedatives to alleviate hunger pain. If it were, patients hungry from, say, pre- and post-operative fasting would be routinely administered narcotics or sedatives as part of their care. As we know, this is not done. Nurses should be rightly suspicious of medical prescriptions directing the administration of potentially lethal doses of narcotics or sedatives to infants who do not have a genuine organic pain syndrome and who are suffering hunger only from not being fed adequately.

A second reason why narcotic or sedative administration is not justified in the case of hungry severely disabled newborns is that there is no clinical basis for preferring a narcotic agent or a sedative agent over a solid bottle of milk for alleviating these infants' so-called 'pain states' and associated distress. As a general rule, narcotics are prescribed only for extreme organic pain states or where other non-narcotic agents are known to be ineffective in alleviating a given type of pain. In less extreme pain states, the tendency is to prescribe non-narcotic agents (such as aspirin or paracetamol), or even to avoid prescribing analgesia altogether, with preference being given to other methods of pain manage-ment such as exercise, change of bodily position, massage, physiotherapy, transneuronal stimulation, the administration of antacids, and, in the case of babies and infants, simply nursing them on one's lap and spending time with them. Since hunger is not generally regarded as an extreme pain state (in fact hunger is not even listed as a pain state in general analgesic guidelines and manuals), it is again highly suspect that narcotics should be chosen as a preferred 'treatment' option over the simple administration of a bottle of warm milk. Similarly, sedatives are usually prescribed for children only as a last resort. Where children's distress can be easily resolved by feeding them and/or nursing them on one's lap, there seems little to justify the administration of potentially lethal doses of a given sedative or narcotic analgesic.

It is, I think, fairly obvious that 'nursing care only' orders, as given by doctors in the case of severely disabled newborns, are prescriptions for euthanasia. It is also clear that, by so ordering 'nursing care only', doctors are placing nurses in a position of legal negligence and possibly of even committing homicide. Obvious as these points are, however, they have been conveniently ignored by some courts. In the case of Dr Leonard Arthur, the suggestion that John Pearson had been killed by the *nursing care only* order was dismissed. Significantly, the defence council's success was largely based on showing that ordering 'nursing care only' was *proper medical practice* (Kuhse and Singer 1985, p. 9). In this case, the judge ignored any thought that the attending nurses had acted negligently by giving 'water only' to a hungry infant otherwise capable of feeding, and had effectively committed homicide by giving potentially lethal doses of narcotics to an infant who did not have a genuine organic pain syndrome (see also Gunn and Smith 1985). Following his trial at Leicester in November 1981, Dr Arthur was acquitted of the criminal charges brought against him. His acquittal is reported to have sparked 'public rejoicing' (Kuhse and Singer 1985, p. 10).

The Danville case

On 6 May 1981, Siamese twins were born at a hospital in Danville, Illinois. The babies were joined at the waist with three legs. Upon seeing the deformity, the attending anaesthetist passed the order: 'Don't resuscitate, let's just cover the babies' (Robertson 1981, p. 5; Horan 1982). The father of the twins, also a doctor, gestured support for the anaesthetist's decision. It was later revealed that the decision to let the infants die had been made on little more than a visual impression of the infants' condition. Robertson (1981) writes that in fact no assessment was made to check whether there was any brain damage, whether the twins could be separated, or what their prognosis was. No effort was made to explore either adoption or institutional alternatives for the babies. The decision was made in total ignorance, and furthermore was made at the most stressful point in time — at delivery. Nevertheless, an order was written in the medical notes not to feed the babies, and they were taken to the newborn unit to die.

Nurses involved in caring for the twins, not surprisingly, became increasingly uncomfortable with the decision to withhold feeds from the babies. And it is claimed that at least one of the nurses 'fed the babies several times' (Robertson 1981, p. 5). The case received public attention after an anonymous caller reported it to the Illinois Department of Children and Family Services. Upon receiving the call the department immediately investigated the caller's claim, and the babies were transferred to another hospital for assessment and care. Later, in an unprecedented step, criminal charges were filed against both the parents and the doctors for 'conspiracy to commit murder and endangering the life and health of children' (Robertson 1981, p. 5). In the legal case that followed, nurses described how the twins 'cried in pain because they were hungry; how the cries dwindled down to whimpers as they were starved to death, how the skin started to wrinkle . . .' (Robertson 1981, p. 6; Horan 1982).

As in the Dr Arthur case, nurses were once again placed in a legally and morally intolerable position on account of a 'routine' medical order to withhold nourishment. Curiously, because the nurses were unable 'to link the parents and the physicians directly with the orders to withhold food and fluids from the twins', the judge hearing the case dismissed the charges on grounds of lack of evidence (Robertson 1981, p. 5). It seems that either the nurses' expert testimony was not admitted, or, if it was admitted, it was considered insignificant. Either way, the universal euphemism for euthanasia, viz 'nursing care only', remained intact.

Issues and recommendations

Severely disabled newborns are not, of course, the only ones subjected to letting die or euthanasia decisions. Chronically and terminally ill adults are also the subjects of such decisions, as examples already given in this text make plain. And the dilemmas posed for nurses by withdrawing or withholding life-prolonging or life-supporting measures from adult patients are just as perplexing and as intense as those posed in the case of severely disabled infants. The question still remains: is killing or letting die morally impermissible?

There are clearly many types of cases where prolonging an individual's life would be cruel, inhumane and immoral. Furthermore, given the demands of a sound, critically reflective morality, it is likely that *allowing a person to die* — for example, by not resuscitating them in the event of a cardiac arrest, or by withholding fluids at the end stage of terminal disease (see also Zerwekh 1983) — *or assisting a person to die* — for example, by giving them a lethal drug dose — may well be the morally best thing to do in some cases. However, in equally as many types of cases, a failure to administer certain life-supporting measures would be cruel and inhumane and even immoral, just as withdrawing a life-supporting measure in a particular manner would be morally indefensible.

It is not being argued here that hastening or directly causing a patient's death is always morally indefensible. The contrary is true: in cases of considered preferences and intractable and intolerable suffering, the demand for euthanasia (as defined by Beauchamp and Davidson, cited earlier) is compelling, and it would be cruel and inhumane to deny people a 'good death' in such cases (see also Battin 1983; Humphrey 1991; Voluntary Euthanasia Society [UK] 1992). Rather, it is being argued that we need to be much more honest about the nature of death-inducing acts being performed in our hospitals, and be considerably more careful about the grounds upon which, and the ways in which, these are performed. It is not acceptable that euthanasia is disguised under the euphemism 'nursing care only'. Neither is it acceptable that doctors and the courts uphold the euphemism as a means of avoiding the euthanasia debate, or as a means of side-stepping the need to formulate a substantive legal position on the matter.

The law must confront the question of euthanasia. The law must also confront and appropriately deal with the plight faced by nurses who are forced into a position of having to perform the death-hastening acts that doctors do not — and, in some instances, will not — otherwise bring themselves to perform. It is essential that nurses have the legitimated freedom and authority to practise nursing as they have been educationally prepared to practise it. They must be free psychologically, as well as legally, from the implied restrictions of the currently legally protected medical prerogative to prescribe 'nursing care only' in cases where nothing more, medically speaking, can be done (or will be done) for a patient.

Meeting the basic health needs of patients is just as much a nursing prerogative as it is a medical one, and it is always the patients' prerogative. It is a matter to be shared, not dominated. Until this simple point is understood, the power to terminate life will always be concentrated in the hands of one dominant group (notably the medical profession), and thus will always be open to misuse and abuse. The legislation that is required is not that which concentrates the power of one particular group to terminate life, but that which diffuses or dissipates the power that one particular group — the medical profession — already firmly has.

The question society needs to answer is not: is euthanasia morally permissible? (it has already tacitly conceded that it is), but which type of euthanasia is permissible, and under what conditions? And, further, what kinds of methods can decently be employed to end a person's life? The nursing profession must also confront these questions, and must articulate a formal and substantive position on the extent to which it does or does not support certain methods popularly used to hasten death or to end a patient's life. And it must also formulate a stated position on the extent to which nurses can be decently expected to perform acts which are aimed at hastening a patient's death but which others cannot and will not bring themselves to do. Needless to say, these are issues that only morality can decide, not law, nor public opinion — nor, indeed, medical etiquette.

References

Admiraal, P. V. (1991). Is there a place for euthanasia? *Bioethics News* 10 (4), pp. 10–23.

Amato, J. A. (1990). *Victims and values: a history and a theory of suffering.* Praeger, New York.

Athersmith, F. (1986). Euthanasia could be abused by selfish relatives, says doctor. *The Age*, 3 July, p. 10.

Australasian Nurses Journal (1912). The right to die. 19 (9), 16 September, pp. 304–8.

Australian Dr Weekly (1990). Mercy killing survey, 10 August, p. 10.

Australian Nursing Federation (1987). Assuring quality care for those who are dying. In *Ethics nursing perspectives*, vol. 1, Royal Australian Nursing Federation (Federal Office), Melbourne, pp. 112–14.

Battin, M. Pabst (1983). The least worst death. *Hastings Center Report* 13(2), April, pp. 13–16.

Beauchamp, T. L. and Davidson, A. I. (1979). The definition of euthanasia. *Journal of Medicine and Philosophy* 4(3), pp. 294–312.

Beauchamp, T. L. and Perlin, S. (1978). *Ethical issues in death and dying.* Prentice Hall, Englewood Cliffs, New Jersey.

Beloff, J. (1992). Do we have a duty to die? In Voluntary Euthanasia Society (1992), pp. 52–6.

Birnbauer, B. (1983). Report calls for laws governing right to dignified death. *The Age*, 9 September, reprinted in *The Age Reprint Booklet, no 44: Euthanasia*, The Age Education Unit, Melbourne, p. 1.

British Medical Association (1986). *News Review* 11 (1), pp. 22–3.

Browne, A. (1990). Assisted suicide and active voluntary euthanasia. *Bioethics News* 9 (4), pp. 9–38.

Burchill, T. (1989a). There is no right to die, court rules. *The Age*, 19 January, p. 1.

Burchill, T. (1989b). Law body warns on 'killings'. *The Age*, 20 January, p. 4.

Campbell, C. S. (1992). Religious ethics and active euthanasia in a pluralistic society. *Kennedy Institute of Ethics Journal* 2 (3), pp. 253–77.

Carrick, P. (1985). *Medical ethics in antiquity.* D. Reidel, Dordrecht.

Cassell, E. J. (1982). The nature of suffering and the goals of medicine. *New England Journal of Medicine* 306, pp. 639–45.

Cattanach, J. F. (1985). The distinction between membership of the human species and characteristics of the human being. *Bioethics News* 5 (1), October, pp. 28–30.

Chopra, D. (1989). *Quantum healing: exploring the frontiers of mind/body medicine*. Bantam Books, New York.

Cossar, L. (1986). AMA: don't change law on euthanasia. *The Herald* (Melbourne), 14 July, p. 4.

de Beauvoir, S. (1964 [1987 edn]). *A very easy death*. Penguin, Harmondsworth, Middlesex.

de Wachter, M. A. M. (1992). Euthanasia in the Netherlands. *Hastings Center Report* 22 (2), pp. 23–30.

Donovan, M., Dillon, P. and McGuire, L. (1987). Incidence and characteristics of pain in a sample of medical–surgical inpatients. *Pain* 30, pp. 68–78.

Dossey, L. (1991). *Meaning & medicine*. Bantam Books, New York.

Ewing, T. (1994). Spinal damage: scientists cross the frontier. *The Age*, 13 January, p. 1.

Fletcher, J. (1973). Ethics and euthanasia. *American Journal of Nursing* 73 (4), April, pp. 670–5.

Gibbs, N. (1990). Dr Death's suicide machine. *Time Magazine*, 18 June, pp. 70–1.

Gibbs, N. (1993). Death giving. *Time Magazine*, 31 May, pp. 49–53.

Glaser, R. J. (1975). A time to live and a time to die: the implications of negative euthanasia. In J. A. Behnke and S. Bok (eds), *The dilemmas of euthanasia*, Anchor Books, Anchor Press/Doubleday, Garden City, New York, pp. 133–50.

Glover, J. (1977). *Causing death and saving lives*. Penguin Books, Harmondsworth, Middlesex.

Green, O. H. (1980). Killing and letting die. *American Philosophical Quarterly* 17 (3), July, pp. 195–203.

Gruzalski, B. (1981). Killing by letting die. *Mind* 90, pp. 91–8.

Gunn, M. J. and Smith, J. C. (1985). *Arthur*'s Case and the right to life of a Down's Syndrome child. *Criminal Law Review*, November, pp. 693–756.

Harari, F. (1987). Death can't be legislated, euthanasia committee finds. *The Age*, 1 May, p. 1.

Harari, F. and Clarke, S. (1987). Criticism for bill on rights of dying. *The Age*, 14 October, p. 3.

Hawley, J. (1983). Live or let die. *The Age*, 30 June, reprinted in *The Age Reprint Booklet, no 44: Euthanasia*, The Age Education Unit, Melbourne, pp. 5, 13.

Hill, C. Stratton (1992). Suffering as contrasted to pain, loss, grief, despair, and loneliness. In Starck and McGovern (1992), pp. 69–80.

Hirschler, B. (1993). Dying with dignity in Holland. *The Age*, 11 February, p. 7.

Horan, D. J. (1982). Infanticide: when doctor's orders read 'murder'. *Registered Nurse* 45 (1), pp. 75–82.

Humphries, D. (1983). Poll shows most favor voluntary euthanasia. *The Age*, 26 November, reprinted in *The Age reprint booklet, no 44: Euthanasia*, The Age Education Unit, Melbourne, p. 14.

Humphry, D. (1991). *Final exit: the practicalities of self-deliverance and assisted suicide for the dying*. Penguin, Ringwood, Victoria, Australia.

Johnstone, M.-J. (1988). Quality versus quantity of life: who should decide? *Australian Journal of Advanced Nursing* 6 (1), September–November, pp. 30–7.

Kamisar, Y. (1978). Euthanasia legislation: some nonreligious objections. In Beauchamp and Perlin (1978), pp. 220–31.

Kanitsaki, O. (1993). Transcultural human care: its challenge to and critique of professional nursing care. In D. A. Gaut (ed.), *A global agenda for caring*, National League for Nursing Press, New York, pp. 19–45.

Kanitsaki, O. (1994). Cultural and linguistic diversity. In J. Romanini and J. Daly, *Critical care nursing: Australian perspectives*, W. B. Saunders/Baillière Tindall, Sydney, pp. 94–125.

Kass, L. (1993). Is there a right to die? *Hastings Center Report* 23 (1), pp. 34–43.

Keown, J. (1992). On regulating death. *Hastings Center Report* 22 (2), pp. 39–43.

Kilner, J. F. (1990). *Who lives? Who dies? Ethical criteria in patient selection.* Yale University Press, New Haven and London.

Klemke, E. D. (ed.) (1981). *The meaning of life.* Oxford University Press, New York.

Kuhse, H. (1982). Commenting on David B. Allbrook's paper, 'Medicine and the prolongation of life: does "can" imply "ought"?' *Issues in ethics. Proceedings of the Conference on Medical Science and the Preservation of Life: Ethical and Legal Dilemmas*, November 1981, Centre for Human Bioethics, Monash University, Melbourne, pp. 35–44.

Kuhse, H. (1984). A modern myth. That letting die is not the intentional causation of death: some reflections on the trial and acquittal of Dr Leonard Arthur. *Journal of Applied Philosophy* 1 (1), pp. 21–38.

Kuhse, H. (1987). *The sanctity-of-life doctrine in medicine: a critique.* Clarendon Press, Oxford.

Kuhse, H. (1991). Introduction to the Australian edition. In Humphry (1991), pp. xi–xv.

Kuhse, H. (1993). Time has come for assisted euthanasia. *The Age*, 18 February, p. 13.

Kuhse, H. and Singer, P. (1985). *Should the baby live?* Oxford University Press, Oxford.

Kuhse, H. and Singer, P. (1988). Doctors' practices and attitudes regarding voluntary euthanasia. *Medical Journal of Australia* 148 (20), pp. 623–7.

Kuhse, H. and Singer, P. (1992). Euthanisia: a survey of nurses' attitudes and practices. *Australian Nurses Journal* 21 (9), pp. 21–2.

Maslen, G. (1986). Should the baby die? *The Age*, 28 June, Saturday Extra, p. 7.

McGuire, C. (1987). Euthanasia without consent. *The Age*, Letter to the Editor, 19 October, p. 12.

Muirden, N. (1993). Palliative care and the terminally ill. *St Vincent's Bioethics Centre Newsletter* 11 (1), pp. 13–19.

New South Wales Health Department (1993). *Dying with dignity: interim guidelines on management.* New South Wales Health Department, Sydney.

Nursing Times (1969). Switching off the respirator. 65 (24). 12 June, p. 739.

Nursing Times (1987). Dutch nurses in euthanasia drama. 83 (12), 25 March, p. 8.

Rachels, J. (1975). Active and passive euthanasia. *New England Journal of Medicine* 292, pp. 490–7.

Radic, L. (1982). Most support the right to die. *The Age*, 23 August, reprinted in *The Age Reprint Booklet, no. 44: Euthanasia*, The Age Education Unit, Melbourne, p. 3.

Reiser, S. J. (1975). The dilemma of euthanasia in modern medical history: the English and American experience. In J. A. Behnke and S. Bok (eds), *The dilemmas of euthanasia*, Anchor Books, Anchor Press/Doubleday, Garden City, New York, pp. 27–49.

Robertson, J. A. (1981). Dilemma in Danville. *Hastings Center Report* 11 (5), October, pp. 5–8.

Schwartz, R. L. (1993). Autonomy, futility and the limits of medicine. *Bioethics News* 12 (3), pp. 31–6.

Scott, R. (1991). Euthanasia: murder or mercy? *The Bulletin*, 13 August, pp. 46–9.

Social Development Committee, Parliament of Victoria (1987). *Inquiry into options for dying with dignity, second and final report*. Government Printer, Melbourne.

Starck, P. and McGovern, J. (1992). *The hidden dimension of illness: human suffering*. National League for Nursing Press, New York.

Steinbock, B. (1983). The intentional termination of life. In S. Gorovitz, R. Macklin, A. Jameton, J. O'Connor and S. Sherwin (eds), *Moral problems in medicine*, 2nd edn, Prentice Hall, Englewood Cliffs, New Jersey, pp. 290–5.

ten Have, H. A. M. and Welie, J. V. M. (1992). Euthanasia: normal medical practice? *Hastings Center Report* 22 (2), pp. 34–8.

The Age (1983). A right to die? 13 July, reprinted in *The Age Reprint Booklet, no. 44: Euthanasia*, The Age Education Unit, Melbourne, pp. 8–9.

The Age (1986a). AMA chief opposes active euthanasia. 4 August.

The Age (1986b). Euthanasia. 1 July, 31 December.

Tooley, M. (1980). An irrelevant consideration: killing versus letting die. In B. Steinbock, *Killing and letting die*, Prentice Hall, Englewood Cliffs, New Jersey, pp. 56–62.

Trammell, R. L. (1978). The presumption against taking life. *Journal of Medicine and Philosophy* 3 (1), pp. 53–67.

Turton, P. (1987). Last rights. *Nursing Times* 83 (17), 29 April, pp. 18–19.

Turton, P. (1992). Euthanasia and the nurses: last rights. In Voluntary Euthanasia Society (1992), pp. 92–4.

Twycross, R. G. and Lack, S. A. (1984). *Therapeutics in terminal cancer*. Churchill Livingstone, Edinburgh.

Vatican (1980). *Declaration on euthanasia*. Vatican Polygot Press, Vatican City, Rome.

Veatch, R. M. and Fry, S. (1987). *Case studies in nursing ethics*. J. B. Lippincott, Philadelphia.

Vervoorn, A. (1987). Voluntary euthanasia in the Netherlands: recent developments. *Bioethics News* 6 (2), pp. 19–26.

Voluntary Euthanasia Society (ed.) (1992). *Your ultimate choice: the right to die with dignity*. Souvenir Press, London.

Wallace, M. (1991). *Health care and the law: a guide for nurses*. The Law Book Company, North Ryde, Sydney.

Weinryb, E. (1980). Omissions and responsibility. *Philosophical Quarterly* 30 (118), January, pp. 1–18.

Zerwekh, J. V. (1983). The hydration question. *Nursing 83* 13 (1), January, pp. 47–51.

Chapter

11

Matters of life and death: III

Suicide

In 1992, it was estimated that the overall suicide rate in Australia was approximately eleven per 100 000 of population per year (Davis 1992, p. 93); in 1994 this figure was reported to have increased to thirteen per 100 000 (Middleton 1994, p. 3). These figures do not include attempted suicide rates; while reliable data on the incidence of attempted suicide are difficult to obtain, Davis (1992, p. 92) contends that 'for every youth suicide there are 50–100 suicide attempts'. Alarmingly, suicide is now the second most common cause of death among young Australians (Davis 1992, p. 90). The reality of this trend was underscored in 1992 with the revelation that twenty young people had suicided over a two-year period in the small Victorian township of Kyneton. The suicides were reported to have left the local community feeling stunned, alarmed, and extremely concerned about the welfare of its youth (Kennedy 1992, pp. 4–6; Deane 1992, p. 81; The Leader 1992, p. 8). In the following year, 1993, again in the State of Victoria, suicide deaths were reported to have outnumbered the State's road fatalities (Ryle 1993). The probability that some of these road fatalities were also 'autocides' (deaths as the result of premeditated [suicidal] automobile accidents [Donnelly 1990, p. 8]) merely exacerbates the significance of these statistics. In 1993, a United Nations study showed that 'Australia had the highest suicide rate in the industrialised world among males aged 16–30' (Middleton 1994, p. 3).

Suicide figures in the United States of America are comparable with those in Australia (Davis 1992, p. 92). In 1987, the incidence of suicide in that country was estimated at 12.7 deaths per 100 000 (Donnelly 1990, p. 9). Youth suicide rates in the United States are also alarmingly high (Davis 1992, p. 92; Donnelly 1990, p. 9). The magnitude of the suicide problem in the United States was highlighted recently with the reported suicide of a six-year-old girl, believed to be the youngest recorded suicide in the State of Florida (Power 1993, p. 9). The child was killed after she deliberately placed herself in front of an oncoming train. Her death was witnessed by three other children aged six, seven, and eight years old respectively — all of whom 'tried to move her as the train approached' (Power 1993, p. 9). The engineer was unable to stop the train 'until nearly a kilometer after impact' (Power 1993, p. 9). It is believed that the little girl wanted to die so that she could 'become an angel and be with her mother', who was dying of cancer (Power 1993, p. 9).

Suicide, by its very nature, is an extremely difficult and complex issue to address. At a personal level, the suicide of a loved one, a friend or an associate can be a devastating experience. Those 'left behind' may find themselves struggling 'to make sense of the suicidal act and the causes of suicidal behaviour' (Davis 1992, p. 90); they may also find themselves overwhelmed by feelings of grief, shame, remorse, anger, despair, and possibly even guilt at the thought that 'perhaps they could have done more' or that 'if only they had been there . . . it might never have happened'.

Suicide is also difficult to address at a professional/therapeutic level. Even the very best of psychotherapies may still fail to prevent a person suiciding; and even the very best of medical and nursing care may still fail to restore someone who has attempted suicide to a life that is 'worthwhile' and worth living. Equally if not more problematic are the difficulties of addressing the suicide issue at a moral level. Included among these difficulties is the challenge suicide and attempted suicide pose to fundamental moral notions about the value, sanctity and meaning of life. An important question here is not 'how to achieve a better more fruitful [good] life' — a central question in Western moral philosophy — but, as Heyd and Bloch (1981, p. 185) point out, 'whether to live at all'. More seriously, suicide challenges morality itself, and not least the values, standards and principles comprising it which might otherwise be appealed to for guiding deliberation on such issues as the entitlements and responsibilities of people contemplating suicide; the moral permissibility and impermissibility of suicide prevention; the entitlements and responsibilities of others toward those contemplating or attempting suicide; and other similar issues. Compounding the moral complexity of these issues is the additional consideration that, unlike other causes of death, suicide (or, more specifically, death from suicide) is relatively preventable (Baume 1988, p. 43).

Nurses who have either cared for a person who has attempted suicide, or who have been involved in the care of family members and friends of someone who has attempted suicide or succeeded in suiciding, will be only too familiar with the deep emotional agony that inevitably comes with this kind of situation. They will also be very aware of the complex moral problems that are commonly associated with implementing interventions aimed at preventing suicide, with caring for those who have attempted unsuccessfully to suicide, and with the difficulties of addressing these problems in a satisfying and helpful way.

It is not the purpose of this discussion to examine or present a treatise on the clinical aspects of suicide (its underlying causes, and means of prevention), or, indeed, on the philosophy or sociology or anthropology of suicide. Such a task would require major works in their own right — as has already been undertaken (see, for example, Durkheim 1952; Stengel, 1970; Farberow 1975a; Battin and Mayo 1980; Battin 1982; Clemons 1990; Colt 1991; Kaplan and Schwartz 1993). Rather, the task here is to assist nurses to gain an understanding of the moral aspects of suicide and suicide prevention, and the nature of nurses' moral obligations when caring for people who are contemplating or who have attempted suicide. In undertaking this task, attention will be given to examining briefly:

1. the history of suicide in different cultures and societies;
2. definitions of suicide, and possible criteria which must be met in order for an act to count as suicide; and
3. some important moral concerns which are raised by the suicide question, and which have significant implications for the profession and practice of nursing.

Socio-cultural attitudes to suicide: a brief historical overview

Concepts of and attitudes toward suicide have varied enormously across different cultures and throughout time (see in particular Farberow's [1975a] *Suicide in different cultures*, University Park Press, Baltimore). Just what was regarded as an act of suicide and whether suicide was approved or disapproved depended on a range of factors, including cultural norms and mores, religion, law, politics, and personal and social morality (Stengel 1970, pp. 65–73; Farberow 1975b, pp. 1–13; Beauchamp and Perlin 1978, pp. 88–92; Alvarez 1980, pp. 7–32; Battin 1982, pp. 27–75; Amundsen 1989, pp. 77–153; Brody 1989b, pp. 39–75; Beauchamp 1989, pp. 183–219; Cooper 1989, pp. 9–38; Ferngren 1989, pp. 155–81). These factors have seen Western attitudes toward suicide shift dramatically from those of socio-cultural approval through to religious prohibition, criminalisation, and ultimately the medicalisation of suicide (see figure 11.1).

Socio-cultural acceptance of suicide, 600 BC–4 AD

In the introduction to *Suicide: the philosophical issues*, Battin and Mayo (1980, p. 1) note that 'suicide has not always been assumed to be tragic or a phenomenon that is always to be prevented'. They go on to point out that, in both the early Greek and the Hebrew cultures, 'suicide was apparently recognized as a reasonable choice in certain kinds of situations', and that for some early North African Christians, 'suicide — like martyrdom — was a mark of religious devotion practiced as a way of insuring attainment of immediate salvation' (Battin and Mayo 1980, p. 1).

In Ancient Greece and Rome, suicide was viewed as permissible (at least for the upper classes*) if it was chosen for 'the best possible reason' (Alvarez 1980, p. 18). The 'best possible reasons' included to preserve honour; to avoid dishonour or ignominy; as an expression of grief or bereavement; and for high patriotic principle or for a patriotic cause (Farberow 1975b, p. 5; Alvarez 1980, p. 18). There are many famous examples of suicide deaths in the history and mythology of ancient Greece and Rome. Notable among these are the Greek mythological character Jocasta (the mother of Oedipus, King of Thebes), who hanged herself to avoid the grief and shame she felt upon learning of her unwitting complicity in the sins imposed on her by fate (Sophocles 1911 edn,

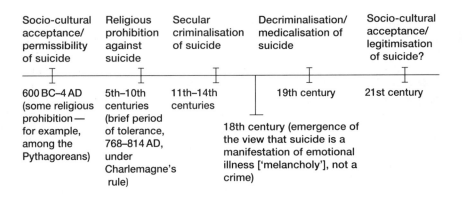

Figure 11.1 The transformation of attitudes to suicide.

---

* Initially, suicide was prohibited on religious grounds. As religious forces weakened, however, attitudes to suicide changed. Farberow (1975b, p. 4) explains: 'while the attitudes of horror and condemnation for suicide were preserved in the lower classes, the upper classes seemed to develop a different religion and different morals, expressing tolerance and aceptance [of suicide]'.

vv. 1213–86); Socrates, the famed ancient Greek philosopher, who killed himself patrioticaly by drinking hemlock after he was sentenced to death for corrupting the minds of the youth of Athens with his philosophical ideas (see Plato's *Euthyphron*, *Apology*, *Crito*, and *Phaedo* in Church's [1903] translation *The trial and death of Socrates*, and in Tredennick's [1969] translation *The last days of Socrates*); and the Roman matron Portia, who, upon learning of the death of Brutus at Philippi, killed herself by swallowing red-hot coals in what French (1985, p. 142) suggests was a kind of *suttee*. Zeno, the founder of Stoic philosophy (who apparently supported Seneca's view that suicide was permissible, but only as a last resort in the case of intractable suffering), also suicided. He apparently hanged himself in disgust at the age of 98 after falling and dislocating a toe! (Farberow 1975b, p. 5). The Roman view of suicide was perhaps among the most liberal during this period. Alvarez comments:

> the Romans looked on suicide with neither fear nor revulsion, but as a carefully considered and chosen validation of the way they had lived and the principles they had lived by [. . .]. To live nobly also meant to die nobly and at the right moment. Everything depended on the dominant will and a rational choice.
>
> (Alvarez, 1980, p. 23)

Not all the ancient Greeks and Romans had a permissive attitude to suicide, however. The Pythagoreans, for example, were vehemently opposed to suicide on religious grounds (Wennberg 1989, p. 41). And both the famed ancient Greek philosophers Plato and Aristotle opposed suicide, on religious and secular grounds respectively (Wennberg 1989, p. 42). While Plato was sympathetic to suicide 'when external circumstances became intolerable' (Alvarez 1980, p. 20), Aristotle was opposed even to this, on the grounds that:

> to kill oneself to escape from poverty or love or anything else that is distressing is not courageous but rather the act of a coward, because it shows weakness of character to run away from hardships, and the suicide endures death not because it is a fine thing to do but in order to escape from suffering.
>
> (Aristotle 1976 edn, p. 130 [1116a 12–15])

Aristotle also opposed suicide on the economic grounds that it deprived 'society of one of its productive members' (Wennberg 1989, p. 42). Interestingly, extant taboos against suicide in the city of Athens saw the corpse of the suicide victim 'buried outside the city, its hand cut off and buried separately' (Alvarez 1980, p. 17). Alvarez points out, however, that suicide taboos and the treatment of corpses in these instances were linked not so much as might be thought to religious prohibition or to Aristotelian notions of one's duty to contribute productively to the state. Rather, they were linked 'with the more profound Greek horror of killing one's own kin. By inference, suicide was an extreme case of this, and the language barely distinguishes between self-murder and murder of kindred' (Alvarez 1980, p. 18).

In Rome, on the other hand, while permissive attitudes towards suicide were enshrined in law (Alvarez 1980, p. 22), there were exceptions based on practical and economic grounds. For example, it was a criminal offence for a slave to suicide, since it deprived the master of his capital investment (if this offence was committed within the first six months of a slave being purchased, he could be returned dead or alive to the original master and a refund obtained) (Alvarez 1980, p. 23). Soldiers who suicided were also deemed to have committed a serious offence — 'desertion'. This was because a soldier was 'considered to be the property of the state [a chattel] and his suicide was tantamount to desertion' (Alvarez 1980, p. 23). Finally, it was considered an offence for a criminal to suicide 'in order to avoid trial for a crime for which the punishment would be forfeiture of his estate' (Alvarez 1980, p. 23). Relatives were, however, entitled to defend the accused in his absence. If successful, they would retain property rights to the deceased's estate; if unsuccessful, they would forfeit all property rights, and the deceased's estate would go to the state. Thus, as Alvarez concludes:

> suicide was an offense against neither morality nor religion, only against the capital investments of the slave-owning class or the treasury of the state.
>
> (Alvarez 1980, p. 23)

There are many other examples of old and ancient cultures in which suicide was tolerated, permitted and even esteemed: the Druids, for example, viewed suicide as a passport to paradise, and as a means of accompanying their departed friends (Alvarez 1980, p. 13); in Japan, suicide was ritualised in the form of *seppuku* or *hara kiri* (more commonly known in the variant spelling *harikari*) (Farberow 1975b, p. 3; Smith and Perlin 1978, p. 1622); and in India and China, the ceremonial sacrifice of widows (of which the Hindu custom of *suttee* is an example) was also common (Wennberg 1989, p. 39). (Whether this 'ceremonial sacrifice' should be viewed as *suicide* rather than *homicide* is, however, a contentious point — see, for example, Daly 1978, pp. 114–33.)

Perhaps some of the most poignant examples of the tolerance, if not the permissibility, of suicide can be found in the early Jewish and Christian traditions.

Suicide in the orthodox Jewish tradition has been and continues to be viewed as an abhorrent and heinous sin, and is expressly forbidden (Smith and Perlin 1978, p. 1622; Kaplan and Schwartz 1993). Historically, suicides in Jewish communities have resulted in the people who have suicided being denied full burial honours and other associated rituals, for example, mourning (Farberow 1975b, p. 4; Wennberg 1989, p. 48). There have, however, been some interesting and heart-rending exceptions to this attitude of prohibition. Possibly one of the most famous of these was the mass suicide in 73 AD of 960 Zealots (men, women and children) at Masada, on the western shore of the Dead Sea. In this instance, the Zealots preferred to die at their own hands rather than submit to the Roman legions surrounding their sanctuary (Wennberg 1989, pp. 49–50; Battin 1982, p. 166; Alvarez 1980, p. 17; Farberow 1975b, p. 4). Significantly, the Masada victims are honoured, not condemned in the Jewish tradition (Wennberg 1989, p. 50). In more recent history, in what has been referred to as 'the incident of the ninety-three maidens' (Wennberg 1989, p. 50), ninety-three Jewish female students and teachers (including the head teacher) chose to suicide rather than to submit themselves to the infamous Gestapo for 'immoral purposes'. Describing the incident, Battin writes:

> During the Second World War, the directress of an orthodox Jewish girls' school in a Nazi-occupied city came to understand that her girls, ranging in age from twelve to eighteen, had been kept from extermination in order to provide sexual services for the Gestapo. When the Gestapo announced its intention to avail themselves of these services — ordering the directress to see that the girls were washed and prepared for defloration by 'pure Aryan youth' — she called an assembly and distributed poisons to each of the students, teachers and herself. The ninety-three maidens, as they came to be called, swallowed the poison, recited a final prayer, and died undefiled.
>
> (Battin 1982, p. 166)

Commenting on this mass suicide, Wennberg (1989, p. 50) explains that, like the suicide of the four hundred children facing defilement in the Talmud (Gittin 57b), rather than this act being viewed as a sin, it would be viewed as 'an act of faithfulness to God'; that is, of the victims submitting themselves to God's purpose, rather than to the immoral purposes of the men who would violate them.

The Christian religion, and more specifically its sacred writings, the Bible, also offers some interesting examples of tolerant if not permissible attitudes toward suicide (Wennberg 1989, p. 47;

Rauscher 1981, pp. 105–7; Farberow 1975b, p. 4; Smith and Perlin 1978, p. 1622). The first and perhaps most poignant example of all is what Wennberg (1989, p. 45) describes as the Bible's 'curious silence' on the subject of suicide. Indeed, as Smith and Perlin (1978, p. 1622) also observe, 'the Bible contains neither an explicit word for suicide nor an explicit prohibition of the act'.

Despite the apparent omission of an explicit condemnation of suicide, there are a number of significant and famous incidents of suicide mentioned in the Bible:

- Samson, who pleaded 'Let me die with the Philistines' as he toppled the temple filled with God's enemies and was crushed to death (Judges 16: 30);

- Saul, who 'took a sword and fell on it' (1 Samuel 31: 4);

- Saul's armour-bearer, who 'also fell on his sword' (1 Samuel 31: 5);

- Ahithophel, who 'hanged himself, and died' (2 Samuel 17: 3);

- Zimri, who 'burned the King's house down upon himself with fire, and died' (1 Kings 16: 18);

- Judas, who 'went and hanged himself' (Matthew 27: 5).

Another (although less certain) Biblical example of suicide (contrary to popular thought, it may in fact be more an example of euthanasia) is the case of Abimelech (Judges 9: 52), who, in the course of attempting to set fire to a tower in which men and women had locked themselves for protection, was seriously injured after a woman in the tower 'dropped an upper millstone on Abimelech's head and crushed his skull' (Judges 9: 53). Fearing that his manner of death would tarnish his posthumous reputation, he begged his young armour-bearer:

'Draw your sword and kill me, lest men say of me, "A woman killed him." ' So his young man thrust him through, and he died.

(Judges 9: 54)

Some even suggest that the death of Jesus Christ is an example of suicide (Alvarez 1980, p. 12; Rauscher 1981, p. 107). Whether Jesus' death can be regarded as suicide, however, depends entirely on how suicide is defined.

The Bible's apparent failure to prohibit or condemn suicide explicitly, while significant, should not be taken as implying

Christian approbation of the act. As Wennberg (1989, p. 46) points out, acts of suicide are — and have long been — incompatible with Christian theology (see also Amundsen 1989, pp. 77–153; Ferngren 1989, pp. 155–81; Beauchamp 1989, pp. 183–219; Boyle 1989, pp. 221–50; Kaplan and Schwartz 1993). The only apparent exception to this prohibition, at least until the teaching of St Augustine, was if suicide was the only option available in order to 'protect one's virginity or to avoid forced apostasy' (Battin 1982, pp. 3, 70–1).

Attitudes of religious prohibition against suicide

Until about 250 AD, attitudes towards suicide were largely permissive, and suicide was common even among the early Christians (Farberow 1975b, p. 6; Alvarez 1980, p. 12; Battin 1982, p. 71). In fact, the rise of Christianity as a persecuted religion brought with it an 'almost epidemic rate of self-destruction', justified as martyrdom (Heyd and Bloch 1981, p. 191). The reasons for this martyrdom are said to have included:

> pessimism, longing for a better life, a struggle for redemption, and a desire to come before God and live there forever.
>
> (Farberow 1975b, p. 6)

The religious fathers of the day were, however, appalled by the 'squandering of human life', and sought to halt it immediately by making it the subject of explicit and absolute religious prohibition (Wennberg 1989, p. 54). Thus, writes Farberow:

> As the 4th century began, changes appeared, with the Church adopting a hostile attitude that progressed from tentative disapproval to severe denunciation and punishment. Antagonism toward suicide developed. Suicide became proof that the individual had despaired of God's grace, or that he [sic] lacked faith and was rejecting God by rejecting life, God's gift to man.
>
> (Farberow 1975b, p. 6)

The Church's emphatic and official prohibition saw a marked decline in the incidence of suicide, with one writer commenting that, by the twelfth century, 'while the Catholic Church held sway in Europe, suicide became practically unknown' (Farberow 1975b, p. 6).

Two highly influential figures in the fight against suicide/martyrdom were the Christian theologians St Augustine (354–430 AD) and St Thomas Aquinas (1225–74). St Augustine's principal theological argument against suicide rested on his interpreting the sixth commandment ('thou shalt not kill') as applying not only to *homicide* (the killing of another), but to *suicide* (the killing of the self) (Heyd and Bloch 1981, p. 191). Rejecting the popular view at the time that suicide was a way of avoiding sin and gaining a passport to eternal paradise, St Augustine countered that 'suicide is itself the gravest sin' (Heyd and Bloch 1981, p. 191). Thus St Augustine denounced suicide 'as a crime under all circum-stances' — a view that was quickly ratified as the official view of the Church (Stengel 1970, p. 68). In 452 AD, for example, the Council of Arles declared the act of suicide to be 'an act inspired by diabolical possession'; one century later, the Church set another disincentive to suicide, this time by ordaining that 'the body of the suicide be refused a Christian burial' (Stengel 1970, p. 69).

St Thomas Aquinas' views against suicide were as absolute and as uncompromising as were St Augustine's (Wennberg 1989, p. 65). His arguments were, however, more systematic (Heyd and Bloch 1981, p. 191) and less vulnerable to criticism (Wennberg 1989, p. 66). Central to Aquinas' position were the arguments that suicide constituted an offence to and a violation of one's duty to oneself, the community, and God; he also regarded suicide as 'contrary to the natural law and to charity', and hence wrong (St Thomas Aquinas 1978 edn, pp. 103–4). Whether suicide is, in fact, any of these things has been and remains the subject of much con-troversy, which will not be settled here (see, for example, Szasz 1977; Beauchamp 1978a, 1978b; Brandt 1978, 1980; Margolis 1978; Battin and Mayo 1980; Battin 1982; Barrington 1983; Hume 1983 edn; Kant 1983 edn; Brody 1989a; Wennberg 1989; Donnelly 1990).

As Christian religious prohibition against suicide spread across Europe, so too did 'the acts of violence and indignity perpetrated against the dead body' — partially, at least, because of 'fears of evil spirits released by the suicide' (Stengel 1970, p. 69). In some countries, for example, 'a stake was driven through the body and it was buried at the crossroads' (Stengel 1970, p. 69; Farberow 1975b, p. 7); an alternative to skewering the body with a stake was to place a stone on the face of the corpse, which would have the same effect as a stake — namely, it would prevent the victim from 'rising as a ghost to haunt the living' (Alvarez 1980, p. 8). The last degradation of the corpse of a person who had suicided occurred as recently as 1823 in England, when a Mr Griffiths was buried at the crossroads of Grosvenor Place and King's Road, Chelsea (Stengel 1970, p. 69; Alvarez 1980, p. 8). For fifty years after this, however, the bodies of suicide victims were still not treated with full respect, and, if unclaimed, were donated legitimately to schools of anatomy for dissection (Alvarez 1980, p. 8).

In France, as in England, it was also common practice to treat the corpse of a suicide victim in a violent and undignified way. Alvarez writes, for example, that:

varying with local ground rules, the corpse was hanged by the feet, dragged through the streets on a hurdle, burned, thrown on the public garbage.

(Alvarez 1980, p. 9)

As well as this, as in other European countries, the property of suicide victims was legally confiscated, and their memories legitimately defamed (Alvarez 1980, p. 9; Stengel 1970, p. 69). Perhaps worst of all, especially for followers of the Christian faith, was the punishment of being denied a proper Christian burial within the consecrated grounds of the church — a punishment which existed around the world right up until the 1960s and 1970s, and which may still exist in some countries even today. In 1968, for example, a United States study of Roman Catholic and Greek Orthodox priests in Los Angeles found that suicide victims were still sometimes — albeit rarely — denied Christian burial (Demopolous 1968, cited in Farberow 1975b, p. 12). Apparently the many sympathetic priests who were burying suicide victims essentially overcame canonical prohibitions against providing Christian burials to suicide victims by accepting that the deaths in question were either 'accidental', 'natural', or the 'irresponsible act of an unsound mind', and hence not a culpable sin (Farberow 1975b, pp. 12–13; Donnelly 1990, p. 9). In the mid-1970s, a similar situation existed in Catholic Italy. In an article examining the psycho-cultural variables in Italian suicide, Farber noted:

Suicide is more severely disapproved and regarded with more horror than in many other countries. A suicide cannot be buried in sacred ground; the family is grievously shamed. On a practical level, for example, an applicant will be rejected by the police force if there has been a suicide in the family. It is understandable, therefore, that a sympathetic doctor, priest, or police official will collaborate in having a suicide reported as a death from some other cause. Such behaviour is widely accepted in the Italian culture, in which family loyalty outweighs the value of civic responsibility.

(Farber 1975, p. 179)

Significantly, this collaboration has resulted in what Farber (1975, p. 179) describes as a 'severe distortion of official statistics on suicide and the reasons for suicide', with 'mental illness' being cited as the main reason. This is because:

in the eyes of the Church, only suicide by a sane person, who is responsible for his [sic] decision, is a sin. The label of mental illness allows for normal, religious burial and provides a shield for the family.

(Farber 1975, p. 180).

The criminalisation of suicide

Prohibitions against and punishments for suicide were not only enshrined in and made a part of canon law. Under the influence of religious views, sanctions against suicide were also enshrined in (secular) common law (Stengel 1970, p. 70). Opinion varies on when suicide was first deemed a crime in England; some suggest that it could have been as early as the tenth century, while others contend that it was not until as late as 1485 (Stengel 1970, p. 70). By around 1554, however, suicide was definitely 'equated with murder as a criminal offence (*felo de se*) and attempted suicide a misdemeanour' (Stengel 1970, p. 71). Legislation in other European countries also viewed suicide as a crime equivalent to murder, and worse. In 1670, for instance, pressure from the Church saw secular legislation enacted making suicide 'not merely murder but high treason and heresy' (Farberow 1975b, p. 9).

Anti-suicide legislation, like its counterpart in canon law, brought with it inordinate prejudice and penalties against suicide. This resulted in bizarre treatment of those unfortunate enough to be caught surviving a suicide attempt. An example of the gross inhumanity that anti-suicide legislation could both prescribe and enforce can be found in what was probably a public execution held some time during the 1860s in London and reported in the contemporary press. (Note: executions in England were public until 1868 [Carr 1961, p. 336].) Nicholas Ogarev, a Russian exile staying in London at the time, described the incident in a letter to his beloved, Mary Sutherland:

> A man was hanged who had cut his throat, but who had been brought back to life. They hanged him for suicide. The doctor had warned them that it was impossible to hang him as the throat would burst open and he would breathe through the aperture. They did not listen to his advice and hanged their man. The wound in the neck immediately opened and the man came to life again although he was hanged. It took time to convoke the aldermen [sic] to decide the question what was to be done. At length the aldermen [sic] assembled and bound up the neck below the wound *until he died*. Oh my Mary, what a crazy society and what a stupid civilisation.

(quoted in Carr 1961, pp. 336)

This example of gross inhumanity and absurdity — and the 'weird vindictiveness [of] condemning a man to death for the crime of having condemned himself to death' (Alvarez 1980, p. 8) — was sanctioned by both the church and the state. Further, this 'weird vindictiveness', as Alvarez (1980, p. 8) describes it, did not end until almost a hundred years after this incident occurred. Stengel (1970, p. 71) comments, for example, that even as late as 1946–55 in England and Wales, 5794 people were brought to trial for attempting suicide. Of these, 5447 were found guilty; and of these, 5138 were fined or put on probation, and 308 were sentenced to prison without the option of a fine or probation (Stengel 1970, p. 71). The capricious way in which the law was implemented is exemplified by a 1955 English case in which a 'sentence of two years' imprisonment was imposed on a man for trying to commit suicide in prison' (Stengel 1970, p. 71).

As religious and social opponents of suicide began to lose their influence, the old, cruel, prejudicial, religiously based superstitious attitudes against suicide and attempted suicide gradually changed. Medical dogma replaced religious dogma, and suicide came to be viewed as the act of a 'diseased mind', rather than a diseased ('diabolically possessed') soul. Laws prescribing the desecration of corpses and the confiscation of property were abolished (Farberow 1975b, p. 12). In 1961, England decriminalised suicide (Stengel 1970, p. 71; Glover 1977, p. 170; Browne 1990, p. 10). In Canada, suicide was decriminalised in 1972; and in the United States, while attempted suicide continues to be illegal in some States, suicide itself 'is not illegal in any state' (Browne 1990, p. 10).

Just over two hundred years ago, in 1790, France emerged as the first country to repeal its anti-suicide legislation (Stengel 1970, p. 71). Two centuries later, 'both suicide and attempted suicide are not criminal events in any civilized society' (Browne 1990, p. 10).

The medicalisation of suicide

The pressure to reform anti-suicide legislation came mainly from doctors, followed by sympathetic magistrates, and lastly members of the clergy (Stengel 1970, p. 71). However, the medical profession's political lobbying in this instance achieved considerably more than mere legislative reform; it also achieved legitimation of the medicalisation of suicide. In England, for example, soon after the 1961 *Suicide Act* was passed, the Ministry of Health in London advised all doctors and relevant health authorities that:

> attempted suicide was to be regarded as a medical and social problem and that every such case ought to be seen by a psychiatrist.

> (Stengel 1970, p. 72)

Whether this 'reform' has been, as Stengel (1970, p. 72) claims, a less 'moralistic and punitive reaction' than that expressed in former legislation remains to be seen. Those who attempt suicide are still frequently the subject of 'negative attitudes', even on the part of attending health care professionals (Baume 1988, p. 44; Donnelly 1990, p. 10; Lindars 1991, p. 30; Knight 1992, p. 260; Bailey 1994); further, they can still find themselves incapacitated involuntarily by the law. As Beauchamp and Childress (1989) point out:

> Although the act of suicide has been decriminalised, a suicide attempt, irrespective of motive, almost universally gives a legal basis for intervention by public officers and for involuntary hospitalization. In most jurisdictions involuntary hospitalization is permitted to establish whether a person is mentally ill and a threat to his or her own person or to others.
>
> (Beauchamp and Childress 1989, p. 225)

As well, social and religious taboos still necessitate a degree of secrecy about the circumstances of a person's 'unexpected illness' or 'accidental death'. Donnelly (1990, p. 9) claims that the legacy of past taboos concerning suicide still sees doctors and coroners pressured into using euphemisms when officially certifying or describing the cause of death of a suicide victim. In one notable example, a British report described as 'accidental' the death of a man 'who just happened to shoot himself while cleaning the muzzle of his gun with his tongue!' (Donnelly 1990, p. 9).

The 'medical gaze' of Foucault's (1973) *la clinique* ('the clinic') may well prove ultimately to be a more humane alternative than the punitive gaze proposed by Jeremy Bentham's penitentiary panopticon, thought to be justified as a system of 'moral account-ing' (Foucault 1977, p. 250). There is, however, no way of predicting this with certainty — or even agreeing about its possibility or probability (see also Heyd and Bloch 1981, p. 193).

When I think of the many people — young and old, vulnerable and desperate — who have been admitted to hospital following a failed suicide attempt, and in whose care I have been involved (mostly in accident and emergency departments or intensive care units), I am inclined to think that the anti-suicide law reforms we have inherited in the twentieth century have not really changed the status quo. These law reforms have resulted not so much in the *decriminalisation of suicide* as in the *medicalisation of the law*: where once suicide victims and their families were made to account to the law, now they must account to medicine (psychiatry); where once suicide victims were made to prove their innocence before the law, now they must prove their competence; and where once those who attempted suicide were imprisoned for the crime of stealing the gift of life from God, now they are hospitalised involuntarily for violating the gift of civil liberty from society. As Alvarez observes:

> modern suicide has been removed from the vulnerable, volatile world of human beings and hidden safely away in the isolation wards of science. I doubt if Ogarev [the Russian exile] and his [. . .] mistress would have found much in the change to be grateful for.
>
> (Alvarez 1980, p. 31)

Over the past few decades there has been a renewed interest in the moral aspects of suicide, prompted largely by the euthanasia/euthanatic suicide (assisted suicide) debate (discussed in chapter 10 of this text), and increasing public demand for the 'right to die' to be enshrined in law. This renewed interest has, arguably, marked the beginning of a trend back (rightly or wrongly) to permissive attitudes toward suicide and, more specifically, the socio-cultural normalisation of suicide — particularly in cases of intolerable and intractable suffering (see figure 11.1). It is no small irony, however, that whereas in the ancient world economic considerations provided the grounds for the legal prohibition of suicide (particularly among the poor and working classes) and for the just punishment of those who attempted suicide, in the modern world economic considerations will probably provide many of the grounds for legalising suicide (and more particularly, euthanasia/ assisted suicide), and for abandoning legal punishments against those who assist people to die before they become — or even *because* they have already become — a financial and material burden, not just on their primary care-givers but on the state (see also Battin 1982, pp. 96–106).

Defining suicide

Before examining some of the moral issues raised by the suicide question, it is necessary first to establish at least a working definition of *suicide* — a term which, incidentally, entered the English language only in 1651 (Wennberg 1989 p. 17; Battin 1982, p. 22–58).

The word *suicide* comes from the Latinate *sui*, 'of oneself' and *cidium*, 'a slaying' (from *caedere*, 'to kill'). Like many other terms used in moral discourse, *suicide* is not easy to define; indeed, there is no universally agreed definition of what suicide is, or of what criteria should be met in order for an act to count as an instance of suicide. As Margolis (1978, pp. 92–3) explains, the 'culturally variable character of suicide' has given rise to many competing views on what it is, with the unhelpful consequence that some acts have been included as suicide and others firmly excluded. This, in turn, has had some important practical consequences, including the difficulty of ascertaining accurate and comparable statistics on the incidence and causes of suicide (Beauchamp 1980, pp. 68–9).

For Wennberg (1989, p. 17), wrestling with the problem of defining *suicide* is to be taught a lesson in 'linguistic humility'. Nevertheless, our commonsense notions of what suicide is, our ability to recognise instances of suicide and to distinguish these from other kinds of death (for example, homicide, patricide, matricide, fratricide, sororicide, infanticide, regicide, and euthanasia or euthanatic suicide [Battin 1982, p. 20]), and the very existence of terms in our language which make it possible to speak of suicide as a distinctive kind of death, all provide considerable grounds for optimism about our ability to achieve at least a working — if not a universal — definition of suicide.

According to Stengel, a commonsense notion of suicide can be expressed in the following terms:

> A person, having decided to end his [or her] life, or acting on a sudden impulse to do so, kills himself [or herself], having chosen the most effective methods available and having made sure that nobody interferes. When he [or she] survives he [or she] is said to have failed and the act is called an unsuccessful suicide attempt. Death is the only purpose of this act and therefore the only criterion of success. Failure may be due to any of the following causes: the sense of purpose may not have been strong enough, or the act may have been undertaken half-heartedly because it was not quite genuine; the subject was ignorant of the limitations of the method; or he [or she] was lacking in judgement and determination through mental illness.
>
> (Stengel 1970, p. 77)

This definition is not, of course, without controversy. For example: what constitutes a 'genuine' suicide attempt? and when is a suicide attempt to be regarded as 'half-hearted' as opposed to 'whole-hearted'? (see also Knight 1992). Further, as Stengel himself points out, the definition may not do justice to what has become 'a very common and varied behaviour pattern' (1970, p. 77). Nevertheless, it provides an important insight into the kinds of criteria that should be met in order for an act to count as suicide. One such criterion is that of *intention*—specifically, the *intention to end one's life* (Margolis 1975, reprinted in Beauchamp and Perlin 1978, p. 95). As Beauchamp points out, central to what is called the 'prevailing definition' of suicide is the following premise:

Suicide occurs if and only if there is an intentional termination of one's own life.

(Beauchamp 1980, p. 70)

Beauchamp (1980, pp. 73–9) suggests that other criteria that should be met in order for an act to count as suicide include the following:

1. death is chosen voluntarily (that is, is free of coercive or manipulative influences);
2. an active means of death is chosen;
3. death is caused by the person desiring death (one dies by 'one's own hand', as it were);
4. death is *self-regarding* (rather than altruistic or *other-regarding*); and
5. the person seeking death does not have a fatal or terminal illness.

Windt suggests similar criteria (all of which have been mentioned in the suicide literature) of suicide. These are:

1. death [must be] caused by the actions or behaviour of the deceased;
2. the deceased wanted, desired, or wished death;
3. the deceased intended, chose, decided or willed to die;
4. the deceased knew that death would result from his [or her] behaviour; and that
5. the deceased was responsible for his [or her] own death.

(Windt 1980, p. 41; tabulations added)

At first glance, these and similar criteria of suicide appear helpful. On closer analysis, however, a number of problems quickly become apparent — not least the problem of so-called 'exceptional cases', and whether the criteria listed are relevant to or can be applied appropriately and meaningfully to these cases. Consider, for example, the cases of people engaging in dangerous and potentially life-threatening ('suicidal') sports (for instance, bungey jumping, mountain climbing, racing car driving, hang gliding); dangerous work activities (being a member of a bomb disposal squad or a combat soldier are paradigm examples here); or other life-threatening activities such as cigarette smoking, eating and drinking excessively, illicit drug taking, and so on (see also Glover 1977, p. 173; Beauchamp and Perlin 1978, p. 88; Beauchamp

1980, p. 72). In all these cases, it is probably true that the people concerned chose the activities in question; were aware of the potential threats the activities posed to their lives and well-being; voluntarily engaged in the activities chosen; and, were they to die as a result of engaging in these activities, were 'responsible for their own deaths', in so far as they were witting accomplices to the activities and the associated risks. Further, while the people concerned might not have *intended* their own (accidental) deaths, they nevertheless foresaw their deaths as a possibility associated with the risky activities they had engaged in, and thereby, ipso facto, can be said to have intended their own demise. Given the criteria for suicide outlined above, it seems we are committed to accepting that people who die as a result of their deliberately engaging in dangerous sporting activities, work activities or life-styles have, in essence, suicided. Yet, this does not seem to accord with our intuitions on the matter — nor does it sit comfortably with what we would perhaps ordinarily regard as suicide. Let us examine another example to see if this will clarify the matter.

In 1982, Barney Clark, aged 62, became the first human being to receive an artificial (mechanical) heart (Beauchamp and Childress 1989, p. 222). Recognising that this medical experiment had the potential to make Barney Clark's life burdensome, his doctor, Willem Kolf, gave him a key that could be used to turn off the compressor sustaining the artificial heart's action. Defending his decision to supply this key, Dr Kolff argued that if Barney Clark:

> suffers and feels it isn't worth it any more, he has a key that he can apply. [. . .] I think it is entirely legitimate that this man whose life has been extended should have the right to cut it off if he doesn't want it, if life ceases to be enjoyable.
>
> (cited in Beauchamp and Childress 1989, p. 223)

The conceptual dilemma which arises here is this: if Barney Clark had chosen to use the key he had been given, and had turned off the compressor driving his artificial heart, which of the following statements would have been the most accurate description of his action and the cause of his death:

1. forgoing extraordinary means of life-sustaining treatment;
2. withdrawing from an experiment;
3. letting nature take its course;
4. natural death;
5. euthanasia;
6. suicide.

To complicate the issue, as Beauchamp and Childress point out:

> If Clark had refused to accept the artificial heart in the first place, few would have characterised his act as one of suicide, because of his overall condition and the experimental nature of the artificial heart, but if he had shot himself while on the artificial heart, it would have been difficult to avoid characterising the act as one of suicide.
>
> (Beauchamp and Childress 1989, p. 223)

And, to complicate the issue still further, what if Barney Clark had consented to receiving the heart in the belief that the risks associated with the experiment were so great that a hastened death would be assured? Could this be classified as a kind of suicide?

Part of the difficulty in sorting out the conceptual confusion surrounding the development of an adequate definition of and criteria for suicide can be linked to the lingering legacy of varying socio-cultural historical and religious taboos against suicide. Beauchamp and Childress (1989, p. 223) suggest, for example, that we often shield acts of which we approve (or at least acts of which we do not disapprove) from the stigmatising label of 'suicide' — preferring instead to use terms that are more socially acceptable, such as 'euthanasia' or 'withdrawing extraordinary life-saving treatment', and similar notions. If this is correct, it is ironic, considering that the term 'suicide' was first adopted in the seventeenth century as a more 'acceptable' alternative to the then contemporary usages 'self-murder' and 'self-slaughter', which were regarded by more liberal-minded people of the day as having unacceptably negative connotations (Battin 1982, pp. 22, 58).

In the light of these considerations, perhaps an important first step in developing a workable definition of and criteria for suicide is to demystify suicide, and to strip it of the taboos and stigmatisations which still seem to linger around it — and which may encourage people to be less than intellectually honest when speaking of its incidence and cause. A second and related step is to modify the negatively connoted language that tends to be used in referring to and discussing suicide. In this instance, the problem of language is highly significant, and should not be underestimated. As Wennberg explains:

> 'suicide' is not a neutrally descriptive term like 'cat', 'car', or 'flower'. Rather, it carries with it a strong negative connotation, especially when it is part of the phrase 'commit suicide'. For one typically does not *commit* X where X is either something approved or something of neutral standing (cf. 'commit murder', 'commit a

felony', 'commit a crime', 'commit adultery', 'commit a sin', 'commit treason', 'commit a *faux pas*', etc.).

(Wennberg 1989, p. 17)

The lesson here is important and obvious: the use of the phrase 'committed suicide' (as opposed to using the term *suicided*) is misleading and unhelpful — not least because it seems to imply the commission of a crime, or even a sin, when clearly there has been none.

A third and final step toward developing a working definition of and criteria for suicide is to reinstate the authority of our own ordinary commonsense experience of the world, and our collective experience-based knowledge of what is and is not an act of suicide or attempted suicide. One reason for this is that, in the ultimate analysis, the distinction between suicide and other types of death (for example, euthanasia) may rest not on sophisticated philosophical criteria, but on our fine intuitions informed by life-experience. I suspect, however, that in the main, conceptual clarity in regard to what is and is not an act of suicide will rest on something far more substantial than abstract criteria or even well informed intuition. Rather, the matter will be decided by appealing to:

1. the known intentions and motivations of the person who has died (for instance, whether the death was pursued as 'an alleged solution for the ills of dying' [euthanasia], or pursued as an 'alleged' cure for the ills of living [suicide] [Donnelly 1990, p. 9];

2. the context in which the person died;

3. whether the person who died genuinely believed there was no other alternative besides death in order to alleviate his or her suffering, or to transcend the life circumstances which for him or her had become unbearable.

The problem remains, however, that ascertaining these things may be just as difficult as establishing reliable criteria for suicide. Nevertheless, it is important that suicide be defined. One reason for this is that without an adequate definition of suicide it will remain extremely difficult to assess accurately the incidence, cause and appropriate means of preventing suicide. It will also be difficult to eradicate the spurious distinction which is sometimes drawn between 'genuine' and 'non-genuine' suicide attempts, with the tragic consequence that some who are suffering and needing help will be dismissed as malingerers, and worse, as not suffering or needing help at all. (See also Knight's [1992] discussion on the suffering of suicide.) Finally, it will make it difficult to engage in substantive moral debate on the ethical aspects of suicide, and to respond effectively and appropriately to the many moral problems raised by the suicide question, some of which are now considered.

Suicide: some moral considerations

As discussed under the earlier subheading 'Socio-cultural attitudes to suicide: a brief historical overview', the Judaeo-Christian traditions have, for the most part, regarded suicide as the gravest sin imaginable, and as constituting the most serious violation of one's duties to oneself to others and to God. These views have been extremely influential and, not surprisingly, the subject of much philosophical debate. Today, however, as Knight (1992, p. 262) correctly points out, 'religiously speaking, the notion of suicide as an unforgivable sin has few, if any, defenders in contemporary moral philosophy'. Further, unlike the days when religious prohibition saw suicide condemned as a grossly immoral act, it is difficult today to find tenable moral arguments against the suicide of people who are able to choose autonomously to end their own lives (Knight 1992, p. 262). Nevertheless, a number of troubling questions remain about the ethics or morality of suicide, such as: is there a right to suicide? If so, what conditions must be satisfied before this right can be claimed? What are the obligations of others in regard to those contemplating or attempting suicide? Is there a duty to prevent suicide? If so, under what conditions should a suicide be prevented? It is to briefly answering these questions that the remainder of this discussion now turns.

Autonomy and the right to suicide

Fundamental to Western moral thinking is the principle of autonomy. As discussed in chapter 3 of this text, the moral principle of autonomy prescribes that a person's considered choices should be respected — even if others disagree with them or regard them as foolish — provided they do not interfere with or harm the significant moral interests of others. If we accept this principle, we must also accept that people who choose autonomously to suicide are entitled to have their choices respected, and further, that it would be morally indefensible to prevent these people from exercising their choices. By this view, as Beauchamp explains:

> If people are autonomous, then they have the right to be left alone and to do with their lives as they wish, so long as they are sufficiently free of responsibilities to others. From this perspective, the intervention in the life of a suicide is simply an unjust deprivation of liberty.
>
> (Beauchamp 1980, p. 100)

Jonathan Glover argues along similar lines, explaining that once it is admitted that suicide need not always be regarded as an 'irrational symptom of mental disturbance' (see also Wennberg 1989, p. 39), then:

> [it] is a matter for each person's free choice: other people should have nothing to say about it, and the question for someone contemplating it is simply one of whether his [or her] future life will be worth living.
>
> (Glover 1977, p. 171)

It is far from certain, however, that people contemplating or attempting suicide are, in fact, entitled to be 'left alone and to do with their lives as they wish' (Beauchamp 1980, p. 100), or that 'other people should have nothing to say about it' (Glover 1977, p. 171). There are a number of reasons for this. First, an act of suicide is never without moral consequences: not only does it have an impact on the significant moral interests of the person suiciding, but it can significantly affect the important moral interests of others. As experience tells us, suicide can shatter, injure and destroy the lives of other people; it can also cause substantial loss to society (see also Battin 1982). Where suicides do affect the significant moral interests of others, there are at least prima facie grounds for justifying paternalistic intervention to prevent those suicides occurring. As well as this, where other people's significant moral interests are at stake, there may even be an obligation on the part of people contemplating suicide not to proceed with planned actions aimed at ending their own lives (Brandt 1978, p. 128) —although it is an open question just how realistic this demand is in the case of people suffering severe psychological distress.

In the light of these circumstances, it is evident that claims to autonomy *alone* are not sufficient to justify an unequivocal acceptance of a person's decision to suicide, or to justify non-intervention or 'non-postvention' (counselling and therapy after a suicide attempt [Battin 1982, p. 16]) in the case of contemplated or attempted suicide. Of course, there is always the possibility that the concerns or interests of others may not be strong enough to override a person's autonomous choice to suicide. This, however, is something which must be determined by careful evaluation and a 'balancing of considerations' of all the moral interests involved (Beauchamp and Perlin 1978, p. 91), not just by an uncritical deontological acceptance of the moral principle of autonomy. Such a calculation might even show that a contemplated suicide, once carried out, should indeed be permitted in the interests of others. For example, the suicide of a long-term abusing spouse might be shown to be more permissible morally than the homicide of his abused wife and children. Whether this would really be a morally desirable outcome, however, is a contentious point and unfortunately one which is beyond the scope of this work to address.

A second reason why it is not clear that people contemplating or attempting suicide should not have their choices interfered with is that the *quality* of the autonomy behind the choice may not be optimal. As discussed in chapter 3 of this text, as a *concept* (to be distinguished here from a *principle*), autonomy refers to a person's independent and self-contained ability to decide. At issue in the case of suicide is the question of whether a person contemplating suicide is really capable of making the evaluative, deliberative and reflective choices that are fundamental to a 'rational' and autonomous decision to suicide. While it is true that even so-called 'incompetent' people are still capable of making self-interested choices (see, for example, the discussion on competency in chapter 7 of this text), the extent to which the choices of these people should be respected is not something that can be decided solely on the basis of the demands prescribed by the moral principle of autonomy; there are other moral considerations that need to be taken into account — including the moral demand to prevent otherwise avoidable harm to people, which an unnecessary and senseless suicide-death could cause.

The issue of the quality of a suicidal person's autonomous choice to kill himself or herself is an important one, and, even when considered from a clinical as opposed to a philosophical perspective, has an important bearing on deciding the ethical acceptability of paternalistic interventions aimed at preventing people from suiciding.

It has been suggested that depression 'is a substantial part of the picture of at least 50 per cent of suicides' (Knight 1992, pp. 249–50). While depression alone may not result in suicide, when it is coupled with abiding and intolerable feelings of hopelessness about the future, the risk of suicide is extremely high (Knight 1992, p. 250). Of importance to the discussion at this point is the consideration that feelings of depression, hopelessness and despair can have a significant and far-reaching impact on a person's ability to make 'truly' autonomous choices. As has long been recognised in the bioethics literature, these feelings can:

- restrict people's abilities to evaluate and calculate correctly the range of possibilities and probabilities available when planning and making judgments about their lives and future prospects (Brandt 1978, p. 131; Beauchamp 1980, p. 101);

- skew calculations of the probable harms and benefits that may flow from suicide (as Beauchamp [1980, p. 101] points out, 'without depression, persons might make quite different calculations even when their situation is dire');

- result in suicidal people overestimating the magnitude and insolubility of their problems (Knight 1992, p. 266);
- result in impulsive and imprudent choices which might otherwise not have been made (Heyd and Bloch 1981, p. 187).

In short, feelings of depression, hopelessness and despair can undermine in very significant ways a person's ability to make sound autonomous choices. The question remains, however, of whether these feelings and a possible associated diminution in the ability to make sound autonomous choices are of a nature that justifies paternalistic intervention to prevent a person suiciding — including using invasive procedures to resuscitate someone who has attempted suicide. Or would such intervention — no matter how benevolent — still constitute an unacceptable violation of the moral principle of autonomy?

The short answer to these questions is that intervention may not only be justified, but may even be required, in the interests of both promoting a person's autonomy and saving a worthwhile life. On this point, Jonathan Glover explains:

> Where we think someone bent on suicide has a life worth living, it is always legitimate to reason with him [or her] and to try and persuade him [or her] to stand back and think again. There is no case against reasoning, as it in no way encroaches on the person's autonomy. There is a strong case in its favour, as where it succeeds it will prevent the loss of a worth-while life. (If the person's life turns out not to be worth-while, he [or she] can always change his [or her] mind again.) And if persuasion fails, the outcome is no worse than it would otherwise have been.
>
> (Glover 1977, pp. 176–7)

Glover (1977, p. 178) goes on to contend that where suicidal tendencies are the product of temporary depressive mood-swings — for instance, where the person 'alternates between very much wanting to go on living and moods of suicidal depression' — then intervention aimed at overriding a decision to suicide 'is less disrespectful of autonomy than overriding a preference that plays a stable role in a person's outlook'. If, for example, a person repeatedly and persistently attempts suicide, and the underlying preference (that is, to die) informing these attempts remains constant, then the onus is on would-be 'rescuers' or interveners to reconsider their own judgments about whether the life of the person attempting suicide is, in fact, worthwhile and worth living, or whether they have been mistaken in their views. Unpleasant as it may be, the demand in the latter instance may be an overriding one in favour of *not* intervening to save the person's life (Glover 1977, p. 178). Before this position is accepted, however, there are at least prima facie grounds for asserting that the following five conditions must be met:

1. that the decision to suicide is based on a realistic assessment of the life-circumstances or situation at hand (Motto 1983, pp. 443–6; Knight 1992, p. 254);

2. that the person contemplating suicide has made an 'exhaustive examination' of all available options and has taken into account the 'various possible "errors" and [made] appropriate rectifications of his [or her] initial evaluation' (Brandt 1978, p. 132);

3. that the thought processes used in reaching the decision to suicide have not been impaired by severe emotional distress, feelings of hopelessness and despair, mental illness or the adverse side-effects of drugs (Knight 1992, p. 254);

4. that the degree of ambivalence between wanting to live and wanting to die is minimal (Motto 1983, pp. 443–6; Glover 1977, p. 178; Donnelly 1990, p.8); and

5. that the desire and motivation to suicide is of a nature that 'uninvolved observers from their community or social group [would find] understandable' (Knight 1992, p. 254).

While the satisfaction of these criteria may not always result in the prevention of morally undesirable consequences in situations involving people wanting to suicide, it may nevertheless result in more appropriate assessments of when it is right and when it is not right to paternalistically override a person's autonomous choice to suicide.

One problem which emerges here, however, is that, even if these criteria are not satisfied, does that necessarily justify paternalistic intervention to prevent a person suiciding? What if the suicidal person in quesion is in a state of intolerable suffering (see Knight 1992; Slater 1980)? Here the additional question arises: can those who are suffering intolerably and intractably (whether on account of physical or mental illness or some other state of physical or psychogenic distress) be expected decently to go on living? Or should people in these situations be released from the 'obligation to live' — if, indeed, it is an obligation — irrespective of their ability to decide autonomously what is in their own best interests? Are others entitled morally to force a person to go on living a life characterised by excruciating feelings of depression, hopelessness, despair and a sense that life has lost all meaning and purpose?

It is not unreasonable to hold that a person in this state would prefer death to life. As Glover points out:

> Most of us prefer to be anaesthetized for a painful operation. If most of my life were to be on that level, I might opt for a permanent anaesthesia, or death.
>
> (Glover 1977, p. 174)

Margolis (1978, p. 96) argues, however, that while prolonged anaesthesia may indeed be 'prudentially preferable to enduring pain', the desire to reduce pain in itself 'cannot justify suicide to end pain as a decision of a prudential sort'. One reason for this is that enduring even intolerable pain may, in the ultimate analysis, still be preferable to no life at all (Margolis 1978, p. 96; see also Glover 1977, p. 174). Another reason is that to allow suicide as a means of alleviating suffering is to compound the hopelessness underpinning the suffering of suicide; it is also to abandon as hopeless those who have abandoned themselves as hopeless, and thereby to violate a fundamental professional ethic of care and responsibility to aid the distressed (see also Murphy 1983, p. 442).

If suicide is viewed as a 'violent statement about human connections, broken and maintained' (Lifton 1979, p. 239), and not simply as a matter of exercising an autonomous choice (as Hauerwas [1986, p. 107] reminds us, 'life has a purpose beyond simply being autonomous'), perhaps our moral obligations toward those contemplating or attempting suicide will become clearer. In particular, as Knight's (1992) discussion on the suffering of suicide clarifies, there needs to be a much greater understanding of the excruciating sense of hopelessness and despair that underlies and motivates many a decision to suicide. Once this is understood, it may become clearer that the way to remedy the suffering underlying a decision to suicide is not to do away with the sufferer, but to do away with the sense of hopelessness and despair fuelling the suffering. This, however, requires great compassion and commitment on the part of those intervening and preventing people suiciding. As Knight puts it:

> Intervention in suicide involves walking down that 'dark road' and immersing oneself into that world in which the suicidal person is living. One soon discovers that most suicidal persons have a predisposition to overestimate the magnitude and insolubility of their problems. Coupled with this, as has been emphasised by those 'who have been there', is an exaggerated negative view of the outside world, of themselves, and of the future. An awareness of what and how a suicidal person is thinking and feeling may

lead those intervening to see quickly that the suicidal person's plight has a way out, and soon hope begins to dawn.

(Knight 1992, p. 266)

Suicide prevention: some further considerations

It is probably true that most health care professionals feel obliged to:

1. try and persuade people contemplating suicide to change their minds;

2. counsel those who have lost their sense of hope, purpose and meaning in life, in order to modify their perceptions and regain a more optimistic outlook on the future;

3. resuscitate people who have attempted suicide and who are on the brink of death; and

4. treat the injuries of people whose suicide attempts have failed.

Whether health care professionals do, in fact, have these obligations may, in the end, be a matter to be decided not by moral theory, or even by law, but by empathy, compassion, kindness, and wisdom, informed by a profound understanding of human vulnerability and suffering, together with a commitment to take each case on its own unique and individual merit. Either way, it is important not to forget that our obligation to render aid to a person contemplating or attempting suicide is as strong as it would be to aid any person in distress (Brandt 1980, pp. 129–31), and that this may require more than merely protecting a person's autonomy; it may require the more substantive task of protecting a person's genuine human welfare, and restoring in them a sense of hope that, often due to circumstances quite beyond their control, has abandoned them.

Issues and recommendations

Some may find it attractive to view suicide as the manifestation of a mental illness, and hence something that is 'irrational' and 'irresponsible' and ipso facto quite beyond the realms of moral inquiry (see, for example, Stengel 1970, p. 58; Margolis 1978, p. 96; Heyd and Bloch 1981, pp. 193–4; Beauchamp and Childress 1989, p. 224; Wennberg 1989, p. 18). This discussion has shown, however, that even if suicide is the product of mental illness or extreme emotional distress, depression, or other psychogenic pain states, it still has a profound moral dimension, and still requires those involved in suicide prevention and intervention to justify their views and actions, and not to merely assume that these are in themselves morally correct just because they have as their end the preservation of life or the maximisation of autonomy.

Suicide and attempted suicide is an issue of importance and concern to *all* nurses, not just to those working in the area of mental health. How well nurses and others repond to the moral issues raised depends, however, on a variety of factors —including the success with which suicide is stripped of the taboos which still surround it, and the degree to which suicide is demystified as a desperate act aimed at transcending a situation which a distressed person has come to perceive as hopeless (Knight 1992).

Some years ago I was involved in the care of a woman who had attempted suicide by pouring a can of petrol over herself and setting fire to it. She arrived in casualty with 100 per cent burns to her body. Incredibly, despite the horrendous injuries her body had sustained, her eyes were unharmed. The extent of her burns made it impossible to insert an intravenous line in the usual way, and a cut-down (which involves a surgical incision to expose a deeply situated vein) had to be performed. I remember the doctor looking at me while he was performing the cut-down, and gasping in horror as the woman's burnt flesh parted in his hands. Nevertheless, this compassionate man succeeded in inserting the intravenous line, and consoled the woman as he did so. As we all worked diligently to retrieve this injured life, the woman looked on smiling, and reassuring us all with the words, 'Don't worry dears, I will be all right.' I remember looking up at this woman and, on observing her terrible injuries, thinking how desperate she must have been to have engaged in such an act. She, however, looked back at me with eyes that were clear and shining, and, bizarre as this whole scene was, I could see that she had found incredible peace within herself. The image of her burnt and tortured body did not sit well with the peace expressed in her eyes, but I knew that she had achieved her goal, and that it would be only a matter of time before she would be released from the suffering that had motivated her to undertake such a desperate act. Her death a day or two later was no surprise. Yet I still cannot help thinking that that woman paid a terrible price for the peace she eventually found in death, and could not find in life.

During the same year, I was involved in the care of a man who had also attempted suicide, in this instance by placing the muzzle of a gun in his mouth and shooting himself. He failed in his attempt to kill himself, however, and succeeded only in destroying one side of his face. After receiving plastic surgery to repair the serious gunshot wound sustained, he was admitted to intensive care. Unlike the woman who had set fire to herself, however, he was not at peace within himself. As he lay corpse-like on his bed, I

remember noting that his eyes were like the eyes of a dead man —
fully dilated, dull, and unresponsive to light. It was as though his
soul had died, and nothing mattered any more. Once, when his
plastic surgeon visited to check his wounds, the man handed the
doctor a note. Written on the note were the words: 'Dear Dr X — did
you do this [the surgical repair] for your sake or mine?' Understandably, this very compassionate and gentle surgeon was
devastated. Shortly after being transferred out of the intensive care
unit, the man climbed out through a toilet window and plunged to
his death several storeys below. Many of the staff were left feeling
that they had failed this man. The circumstances motivating his
initial suicidal attempt had not seemed insurmountable to them,
and they sincerely believed he was 'getting better'. But he was not
getting better, and eventually he too achieved his goal of death. As
I recall the case of this desperate and hopeless man, I cannot forget
the costly suffering and distress of those he left behind — especially
his wife and young children. How different things would have been
if he, like the people caring for and about him, could have perceived
that his problems were not as overwhelming as he thought, and
that it was not necessary to take the desperate action that he
ultimately took. To this day, I am reminded by this case of the
importance of never underestimating the capacity of human beings
to feel deeply and to suffer profoundly on account of things which
seem (though they may not necessarily be) insurmountable, and of
how feelings of desperation and hopelessness associated with
problems perceived as insurmountable can so easily override the
desire to go on living.*

In June of 1993, a Victorian coroner's court was reported to have
found that the suicide of five severely depressed patients at
Larundel Hospital was, among other things, a regrettable consequence of a well intended but nevertheless misguided priority being
given to upholding patients' rights to confidentiality (i.e. the 'right'
not to be observed too closely) at the expense of patient care;
further there had been a less than optimal level of commitment to
'patient-centred *continuity of care* rather than changes in treating
medical personnel due to patient progress [emphasis added]'
(Pegler 1993, p. 26). The coroner is reported to have also found that
'the most important issue arising from the inquests was family and
carer involvement in treatment', and that 'a policy needed to be
developed on the conflict between patient rights and patient care'
(Pegler 1993, p. 26).

Whether matters such as these can — or, indeed, should be — the
subject of institutional policy is a debatable point. As experience

---

* Names and details of times and places have been suppressed, but these are
true stories that reflect the experience of all nurses everywhere.

tells us, even the very best of policies may still fail to prevent this kind of situation from occurring. Nevertheless, it is clear that there is room for improvement in the care and treatment of those contemplating or attempting suicide, and, more importantly, in understanding the moral issues involved in caring for those who, for whatever reason, are unable to care about themselves. It is also clear that, in securing these improvements, nurses must ensure that, in attempting to uphold the moral rights of their emotionally distressed, severely depressed and mentally unwell patients, they do not lose sight of the importance of also protecting and promoting their patients' *welfare and well-being* — something which may not always be secured by paying homage to abstract moral rights and principles. By doing this, nurses, and others involved in caring for people who are contemplating suicide or who have already attempted suicide, may well succeed in helping to prevent and remedy the terrible sufferings and tragedies that have become so characteristic of the whole phemonemon of suicide in the world.

References

Alvarez, A. (1980). The background. In Battin and Mayo (1980), pp. 7–32.

Amundsen, D. (1989). Suicide and early Christian values. In B. Brody (ed.), *Suicide and euthanasia: historical and contemporary themes*, Kluwer Academic Publishers, Dordrecht, pp. 77–153.

Aquinas, St Thomas (1978). Whether it is lawful to kill oneself. Reprinted from *Summa Theologica* in Beauchamp and Perlin (1978), pp. 102–5.

Aristotle (1976 edn). *Nicomachean ethics* (translated by J. A. K. Thomson). Penguin, Harmondsworth, Middlesex.

Bailey, S. (1994). Critical care nurses' and doctors' attitudes to parasuicide patients. *Australian Journal of Advanced Nursing* 11 (3), pp. 11–17.

Barrington, M. (1983). Apologia for suicide. In S. Gorovitz, R. Macklin, A. Jameton, J. O'Connor and S. Sherwin (eds), *Moral problems in medicine*, Prentice Hall, Englewood Cliffs, New Jersey, pp. 472–6.

Battin, M. Pabst (1982). *Ethical issues in suicide*. Prentice Hall, Englewood Cliffs, New Jersey.

Battin, M. Pabst and Mayo, D. (1980). *Suicide: the philosophical issues*. Peter Owen, London.

Baume, P. (1988). Perspectives on youth suicide. *Australian Journal of Advanced Nursing* 5 (3), pp. 40–8.

Beauchamp, T. (1978a). What is suicide? In Beauchamp and Perlin (1978), pp. 97–102.

Beauchamp, T. (1978b). An analysis of Hume and Aquinas on suicide. In Beauchamp and Perlin (1978), pp. 111–22.

Beauchamp, T. (1980). Suicide. In T. Regan (ed.) (1980), *Matters of life and death: new introductory essays in moral philosophy*, Random House, New York, pp. 67–108.

Beauchamp, T. (1989). Suicide in the age of reason. In B. Brody, pp. 183–219.

Beauchamp, T. and Childress, J. (1989). *Principles of biomedical ethics*, 3rd edn. Oxford University Press, New York.

Beauchamp, T. and Perlin, S. (eds) (1978). *Ethical issues in death and dying*. Prentice Hall, Englewood Cliffs, New Jersey.

Boyle, J. (1989). Sanctity of life and suicide: tensions and developments within common morality. In Brody (1989a), pp. 221–50.

Brandt, R. (1978). The morality and rationality of suicide. In Beauchamp and Perlin (1978), pp. 122–33.

Brandt, R. (1980). The rationality of suicide. In Battin and Mayo (1980), pp. 117–32.

Brody, B. (ed.) (1989a). *Suicide and euthanasia: historical and contemporary themes.* Kluwer Academic Publishers, Dordrecht.

Brody, B. (1989b). A historical introduction to Jewish casuistry on suicide and euthanasia. In Brody (1989a), pp. 39–75.

Browne, A. (1990). Assisted suicide and active voluntary euthanasia. *Bioethics News* 9 (4), pp. 9–38.

Carr, E. H. (1961). *The romantic exiles: a nineteenth-century portrait gallery.* Beacon Press, Boston.

Clemons, J. (ed.) (1990). *Perspectives on suicide.* Westminster/John Knox Press, Louisville, Kentucky.

Colt, G. Howe (1991). *The enigma of suicide.* Simon & Schuster, New York.

Cooper, J. (1989). Greek philosophers on euthanasia and suicide. In Brody (1989a), pp. 9–38.

Daly, M. (1978). *Gyn/ecology: the metaethics of radical feminism.* The Women's Press, London.

Davis, A. (1992). Suicidal behaviour among adolescents: its nature and prevention. In R. Kosky, H. Eshkevari and G. Kneebone (eds), *Breaking out: challenges in adolescent mental health in Australia.* Australian Government Publishing Service, Canberra.

Deane, J. (1992). Teen suicide. *Sunday Herald-Sun* [Melbourne], 2 February, p. 81.

Demopolous, H. (1968). Suicide and Church canon law. Unpublished doctoral dissertation, Claremont School of Theology, California.

Donnelly, J. (ed.) (1990). *Suicide: right or wrong?* Prometheus Books, Buffalo, New York.

Durkheim, E. (1952). *Suicide.* Routledge & Kegan Paul, London.

Farber, M. (1975). Psychological variables in Italian suicide. In Farberow (1975a), pp. 179–84.

Farberow, N. (ed.) (1975a). *Suicide in different cultures.* University Park Press, Baltimore.

Farberow, N. (1975b). Cultural history of suicide. In Farberow (1975a), pp. 1–15.

Ferngren, G. (1989). The ethics of suicide in the Renaissance and Reformation. In Brody (1989a), pp. 155–81.

Foucault, M. (1973). *The birth of the clinic.* Tavistock Publications, London.

Foucault, M. (1977). *Discipline and punish: the birth of the prison.* Penguin, London.

French, M. (1985). *Beyond power: on women, men and morals.* Abacus, London.

Glover, J. (1977). *Causing death and saving lives.* Penguin, Harmondsworth, Middlesex.

Hauerwas, S. (1986). *Suffering presence.* University of Notre Dame Press, South Bend, Indiana.

Heyd, D. and Bloch, S. (1981). The ethics of suicide. In S. Bloch and P. Chodoff (eds), *Psychiatric ethics*, Oxford University Press, Oxford, pp. 185–202.

Holy Bible (new King James version). Thomas Nelson, Nashville, Tennessee.

Hume, D. (1983 edn). Essay on suicide. In S. Gorovitz, R. Macklin, A. Jameton, J. O'Connor and S. Sherwin (eds), *Moral problems in medicine*, Prentice Hall, Englewood Cliffs, New Jersey, pp. 437–42.

Kant, I. (1983 edn). Suicide. In S. Gorovitz, R. Macklin, A. Jameton, J. O'Connor and S. Sherwin (eds), *Moral problems in medicine*, Prentice Hall, Englewood Cliffs, New Jersey, pp. 434–7.

Kaplan, K. and Schwartz, M. (1993). *A psychology of hope: an antidote to the suicidal pathology of Western civilization.* Praeger, Westport, Connecticut.

Kennedy, H. (1992). Why do the kids suicide? Kyneton stunned by youth suicides. *Sunday Herald-Sun*, Melbourne, 16 August, pp. 4–5.

Knight, J. (1992). The suffering of suicide: the victim and family considered. In P. Starck and J. McGovern (eds), *The hidden dimension of illness: human suffering*, National League for Nursing Press, New York, pp. 245–68.

Lifton, R. (1979). *The broken connection.* Simon & Schuster, New York.

Lindars, J. (1991). Holistic care in parasuicide. *Nursing Times* 87 (15), pp. 30–1.

Margolis, J. (1975). Suicide. Reprinted in Beauchamp and Perlin (1978), pp. 92–7.

Middleton, K. (1994). Act on suicide's tragic toll: expert. *The Age*, 1 March, p. 3.

Motto, J. (1983). The right to suicide: a psychiatrist's view. In S. Gorovitz, R. Macklin, A. Jameton, J. O'Connor and S. Sherwin (eds), *Moral problems in medicine*, Prentice Hall, Englewood Cliffs, New Jersey, pp. 443–6.

Murphy, G. (1983). Suicide and the right to die. In S. Gorovitz, R. Macklin, A. Jameton, J. O'Connor and S. Sherwin. (eds), *Moral problems in medicine*, Prentice Hall, Englewood Cliffs, New Jersey, p. 442.

Pegler, T. (1993). Coroner urges tight surveillance of psychiatric patients. *The Age*, 19 June, p. 26.

Plato (1903 edn). *The trial and death of Socrates, being The Euthyphron, Apology, Crito, and Phaedo of Plato* (translated by F. J. Church). Macmillan, London.

Plato (1969 edn). *The last days of Socrates* (translated by H. Tredennick). Penguin, Harmondsworth, Middlesex.

Power, T. (1993). Mother's illness drove six-year-old to commit suicide. *The Age*, 17 June, p. 9.

Rauscher, W. (1981). *The case against suicide.* St Martin's Press, New York.

Ryle, G. (1993). Suicide deaths outstrip state's road fatalities. *The Age*, 8 January, p. 3.

Slater, E. (1980). Choosing the time to die. In Battin and Mayo (1980), pp. 199–204.

Smith, D. and Perlin, S. (1978). Suicide. In W. T. Reich (ed.), *Encyclopedia of bioethics*, The Free Press, New York, pp. 1618–27.

Sophocles (1911 edn). *Oedipus King of Thebes* (translated by G. Murray), George Allen & Unwin, London.

Stengel, E. (1970). *Suicide and attempted suicide.* Penguin Books, Harmondsworth, Middlesex.

Szasz, T. (1988). The ethics of suicide. In T. Szasz, *The theology of medicine*, Syracuse University Press, New York, pp. 68–85.

The Leader (1992). Save young lives. 19 August, p. 8.

Wennberg, R. (1989). *Terminal choices: euthanasia, suicide, and the right to die.* William B. Eerdmans Publishing Company, Grand Rapids, Michigan, and The Paternoster Press, Exeter, UK.

Windt, P. (1980). The concept of suicide. In Battin and Mayo (1980), pp. 39–47.

Chapter

12

Matters of life and death: IV

Our discussion on matters of life and death would not be complete without some consideration being given to three additional ethical issues which, in recent years, have assumed increasing importance for nurses: quality of life, 'Not for Resuscitation' (NFR) orders, and organ transplantation. As with abortion, euthanasia and suicide, unless nurses are well informed about the nature and moral implications of the issues of quality of life, 'Not for Resuscitation' (NFR) orders, and organ transplantation, they will not be in a good position from which to contribute to community and professional debate about them. It is to examining these three issues and their moral implications for nurses and nursing practice that this chapter now turns.

Quality of life

The notion of quality of life is a popular one; many see it as a highly important if not central consideration when making life and death decisions. Like other terms and concepts in the health care repertoire, however, the notion of quality of life is not entirely unproblematic, and is vulnerable to criticism. Part of the difficulty here is that 'quality of life' is not a term that can be easily defined. As Welch-McCaffrey (1985, p. 151) correctly points out: 'Quality of life is not a term that has unequivocal meaning nor is it unambiguously determinable in any given case'.

Despite the difficulties associated with trying to define quality of life, nurses and allied health professionals continue to use the term as if it has an objective and clear-cut commonsense meaning, and, further, they also take it as implying binding prescriptions and proscriptions in relation to how a given individual human life ought and ought not to be regarded. What is troubling about this is that people (particularly those with significant life-threatening diseases) may find themselves being subjected to a quality of life view which is not only inappropriate for them, but also wholly and dangerously misleading in terms of guiding the choices which are critical to both the realisation and the maximisation of their significant moral interests. This raises two very important questions. First, if it is possible to define quality of life, how should it be defined? Second, in what way and to what extent ought a given quality of life view influence decision making in health care domains?

Defining quality of life

The question of how to define quality of life is complex and difficult, and might never find a wholly satisfactory answer. Nevertheless, the question deserves serious attention by nurses. It is hoped that the comments given in this chapter will help to shed some light on how the issue might be meaningfully approached.

In examining discussions in both nursing and bioethical literature, it quickly becomes evident that there are as many different interpretations of 'quality of life' as there are authors. It also quickly becomes evident that different authors have quite different views on how and the extent to which quality of life considerations should be permitted to influence therapeutic decision making. Consider the examples which follow.

Foltz (1987) argues that an individual's quality of life is interdependent with that individual's self-concept. Describing the influence that cancer and cancer treatment can have on a person's self-concept (taken here as comprising four fundamental components, notably the body self, the interpersonal self, the achievement self and the identification self), Foltz goes on to suggest that, where an individual's self-concept is diminished or undermined, so too is that individual's quality of life. She concludes that one way of enhancing quality of life is to intervene in a way that bolsters or promotes self-concept, whichever aspect (or aspects) of it is warranting attention.

Germino (1987) takes a slightly different view. She argues that quality of life is linked in an important way to symptom distress. She goes on to suggest that improving quality of life thus becomes very much a matter of improving symptom control. Germino also points out that improved symptom control stands to improve not only quality of life but also its quantity or survival (Germino 1987, p. 300). Another important point which Germino makes is that a balance needs to be achieved between what a *health professional* might regard as 'effective and reasonable' in terms of symptom management, and what the *patient* might regard as being so. She gives the example of how a patient and a nurse might agree that comfort is a mutual goal, but that 'the meaning of comfort to each and the cost each is willing to pay may differ' (Germino 1987, p. 300). She writes:

For instance, decreasing mental alertness or awake time to achieve total freedom from pain may not be agreeable to the patient while the nurse sees it as worthwhile . . . Quality of life [thus] becomes a personal decision with choices to be made about the extent to which symptom distress outweighs the actual or potential distress of unmet or frustrated needs.

(Germino 1987, p. 300)

Other authors, however, seek to define quality of life in quite different terms. Fredette and Beattie (1986, p. 315), for example, in researching the need for patient education programs to address the informational and emotional concerns of cancer patients and their families, found 'unexpectedly' that *hope* emerged as an important measure of quality of life. Graham and Longman (1987, p. 339), on the other hand, viewed quality of life more in terms of 'the degree of satisfaction with present life circumstances, as perceived by the patient'.

Still other authors define quality of life in quite different terms again; for example, as 'a combination of minimal anxiety, a purpose in life, and adequate self-esteem' (Germino 1987, p. 299); as a 'complex of physical function, personal attitudes, perceived well-being, and support' (Germino 1987, p. 299); as a 'perceived control over one's life' (Graham and Longman 1987, p. 339); or, more simply, as a person's ability to lead an 'independent and minimally satisfying' life (Kuhse 1987, p. 6).

There are many more views which could be considered here, but these few examples show the difficulties likely to be encountered in attempting to formulate a universal view on how quality of life should be defined and used to guide important life and death decisions in health care domains. It is probably fair to argue that quality of life essentially defies precise definition, or at least a definition which could be regarded as being universally acceptable. Even so, as Downie and Calman (1987) argue:

Most . . . would agree that quality of life relates to the individual person, that it is best perceived by that person, that conceptions of it change with time, and that it must be related to all aspects of life.

(Downie and Calman 1987, p. 190)

The message that quality of life is a concept which lends itself overwhelmingly to subjective interpretation is an important one. However, whether given views are in themselves reliable in terms of their ability to guide important moral choices in health care domains is quite another question, and one which is now briefly addressed.

In reaching a position on how best to interpret and use the term quality of life, it is important first to carefully distinguish the different philosophical senses in which the term might be meaningfully employed. Reich (1978), for example, argues that 'quality of life' may be used in at least three different ways: *descriptively*, *evaluatively*, and/or *prescriptively* (that is, morally).

Reich (1978, p. 830) explains that where the term quality of life is used as a descriptive statement, an observation is being made merely about the properties or characteristics of a human individual. In other words, quality of life in this sense simply refers to a *factual description* about certain features or traits a person might have, and thus is morally neutral. An example of a descriptive quality of life statement would be: 'this person has pain', or 'this person has lost her or his functional ability', or 'this person is totally dependent on others for care'. By this view, to say someone has lost quality of life would be to say nothing more than that she or he has lost a particular property or characteristic (or set of characteristics) of life, not the value of life itself.

Quality of life in the evaluative sense, however, is quite different. Here a quality of life statement would express that 'some value or worth is attached to the characteristic of a given individual or to a kind of human life' (Reich 1978, p. 831). For example, an evaluative quality of life statement might assert that 'the pain suffered by this person is bad' and 'the absence of pain in this person is good', or that 'the loss of functional ability experienced by that person is bad' and 'the regaining of function by this person is good', or that 'this person's dependency on others for care is bad' and the 'regaining of independence by this person is good', and so on. To say a person has lost quality of life in this sense would be to assert merely that some property or aspect of her or his life has lost value, not that life itself has lost value — although the attachment of value to certain qualities or characteristics, in this instance, often becomes the very basis upon which an individual human life might be judged worth living or not worth living, as the case may be.

Quality of life in the morally normative or prescriptive sense, on the other hand, is quite different again. Here, a quality of life statement would entail a *moral judgment* on a given (already evaluated) quality or set of qualities of an individual human life. Quality of life expressed as a moral judgment in this instance would seek to prescribe what would be a good or bad, right or wrong way of regarding a given individual human life or, more specifically, on the basis of its qualities, what ought and ought not to be done 'to support and protect' it. An example of a morally prescriptive quality of life statement would be: 'a life marked by intense pain is a life which it is not in an individual's best interests to go on living; ending such a life would thus be a morally just thing to do'; or 'a life free of pain is a minimally decent life, and thus one worth living; to take such a life would be morally objectionable'; or 'a life which cannot be lived independently is a life not worth living; therefore, ending such a life would be a morally decent thing to do'; or 'a life which can be lived independently of others is a minimally decent life and therefore a life worth living; taking such a life would be morally objectionable'. In this instance, a statement concerning the loss of quality of life could most certainly be interpreted as indicating that the life in question no longer has worth and thus is dispensable. Alternatively, a statement concerning an increase in quality of life could most certainly be interpreted as indicating that the life in question has improved worth and thus warrants preservation and protection.

In the light of these three different senses of quality of life, it can be seen that there is enormous potential for making moral errors when deciding quality of life matters in health care domains. This observation raises a number of important points. First, it wisely instructs the need for nurses to distinguish carefully the senses in which they might be using, or rather misusing, quality of life statements. This is particularly important in situations where decisions need to be made about which interventions should be implemented in order to enhance or promote the objective qualities of a person's life, and, further, about which quality or qualities ought to be enhanced or restored over others. For example, once it is identified that a person is in a state of pain which can be described factually and that the pain in question is evaluated negatively by that person, an attending nurse will be in a relatively strong position to assert that interventions aimed at alleviating pain ought to take priority in that situation. If, however, it is determined that the person in question does not regard the pain as a disvalue, or at least regards its relief as being less valuable than, say, maintaining mental alertness, an attending nurse might be in quite a different position. Chosen interventions aimed at alleviating pain might assume quite a different priority, and indeed might take on quite a different form.

A second important point here is that, by distinguishing the different senses in which the term quality of life can be used, the nurse may become more aware of the logical leap between making a *descriptive* judgment on the quality or qualities of a person's life and then making a *prescriptive* judgment (on the basis of that descriptive judgment) concerning what ought or ought not to be done in relation to that person's life. For example, if we distinguish between the different senses of 'quality of life', it soon becomes apparent that it is one thing to say a given person has lost one or two objective (descriptive) qualities or properties of their life, but it is quite another to say that, on the basis of those lost properties or qualities, the life of the person in question has less moral value or ought to be treated in one particular way rather than another. If such a judgment is to be made, this should be done on the basis of sound critically reflective moral standards, not on the basis of mistaken deductive reasoning.

Lastly, when we examine the fragile connection between the descriptive, evaluative and morally prescriptive senses of quality of life, the fundamental questions emerge of *who should decide* which values ought to be given to certain qualities or properties of life, and, further, on the basis of these ascribed values, of whether an individual human life in a particular context ought to be regarded as having one type or degree of moral value rather than another.

In relation to this last point, there is little doubt, at least from a moral point of view, that only the people whose lives are in question can decide what values to ascribe to their properties or qualities of life and which moral value to ascribe to their lives generally. For example, only those people can know what pain or dependency levels they can tolerate, and accordingly only they can identify the boundaries within which their pain or dependency states will be ascribed either positive or negative value. Only those people can know the point beyond which pain or dependency on others would render their life intolerable, and the point at which they would judge their life as being either morally less or morally more worthwhile. Bear in mind here that, while some might view pain as diminishing life's worth, others might view it as their passport to salvation. Likewise, some might consider dependency on others as diminishing their life's worth, while others might consider it quite irrelevant to either the meaning or value of their life — as Kanitsaki (1988) makes abundantly clear in her informative article 'Cancer and informed consent: a cultural perspective'. What is important to understand is that, no matter how well intentioned a nurse might be, or how knowledgeable or experienced, this probably will never be enough to enable that nurse to judge correctly either the evaluative or the morally prescriptive aspects of another person's (that is, that patient's) 'quality of life'. Even the descriptive aspect, for that matter, is difficult to judge, given the highly subjective nature of some so-called 'objectively observable' qualities, such as pain or loss of function. Since describing qualities is also very much a matter of interpreting them, there is always room for making judgment errors. It is for this reason that the people whose quality of life is at issue must be respected as the only ones who really are the best judges of what is to count as being in their best interests, and, further, as the only ones who are able to judge correctly what is to count as being their quality of life. In instances where people are unable to judge their own quality of life or best interests, this task should rightly fall to those (for example, close family members and/or friends) who intimately know the person in question and who know thoroughly their world views.

It can be seen that in using the notion of quality of life, nurses must be very careful to distinguish the exact sense in which they are using it. They must also be very aware of how easy it is to leap from a *descriptive statement* concerning a person's qualities of life to a *prescriptive statement* on what should be done for that life — morally, medically, or otherwise. Furthermore, they must take steps to guard against making this leap in judgment, particularly in instances where doing so might result in another not only losing a minimally decent level of life, but losing life itself.

'Not For Resuscitation' (NFR) orders

At some stage during their careers, nurses will be confronted with the difficult moral choice of whether to follow a *Not For Resuscitation* (NFR) order (also referred to as *Do Not Resuscitate* [DNR], and *No Code*). This type of order is usually given by a doctor in an attempt to 'avoid over-treatment and CPR (cardiopulmonary resuscitation) abuses', particularly in cases involving hopelessly ill patients 'who would be otherwise hopelessly revived' (Humphry and Wickett 1986, p. 209). Typically, an NFR order directs that: 'in the event of a cardiac arrest, neither basic nor advanced life support measures will be instituted by physicians, nurses, or other hospital staff' (Cushing 1981, p. 22; Honan et al. 1991, p. 54).

A decision not to resuscitate a person is popularly thought to flow from a medical judgment concerning the irreversible nature of that person's disease and their probable poor or hopeless prognosis (see, for example, Haines et al. 1990, p. 228). This popular view is, however, a highly controversial one. Yarling and McElmurry (1986), for example, persuasively argue that the NFR decision is not a *medical* decision per se, nor is it a legal or nursing decision. Rather, they contend, the NFR decision is fundamentally a *moral* decision, since it is based primarily on *moral values*, such as those concerning 'the meaning, sanctity, and quality of life' (p. 125).

Despite its serious moral and indeed legal implications, the issue of NFR orders has, on the whole, been poorly addressed by the nursing profession in Australasia — not only in academic terms (as suggested by the surprising paucity of nursing literature on the subject), but also in practical terms (as evidenced by the lack of explicit guidelines and policies governing NFR procedures and practices in most Australasian hospitals).

Just why this state of affairs has occurred is a matter for specu-lation. It may be that nurses have come to view the NFR order as absolutely constituting a lawful and reasonable medical order, and thus not something warranting any special or particular concern. Or it may be that nurses *are* troubled by current practices in this area but say or do nothing out of fear that their employment or career prospects may be hampered in some way if they speak out. Or it may be that nurses are troubled by current practices and do wish to speak out, but genuinely do not know how to go about articulating their concerns.

Whatever the reasons for the nursing profession's failure to address the NFR issue, the fact remains that nurses can no longer ignore the serious moral, legal and professional questions which current NFR practices raise, much less their implications for clinical nursing practice, nursing education and administration. Neither can the nursing profession ignore the point that, while the practice of prescribing NFR for seriously ill patients is a commonly *accepted* one in most Australasian hospitals and residential care agencies (as it is in many hospitals and residential care agencies worldwide), it is nevertheless open to serious question whether the practice is wholly *acceptable*. A whole range of important moral, legal and professional considerations must be taken into account, as it is hoped the following discussion will show. Two central questions are involved: What is the nature of NFR (DNR/No Code) orders? And what are the implications of NFR (DNR/No Code) orders for members of the nursing profession? Possible answers to these questions are considered now in relation to two cases, those of Mr H and Mr X. These cases both occurred in Australia.

Case 1: Mr H

Mr H*, 60 years old, was admitted to the intensive care unit of a major city hospital with a provisional diagnosis of septicaemia. At the time of admission he was pale, markedly short of breath, and had an axillary temperature of 40° C. Mr H's past medical history included severe coronary artery disease and a malignant condition. The malignant condition had, however, been successfully treated with chemotherapy, and Mr H was presently in a state of remission. In the light of his provisional diagnosis, a regime of intravenous antibiotics was commenced.

A few hours after Mr H's admission, the on-coming nursing staff for the afternoon shift gathered for 'hand-over'. During hand-over, the charge nurse informed the nursing staff present that she had just received a telephone call from Mr H's physician confirming that the patient was not for resuscitation (NFR). As she proceeded to give the afternoon report, a second consulting physician — also involved in Mr H's medical care — approached the assembled nursing staff and reaffirmed her colleague's initial NFR order. The physician then wrote up her clinical assessment of Mr H and

---

*Details of this case have been altered to disguise the identity of the patient, the staff and the hospital concerned. Any resemblance the case of Mr H might have to an actual case is therefore purely coincidental.

made other important documentations on his medical history chart. She did not, however, make any attempt to document the NFR order which she had just given to the nursing staff. This 'oversight' was later dealt with by the nursing staff writing the initials 'NFR', in pencil, on the top left-hand corner of Mr H's nursing care plan, which was held in his medical history chart.

A short time later, a nurse who had been sent to help in the unit became involved in a deep conversation with Mr H. During the conversation, Mr H spontaneously and emphatically exclaimed: 'Oh, I wish they would operate on me!' (referring to coronary artery bypass surgery, the opportunity for which he had recently been denied). In response to this the nurse gently asked Mr H whether he had discussed the possibility of bypass surgery with his doctor.

To this Mr H replied quite openly: 'Sure I have, many times, but they won't do it because they say there's only a 50–50 chance of success...' He went on to say: 'What can you do? You can't hit them over the head with a bottle and make them do it, can you?' The nurse enquired further: 'So even though you'd only have a 50–50 chance — you'd still want this coronary bypass surgery?'

Mr H replied, sombrely: 'Oh, yes. I'd do anything to buy some time. You see, my wife's very ill at home. She has cancer which can't be operated on. She's always been totally dependent on me — even more so since she's been sick. She doesn't have very long to live, and all I want is to live long enough for her, because she's so afraid of being left alone. We can't do much, and we each stay in separate rooms at home. But at least we're reasonably independent and together. I can bring her a cup of tea when she wants it and things like that. I don't care about me, but I want to live long enough for her... she's so afraid of being left alone...' Smiling, Mr H concluded: 'It's such a comfort knowing that you and the doctors are doing all that you can for me here...'

Realising that Mr H clearly had no knowledge of the NFR order against him, the nurse went immediately to discuss the matter with the other nurses, who were still in the nurses' bay, having not yet moved to care for their respective patients. There, she discreetly asked whether Mr H or his relatives had been involved in making the NFR decision. To this question one nurse replied: 'Oh! Surely that's silly to include the patient or the relatives...' And, almost simultaneously, another nurse replied: 'No. We don't do that in this hospital. It's the doctors' decision, and we're obliged to obey their orders...'

The nurse caring for Mr H then attempted to point out that her patient had indicated that he very definitely wished to risk the odds of active resuscitation. She then asked further whether the doctors were aware of Mr H's desires. To this, the nurse in charge replied sternly: 'Of course the doctors know! It's their decision, and it's the policy of this hospital to follow such orders.'

As the afternoon shift progressed, Mr H experienced a number of bradycardiac episodes, with the cardiac monitor showing his heart rate dropping to as low as 34 in some instances. The arrhythmia could have been treated relatively easily by the attending nurse administering a prescribed bolus dose of intravenous atropine. When the nurse caring for Mr H went to have the drug checked with the nurse in charge (as was required by unit policy), she was told: 'You don't need to worry about that, he's NFR . . .' Despite the attending nurse's protests, the nurse in charge still refused to check the atropine. Fortunately, during the time of intense debate between the attending nurse and the nurse in charge, Mr H's cardiac rhythm reverted spontaneously to a rate of between 80 and 90 beats per minute. Mr H had several more bradycardiac episodes throughout the shift, but each time spontaneously reverted to a safe rate of 80–90 beats per minute.

A few days later, Mr H's temperature dropped significantly to within normal limits. He stated that he felt better and was looking forward to going home. His blood cultures came back negative (negating his provisional diagnosis of septicaemia), his heart rate was more stable, and his breathing continued to improve. Despite this, however, the NFR order was not rescinded. Mr H's condition dramatically improved even further one afternoon when he was given a stat dose of intravenous lasix (a diuretic). Following this, it was decided that the presenting medical condition had not, in fact, been septicaemia but pulmonary congestion (secondary to his heart disease) and pneumonia.

Just six days after his initial admission into the intensive care unit, Mr H was judged sufficiently well recovered to be discharged home. He left, happy, thanking the nursing staff for all that they had done and expressing his eagerness to leave and be reunited with his dying wife.

Rightly troubled by the incident, the nurse made an appointment to discuss the matter with the then director of nursing. During the conversation, the nurse indicated that in future she would override any nurse in charge and would contact the prescribing doctor to clarify an existing NFR order. To this the director of nursing replied:

> Well, of course, if you had contacted the doctors involved in this case, you would probably have found that they wouldn't be very forthcoming anyway. In fact, they would probably have told you it was not your concern. You will find here that it is really the doctor's decision in cases like these, since it is *they* who have the contract with the patient, not the nurses . . .

After many days' deliberation and discussions with trusted friends and colleagues, the nurse resigned from her position, since she believed this was the only way of avoiding the kinds of dilemmas that would be posed when she had to care for patients who had been deemed 'Not For Resuscitation' without their knowledge or informed consent, or against their express wishes.

Case 2: Mr X

The second case to be considered here is taken from the Victorian State Government Social Development Committee's *Inquiry into options for dying with dignity: second and final report* (1987). It involves the case of Mr X, who was also cared for in a major city hospital.

Mr X, 78 years old, was admitted to hospital with a provisional diagnosis of 'Transitional Cell Carcinoma, with metastatic spread to the lungs, liver and spinal cord and brain' (Social Development Committee 1987, p. 111). On admission, Mr X was observed to be lethargic, disorientated and suffering a greater degree of pain than on previous admissions. He had lost weight and admitted to having lost his appetite. The nurse relating the case stated that:

> it was apparent to me that Mr X's disease process had insidiously created a decline in his overall well-being, to a point where it had now affected his quality of life.

> (Social Development Committee 1987, p. 112)

On Friday morning, upon consultation with the ward's resident medical officer, it was stated that Mr X 'had now reached the terminal stage of his illness' and that, apart from keeping him comfortable, nothing more could be done for him, medically speaking. On Friday evening, Mr X's deteriorating condition was discussed with his relatives. It was reported that:

> His relatives were distressed over the deterioration they had observed over the past few weeks in Mr X's condition and well-being. At this time they emphatically expressed their wish that should Mr X arrest while in hospital, they in no way wanted an emergency procedure of resuscitation performed on him, and wished for him to be allowed to die peacefully with a degree of dignity assured.

> (Social Development Committee 1987, p. 112)

Later that same evening, Mr X himself requested (via the hospital chaplain) that 'should he die that evening he had no wish to be actively resuscitated and would prefer to die peacefully' (Social Development Committee 1987, p. 113).

Mr X's condition continued to deteriorate. On Saturday morning, the nurse in charge called the covering resident medical officer to examine Mr X medically so that it could be formally established that Mr X 'would not be for resuscitation' in the event of his suffering a cardiac arrest. The Social Development Committee (1987) further reports:

> The doctor examined Mr X, and agreed that he should not be for cardiopulmonary resuscitation. However, he also stated that he could not instigate that decision until Monday morning, until he had consulted the Registrar and Consultants of the unit, thereby allowing his decision to be reached as a team decision. On this note, Mr X was still for resuscitation should he arrest, in spite of his and his relatives' wish to allow him to die with peace and dignity.
>
> (Social Development Committee 1987, p. 113)

Over the next 24 hours, Mr X's condition declined even further, and at 5 pm on Sunday, in the presence of his relatives, he suffered a cardiac arrest. As the covering resident medical officer had requested that Mr X should still be resuscitated — at least until the matter could be discussed with the unit team — an immediate resuscitation code was called. Full resuscitation procedures were instigated and continued for approximately 20 minutes. No positive outcome was achieved, however, and Mr X was declared clinically dead. Understandably, Mr X's relatives were very distraught about the incident and 'even more so', as the report goes on to quote, 'about the fact that Mr X had been resuscitated both against his and their wishes' (Social Development Committee 1987, p. 113).

Raising the issues

The cases of Mr H and Mr X are just two among many — possibly even thousands — which serve very well to illustrate the moral dangers of permitting misguided (or indeed unguided and/or ethically unconstrained) medico-nursing decision making in life and death situations in the clinical setting. In short, ethically unconstrained or misguided decision making in arrest situations could result in the undesirable moral consequence of patients either *not being resuscitated* when they otherwise wish to be (as in the case of Mr H) or, alternatively, of *being resuscitated* when they have clearly indicated a preference to die peacefully and without the undignified intrusion of active resuscitation interventions (as occurred in the case of Mr X).

In most Australasian hospitals and residential care agencies, NFR policies are tacitly assumed rather than clearly stated. Actual practices are, on the whole, covert rather than overt, and may vary from hospital to hospital, agency to agency, or doctor to doctor and nurse to nurse. This is certainly the case in Victoria, as the *Inquiry into options for dying with dignity: second and final report* makes clear (Social Development Committee 1987, p. 108). In fact, the Social Development Committee was so disturbed by its findings with regard to current practices in Victorian hospitals and related health care agencies that it made the following formal recommendation:

> that the Health Department Victoria as a matter of urgency obtain all relevant health care institutions' 'not-for-resuscitation' (NFR) guidelines in order:
>
> • to review current practices in this area, and that such information be referred to the National Health and Medical Research Council (NH & MRC) by the Minister for Health at the next Health Ministers' Conference; and
>
> • that the NH & MRC develop a commonly accepted set of standards and practices that can be incorporated into guidelines, and observed.
>
> (Social Development Committee 1987, p. v)

At the time of writing, the Health Department Victoria has still not undertaken any action to improve NFR practices in Victorian hospitals and residential care homes. This non-action compares poorly with the initiative of the NSW Health Department, which has recently issued guidelines on prescribing and implementing CPR/NFR orders (NSW Health Department 1993, Section 5).

For many who have uncritically followed institutional NFR practices, and who have done so 'for years', this debate might seem somewhat irrelevant and even unnecessary. After all, they might argue, these practices have worked well for the past thirty years; why worry about them now?

What such a view ignores, however, is that, if there are no carefully formulated and clearly documented guidelines and policies governing NFR procedures and practices, a number of otherwise avoidable harmful consequences might occur — and have already occurred, as literature on the subject painfully reminds us. The kinds of morally undesirable outcomes that might occur include, among others:

1. patients' rights and interests being unjustly violated (particularly in instances where an NFR/CPR decision does not accord with a patient's considered preferences);

2. nurses being left to carry a disproportionate burden (in moral, legal, professional and personal terms) with regard to actually carrying out NFR/CPR orders;

3. other allied health workers (including less senior doctors) carrying disproportionate legal, moral, professional and personal burdens on account of the dilemmas posed by administering uncertain and ambiguous NFR/CPR procedures and practices.

These and similar considerations, needless to say, raise two further questions: What exactly is wrong with current NFR practices and procedures? And what can and should the nursing profession do in order to ensure that morally just NFR policies and guidelines are formulated and implemented in hospitals and related health care agencies?

The difficulties surrounding current NFR practices can be roughly categorised under three general headings:

1. problems concerning NFR decision-making criteria, guidelines and procedures;

2. problems concerning the documentation and communication of NFR orders;

3. problems concerning the implementation of NFR orders.

1. Problems concerning NFR decision-making criteria, guidelines and procedures

A. CRITERIA AND GUIDELINES USED

As already briefly mentioned, most hospitals and related health care agencies lack clear guidelines on how NFR decisions should be made and implemented, or, if they do have guidelines, their practices do not always conform with them (Lipton 1989, p. 112; *Bioethics News* 1992, p. 4). As a result, patients have very often been subjected to arbitrary and at times haphazard and even whimsical decision making with regard to their being resuscitated or not resuscitated in life-threatening situations. Different doctors and nurses may appeal to different *criteria* (to be distinguished here from *procedures*) for making an NFR/CPR decision (see also Stewart and Rai 1989; Thom 1988). For example, some doctors and nurses might appeal to *quality of life* criteria (such as age, mental competence, pain states, chronicity of disease, poor prognosis, and so forth) when making an NFR/CPR decision. An NFR decision based on such criteria might well be in accordance with a patient's preferences, but it might equally as well be thoroughly opposed to them, as occurred in the Fred Walker case (Hastings Center 1982). Fred Walker was a previously fit 90-year-old who required admission to hospital for multiple medical problems. While in hospital Mr Walker suffered a cardiac arrest and was not resuscitated, even though both he and his wife had clearly indicated that they wished 'everything possible' to be done to try and preserve his life (Hastings Center 1982, pp. 27–8).

Alternatively, some doctors and nurses might appeal to *sanctity of life* criteria (which essentially demand that life be preserved, whatever the cost) when making an NFR/CPR decision. Doctors' or nurses' decisions in this instance might well accord with patients' expressed wishes, but, as with the previous example, they could also be violatory of them. Annas (in Bandman and Bandman 1985), for example, cites the case of a 70-year-old woman 'who was resuscitated over 70 times within a few days' (p. 236). And Dolan (1988) cites the case of a patient who was resuscitated 52 times before 'family members literally threw themselves across the crash cart to prevent the team from reaching the patient' for the fifty-third time (p. 47).

Still others, however, may appeal to nothing more than a personal sense or 'gut feeling' of right and wrong when making NFR/CPR decisions. What is troubling about this is that, while attending doctors or nurses might 'feel' that a particular NFR or CPR decision is right (or wrong, as the case may be), it does not follow that the decision in question is, as a matter of fact, morally sound. Whether an NFR/CPR decision is morally sound can and should be decided only by critical reflection and appeal to sound moral standards, not, as some might contend, by appealing solely to the dictates of 'gut response', for reasons considered previously in this text.

Even more troubling is the practice of deeming patients NFR on the basis of an NFR decision made during a previous hospital admission. For example, if a patient is made NFR during an admission to hospital in March, is discharged, but comes back into hospital in April, the patient can be made NFR again on the basis of the March hospital admission decision. The rationale behind this is not entirely clear.

Equally disturbing is the over-reliance on *age* as a decisional criterion when making NFR/CPR decisions. Many residential care homes for the aged, for example, have a blanket (unwritten) policy of not resuscitating their residents. As discussed earlier (in chapter 6), persons entering these homes are asked 'whether they wish to be cremated and where they wish to be buried, but not whether they wish to be resuscitated' if and when they should cardiac arrest (Johnstone 1988, p. 8). This practice is disturbing for two main reasons: first, it totally violates the residents' autonomy; second, it relies on what recent research has shown to be an unreliable and invalid decisional criterion — notably *age* (see in particular Sage et al. 1987).

As a point of interest, one American study investigating the implementation of a 'Do-Not-Resuscitate' (DNR) policy in a nursing home found that, of the 48 residents (mean age 81.7 years) who were deemed capable of deciding whether they wanted CPR/DNR, 30 (63.5 per cent) 'chose to be resuscitated in the event of a cardiopulmonary arrest', compared with only 18 (37.5 per cent) who 'decided in favour of DNR' (Fader et al. 1989, p. 545).

B. THE EXCLUSION OF PATIENTS FROM DECISION MAKING

Some doctors and nurses genuinely believe that patients or their relatives should not be included in the process of making NFR decisions (see also Perry et al. 1986; Schade and Muslin 1989; Loewy 1991). Responding to the Fred Walker case (mentioned above), Professor Carson (1982) points out that the admitting hospital in that case had an official policy which effectively took the position 'that entering patients should not be bothered with the details of resuscitation policy but should assume that they will be well cared for and coded if necessary' (p. 28).

Also commenting on the Fred Walker case, Mark Siegler (an associate professor of medicine) goes even further, and argues that where a physician knows ('within limits of uncertainty that characterize all medical knowledge') that CPR would be of no possible benefit to the patient, it should not be initiated — *regardless* of a patient's preferences to the contrary (Siegler 1982, p. 29).

Carson's and Siegler's comments on the Walker case alert us to some of the moral dangers of uncritically following institutional policies, norms, etiquette and the like when making important life and death decisions, as well as to the unnecessary suffering which can be caused by an unthinking and dogmatic application of them. The unnecessary suffering caused in this case is summed up very well by Mrs Walker's comments upon being informed that no attempt had been made to resuscitate her husband. The *Hastings Center Report* (1982) describes her response in the following terms:

> Upon being informed that no emergency measures were taken in her husband's case, Mrs Walker said that that decision was against her wishes. 'Doing everything,' she says, 'is the difference between life and death. The doctor was playing God when he decided he should not try to save my husband. You're not playing God when you've tried everything and exhausted all methods. All I wanted was for them to try. My husband knew how to love and be loved. That was his quality of life. That suited him and it suited me.

> (Hastings Center 1982, p. 28)

Many doctors believe that patients should not be 'burdened' with having to decide whether they should be resuscitated in the event of a cardiac arrest — particularly if the patient's condition is 'medically hopeless' and any further treatment — including CPR — would be 'futile' (Perry et al. 1986; Schade and Muslin 1989; Haines et al. 1990; Tomlinson and Brody 1990; Scofield 1991; Lo 1991; Loewy 1991). This has resulted in patients often not being consulted about an NFR/DNR order that has been made against them. In one American study, for example, it was revealed that only 22 per cent of patients surveyed had been involved in the DNR decision in their case (Lipton 1989, p. 108). Another study found that, while fewer than 50 per cent of nurses and doctors surveyed agreed that patients should be given information about 'No Codes' on admission to hospital, 75 per cent of lay persons surveyed 'believed this information should be available' (Honan et al. 1991, p. 60). And another study revealed that 68 per cent of respondents surveyed indicated their wish to discuss the use of life-sustaining treatment, yet only *six per cent* had been given the opportunity to do so (Lo et al. 1986). While these and other findings (see, for example, Council on Ethical and Judicial Affairs, American Medical Association, 1991) cannot be generalised as applying universally, it is nevertheless possible to speculate that, were these studies to be duplicated in Australia, New Zealand, England and other Western countries, they would probably yield very similar results.

C. MISINTERPRETATION OF ORDERS AND QUESTIONABLE OUTCOMES

Another major difficulty associated with current NFR guidelines and procedures is that they are essentially inadequate for ensuring that given NFR orders are interpreted in a precise, reliable and uniform manner. Consider, for example, the case of Mr H, described at the beginning of this discussion. In this case the NFR order was interpreted, controversially, as also including the non-treatment of a potentially fatal but relatively easily treatable cardiac arrhythmia. This interpretation becomes even more troubling, and the appropriateness of the NFR decision more questionable, when it is considered that the patient was, after all, being cared for in an *intensive care unit*. What clearly needs to be questioned here (particularly in cases involving patients who have been admitted to intensive care units) is that, if a patient's condition is so medically hopeless, and an NFR order is therefore medically justified, why is that patient being cared for in an intensive care unit, where the imperative 'to treat' is usually considered to be both foremost and overriding? There is surely something seriously questionable — and, indeed, inconsistent and contradictory — in caring for patients in an intensive care situation (or any other ward), having their heart beat monitored, observing and recording presenting cardiac arrhythmias, having a standing prescription for drugs to treat given arrhythmias, and yet doing absolutely nothing when and if that patient cardiac arrests. Such a situation reveals not only moral confusion but moral negligence.

Another disturbing example of the way in which an NFR/DNR order can be misinterpreted can be found in the case of a dying patient who had pulmonary congestion and pneumonia, and, associated with these two conditions, copious mucus production. In this case, the nurses (mis)interpreted the NFR order to include withholding oropharyngeal/nasopharyngeal sunctioning. As a result, the patient was left, quite literally, to drown in his own secretions — until another nurse detected the error and took immediate action to correct the other nurses' misinterpretation of the order. The lesson to be learned from this case — and others like it — is that 'No Code' does not mean 'no care' (Saunders and Valente 1986; see also Lo 1991).

D. 'GO SLOW' CODE

Another common but questionable NFR practice which prevails in some institutions is the 'go slow' code or 'slow code' (Social Development Committee 1987, p. 108; Bandman and Bandman 1985, p. 235; Honan et al. 1991, p. 55) — loosely defined here as 'responding to a code slowly or not using every available lifesaving measure' (Humphry and Wickett 1986, pp. 210–11):

> Here attempts are made to revive the patient, but only after a delay, usually long enough to ensure that the patient won't respond. In this way, the patient's wishes — or so the physicians can claim — have been honoured, while the hospital is protected from litigation.
>
> (Humphry and Wickett 1986, p. 211*)

Citing the comments of a nurse, these authors go on to point out, however, that:

> resuscitation, even when delayed, is rarely done for the patient's benefit: 'Resuscitation is more for the benefit of the living than helpful to the dead or dying patient. The family can say they tried everything, but [the loved one] was too far gone to bring him [sic] back, and the act of resuscitation makes the professional staff look efficient'.
>
> (Humphry and Wickett 1986, p. 211*)

The practices of formulating and following 'go slow' codes, while common, are nevertheless vulnerable to a number of criticisms. First, those who uphold 'go slow' codes seem erroneously to presume that a morally valid distinction exists between 'going slow' (as in the case of 'go slow' orders) and 'doing nothing' (as in the case of NFR orders). On closer analysis, it can be seen that in essence there is very little distinction between the two, for the following reasons.

1. Both entail intentional omission (in this instance, doctors, nurses, and allied health workers deliberately refraining from performing CPR when they have both the ability and opportunity to do so) at a point in time otherwise critical to the achievement of positive therapeutic outcomes — that is, the actual resuscitation or revival of the patient in question. (For further insight into the problem of 'intentional omission', see the preceding discussion on euthanasia (chapter 10), as well as Kuhse 1987, p. 43.)

2. The intentional omission of CPR or other basic resuscitation measures by doctors, nurses and allied health workers (whether in response to a 'go slow' or an NFR code) results in the same foreseeable and intended outcome — notably, the irreversible death of the patient.

3. Given the intentionality of 'go slow' and NFR codes (notably, the *intention* of bringing about or hastening death by deliberately withholding certain cares and treatments), both of these orders unquestionably stand as acts of passive euthanasia. (See the discussion on euthanasia in chapter 10.)

A second criticism here relates to the legal aspect of 'go slow' codes. Proponents of 'go slow' codes, for example, seem to assume that such codes are legally permissible and thus preferable.

Cushing (1981) writes, however, that it is doubtful 'that a court would legitimize a partial code order' (p. 27), since such a code generally means 'that the procedure is not to be carried out according to acceptable practice standards' (p. 27). In short, those upholding 'go slow' codes or 'partial codes' could be held legally negligent for their outcomes (Cushing 1981).

---

* Reprinted with permission of Angus & Robertson/Collins.

2. Problems concerning the documentation and communication of NFR orders

A second major area of concern in the NFR debate involves the means by which NFR orders are documented and communicated to health care providers generally, and to nurses in particular.

Modes of communicating NFR orders are, for the most part, disturbing. Common practices include the following.

1. NFR orders are given verbally only (i.e. they are not formally documented in the patient's medical or nursing notes). This practice has come about largely because doctors are 'loathe to indicate in written notes in patient records that a patient is not for resuscitation' (Social Development Committee 1987, p. 108).

2. NFR orders are 'confirmed' by sticking coloured dots (usually black ones) or scribbling an asterisk either on the patient's medical history chart and/or by the patient's name on the ward's bed allocation board. As a point of interest, in 1988 the Association of Medical Directors of Victorian Hospitals recommended to the Victorian Hospital Association that 'a round white sticker with "sky" blue border and an oblique "sky" blue stripe be adopted by hospitals to denote Not for Resuscitation. They advised that the sticker should be placed on the front of the patient record, on the bed card and on the patient's wristband' (*Victorian Hospital Association Report* 1988, p. 3). (Whether the colour sky blue is significant or not is anyone's guess!)

3. NFR orders are 'confirmed' by pencilling the initials 'DNR' or 'NFR' or some other equivalent in an inconspicuous place on the patient's medical history or nursing care plan, or both.

4. NFR orders are written euphemistically as 'routine nursing care only', or 'cares for comfort only' (Cushing 1981, p. 24).

These types of practices may well be commonly *accepted* throughout institutional health care settings, but, as noted earlier, it is far from clear that they are *acceptable*, morally, professionally or legally. As with *any* verbal orders, verbal NFR orders are vulnerable not only to misinterpretation but also to denial, in the sense that doctors could always deny that they ever gave such an order in the event of an intentional omission in relation to a cardiac arrest being discovered. Michael Adams (1984), for example, cites an instructive example of how very serious errors can be made on account of verbal NFR orders being given and, equally instructive, how easily an attending doctor can deny ever giving an NFR order in the first place!

The case in question involved a patient, identified as Mrs M, who suffered a cardiac arrest while being cared for in an intensive care unit. A medical student covering the unit was called. After initiating CPR he is alleged to have stopped, saying: 'What am I doing? She's a no-code,' and then stopped performing cardiac massage (Adams 1984, p. 54). The case was eventually brought before a grand jury after a nurse anonymously informed Mrs M's daughter that 'her mother had died "unnecessarily" because "a no-code was sent out" ' (Adams 1984, p. 55). As a point of interest, the medical student testified that he never made the comment. When the medical student was later asked in an informal situation why he treated Mrs M as a 'no-code', he replied that the order to do so had been given to him verbally by a cardiologist (Adams 1984, p. 55).

It is popularly but erroneously presumed that a verbal order, in the case of either NFR or 'go slow' codes, will 'convey the directive without attaching any legal liability' (Cushing 1981, p. 27). Cushing warns, however, that: 'while many hospitals allow no code orders to be "unofficial", it is difficult to justify a continuation of this practice. Once the medical decision has been made, the order should be written as any other medical directive' (1981, p. 27).

Also commenting on the legalities of verbal no-code orders, Kellmer (1986) writes that legal liability is in no way diminished by not writing NFR orders: if anything, failure to document a no-code or NFR order adequately would probably increase legal liability (a view shared by Cushing). These two authors are admittedly writing from an American context, but in the Australian State of Victoria, given the Victorian State Government's *Medical Treatment Act 1988*, it is not difficult to imagine that nurses and other health care professionals could be found legally negligent for not initiating full CPR in cases where there is absolutely no written documentation of patients exercising their legal right to refuse orthodox medical treatment. This point was made abundantly clear in the parliamentary debates leading up to the enactment and proclamation of the *Medical Treatment Act 1988*. In the parliamentary session of 3 May 1988, for example, the Hon. D. R. White (the then Minister for Health), citing a hypothetical NFR example, stated that, if a person dies as a result of a doctor (and, it may be presumed, a nurse) failing to initiate CPR in the event of a cardiac arrest, 'a relative can sue the doctor under common law for negligence where there is no evidence that the patient has consented' (Parliament of Victoria, Legislative Council, 3 May 1988, p. 1015). Earlier in the same parliamentary debate, Mr White also commented:

if a person in a hypothetical circumstance — and I repeat that it is hypothetical — has been resuscitated three times and decides not to seek further treatment, or not to be resuscitated a fourth time, under common law the issue is by no means clear. If a medical practitioner decides, in good faith, that he or she wishes to continue resuscitating that patient, the patient must go to court to get a court to uphold the patient's right to refuse medical treatment. This is a difficult process because there is no effective procedure. Moreover, the outcome of the action before the court is by no means certain.

(Parliament of Victoria, Legislative Council, 3 May 1988, p. 1019)

It is also worth noting here the Victorian Nursing Council's (1988) position statement, 'Resuscitation by the nurse', which, among other things, warns that:

Registered Nurses must be aware that acting within a guideline or policy statement of a professional organisation or an employer does not relieve them of responsibility for their own acts and may not provide immunity in case of negligence.

(Victorian Nursing Council 1988, p. 4)

The practice of giving verbal NFR orders has seen the emergence of other questionable methods for communicating given NFR orders, such as the use of coloured dots, asterisks and pencilled initials and abbreviations. Like verbal orders, however, coloured dots, asterisks and pencilled initials and abbreviations are less than adequate in terms of their ability and reliability in guiding sound and defensible practices in arrest or emergency situations. Such methods of communicating NFR orders are, in fact, quite dangerous — not only on account of their *anonymity* (for example, it would be extremely difficult to prove who, in fact, stuck a dot or sketched an asterisk on a patient's chart), but also on account of their being *inarticulate* (they are, after all, merely a symbol of a supposed medical directive, not the carefully worded medical directive itself). For my part, it seems quite inconceivable that important and supposedly competent medical decisions concerning the life and death of a fellow human being could be reduced to something so careless and so vulgar as a simple black dot, an asterisk, or a set of unintelligible initials. It is also almost inconceivable that competent nurses could rely so readily on nothing more than a set of crude symbols for determining whether or not the interventions needed to aid a seriously ill or dying patient should, in fact, be initiated. The additional dangers of dots are, of course, that they can be bought and placed on charts by almost anybody; they can also become dislodged, stick to the wrong chart, or be placed by the wrong person's name on the bed allocation board, and so on (Adams 1984). To further complicate the problematic use of dots, recent anecdotal evidence points to the emergence of yet another questionable practice: the use of dots to identify patients who *are* for resuscitation (that is, on wards or in residential care homes where the number of patients/residents deemed NFR outnumber those who are for resuscitation) (confidential source, personal communication). It is not yet known how widespread this practice is. In the light of such difficulties, I am not convinced that the recommendation of the Association of Medical Directors of Victorian Hospitals that the use of a specially designed sticker will improve the situation. It merely replaces one problem with another; it does not, it seems, resolve it.

The use of initials such as 'NFR' or 'DNR', and variations thereof, is also seriously problematic. In one case, for example, a nurse informed me that a doctor had once ordered her to write the initials 'NFR' on a patient's chart. When she queried this directive, she was politely told: 'Don't worry. If there are any problems, we'll just say it means 'Not for Referral . . .' In another case, the initials 'NFR' were written on a patient's nursing care plan, which was left hanging on the end of his bed. During visiting hours, a family member visiting the patient took the liberty of examining the nursing care plan and noticed the initials 'NFR' on it. She asked a passing nurse what the letters meant. To this question the nurse replied: 'Oh, don't worry about that. It just means 'Nice Fellow Really . . .'

In yet another case, a dietitian writing in a patient's integrated case notes (that is, where all members of the health care team — doctors, nurses, and other allied carers — write up their notes) wrote the initials 'NFR' meaning 'not for referral'. Understandably, the dietitian was very distressed when the significance of what she had written was pointed out to her.

The practice of using *pencilled* abbreviations provokes one more comment. This is done so that the initials can be erased when and if the patient dies or alternatively is discharged; the task almost invariably falls to attending nursing staff.

A last concern to be considered here is the practice of ordering 'nursing care only' or 'cares for comfort only' when it is considered that nothing more medically can be done for the patient. In many respects (as already argued in the discussion on euthanasia) this practice has emerged as an almost universal euphemism for ordering passive euthanasia. The professional — not to mention the moral — acceptability of such practices needs to be seriously questioned, however. Nurses need to realise — and need to make it publicly known — that, contrary to popular medical opinion, writing such orders is not an acceptable medical tactic for refusing to accept responsibility in instances where it is decided on the basis of questionable criteria that 'nothing more (medically) can be done'. For one thing, in situations where all means have not, in fact, been exhausted, there is always room to question whether CPR (or any other life-supporting measure, for that matter) should, in fact, be rightfully withheld from a patient. On this point it is worthwhile to consider Veatch's helpful comments. In his book *Death, dying and the biological revolution*, Veatch writes:

> The question should never be, 'When should we stop treating this patient?' as if the patient were an object to be repaired or discarded. Rather the moral question must be, 'When, if ever, should it be morally and/or legally possible for the patient to decide to refuse medical treatment even if that may mean that dying will no longer be prolonged?'
>
> (Veatch 1977, p. 8)

Whatever the reasons for permitting verbal NFR orders, and for using dots, asterisks, abbreviations and initials to communicate these, the provocative question remains: **if the practice of ordering NFR is so medically, morally and legally justified, why are doctors so reticent in and so loathe to document their NFR orders formally? Why are nurses so ready to use crude and erasable symbols to communicate such important orders?** Until satisfactory answers to such questions can be given, the practices in question should rightly be condemned as professionally, ethically and legally unsound.

Nurses who continue to use dots and similar symbols to communicate a doctor's NFR order must accept that they alone are the ones responsible for documenting the decisions which doctors otherwise refuse to put in writing (Adams 1984, p. 53). If they do not wish to have this responsibility, clearly they need to stop enforcing and upholding the communication modes currently being employed in this area. They must insist that their medical colleagues take full responsibility for the decisions they make and the directives they give to nursing staff on the basis of those decisions.

3. Problems concerning the implementation of NFR orders

A third major area of concern in the NFR debate involves following or carrying out the NFR order. While at first glance this might seem to be a relatively trivial concern, literature on the subject suggests otherwise (see also *The Regan report on hospital law* 1985).

It is probably true to say that many nurses experience no difficulty whatsoever in carrying out NFR orders — indeed, in some instances, they may be largely responsible for encouraging doctors to prescribe them. Humphry and Wickett (1987), for example, cite a 1984 poll surveying nurses' attitudes towards withholding life-sustaining procedures from dying patients (p. 128). The poll suggested that a staggering majority (70–84 per cent) of those nurses surveyed were in favour of withholding life-support procedures and extraordinary means of life-saving treatment in given situations.

Polls such as these should, however, be treated cautiously. I would argue, for instance, that it is also probably true that many nurses suffer significant hardships on account of covert institutional demands to follow NFR/CPR orders (see also Dolan 1988). The case of the nurse involved in caring for Mr H, cited earlier, stands as an important example of the kinds of difficulties nurses can face, particularly in instances where an informed consent has not been obtained before giving an NFR order. Very often, nurses follow a questionable NFR order simply to avoid the wrath of a prescribing doctor — or even nurse superiors — both of whom have the power to 'make life difficult' for a dissenting nurse.

Conversely, nurses who decide not to initiate resuscitation in the absence of a medical NFR/DNR order can also face enormous difficulties. In one noted English case, for example, a registered nurse 'who chose to let an elderly man die rather than call in a resuscitation team' was dismissed for gross misconduct (*Nursing Times* 1983, p. 20; see also Johnstone 1994, pp. 258–9). The fact that the man was 78 years old, had lung cancer, and essentially died of 'natural causes' apparently had no bearing on the case (Buchanan 1983; Regan 1983).

The issue of carrying out NFR orders is, of course, of particular concern to nurses; quite simply, they are almost invariably left with the ultimate decision whether or not to initiate CPR in an arrest situation. They are also thus invariably left with the burden of having to accept the responsibility for the consequences of both their actions and their omissions in arrest situations — a point which, I believe, is not always fully understood by attending nurse practitioners. Given this, it is nothing short of nonsense to suggest that nurses have no separate moral, legal or professional responsibilities in situations where a patient's life and well-being are hanging in the balance. What such considerations wisely instruct is that nurses, who carry the legal, moral, professional and indeed personal burdens of implementing NFR orders, must take a much stronger stand on ensuring that sound and reliable guidelines and policies are brought into being — not only to protect their own interests, but equally importantly, if not more so, the interests of their patients.

NFR: issues and recommendations

Until now it has been argued that NFR decision making has, on the whole, been:

1. arbitrary, haphazard and even whimsical in nature;

2. based on questionable and unreliable criteria — particularly in instances where doctors and nurses have relied on little more than a personal sense of right and wrong or institutional norms for guiding NFR decisions, rather than on sound moral standards and deliberations;

3. not always respectful of a patient's considered preferences;

4. open to serious misinterpretation as a result of inadequate guidelines;

5. made in a way that serves the interests of attending health care professionals and the health care agency, rather than those of the patient;

6. tantamount to acts of passive euthanasia; and

7. unfairly left to nurses, who then have to carry an enormous share of the burdens associated with doctors prescribing NFR orders.

As a response to some of the weaknesses in current NFR decision making practices, I shall briefly outline a number of important points which I believe ought to be reflected in NFR guidelines.

1. There needs to be a recognition that NFR decisions are *intrinsically moral* in nature, not just medical, nursing or legal, and because of this must be made by appealing to sound moral criteria and standards as well as to relevant factual information.

2. Any NFR decision made ought to reflect the *patient's informed choice* (given informed choice in its most stringent sense here).

3. NFR decisions/orders should be *properly written* on patients' medical and nursing charts, and should include all the relevant factual data upon which the decisions have been based (including descriptions of the patients' statements relevant to their request that given life-saving measures be withheld). Alternatively, an 'NFR authorisation form' could be signed; an example is shown in figure 12.1.

4. Mechanisms must be established to ensure the *correct interpretation* of non-treatment orders.

5. Once an NFR decision has been made, it should be *reviewed and re-affirmed* in writing at intervals which are appropriate to the patient's changing condition (Clinical Ethics Committee 1984).

6. An NFR order should be *able to be revoked* at 'any time at the request of the competent patient, or in the case of the incompetent patient, by the cited next-of-kin or legal representative', or as is morally appropriate (Clinical Ethics Committee 1984).

7. An NFR decision should be carried out only by those who have freely and informedly agreed to carry out such orders. Where nurses or doctors have genuine conscientious objection to following an NFR order, morally they ought to be *permitted to abstain* from being actively involved in caring for the patient in question. (See the discussion on conscientious objection in chapter 13.)

Ordering NFR/DNR on patients is a common and widespread practice in hospitals both in Australia and overseas. In one Australian study, for example, it was found that of the 272 people who had died over a three-month period during 1987 in a major South Australian teaching hospital, 166 (61 per cent) had been the subject of an NFR order (Stanley and Reid 1989, p. 260). This figure was noted by the investigators to be consistent with the findings of other studies (Stanley and Reid 1989, p. 261). Several studies in the United States, meanwhile, have shown that NFR/DNR occurs in 'approximately 3%–14% of [all] hospital admissions' (Lipton 1989, p. 108). In some residential care homes in Australia, however, the percentage of those made NFR is likely to be 100 per cent, because unwritten policies in some homes prescribe that all residents are *automatically* NFR/DNR on admission.

Where, then, does this leave the nursing profession? What can and should the nursing profession do about the NFR/DNR issue? I believe that a number of important activities can and should be carried out. In summary, the nursing profession must actively work to:

- ensure that its members are adequately informed of the issues at stake and are adequately prepared to articulate the important concerns facing them when confronted with NFR decisions and orders during their everyday practice;

- ensure that sound and reliable mechanisms are put in place to protect patients' rights and interests when confronted with a life-threatening or harm-causing situation;

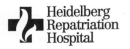

Heidelberg Repatriation Hospital

Banksia Street
Heidelberg West
Victoria 3081 Australia

Surname	Given names	File number

(Affix patient label if available)

PATIENT MANAGEMENT PLAN

In the event of a cardiac arrest ....

UR No. ...., is not to undergo cardiopulmonary resuscitation (CPR)

Name of consultant in charge of patient's care who has given approval ....

....

Reason for decision to withhold CPR ....

....

....

....

Specific treatment to be continued other than CPR (eg. antibiotics, blood transfusion)......................

....

....

Extent of communication with the patient and next of kin (with names) ....

....

....

Staff (medical, nursing, allied health) consulted about the decision to withhold CPR ....

....

....

Staff informed about the decision to withhold CPR (especially nursing staff) ....

....

....

....

Other relevant information (eg. Refusal of Medical Treatment certificate, role of patient's guardian, role of Director of Medical Services) ....

....

....

Signed .... Name ....

Position .... Date ....

Not For Cardio-Pulmonary Resuscitation MR/120

Figure 12.1 An example of a form authorising a 'Not for Resuscitation' order. (Reproduced with permission)

NOT FOR CARDIO-PULMONARY RESUSCITATION GUIDELINES

A decision to withhold CPR should be carefully considered, and only made after investigating all available options.

1. **INDICATIONS**

a) If after being adequately informed about the diagnosis, prognosis and the nature of the procedure, and having had time and adequate counselling to adjust emotionally, a competent patient expresses the seriously considered judgement that he or she not be resuscitated in the event that the current condition results in a cardiac arrest, and there is no reason to believe that the patient is suicidal.

b) If on medical grounds, the procedure is considered futile.

c) If the medical team is reasonably certain that in the event of a cardiac arrest, resuscitation being achieved, the patient would be so severely disabled and have such a poor prognosis that the distress caused by the resuscitation procedures would be disproportionate to the result.

d) The patient may have appointed, whilst competent, an agent with enduring power of attorney (under the Treatment Act 1990) to make decisions regarding treatment in the event that the patient becomes incompetent. An agent may refuse treatment on behalf of the patient.

2. **COMMUNICATION**

If CPR is not considered appropriate it should be discussed with the patient if his or her emotional and cognitive state permits. The clinician in charge should fully outline the diagnosis, prognosis and treatment options available, allow the patient time to review and discuss this information, involve the patient in the decision about CPR and ensure that the patient is informed of the final decision. If the patient is not competent or is emotionally incapable of being involved these discussions should take place with the patient's next of kin.

If the patient presents a Refusal of Treatment certificate issued under the Treatment Act 1990, or if the patient has an enduring power of attorney or a legally appointed guardian then the matter should be referred to the Director of Medical Services.

3. **DOCUMENTATION**

a) The names of the person making the Not for Resuscitation Order and the consultant who approved the order. A Not For Resuscitation Order should not be signed without the approval of the consultant in charge of the patient's care.

b) The reason for the decision.

c) Specific treatment to be continued other than CPR (eg. antibiotics, blood transfusions).

d) The extent of communication about the decision with the patient or the patient's next of kin.

e) The names of other staff consulted about the decision (medical, nursing, allied health).

f) The names of other staff informed of the decision (medical, nursing, allied health).

g) Any other relevant information (eg. Refusal of Medical Treatment Certificate, role of patient's guardian, role of Director of Medical Services, names of those to be contacted if the patient dies).

A Not for Resuscitation Order is not irreversible and should be reviewed at regular intervals. In particular it should be reviewed if there is a change in the patient's prognosis or if a new consultant takes on a significant role in the patient's management (eg. during the immediate post-operative period if the patient undergoes surgery). Wherever possible, this should be discussed with the patient or the patient's next of kin.

- encourage open and honest public debate on the NFR issue and help to promote the community's awareness of what is at stake for its members;

- promote the community's entitlement and duty to participate in any public debate on the NFR issue;

- fight for its entitlement to participate in the development of criteria for NFR policies, and guard against the likelihood of criteria being formulated and imposed that do not ensure the achievement of morally desirable outcomes in arrest or life-threatening situations (personally, I believe there should only be one decisional criterion, and that is the *patient's preferences or expressed wishes*, regardless of what others might think of these);

- ensure that morally sound and reliable policies and guidelines are adopted in the clinical setting for guiding NFR/CPR decisions; and, lastly,

- ensure that provision is made for those of its members who are otherwise conscientiously opposed to a given NFR/CPR order and thus wish to be exempted from caring for a patient who is the subject of such orders.

It is not being argued here that NFR orders have no place among the care/treatment alternatives available to seriously ill patients. To reject the moral acceptability of NFR orders outright — without any regard for the kinds of circumstances under which they might well be justified — would be capricious. What is being argued here, however, is that, if NFR orders are to be formulated, this must be done on the basis of morally sound criteria and decision-making processes.

Responding to the difficulties posed by the use of life-support systems and the NFR issue, the Clinical Ethics Committee of Physicians and Dentists of the Royal Victoria Hospital, Montreal (1984), argues that guidelines must be directed towards:

> defining important ethical principles and their application, recognition of the autonomy of the competent patient, the role of the family, the importance of good communication at all levels, special mechanisms to deal with persistent disagreement, and circumstances in which judicial opinion must be sought.
>
> (Clinical Ethics Committee, Council of Physicians and Dentists 1984, p. 1)

By incorporating these and the many other similar considerations in NFR policies and guidelines outlined in this chapter and elsewhere (see Hickie 1990), nurses and doctors can rest assured that they truly have done all that is possible to ensure that patients' rights and interests have been properly respected in life-threatening situations, and that they have not overstepped their authority as health care providers. Members of the community at large can also rest assured that their assumptions about being well cared for upon coming into hospital or other related health care agencies are not misplaced, and that they can indeed trust and rely on those people who will most probably care for them during those delicate, life-threatening moments which are all too often charac-terised by intense personal need and human vulnerability.

Organ harvesting and transplantation

Headlines celebrating organ transplantation — and the doctors performing them — have become almost commonplace in our world's daily newspapers, not to mention radio and television news reports. These news reports have become so abundant that it is difficult to avoid the impression that the media is not merely informing the public about something it has a right to know, but also engaging in a full-scale publicity campaign aimed at soliciting public support for a highly controversial and emotional issue. Popular headlines, many of them on the front page (and, inciden-tally, breaching the requirements of confidentiality and anonymity of both donors and recipients), include:

- 'The shy pioneer on the frontier of heart surgery' (Pirrie 1988a)
- 'Modern medicines maker of miracles' (Pirrie 1988c)
- 'School girl, 11, undergoes liver transplant' (Reddy 1988)
- 'The man behind our heart-transplant unit' (Lee 1989)
- 'Given new heart, Michael is set to take on the world' (Pirrie 1988d)
- 'Hospital expects first heart swap by Christmas' (Messina 1988)
- ' "We're happy he gave four lives" — Donor boy's special gift' (Carter 1988)
- 'A sporting chance for transplant patients' (Lahey 1988)
- 'Heart transplant boy fine thanks, and ready for a chat' (Athersmith 1989)
- 'State tries to hasten collection of organs' (Pirrie 1989a)

- 'New cornea offers sight to a child' (Boreham 1989)
- 'Brave Paula waiting in hope: a plea for donors' (Bout 1989)
- 'Department balked at donor-liver flight' (Pirrie 1989b)
- 'Alfred prepares for heart–lung transplant' (Pirrie 1989c)
- 'Boy, 6, is Australia's youngest liver recipient' (Bock 1990)
- 'Heart beats announce a life renewed' (Heath 1991)
- 'A new liver means new life after 10 years of pain' (Heath 1992)
- 'A deep breath of life with new lungs brings hope' (Ryle 1992)

It is significant that, of the numerous newspaper and other media reports devoted to the organ transplantation movement, almost all simply extol the virtues of organ retrieval and transplantation. More general controversies and, concerns, by contrast, are rarely given a mention, let alone prominent headlines, and when they are, they tend to be dismissed by proponents of the movement as manifesting little more than 'transplant hysteria' (Gould 1986), or 'sentimentalism' (Jolliffe 1986).

Australia's medical specialists, law reformers and politicians supporting the organ transplant movement encourage the belief that organ donation and transplantation is now a fairly clear-cut moral, legal and medical issue (see O'Neill 1988; Pirrie 1988b; Svendsen 1988; McCauley 1988; Roper 1984; Scott 1984; Robertson 1984) — or at least more clear-cut than the abortion and euthanasia issues. And the current State laws on tissue donations all seem to offer some reassurance that the proponents of organ transplantation are standing on firm ground. Their position finds even further strength when compared with overseas 'opting-out' or 'contracting-out' laws, which take the extraordinary step of permitting doctors to retrieve organs from any individuals who have died in hospital unless the individuals have explicitly requested that they do *not* wish to be used as organ donors, that is, by registering on a non-donors' register, or by written will (Sommerville 1985; see also *Bioethics News* 1987). 'Opting-out' laws, unlike 'opting-in' laws, do not require doctors to obtain active consent before taking patients' organs, and, further, permit doctors to remove organs even when patients' families have refused consent. It is noteworthy that in 1988, Australia's then Federal Minister for Community Services and Health, Dr Neal Blewett, publicly supported a move towards the introduction of 'opting out' laws in this country (McCauley 1988; see also *Bioethics News*

1988). The debate on this issue is continuing, led by the Australian Health Ethics Committee (AHEC) and the National Health and Medical Research Council (NH & MRC) (Carter 1993, pp. 29–31).

For all the medical, legal, political and media support of the organ transplant movement, the general community remains quietly uneasy about it. While it is conceded that the community does not vociferously oppose the transplant movement, neither does it vociferously support it; for example, there is in the community a general reluctance formally to consent to become donors. Caplan (1983), for example, writes that many people in the United States ignore the National Kidney Foundation's massive publicity campaign aimed at educating the public to become donors. Citing a 1983 Gallup poll surveying the attitudes of Americans toward kidney donations, Caplan further writes that, of the 1500 men and women over the age of 18 surveyed, only 18 per cent had in fact signed donor cards. Hazinski (1987) cites more recent studies which indicate that only '10–20% of suitable patients serve as organ donors following declaration of brain death' (p. 354). The situation in Australia is very similar. A 1989 survey of 1400 people from all Australian State capitals found, for example, that, of those surveyed, 98 per cent were aware of organ donation, and 71 per cent supported organ donation in principle. Yet, only 26 per cent of those surveyed had discussed organ transplantation with their families (*Austopics* 1989, p. 1). More recent estimates show that, despite a 70 per cent acceptance rate of organ donation among the public, only about 45 per cent of drivers have indicated their consent to organ donation on their driver's licence application (Carter 1993, p. 29); it has also been estimated that between 55 per cent and 60 per cent of relatives refuse consent to organ donation when approached to approve organ retrieval (Carter 1993, p. 29). The community's unease here is also shared by some doctors and nurses (examples are given shortly).

Infrequently told but nevertheless unforgettable stories remind us that the organ transplant movement is not as altruistic or as beneficent and as caring as the general public may believe. For example, in August 1988, the world was alerted to a bizarre rumour from Central America which alleged that thousands of Honduran children had been sent to the United States 'to be used as organ donors for children from rich families' (Reuter 1988; Barrett 1988). This rumour surfaced following an alleged rescue of seven babies by Paraguayan police from kidnappers accused of trafficking babies for 'spare parts' (Barrett 1988). The United States Justice Department, the FBI, the Food and Drug Administration, the Department of Health and Human Resources and the immigration service all hotly denied the rumour.

Two years later, media reports alleged that Brazilian babies were 'being sold for organ-transplant rackets in Thailand and Mexico'

(Byrne 1990, p. 8). Two Italian judges who visited northern Brazil to investigate the (adoption) 'baby trade' between Italy and Brazil are reported to have confirmed that 'babies with physical deficiencies had been sold for their organs', and that an organ for transplantation could fetch as much as $42 000 (Byrne 1990, p. 8). The Brazilian Government is reported to have called an immediate investigation into the claims.

On 23 January 1989, the Australian television station, SBS, gave a news report on a Turkish television program in which it was alleged that Turkey's poor were being exploited by British surgeons, and were being asked to sell their kidneys to would-be recipients for up to £4000 each. A British physician interviewed admitted that rumours had been rife in the transplant community (to the effect that kidneys were being bought from third world countries, including the subcontinent of India), but that, until the Turkish television documentary, these had never been substantiated (see also Brahams 1989). One Turkish donor alleged that he had initially been offered £4000 for his kidney, but after he had donated it received only £1800. A week later, on 30 January 1989, SBS presented another report concerning organ transplants; this report featured a German businessman who was setting up a multi-million-dollar business in trading human organs. Meanwhile *Bioethics News* (1989a, p. 2) carried the report of a West German Count (describing himself as a 'specialist in legal loopholes') who had founded an organisation for the purpose of buying organs from bankrupts who were desperate to raise money to pay off their debts. His organisation, called 'Organ Donation and Human Replacement Association for Mutual Benefit', has been condemned by the West German government, but so far 'lawyers have been unable to find any way in which to stop or prosecute the Count' (*Bioethics News* 1989a, p. 2).

Other stories allege that accident victims have had their bodies desecrated by organ-retrieving physicians (dubbed by some as the modern-day 'body snatchers') even before the victim's family members have learned of their loss. One notable case, in Portugal, involved a married man by the name of Mario Meles who was killed on his way home to lunch (Jolliffe 1986). When his wife and children went to inspect his body in the local mortuary they found that his heart, both corneas and one kidney had been removed. They also found that instead of prosthetic devices being used to fill the empty eye sockets, Mr Meles' eyelids had simply been stitched together. The family is reported as saying that, had they been asked, they would not have consented to organ removal. In response to the family's reaction, one of the doctors responsible for transplanting Mr Meles' kidney, Professor Linhares Furtado, is reported to have 'poured scorn on the critics [of the Meles case], condemning them as "pseudo-sentimentalists" and "obscurantists" ' (Jolliffe 1986). The recipient of Mr Meles' kidney, meanwhile, expressed gratitude 'that her life had been extended' (Jolliffe 1986).

Australia has also experienced some notable problems in regard to unconsented organ retrieval. In one case, for example:

> the hearts of two boys killed in a car accident were removed for transplant then disposed of without the knowledge of the boys' parents.

> (Athersmith 1991, p. 1)

Understandably, the respective families involved were greatly distressed upon discovering sixteen months later what had happened to the boys' hearts. In another media report commenting on the case, a professor of forensic pathology was quoted as saying: 'The same situation would not occur today, but even if it did, it would be legal' (Backhouse 1991, p. 4).

It is not only the lay community that has an uneasy concern about the organ transplant movement. For example, in January 1985, Dr Paul Gerber, a Brisbane lawyer and a member of the clinical research ethics committee at the Royal Brisbane Hospital, was reported to have described the Queensland Government's decision to establish a liver transplant unit as 'irresponsible and utterly parochial' (Metherell 1985). He is also reported to have criticised liver transplant operations as 'experimental', 'horrendous' and 'bordering on obscenity' (Wragg 1985), and to have said that, for children receiving organs, anti-rejection drugs caused serious growth retardation to the point that '10-year-old survivors of the operation would look like 3-year-olds' (Metherell 1985). Dr Gerber's views were rejected by two Melbourne medical authorities, however. One of these authorities, Dr Mackay, is quoted as replying: 'I think that growth retardation could not be any more than you would get with kidney transplantation, which has not stopped us doing kidney transplants' (Metherell 1985).

In a provocative newspaper report entitled 'Doubting doctors ask a vital question of life or death', Donald Gould (1986) claims that a number of experienced British physicians have serious concerns about Britain's transplant program — concerns which are of a profoundly moral nature, and not merely sentimental.

Dr David Hill, for example, a consultant anaesthetist at Addenbrooke's Hospital, Cambridge, is reported as questioning the quality of the supposed informed consent that people give when signing organ donor cards. He points out that most people have a 'miserably inadequate' concept of themselves being 'cold and white and slightly stiff — laid out . . .' at the moment of organ removal, as opposed to the reality of being 'pink and perfused and [still] responsive to pain' (Gould 1986). Dr Hill's comments imply that if people knew the realities of organ removal they probably would not sign their cards.

Another medical specialist, Dr Phillip Keep, medical director of the intensive care unit at the Norfolk and Norwich Hospital, is reported as having a different set of concerns, most notably about the way in which a potential donor's relatives are dealt with. He is quoted as saying:

> You have to lie to them a bit. You say 'We're going to take the organs out when he's dead.' They really believe that, and I've never had the courage to tell them anything different, because I'm sure that if you actually told them what was going to happen you'd get no more donors.
>
> (Gould 1986, p. 6)

Commenting further on a family's wish to say 'goodbye properly', Dr Keep is quoted as saying:

> Then you have to say, 'Well — er — there are certain *technical* reasons why you're not going to be allowed to do that.' You mean the patient's going to be wheeled out with his [sic] heart beating and on a ventilator, and you have to take great steps to make sure they don't see this happening.
>
> (Gould 1986, p. 6)

Other medical specialists are reported to be strongly opposed to the use of 'beating heart' donors, on the grounds that the 'brain death' criteria and the tests used to establish these are 'inconclusive' and 'unreliable' (Gould 1986; Chipman 1988; Coulter 1987). The implications are that there can never be any certainty that a person being used as an organ donor is in fact *dead* at the time of organ removal. For example, one controversial opponent of transplant surgery, Dr David Wainwright Evans (a recently retired consultant cardiologist at Papworth Hospital, Cambridge), is reported as arguing:

> However reliable the 'brain-stem death' criteria are for forecasting the patient is going to die, they do not suffice for the diagnosis and certification of death itself.
>
> I would go on treating a patient in that state as a human being deserving of our every care and consideration — I could not regard him [sic] as a corpse with a beating heart.
>
> (Chipman 1988, p. 11)

Interestingly, medical specialists in Australia appear not to share the concerns of their British colleagues, and are reported as having 'no doubts' about Australia's transplant program (McIntosh 1986).

They deny that any 'organ snatching' is going on, and insist that, unlike their British counterparts, transplant surgeons in Australia are 'not calling the shots' (McIntosh 1986). Whatever the truth value of these specialists' claims, the reality is that Australia's transplant program is just as plagued by moral problems as are other transplant programs around the world. And of particular concern to the nursing profession is the further reality that Australia's transplant program has created yet another set of moral burdens for nurses, as is shown shortly. It remains the task here to explain the nature of the organ transplant debate and show why the issue of organ transplantation generates moral controversy.

Blood and organ donorship — a historical overview

Organ, blood and bodily donation and sacrifices are as old as human history itself. The ancient Aztecs, for example, used to make blood sacrifices to the sun god Tezcatlipoca. Priests performing the sacrifices would open the breast of the chosen victim and tear out the beating heart, which was immediately offered to the sun god (*New Larousse encyclopedia of mythology* 1968, p. 437). The ancient Celts also used to perform human sacrifices. Archaeological evidence suggests that they frequently offered human heads to their gods in an attempt to propitiate them (*New Larousse encyclopedia of mythology* 1968, pp. 236–8). There are many other examples of ancient human sacrificing, and their objectives were almost universal: to appease the gods and thereby secure health and prosperity for the people.

Organ donorship and transplantation as we know it today has a relatively short history, and has only become possible in the twentieth century owing to the development of techniques for suturing blood vessels together and the development of anti-rejection drugs (Howard and Najarian 1978). Organ transplants were first performed in animals, but it was not until the early 1950s that transplants were performed in humans. Early kidney transplants failed because of rejection. Success, however, eventually came in a transplant between identical twins, and then improved with the advent of anti-rejection drugs (Howard and Najarian 1978). Heart transplants in humans did not become a reality until 1967, when Dr Christiaan Barnard, a relatively unknown South African surgeon, performed the world's first human heart allotransplant. Four years earlier a doctor had attempted a xenograft using a chimpanzee's heart. This failed, however, and the patient died. Following Dr Barnard's achievements, many surgeons around the world transplanted other organs, for example, lungs, livers, pancreases and, more recently, fetal tissue — including brain tissue (Howard and Najarian 1978; Christopherson 1982; Mandel 1985).

The modern history of organ donation has not been free of controversy, however. Animal liberationists have decried the use of animal parts in the treatment of humans as 'speciesist' and morally indefensible. Egalitarians have condemned the exploitation of the poor, and have publicly declared their suspicion of the world's highly organised publicity machine, which generates not only organ supplies but huge profits for those in the business (Reed 1985). Humanitarians, meanwhile, stand shuddering on the sidelines, well aware of the fact that, if any organ is to be of use for transplant purposes, it 'has to be plucked from the body of the donor while blood is still coursing through the arteries and veins' (Gould 1986).

Proponents of the transplant movement predictably reject such criticisms. Central to their defence is that organ retrieval and transplantation is only ever done under the strictest conditions (McCormick 1978) and that brain-death criteria, if properly applied, are completely reliable (Youngner et al. 1989; Olick 1991). For example, stringent legal laws limit what a person can consent to, and do not permit consent 'to the infliction of death' (such as would occur if patients consented to the removal of their vital organs), or to any other act that would 'seriously incapacitate the donor', as in the case of live donors consenting to the removal of both eyes for cornea transplants or both kidneys (Dukeminier 1978). Another stringent requirement is that the donor (in the case of live donors) or the donor's advocate (in the case of 'brain dead' donors) must give a voluntary, informed and uncoerced consent to the removal of an organ or tissue (a requirement which, against this reassurance, is beginning to be seriously eroded by the opting-out or contract-ing-out laws that are being increasingly adopted around the world). Further to this, in the case of 'dead' cadavers, brain death or 'neurological' death must be conclusively established. Another stringent requirement is that transplantation should be under-taken only where there is 'a reasonable hope of clinical success and with an acceptable therapeutic goal' (McCormick 1978, p. 1172) — a requirement which is also beginning to be seriously eroded as demands for experimental medicine increase. Lastly, the patient–recipient, where possible, is required to be fully informed of the consequences of transplantation. (Whether in fact this happens is another matter.)

Superficially these requirements seem to offer a satisfactory response to many of the moral concerns raised by those opposed to transplantation. On a deeper level, however, they are utterly inadequate, as the remainder of this discussion shows.

Law, medicine and defining death

Legal law aims to protect a potential donor from consenting to an 'infliction of death'. While this may seem a just and defensible provision, its integrity is somewhat weakened when it is considered that the law's (not to mention the medical profession's) conception and definition of death are at significant odds with the lay community's conception and definition of it (Bernat et al. 1982, p. 6). Whereas lay persons typically regard *the permanent cessation of heart and lung function* as determining death, the law and the medical profession regard *the permanent cessation of brain function* ('brain death' or 'neurological death') as determining death. Just which of these two conceptions of death is 'correct' is a question that has sparked enormous philosophical debate. In order to understand why this debate has emerged, it is necessary to examine some of the factors that led to a redefinition of death in the first place.

The concept of 'brain death' first emerged in France in 1959, when French neurologists described 'a condition of irreversible coma associated with irreversible loss of the capacity to breathe' (Lamb 1985, p. 4). The neurologists named this condition *coma dépassé*, literally 'a state beyond coma' and, as it was thought at the time, just before death (Black 1987, p. 368). The term never really caught on in the international medical community; it was not until 1968, after the release of the now internationally acclaimed *Report of the Ad Hoc Committee of the Harvard Medical School on a definition of irreversible coma*, that the term 'brain death' (synonymous with the French *coma dépassé*) achieved international recognition (Lamb 1985, p. 4). There is little doubt that acceptance of this new brain death definition was substantially motivated by a desire to escape the dilemmas posed by the costly prolongation of 'hopeless' life with artificial life-supporting technologies. By adopting the new brain death criteria and, what is more, by having it incorporated into law, doctors could now remove artificial life supports without risk of being accused either of homicide or of performing euthanasia — the presumption being, of course, that an already 'dead' person cannot be killed (Bernat et al. 1982; Pallis 1983, p. 36; Browne 1983, p. 29; Black 1987, p. 369; Moussa and Shannon 1992, p. 35). Some have suggested that both the formulation and the adoption of the Harvard criteria were substantially motivated by what has been termed the 'transplant interest' (Jonas 1982; Lamb 1985, p. 108; Moussa and Shannon 1992, p. 35). Jonas became particularly suspicious of this motivation after hearing Dr Henry K. Beecher, Chairman of the Harvard Committee and author of the Harvard Committee Report, pose the following question:

> Can society afford to discard the tissues and organs of the hopelessly unconscious patient when they could be used to restore the otherwise hopelessly ill, but still salvageable individual?

(Jonas 1982, p. 289)

Whatever the motivations behind this new conception and definition of death, a number of highly significant gains were to be made for the medical profession by doing so: first, the medical profession emerged as society's dominant cultural interpreters of death; second, by redefining death in terms different from those used by the popular lay culture, and by gaining legal support for this definition — gained also through the well established 'reasonable doctor' standard (Gervais 1986, p. 6; Lamb 1985, p. 75) — the medical profession was able to gain ultimate control of life and death in scientific health care contexts, and further was able firmly to cement that control politically, legally, professionally and socially (see also Olick 1991, p. 284). (The 'opting-out' laws cited earlier provide a compelling example of the kind of extraordinary power that a control over the definition of death has given some sections of the medical community.) A third gain for the medical profession was that death could now be used as a justification for a set of behaviours not previously considered justified, such as the removal of life supports and the retrieval of organs (Browne 1983, p. 29). Thus, yet again, the medical profession succeeded in translating an ethical problem into a technical problem to be solved by a clinical solution; that is, the *medical* judgment of death. Lastly, the new definition achieved the gradual erosion of the lay community's ability not only to define death, but also to accept it as a normal part of life. This has seen a trend towards an increasing over-reliance on doctors for a 'quick fix' of health and life, which, in turn, has further cemented the medical profession's hegemony in society. There were also considerable gains for the ideology of rationalism; the widespread acceptance of 'brain death' gave further support to the notion of mind–body dualism, not to mention the rationalistic account of personhood and moral entitlement.

Regardless of the medical profession's (and the law's) acceptance of this new definition of death, the question remains whether 'brain death' is a wholly satisfactory concept of human death (see also Black 1987; Olick 1991; Moussa and Shannon 1992). And even if it is satisfactory, is it substantial enough to provide justifications for removing life supports, retrieving organs, stopping active treatment, and similar actions?

Browne (1988, p. 35) argues that to say a person is dead is to say nothing more than that that person 'lacks a certain property', such as spontaneous heart beat, respiration, whole brain function, brain stem function, or neocortical function. Furthermore, it is not a statement of fact that a person with 'whole brain death' is *dead*; it is merely a statement that a *part* of that person is not functioning. While a person is being maintained on a ventilator, other processes vital to life are still occurring — blood is circulating, wastes are being eliminated, and so on. Neither have the social and cultural meanings of life stopped: human relationships do not stop because of mere unconsciousness or 'brain death'. Browne (1988) goes on to argue that, once we adopt this account of death, then the whole-brain-dead individual on a respirator emerges not as a case of 'simulated life, but of artificially supported life' (p. 37). He warns elsewhere that, once certain conceptions of death are used to justify certain behaviours, pronouncements of death are no longer judgments of *fact*, but rather of *value* (Browne 1983). Once we admit that, we need to be very careful in the judgments we do actually make.

Gervais (1986) discusses a number of other competing views, including the biological, moral and ontological/existential conceptions and definitions of death — none of which appears to share much common ground. The biological view, for example, sees death as fundamentally a biological issue, and rejects moral philosophy's intrusion as a confused attempt to bring in quality of life issues. The moral view, by contrast, asks the question: when is it morally justified to regard a person as dead? The underlying contention here is that death is a moral and social event, and thus not a matter which can be decided by mere biology (p. 105) — a view supported by Olick (1991, p. 277). The ontological view, on the other hand, simply asserts that the 'death of a person is that person's death' (p. 111).

About the only certain thing to emerge from this ongoing philosophical debate is that there is no philosophical certainty on what constitutes human death. Interestingly, the law also partially acknowledges this problem by defining death in two distinct terms, notably as being *either* irreversible cessation of circulation of blood in the body of the person, *or* irreversible cessation of all function of the brain of the person (see also Staunton and Whyburn 1993, pp. 243–67; Wallace 1991, pp. 327–8; Olick 1991).

The question which I think inevitably arises here is not which definition should be chosen, but upon what basis should either be chosen? If we can find an answer, we will all be a step closer to understanding the real motivation and the intentions behind redefining the traditional conception of death. Either way, it is unlikely that a given definition of death will yield a satisfactory solution to the ethical disagreements at hand; at best, to borrow from Clarke and Clarke (1977), it will merely shift the focus of the original ethical disagreement.

Donor consent

Another area in which the restrictions governing organ donations are grossly inadequate is in the area of consent. By all accounts, consent procedures are just as lacking in the case of organ removal as they are in the case of medical treatment generally. Live donors contemplating signing a donor card are not fully informed of the consequences of their decision, nor are families of potential donor cadavers given all the relevant information necessary for making an informed consent to organ donation. As we have already seen from Dr Keep's comments cited earlier, relatives are deceived and manipulated into giving consent. Let us explore these claims further.

Consider the common donor card. A good example is shown in figure 12.2, which reproduces one of the donor cards issued by the Health Department Victoria. This critically important card carries the photograph of a small child, with the caption: 'He's just got the best present of his life. Organ donation . . . The gift of a lifetime.' On the same side are the words:

> With the wish that I may help others by an anatomical gift, I consent to the removal from my body after my death of
>
> * kidneys
> * eyes
> * heart
> * any needed tissue
>
> to be used for
>
> * transplant to the body of a living person
> * other therapeutic, medical, or scientific purposes.

Then, in small print, are written the words: 'Note: Cross out items NOT included in gift (if any) and sign the reverse side'. In the remaining space is a small adhesive red sticker which may be placed on the back of a driver's licence. The would-be donor is then invited to sign the card in the presence of a witness, to tear off the relevant part of the card, and to 'inform your family of your wish to be a donor to ensure their co-operation'. The card concludes by advising that those at risk of having AIDS 'can not identify themselves as organ donors'.

While the card advises that the Health Department Victoria can be contacted for further information, it does not supply a phone number or the name of any person who can be contacted. No other information which might otherwise be considered 'material' to an informed and valid consent is given. For example, no mention is made that before the organs are removed, the donor has to be stabilised, and that this also involves the withholding of drugs (including anaesthetic or pain suppressing drugs) (Wiberg et al. 1986, p. 942). It is pertinent to note here the comments of one nurse who alleged that a cadaver's blood pressure 'rocketed' when the operating surgeon performed his initial surgical incision in a kidney removal operation. She believed this rise in blood pressure indicated that the cadaver was still sensitive to pain and thus was not 'dead'. While some might be quick to dismiss this nurse's claim as 'transplant hysteria' or 'mistaken observation' or 'technical fault involving monitoring equipment', or the like, there is nevertheless a possibility of this happening, particularly if the brain death criteria have not been applied properly or the diagnosing doctors have not had sufficient experience in diagnosing 'brain death' (Black 1987).

The attitude expressed on the card towards a potential donor's family is also highly questionable, and carries overtones of classical objectivism (discussed in chapters 3, 4 and 5) and its rejection of

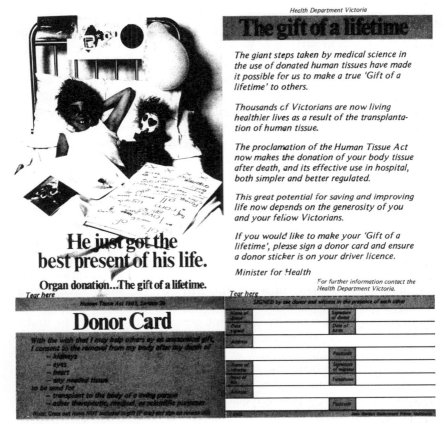

Figure 12.2   Organ donor card from the State of Victoria.
(Reproduced courtesy of the Health Department Victoria)

context and *the particular* (i.e. family relationships and the obligations, feelings, and sentiments incurred therein). It will be noted,
for example, that the card instructs a potential donor to

'*inform* your family of your wish to be a donor to *ensure their
cooperation*' (italics added), rather than to '*discuss* with your family
your wish to be a donor to *seek their support*'. The reason for this
tone of approach is fairly obvious — it will help to reduce the
likelihood of potential donors being persuaded by their families to
change their minds. Once a potential donor has consented via a
donor card to be a donor cadaver, a doctor can, legally speaking, go
ahead and remove the organs. On this, the National Health and
Medical Research Council states in its 1982 *Code of practice for
transplantation of cadaveric organs*:

> If it is known at the death of the patient, without having to ask
> relatives, that the deceased had consented to act as a donor (for
> example, if a patient carries a signed donor card or has otherwise
> recorded his wish to be considered an organ donor) there is no
> legal requirement in any State or Territory to establish lack of
> objection on the part of relatives.

> (National Health and Medical Research Council 1982, 4.1)

In the case of a donor who has no next-of-kin, 'the Designated
Officer may authorise donation, provided the donor has not
expressed an objection' (d'Apice 1984).

Another disturbing feature of the card is the imagery and
language it uses: a small, vulnerable child, and emotive terms such
as 'make a true "Gift of a lifetime" to others', and 'saving and
improving life now depends on the generosity of you and your fellow
Victorians'. Since morality does not generally require us to make
large personal sacrifices on behalf of others, it cannot be claimed
that this language is merely reminding us of our moral duties
toward our fellow humans. It seems, then, that the language used
is deliberately manipulative. In the light of my comments so far, I
would argue that, whatever else the donor card is, it is not the
basis of an informed and valid consent. It might be argued here:
'Well, what does it matter? After all, the patient is dead!' However,
such a response is hardly reassuring, since the question of death is
precisely what is at issue in this debate. Even if *death* is conceded,
there remains the complex question of what kind of respect is due
to a corpse. For example, is it really right to use a corpse as a
source of 'spare parts'? Is it really fair to subordinate deeply
ingrained cultural and social traditions to the demands of science
and scientific medicine? Why should the tragedies of potential
organ recipients be regarded as being any more worthy of attention

than the tragedies of others who are also suffering irreversible (but not so glamorous) disease states? And so on.

Practices for obtaining consent from a potential donor's next-of-kin are also less than adequate, and are morally questionable. Anecdotal evidence suggests, for example, that consent seekers sometimes embark on a campaign of deceit in order to obtain the permission they require for organ retrieval. It is certainly open to question whether those being approached for consent are fully informed about what they are consenting to — for example, the procedures detailed below.

Once brain death has been diagnosed, and consent for organ retrieval received, every effort is made to stabilise patients before they are taken to theatre for organ removal. The stabilisation process generally entails maintaining circulation and ventilation, maintaining fluid and electrolyte balance (aiming for a regular urine output of 50 mL per hour and no abnormalities), keeping the systolic blood pressure above 100 mmHg, and refraining from administering any medication (see also Wiberg et al. 1986; Hazinski 1987). As a point of interest, some nurses caring for these patients have informally alleged to me that, once rigorous stabilisation treatments are administered, the donor's neurological status some-times improves, raising doubts in their minds about whether the patient is, in fact, brain dead. When patients are stabilised, they are then transferred to theatre, and the designated organs (for example, kidneys, lungs, pancreas, eyes, heart) removed. The organ removal operation, as described by Wiberg et al. (1986), generally takes the following form:

> The surgical team prepares the operative site by scrubbing the chest and the anterior abdominal wall, and draping the patient. *Inhalation or intravenous anesthesia is not required because the patient is brain dead* [italics added]. A muscle relaxant (pancuronium bromide injection [Pavulon]) is sometimes necessary to ease occasional abdominal spasms. The surgeon makes a long midline incision from the sternal notch to the pubic bone and the organs are removed in the order agreed upon by the procurement teams . . . A sternal saw or Lebsche knife is needed to divide the sternum in the midline. A retractor is inserted into the chest so the team can view the heart.
>
> (Wiberg 1986, p. 942*)

---

*Reprinted with permission from *AORN Journal* 44, p. 942, December 1986. Copyright © AORN Inc, 1017C East Mississippi Avenue, Denver, Colorado 80231, USA.

Once the other surgical team members have exposed but not excised 'their organs', the cardiac surgeon removes the heart, which is done by cross-clamping the major blood vessels leading to the heart and, after cutting through these vessels, retrieving it from the chest cavity (Wiberg et al. 1986). Skin and bones (including ribs, clavicles, parts of the pelvic bone, and long bones) may also be procured during the procedure.

It can be understood that some doctors would prefer to keep this kind of information secret, particularly if knowledge of it might cause consent to be withheld. This, however, is not in itself a moral justification for withholding the information. If a family does not wish their mother or father or brother or sister to be offered as a 'gift of life', then health professionals are bound to respect that wish. It is unfortunate that someone else may be deprived of a kidney or a heart or a pancreas, but so too is it unfortunate that the potential donor has lost the capacity to function fully as a human being. There is nothing to suggest that the potential donor's tragedy ought to be turned into a benefit for a stranger.

Acceptable therapeutic goals

A final concern about the adequacy of transplant restrictions pertains to the demand that transplantation should only be undertaken when there is a reasonable hope of clinical success and an acceptable therapeutic goal.

One obvious question to be raised about this restriction is: what is to count as a 'reasonable hope of clinical success' and an 'acceptable therapeutic goal'? The next obvious question is: by what standards can *reasonable* be judged and to whom is it *acceptable*? It takes little imagination to realise that what one person might consider 'reasonable' or 'acceptable' another might reject, and vice versa. For example, Dr Bailey, a heart transplant surgeon, considered it medically acceptable and reasonable to implant a baboon's heart into a 12-day-old baby girl. He is reported as arguing in defence of the procedure that the risk of rejection could be reduced in the newborn, since 'a newborn is a gracious host' (Wallis 1984). Bailey's views were not, however, widely shared by members of the medical or the lay communities (Prentice 1985). Baby Fae, as she came to be known, died 21 days after the transplant from the complications of tissue rejection (Capron 1985).

Dr Jack Copeland, who led the team that performed four heart transplants (three of them within 48 hours) on the same patient, also believed that his actions — and those of his operating team — were medically reasonable and acceptable. He also thought it reasonable and acceptable to use an unauthorised artificial heart in the process of trying to 'save the life' of Thomas Creighton, the first person ever to have been the subject of such 'desperate' medical measures (Reed 1985). Dr Copeland was criticised for his actions — but not on account of his transplanting four hearts into the same person over a matter of a few days, and thereby subjecting that person to an undignified death; rather, he was criticised because he had used an *unauthorised* artificial heart.

In 1992, surgeons at the University of Pittsburgh who transplanted a baboon's heart into a man dying of hepatitis B also believed their actions to be reasonable and acceptable (Altman 1992, p. 1). Further, their actions were approved by the human experiment ethics committee at the university where the organ transplantation program was based. The transplant specialist, Dr Thomas Starzl, is reported to have been severely criticised by animal-rights activists, who argued that 'animals are not spare parts' and that 'one species [should not be sacrificed] for another' (AP, New York Times, 1992, p. 7).

Admittedly these are extreme examples, but they are modern examples nevertheless. And they are enough to warn us about the inadequacy of parochial definitions of 'reasonable' and 'acceptable', and about parochial standards of conduct.

Organ transplantation and its implications for nurses

As with most bioethical issues, the nursing perspective on organ transplantation has been all but totally ignored. So much so that, in 1987, nurses in the Australian State of Victoria were not even informed, let alone invited to speak on, a proposed amendment to the Victorian Human Tissue Bill which would effectively allow nurses to be authorised to enucleate the eyes of cadavers in a bid to increase the numbers of corneas retrieved for transplanting. The Australian Nursing Federation (Victorian Branch) discovered the amendment 'quite by accident'. Upon investigating the matter further, the ANF found that in fact 'none of the bodies representing nurses had been notified much less consulted' — neither the Victorian Nursing Council, the Director of Nursing of the Royal Victorian Eye and Ear Hospital, nor the Nursing Division of the Health Department had been notified of the proposed amendment (*Nurses' Action*, April 1987, p. 3).

What is often not appreciated is that nurses are fundamentally involved in transplantation work. They care for and 'stabilise' the donor-patients, assist in operating theatre (in both organ retrieval and transplantation work), and care for the patient-recipients after transplantation. They also care for grieving and bereaved relatives, and must sometimes deal with the conspiracy of deceit aimed at securing consent for organ donation (see also Hazinski 1987).

Not all nurses favour being involved in transplant work, however, and in one reported case some have even conscientiously refused to be involved (Miller 1988; see also Wiberg et al. 1986,

p. 943). Significantly, the responses of these nurses were not supported, and they were allegedly told by a nursing supervisor that 'they could not avoid transplant "duties" because of severe staff shortages, regardless of their qualms' (Miller 1988). The nurses were also reported to have been denied conscientious objectors' status, and to have had their job security threatened. Thus, once again, the nursing perspective was trivialised and nurses were forced to bear intolerable moral and personal burdens.

Organ transplantation — issues and recommendations

I have not attempted here to raise and examine popular arguments for and against organ transplantation. Neither have I attempted to consider other controversial issues arising from the transplant movement — for example, the use of prisoners as cadavers after they have been executed as capital punishment for criminal offences; the cancer risks associated with long-term ingestion of anti-rejection drugs (Ewing 1993, p. 1); the use of anencephalic infants and fetuses as organ donors (*Bioethics News* 1989b, p. 5; Engelhardt 1989; Gillam 1989; Meinke 1989; Sanders and Moore 1991); and the possibility of 'special units' being set up to which 'brain dead' donors can be admitted for stabilisation and maintenance, thus taking the pressure off hospitals' already over-stretched intensive care units. Nor have I tried to defend a particular concept or definition of death. These are tasks which require a book of their own. Instead, I have tried to show that organ transplantation is not a morally clear-cut issue, so there are no clear-cut grounds upon which nurses can be decently expected to assist with organ transplantation work or decently compelled to do so against their moral will. I have also tried to show that legal and medical definitions of death are not free of controversy, so that any decision which rests on them is open to question. The consider-ations raised, at the very least, lead to the conclusion that provisions must be made for permitting conscientious objection — as has, in fact, been provided for by legislation in the American State of New Jersey (Olick 1991); they may also dictate the more serious conclusion that 'beating heart' organ donation should perhaps be abandoned altogether.

Another important consideration which I have tried to draw out is that donors are not mere 'objects' or 'dead things', to be dis-carded at will, but are human beings — albeit impaired ones — who are still recognised as an integral part of an interdependent human group. Just because someone is 'brain dead', they do not cease to be someone's mother or brother or sister or father or friend. As cultural and social traditions show, relationships can continue long after a person is dead (or buried, for that matter). Science is very bold (and arrogant) to try to reduce the cultural and social complexities of the death experience to a matter of biology. The troubling reality is that it has partially succeeded in doing just that, as it has in launching yet another assault on holism and the ideals that holism espouses. Even more troubling, however, is that no one and nothing seems to be capable of stopping it.

As with the abortion and euthanasia issues, it is clear that organ transplantation has not received the attention it should have had in nursing domains. Unless the ethical–legal issues arising for nurse practitioners are identified and fully discussed, the nursing profession will again be quite unable to protect and prevent its members from suffering the intolerable burdens that will be imposed on them by morally controversial organ transplantation practices. Neither will the nursing profession be in a position to protect patients who might otherwise find themselves the victims of transplant zealots. Either way, the consequences promise to be dire. If unhappy consequences are to be avoided, clearly the nursing profession has a moral obligation to confront and effectively deal with the ethical–legal issues arising from organ transplantation, which are posing a serious threat to the integrity of holistic nursing philosophy.

An earlier version of the discussion on 'Quality of life' was included in a paper entitled: 'Ethical issues for the health professional when planning for rehabilitation of patients with advanced cancer', presented at the seminar: Rehabilitation in patients with advanced cancer — a contradiction in terms? *organised by the College of Nursing, Australia in conjunction with the Victoria Association of Hospice Care Programs, Melbourne, 17 October 1988. This segment has been revised for publication in this text.*

An earlier version of the discussion on 'Not for Resuscitation' (NFR) orders was originally presented under the title: 'The nature and moral implications of "Not For Resuscitation [NFR]" orders' at the Nursing law and ethics, First Victorian State Conference. Theme: 'Matters of life and death', *Monash University, Melbourne, 30 September 1988 (organised by the School of Nursing, Phillip Institute of Technology). The paper has been revised for publication in this text.*

References

For the reader's convenience, the references are arranged under the subject headings 'Quality of life', 'Not for Resuscitation (NFR) orders', 'Further reading on NFR', and 'Organ transplantation'.

Quality of life

Downie, R. S. and Calman, K. C. (1987). *Healthy respect: ethics in health care.* Faber & Faber, London.

Foltz, A. T. (1987). The influence of cancer on self-concept and life quality. *Seminars in Oncology Nursing* 3 (4), November, pp. 303–12.

Fredette, S. LaFortune and Beattie, H. M. (1986). Living with cancer: a patient education program. *Cancer Nursing* 9 (6), pp. 308–16.

Germino, B. B. (1987). Symptom distress and quality of life. *Seminars in Oncology Nursing* 3 (4), November, pp. 299–302.

Graham, K. Y. and Longman, A. J. (1987). Quality of life and persons with melanoma. *Cancer Nursing* 10 (6), December, pp. 338–46.

Kanitsaki, O. (1988). Cancer and informed consent: a cultural perspective. Paper presented at Seminar on Controversial Ethical Issues in Patients with Cancer, Heidelberg Repatriation General Hospital, 13 October 1988, Melbourne.

Kuhse, H. (1987). *The sanctity-of-life doctrine in medicine: a critique*. Clarendon Press, Oxford.

Reich, W. T. (1978). Quality of life. In W. T. Reich (ed.), *Encyclopedia of bioethics*, The Free Press, New York, pp. 829–39.

Welch-McCaffrey, D. (1985). Cancer, anxiety, and quality of life. *Cancer Nursing* 8 (3), June, pp. 151–8.

Not For Resuscitation (NFR) orders

Adams, M. (1984). On life . . . and death . . . and dots. *Nursing 84* 14 (6), June, pp. 53–8.

Bandman, E. and Bandman, B. (1985). *Nursing ethics in the life span*. Appleton-Century-Crofts, Norwalk, Connecticut.

Bioethics News (1992). 'Not for resuscitation' orders — Britain. 12 (1), October, p. 4.

Buchanan, F. (1983). Resuscitation procedures. Letter to the Editor, *Nursing Times* 79 (34), p. 7.

Carson, R. (1982). Commentary. *Hastings Center Report* 12 (5), October, p. 28.

Clinical Ethics Committee, Council of Physicians and Dentists (1984). *Use of life support systems: ethical guidelines relating to use of life support systems*. Royal Victoria Hospital, Montreal, Quebec.

Council on Ethical and Judicial Affairs, American Medical Association (1991). Guidelines for the appropriate use of Do-Not-Resuscitate orders. *Journal of the American Medical Association* 265 (14), pp. 1868–71.

Cushing, M. (1981). No code orders: current developments and the nursing director's role. *Journal of Nursing Administration* 11 (26), April, pp. 22–9.

Dolan, M. B. (1988). Coding abuses hurt nurses, too. *Nursing 88* 18 (12), December, p. 47.

Fader, A. M., Gambert, S. R., Nash, M., Gupta, K. L. and Escher, J. (1989). Implementing a 'Do-Not-Resuscitate' (DNR) policy in a nursing home. *Journal of the American Geriatrics Society* 37 (6), pp. 544–6.

Haines, I. E., Zalcberg, J. and Buchanan, J. D. (1990). Not-for-resuscitation orders in cancer patients — principles of decision-making. *Medical Journal of Australia* 153 (4), pp. 225–9.

Hastings Center (1982). Does 'doing everything' include CPR? *Hastings Center Report* 12 (5), October, pp. 27–8.

Hickie, J. B. (1990). Guidelines for the decision making process for treatment with cardiopulmonary resuscitation. *Reflections* (an occasional publication of the Bioethics Committee of St Vincent's Hospital, University Campus, Sydney), November, p. 1.

Honan, S., Helseth, C., Bakke, J., Karpiuk, K., Krsnak, G. and Torkelson, R. (1991). Perception of 'No Code' and the role of the nurse. *Journal of Continuing Education in Nursing* 22 (2), pp. 54–61.

Humphry, D. and Wickett, A. (1986). *The right to die: understanding euthanasia*. Collins/Harper & Row, Sydney.

Johnstone, M.-J. (1988). A critical bioethical issue. *Australian Nurses Journal* 8 (1), July, p. 8.

Johnstone, M.-J. (1994). *Nursing and the injustices of the law.* W. B. Saunders/Baillière Tindall, Sydney.

Kuhse, H. (1987). *The sanctity-of-life doctrine in medicine: a critique.* Clarendon Press, Oxford.

Kellmer, D. (1986). No code orders: guidelines for policy. *Nursing Outlook* 34 (4), July/August, pp. 179–83.

Lipton, H. L. (1989). Physicians' Do-Not-Resuscitate decisions and documentation in a community hospital. *Quarterly Review Bulletin*, April, pp. 108–13.

Lo, B. (1991). Unanswered questions about DNR orders. *Journal of the American Medical Association* 265 (14), pp. 1874–5.

Lo, B., McLeod, G. A. and Saika, G. (1986). Patient attitudes to discussing life-sustaining treatment. *Archives of Internal Medicine* 146, pp. 1613–15.

Loewy, E. H. (1991). Involving patients in Do Not Resuscitate (DNR) decisions: an old issue raising its ugly head. *Journal of Medical Ethics* 17 (1), pp. 156–60.

New South Wales Health Department (1993). *Dying with dignity: interim guidelines on management.* NSW Health Department, Sydney.

Nursing Times (1983). RCN slams 'life and death' choice. 79 (24), p. 20.

Parliament of Victoria, Legislative Council, 50th Parliament, 2nd Session (1988). *Parliamentary Debates (Hansards)* 6 (3, 4, 5 & 6), May. See in particular the debate on the Medical Treatment Bill (no 2), 3 May 1988, pp. 1012–44.

Parliament of Victoria, Social Development Committee (1987). *Inquiry into options for dying with dignity: second and final report,* April. Government Printer, Melbourne.

Perry, S. W., Schwart, H. I. and Amchin, J. (1986). Determining resuscitation status: a survey of medical professionals. *General Hospital Psychiatry* 8, pp. 198–202.

Regan, K. M. (1983). Life at all costs? Letter to the Editor, *Nursing Times* 79 (26), p. 6.

Sage, W. M., Hurst, C. R., Silverman, J. F. and Bortz, W. M. (1987). Intensive care for the elderly: outcome of elective and nonelective admissions. *Journal of the American Geriatrics Society* 35 (4), April, pp. 312–18.

Saunders, J. M. and Valente, S. M. (1986). The question that won't go away. *Nursing 86* 16 (3), pp. 61–4.

Schade, S. G. and Muslin, H. (1989). Do not resuscitate decisions: discussions with patients. *Journal of Medical Ethics* 15 (4), pp. 186–90.

Scofield, G. R. (1991). Is consent useful when resuscitation isn't? *Hastings Center Report* 21 (6), pp. 28–36.

Siegler, M. (1982). Commentary. *Hastings Center Report* 12 (5), October, pp. 28–9.

Stanley, D. P. and Reid, D. P. (1989). Withholding cardiopulmonary resuscitation: one hospital's policy. *Medical Journal of Australia* 151, 4 September, pp. 257–62.

Stewart, K. and Rai, G. (1989). A matter of life and death. *Nursing Times* 85 (35), pp. 27–9.

The Regan Report on Hospital Law (1985). Institution — 'no CPR policy': Constitutional Issue 25 (12) May, p. 1.

Thom, A. (1988). Who decides? *Nursing Times* 85 (2), pp. 35–7.

Tomlinson, R. and Brody, H. (1990). Futility and the ethics of resuscitation. *Journal of the American Medical Association* 264 (10), 12 September, pp. 1276–80.

Veatch, R. (1977). *Death, dying, and the boiological revolution.* Yale University Press, New Haven.

Victorian Hospital Association Report (1988). 'Stickers recommended', 42, August–September, p. 3.

Victorian Nursing Council (1988). Resuscitation by the nurse. *Position Statements*, Victorian Nursing Council, Melbourne.

Yarling, R. and McElmurry, B. (1986). Rethinking the nurse's role in 'Do Not Resuscitate' orders: a clinical policy proposal in nursing ethics. In P. Chinn (ed.), *Ethical issues in nursing*, Aspen Systems, Rockville, Maryland, pp. 123–34.

Further reading on NFR

Annas, G. (1982a). CPR: the beat goes on. *Hastings Center Report* 12 (4), August, pp. 24–5.

Annas, G. (1982b). CPR: when the beat should stop. *Hastings Center Report* 12 (5), October, pp. 30–1.

Cowles, K. (1984). Definitions of life and death continue to elude us. *Nursing Outlook* 32 (3), May/June, pp. 169–72.

Curtin, L. (1979). CPR policies: the art of the possible — optimal care vs maximal treatment. *Supervisor Nurse* 10, August, pp. 16–18.

Freeman, J. and McDonnell, K. (1987). *Tough decisions: a casebook in medical ethics.* Oxford University Press, New York.

Kroeger Mappes, E. (1985). Ethical dilemmas for nurses: physicians' orders versus patients' rights. *Bioethics Reporter* 6/7, pp. 408–13.

Pellegrino, E. (1985). Moral choice, the good of the patient, and the patient's good. In J. Moskop and L. Kopelman (eds), *Ethics and critical care medicine*, D. Reidel, Dordrecht, pp. 117–38.

Rabkin, M. T., Gillerman, G. and Rice, N. R. (1979). CPR policies: the art of the possible — orders not to resuscitate. *Supervisor Nurse* 10, August, pp. 26, 29–30.

Rachels, J. (1986). *The end of life: euthanasia and morality.* Oxford University Press, Oxford.

Organ transplantation

Altman, L. (1992). Liver of a baboon transplanted into dying man. *The Age*, 30 June, p. 1.

Athersmith, F. (1989). 'Heart transplant boy fine thanks, and ready for a chat', *The Age*, 27 January, p. 3.

Athersmith, F. (1991). Coroner to investigate heart use. *The Age*, 1 February, p. 1.

AP, New York Times (1992). Doctor defends transplant. *The Age*, 2 July, p. 7.

Austopics (1989). A gift of life. July, pp. 1–2. (*Austopics* is a publication of Austin Hospital, Heidelberg, Victoria.)

Backhouse, M. (1991). Law allows removal of heart: pathology chief. *The Age*, 2 February, p. 4.

Barrett, G. (1988). The phantom baby trade. *The Age*, 19 August, p. 13.

Bernat, J. L., Culver, C. M. and Gert, B. (1982). Defining death in theory and practice. *Hastings Center Report* 12 (1), February, pp. 5–9.

Bioethics News (1987). Organ transplants in Belgium — a policy of opting out. 6 (4), July, p. 9.

Bioethics News (1988). New laws on organ donations? 8 (1), pp. 6–7.

Bioethics News (1989a). Pay your debts with a kidney. 8 (2), p. 2.

Bioethics News (1989b). Working party on organ transplantation in neonates. 8 (1), p. 5.

Bioethics News (1989c). Sale of human kidneys. 8 (4), p. 8.

Black, P. McLaren (1987). Clinical problems in the use of brain-death standards. In D. H. Cowan, J. A. Kantorowitz, J. Moskowitz and P. Rheinstein (eds), *Human organ transplantation: societal, medical–legal, regulatory, and reimbursement issues*, Health Administration Press, Ann Arbor, Michigan, pp. 367–73.

Bock, A. (1990). Boy, 6, is Australia's youngest liver recipient. *The Age*, 28 August, p. 5.

Boreham, G. (1989). New cornea offers sight to a child. *The Age*, 14 February, p. 1.

Bout, T. (1989). Brave Paula — waiting in hope: a plea for donors. *Herald* (Melbourne), 9 March, p. 4.

Brahams, D. (1989). Kidney for sale by live donor. *Lancet* 1 (8632), 4 February, pp. 285–6.

Browne, A. (1983). Whole-brain death reconsidered. *Journal of Medical Ethics* 9, pp. 28–31.

Browne, A. (1988). Defining death. *Bioethics News* 7 (3), April, pp. 31–49.

Byrne, L. (1990). Brazil probes claim 'babies for organs'. *The Age*, 22 September, p. 8.

Caplan, A. L. (1983). Organ transplants: the costs of success. *Hastings Center Report* 13 (6), December, pp. 23–32.

Capron, A. M. (1985). When well-meaning science goes too far. *Hastings Center Report* 15 (1), February, pp. 8–9.

Carter, H. (1988). 'We're happy he gave four lives' — donor boy's special gift. *The Sun* (Melbourne), 16 December, p. 1.

Carter, M. (1993). Organ donation. *Health issues* 34, March, pp. 29–31.

Chipman, L. (1988). A tale from the other side. *The Age*, 21 October, p. 11.

Christopherson, L. K. (1982). To mend the heart: ethics of high technology. Heart transplants. *Hastings Center Report* 12 (1), February, pp. 18–21.

Clarke, D. D. and Clarke, D. M. (1977). Definitions and ethical decisions. *Journal of Medical Ethics* 3, pp. 186–8.

Coulter, D. L. (1987). Neurological uncertainty in newborn intensive care. *New England Journal of Medicine* 316 (14), 2 April, pp. 840–4.

d'Apice, T. (1984). The law and cadaveric organ donation. *Organ-Tissue Transplantation Resource Kit, no 2*, Centre for Human Bioethics, Monash University, Melbourne.

Dukeminier, J. (1978). Organ donation: legal aspects. In W. T. Reich (ed.), *Encyclopedia of bioethics*, The Free Press, New York, pp. 1157–9.

Engelhardt, H. Tristram (ed.) (1989). *Harvesting cells, tissues, and organs from fetuses and anencephalic newborns. Journal of Medicine and Philosophy* 14 (1) (special issue).

Ewing, T. (1993). Cancer awaits transplant patients, says scientist. *The Age*, 7 October, p. 1.

Gervais, K. G. (1986). *Redefining death.* Yale University Press, New Haven.

Gillam, L. (ed.) (1989). *Proceedings of the conference: The Fetus as Tissue Donor, Use or Abuse?* Centre for Human Bioethics, Monash University, Melbourne.

Gould, D. (1986). Doubting doctors ask a vital question of life or death. *The Age* (Saturday Extra), 30 August, p. 6.

Hazinski, M. F. (1987). Pediatric organ donation: responsibilities of the critical care nurse. *Pediatric Nursing* 13 (5), September–October, pp. 344–57.

Heath, S. (1991). Heart beats announce a life renewed. *The Age*, 9 March, p. 3.

Heath, S. (1992). A new liver means new life after 10 years of pain. *The Age*, 5 June, p. 3.

Howard, R. J. and Najarian, J. S. (1978). Organ transplantation: medical perspective. In W. T. Reich (ed.), *Encyclopedia of bioethics*, The Free Press, New York, pp. 1160–6.

Jolliffe, J. (1986). Transplant success prompts legal row. *The Age*, 29 March, p. 12.

Jonas, H. (1982). Against the stream: comments on the definition and redefinition of death. In T. L. Beauchamp and L. Walters (eds), *Contemporary issues in bioethics*, 2nd edn, Wadsworth, Belmont, California, pp. 288–93.

Lahey, J. (1988). A sporting chance for transplant patients. *The Age*, 18 November, p. 3.

Lamb, D. (1985). *Death, brain death and ethics*. Croom Helm, London.

Lee, S. (1989). The man behind our heart-transplant unit. *The Herald* (Melbourne), 17 January, p. 4.

Mandel, T. E. (1985). The use of immature pancreas as a source of tissue for transplantation in diabetes. *Bioethics News* 5 (1), October, pp. 14–22.

McCauley, C. (1988). Blewett hints at new laws on organ donations. *The Age*, 15 August.

McCormick, R. A. (1978). Organ transplantation: ethical principles. In W. T. Reich (ed.), *Encyclopedia of bioethics*, The Free Press, New York, pp. 1169–73.

McIntosh, P. (1986). No doubts in Australia. *The Age*, 30 August (Saturday Extra), p. 6.

Meinke, S. (1989). Anencephalic infants as potential organ sources: ethical and legal issues. *National Reference Center for Bioethics Literature: Scope Note 12*, Kennedy Institute of Ethics, Georgetown University, Washington DC.

Messina, A. (1988). Hospital expects first heart swap by Christmas. *The Age*, 27 September, p. 17.

Metherell, M. (1985). Risks of liver transplants too big: doctor. *The Age*, 3 January, p. 4.

Miller, C. (1988). Transplant row: nurses fear sack. *Herald* (Melbourne), 18 July, p. 1.

Moussa, M. and Shannon, T. (1992). The search for the new pineal gland: brain life and personhood. *Hastings Center Report* 22 (2), pp. 30–7.

National Health and Medical Research Council (1982). *Code of practice for transplantation of cadaveric organs*. NH & MRC, Woden, ACT.

New Larousse encyclopedia of mythology (1968). Hamlyn, London.

Nurses' Action (1987). Article entitled 'Human Tissue (Amendment) Bill', April, p. 3 (published by Australian Nursing Federation [Vic.], Melbourne).

Olick, R. (1991). Brain death, religious freedom, and public policy. New Jersey's landmark legislative initiative. *Kennedy Institute of Ethics Journal* 1 (4), pp. 275–92.

O'Neill, G. (1988). Somewhere, somebody dies, saving a man's life. *The Age*, 22 June, p. 4.

Pallis, C. (1983). Whole-brain death reconsidered — physiological facts and philosophy. *Journal of Medical Ethics* 9, pp. 32–7.

Pirrie, M. (1988a). The shy pioneer on the frontier of heart surgery. *The Age*, 24 September, p. 2.

Pirrie, M. (1988b). Medicine takes a quantum leap. *The Age*, 30 September, p. 11.

Pirrie, M. (1988c). Modern medicine's maker of miracles. *The Age*, 14 October, p. 11.

Pirrie, M. (1988d). Given a new heart, Michael is set to take on the world. *The Age*, 28 October, p. 1.

Pirrie, M. (1989a). State tries to hasten collection of organs. *The Age*, 15 February, p. 3.

Pirrie, M. (1989b). Department balked at donor-liver flight. *The Age*, 16 February, p. 5.

Pirrie, M. (1989c). Alfred prepares for heart–lung transplant. *The Age*, 28 February, p. 5.

Prentice T. (1985). Doctors divided over transplant pioneers. *Weekend Australian*, 30–31 March, p. 8.

Reddy, M. (1988). Schoolgirl, 11, undergoes liver transplant. *The Age*, 10 December, p. 4.

Reed, C. (1985). Debate over ethics is the legacy of the four-heart man. *The Age*, 20 March, p. 11.

Reuter (1988). Babies saved from sale of vital organs. *The Age*, 9 August, p. 7.

Robertson, I. F. (1984). Corneal transplantation in Victoria. In *Organ-tissue transplantation resource kit no 2*, Centre for Human Bioethics, Monash University, Melbourne.

Roper, the Hon. T. (1984). Organ donation in Victoria. In *Organ-tissue transplantation resource kit no 2*, Centre for Human Bioethics, Monash University, Melbourne.

Ryle, G. (1992). A deep breath of life with new lungs brings new hope. *The Age*, 23 December, p. 5.

Sanders, K. and Moore, B. (1991). *Proceedings of consensus development conference on anencephalics, infants and brain death treatment options and the issue of organ donation*. Law Reform Commission of Victoria, Australian Association of Paediatric Teaching Centre, and Royal Children's Hospital, Melbourne.

Scott, D. F. (1984). The need and benefits of organ donation. In *Organ-tissue transplantation resource kit no 2*, Centre for Human Bioethics, Monash University, Melbourne.

Sommerville, M. A. (1985). Access to organs for transplantation: overcoming 'rejection'. *Canadian Medical Association Journal* 132 (2), January, pp. 113–17.

Staunton, P. and Whyburn, B. (1993). *Nursing and the law*. 3rd edn, W. B. Saunders/Baillière Tindall, Sydney.

Svendsen, I. (1988). Medical success leaves patients waiting for suitable organs. *The Age*, 22 June, p. 4.

Wallace, M. (1991). *Health care and the law: a guide for nurses*. The Law Book Company, North Ryde, Sydney.

Wallis, C. (1984). Baby Fae stuns the world. *Time Magazine*, 12 November, pp. 56–8.

Wiberg, C. A., Prusak, B. F., Pollak, R. and Mozes, M. F. (1986). Multi-organ donor procurement. *ACRN Journal* 44 (6), December, pp. 936–43.

Wragg, T. (1985). To transplant or not: controversy goes on. *Weekend Herald* (Weekend Extra), 19–20 January.

Youngner, S., Landefeld, C., Coulton, C. Juknialis, B. and Leary, M. (1989). 'Brain death' and organ retrieval: a cross-sectional survey of knowledge and concepts among health professionals. *Journal of the American Medical Association* 261 (15), pp. 2205–10.

Chapter
13

Taking a stand

A TIME INVARIABLY COMES WHEN NURSES must take a stand on what they consider, after careful and critical reflection, to be morally important. Taking a stand can involve either individual or collective action. Individual action may involve a nurse refusing conscientiously to participate in a controversial medical procedure; reporting a troubling incident to a superior or some other authority (including an external statutory authority); seeking nomination on an institutional ethics committee; or, quite simply, speaking out in either a conference or workshop, or some other type of public forum. On rare occasions, a nurse might decide to 'blow the whistle' or approach the media. Collective action, on the other hand, may involve groups of nurses embarking on an organised lobbying campaign aimed at particular target groups. Or, as is becoming increasingly common around the world, it may involve all-out strike action.

Whatever action is taken, it is never free of moral risk. There are many examples of nurses having suffered both personally and professionally because they took a stand on what they deemed to be an important professional or moral issue. Nurses conscientiously refusing to participate in morally controversial medical procedures have lost their jobs or have been made to resign 'voluntarily'. Some of those undertaking strike action have likewise lost their jobs, and have even been threatened with deregistration and charges of criminal negligence for their actions. (Examples are given in the discussion on strike action in the second part of this chapter.)

Despite the associated hazards and risks, nurses have a moral obligation to take a stand on issues that pose a serious threat to their moral integrity. Otherwise, they risk silently condoning the very actions and situations they deplore, and even standing as accomplices to them. Moreover, by doing nothing, nurses might well allow morally deplorable actions and situations to continue unchecked, as happened in the cases of the cervical cancer experiment at Auckland's National Women's Hospital and the deep-sleep therapy (DST) tragedy at Chelmsford Private Hospital in Sydney (see chapter 1).

Where nurses participate knowingly in immoral or illegal acts, they are just as culpable as the primary instigators of the acts. Even when nurses act on the orders of a superior, they cannot escape culpability. Indeed, as the United Nations War Crimes Commission, set up to investigate Nazi war crimes, has made clear (as have a number of other military tribunals), 'the doctrine of the duty of absolute obedience to superior orders today stands largely discredited' (Lewy 1970, p. 119).

Curiously, there are some misconceptions about the options open to nurses for taking a stand, and even about whether it is right to take a stand at all. Some nurses even fear that some of the options open to them (such as conscientious objection, strike action, appealing to an institutional ethics committee, or lobbying) are incompatible with their broader professional obligations as nurses and are therefore 'unprofessional'. For some nurses this has caused enormous personal conflict, and has served more to exacerbate the moral problems they face in the workplace than to help resolve them.

This chapter attempts to clarify some of the confusion sur-rounding the options open to nurses for taking a stand, and to show that these options might not only be compatible with professional nursing obligations, but may even be prima facie pro-fessional nursing obligations in themselves. It is to discussing the options of conscientious objection, strike action, and institutional ethics committees that this chapter now turns.

Conscientious objection

Nurses have for years been 'conscientiously refusing' in private or informal ways. Their objections have sometimes gone beyond informal 'cafeteria' conversation and gained public attention — but only in extreme situations, such as when a nurse has been dismissed or denied employment, or has been threatened in some way. Those who have had the courage to formally voice their conscientious refusal to participate in certain medical procedures, or to carry out certain orders given by a superior, have sometimes done so at great personal and professional cost. In chapter 1, for example, we examined the case of Corinne Warthen, a registered nurse who was successfully dismissed from her employing hospital of eleven years for refusing to dialyse a terminally ill unconscious patient on conscientious grounds — i.e. that the procedure was causing him more harm (see also Johnstone 1988); and in chapter 9 we discussed the case of a New South Wales registered nurse who was allegedly denied employment as a midwife because of her conscientious objection to abortion and sterilisation. We also saw the case involving a group of Victorian registered nurses who were allegedly threatened with dismissal for their conscientious refusal to participate in organ transplantation work. And we saw the case of a registered nurse who 'voluntarily' resigned because she was conscientiously opposed to her employing hospital's unwritten policy on 'Not for Resuscitation' (NFR) orders. (Other examples not included in this text involve nurses who have been dismissed for refusing to assist with electroconvulsive therapy (ECT) or other involuntary psychiatric treatment, such as the forced administration of psychotropic drugs — see, for example, Beardshaw 1982; Parsons 1982; *Nursing Times*, 22 September 1982, p. 1573; Hicks 1982; *Nursing Times*, 20 October 1982, p. 1738; *Nursing Times*, 6 April 1983, p. 17; *Nursing Times*, 10 August 1983, p. 18; *Nursing Mirror*, 20 June 1984, p. 2; Vousden 1985; *Nursing Times*, 31 December 1986, p. 7; Crabbe 1988, p. 18.)

These and similar cases illustrate convincingly that the issue of conscientious objection among nurses is by no means trivial. Nevertheless, despite the threat it poses to the moral integrity of the nursing profession as a whole, the issue of conscientious objection remains poorly addressed in nursing domains, and there is a paucity of nursing literature and nursing research on the subject. Professional nursing position statements rely on ill-defined concepts of conscience, and on poorly stated or inadequate conditions under which conscientious objection can be reasonably and justly claimed. A further problem is that mechanisms for protecting nurses who claim objector status are either wholly lacking or grossly inadequate, making it virtually impossible for nurses to conscientiously refuse to participate in certain procedures without fear of censure or of being discriminated against in some other way. One unfortunate consequence of the nursing profession's neglect of this issue is that it makes it easier for policy makers, employers and others to dismiss the problem of conscientious objection among nurses as either a non-issue or at most only a trivial issue, and therefore one not warranting serious attention or concern.

The issue of conscientious objection by nurses is, however, far from being a trivial matter, and deserves the attention of all concerned. In particular, attention needs to be given to clarifying the nature and authority of conscience, distinguishing between genuine and bogus claims of conscientious objection, and determining the kinds of policy there should be towards those who conscientiously refuse to perform or to participate in morally controversial medical and/or nursing procedures. As well as this, attention needs to be given to the question of when, if ever, a superior can decently order nurses to perform tasks which they are conscientiously opposed to performing. These and other key concerns raised by the conscientious objection debate are addressed in the following sections.

The nature of conscience explained

The *Oxford English dictionary* defines 'conscience' as 'the internal acknowledgement or recognition of the moral quality of one's motives and actions; the sense of right and wrong as regards things for which one is responsible; the faculty or principle which pronounces upon the moral quality of one's actions or motives, approving the right and condemning the wrong'. The *Collins English dictionary* defines 'conscience' as a 'sense of right and wrong that governs a person's thoughts and actions'. These definitions, however, are inadequate to answer questions concerning the legitimacy and power of conscience as a bona fide moral authority. In short, while they help to describe what conscience is, these definitions say nothing about whether individuals should always obey their conscientious senses of right and wrong, or whether others can reasonably be expected to respect another's conscientious claims. Once again, we must turn to moral philosophy for some more substantive answers.

Philosophical accounts of conscience fall roughly into three categories: as *moral reasoning*, as *moral feelings*, and as a *mixture of moral reasoning and moral feelings* (see also Mill 1962 edn, pp. 281–4; Hume 1888 edn, p. 458; Kant 1930 edn, pp. 129–35; Rawls 1971, pp. 205–11, 368–9; Beauchamp and Childress 1989, pp. 385–94).

CONSCIENCE AS MORAL REASONING

A reasonable or rationalistic account of conscience regards rational moral principles and reason as the source of one's moral convictions. Conscientious judgments, by this view, are really critically reflective moral judgments concerning right and wrong (Garnett 1965; Broad 1940). Rational insight can be either religious or non-religious in nature, depending on what a person's world views are. Either way, a rational conscience typically manifests itself as 'a little voice inside one's head saying what one should and should not do'. Or, to put this in moral terms, it tells us what our moral obligations and duties are. Statements of conscientious objection then are, by this view, merely statements of moral duty which individuals recognise and commit themselves to fulfil. Whether the duties or obligations identified impose overriding or absolute demands, or only prima facie demands on the individual is, however, another matter entirely, and one that is considered shortly.

CONSCIENCE AS MORAL FEELINGS

There are two possible versions of a 'moral feelings' account of conscience — emotivist and intuitionist. Both consist of a tendency to spontaneously experience either emotions or intuitions 'of a unique sort of approval of the doing of what is believed to be right and a similarly unique sort of disapproval of the doing of what is believed to be wrong' (Garnett 1965, p. 81).

It is generally recognised that these feelings are quite different from the sorts of feelings we might have when, for example, looking at a beautiful painting (aesthetic approval) or an awful painting (aesthetic disapproval), or eating a favourite food (the feelings of mere liking) or smelling an awful smell (feelings of mere disliking), or witnessing an act of remarkable human achievement (feelings of admiration) or an act of extraordinary human failure (feelings of disdain). By contrast, in the case of wicked acts or the violation of duty, conscience may manifest itself in strong and distinguishable feelings of moral loathing, shame, remorse, or even guilt, or, as Beauchamp and Childress (1989) suggest, the unpleasant feelings of 'a loss of integrity, wholeness, peace, and harmony' (p. 387). To borrow from Fletcher (1966), conscience can manifest itself as 'a sharp stone in the breast under the sternum, which turns and hurts when we have done wrong' (p. 54). In the case of virtuous acts, conscience may manifest itself as strong feelings of reassurance or moral goodness (Fletcher 1966, p. 54; Kant 1930 edn, p. 130), or, as Beauchamp and Childress (1989) suggest, as feelings of integrity, wholeness, peace and harmony (p. 387). Either way, moral feelings instruct individuals on what they ought and/or ought not to do. As with the rationalistic account, statements of conscience emerge as statements of obligation and duty.

CONSCIENCE AS REASON AND FEELINGS

The concept of conscience as a mixture of reason and feelings basically involves an integrated response to moral triggers in the world. It does not rely on 'blind emotive obedience', as Kordig (1976) calls it, nor on an exclusive and blind devotion to reason. Rather, it relies on the mutually guiding and instructive forces of both *moral sensibilities* and *moral reasoning*. This account of conscience is, in my view, the most plausible of the three given, and is thus the one that underpins this discussion.

How conscience works

Now that we have briefly examined the essential nature of conscience, the next question is: how does conscience function as a moral authority?

It is generally recognised that conscience functions as a *personal* (internal) *sanction* and as a *personal moral authority* (Childress 1979; Beauchamp and Childress 1989, p. 388). Claims of conscience typically identify individual people with their self-chosen or autonomously chosen standards and principles of conduct (Nowell-Smith 1954, p. 268); further, they *commit* individual people to act in accordance with those principles. In other words, claims of conscience commit the individual person to act morally (Timms 1983, p. 41). Thus, when conscience is said to be 'personal' or 'one's own', all that is being claimed is that a particular set of autonomously chosen moral standards has authority over a particular person — not, as is sometimes mistakenly thought, that that person has a unique and different set of moral standards from everybody else, and thus is a kind of 'moral freak'.

Conscience can be appealed to both as a kind of 'reviewer' or 'judge' of past acts, and as an 'authority on' or as a 'guide to' future acts. Whether conscience is appealed to as judge or guide, however, it is important to understand that conscience is not *morality itself*, nor is it the *ultimate standard* (or even *a* standard) of morality. Rather, as Gonsalves explains, it is:

> ... only the intellect itself exercising a special function, the function of judging the rightness or wrongness, the moral value, of our own individual acts according to the set of moral values and principles the person holds with conviction.
>
> (Gonsalves 1985, p. 55)

Or, as Childress explains, it is merely 'the mode of consciousness resulting from the application of standards' (1979, p. 319).

Gonsalves' and Childress' views make it plain that statements of conscience are not statements of a unique moral faculty or of unique moral standards. Rather, they are statements of a *particular application of adopted moral standards*. Conscientious objection, by this view, essentially translates into a case of *moral disagreement* in regard to which moral statements apply and what one's moral duty is in a particular situation. If this is so, the case for respecting a conscientious objector's claims becomes compelling — particularly in instances where there are no clear-cut moral grounds for settling a specific disagreement (as sometimes occurs in the cases of abortion, organ transplantation, assisting with the involuntary administration of ECT or psychotropic medication, administering blood to Jehovah's Witness patients, and similar cases).

It should be noted here that, once it is accepted that claims of conscience translate into claims of duty, it is conceptually incorrect to speak of conscientious objection as a *right* (as some nursing position statements on the subject do). To assert this would be to assert that an individual has a 'right to have a duty', which is conceptually incorrect. It is more correct to speak of others being bound to respect another's claim of conscience, just as they are bound to respect another's claim of moral duty.

The problem remains, however, that consciences are fallible and can make mistakes (Seeskin 1978). As Nowell-Smith (1954, p. 247) points out, some of the worst crimes in human history have been committed by people acting on the firm convictions of conscience. Hitler, for example, believed he was fulfilling a supreme moral duty by purging the German race of its 'Jewish disease' (Kordig 1976). Others also point out that, in some instances, what appears to be a claim of conscience may be nothing more than a claim of prudence or self-interest or convenience. This invariably raises the question: 'Should I always obey my conscience?' Further to this, claims of conscience can be insincere or counterfeit, raising the additional questions of: 'How can I distinguish between genuine and bogus claims of conscientious objection?' 'Should I always respect another's conscientious claims?' It is to answering these questions that this discussion now turns.

Bogus and genuine claims of conscientious objection

For a conscientious objection to be genuine, it must satisfy at least five conditions.

1. It must have as its basis a *distinctively moral motivation*, as opposed to the motivations of mere self-interest, prudence, convenience or prejudice. By this is meant:

    a. that the action has as its aim the maintenance of sound moral standards, and the achievement of a moral end (Garnett 1965);

    b. that the person performing the act sincerely believes in the moral characteristics of the action in question, and sincerely desires to do what is right (Broad 1940, p. 75; Childress 1979, p. 334); and

    c. that the desire to do what is right is sufficient to override considerations of fear, cowardice, self-interest, and prejudice.

2. It must be performed on the basis of *autonomous, informed, and critically reflective choice*. By this is meant:

    a. that the action must be the agent's 'own', so to speak — that is, it is not the product of coercion or manipulation; and

    b. that that action has been carefully considered — that is, that the person has taken into account all the relevant factual as well as ethical information pertaining to the situation at hand, possible alternatives to the action being contemplated, and predicted moral outcomes of the action once it is taken (Broad 1940, p. 75).

3. Conscience should be appealed to only *as a last resort* — that is, in defence of one's moral beliefs. A claim of conscientious objection is a last resort when all other means of achieving a tolerable solution to a given moral problem have failed. Here conscientious objection is justified on grounds analogous to those justifying self-defence, which permit people to use reasonable force in order to preserve their integrity (in this case, their moral integrity) (Machan 1983, pp. 503–5).

4. The conscientious objector must admit that *others might have an equal and opposing claim of objection.* For example, a nurse refusing on conscientious grounds to assist with an abortion procedure must be prepared to accept that the aborting surgeon may feel obliged as a matter of conscience to go ahead with the abortion; to quote from Broad: "What is sauce for the conscientious goose is sauce for the conscientious ganders who are his [sic] neighbours or his [sic] governors' (Broad 1940, p. 78).

5. *The situation in which it is being claimed must itself be of a nature which is morally uncertain;* that is, there are no clear-cut moral grounds upon which the matter at hand can be readily and satisfactorily resolved.

If we accept these criteria, the task of distinguishing bogus from genuine claims of conscientious objection becomes considerably easier. To illustrate this, consider four types of situations in which nurses commonly claim conscientious objection: the lawful but morally controversial orders of a superior; a conflict of personal values between a nurse and a patient; personal fear of contagion; and unsafe working conditions.

CONSCIENTIOUS OBJECTION TO THE LAWFUL BUT MORALLY CONTROVERSIAL ORDERS OF A SUPERIOR

Nurses as employees are compelled by the principle of employment law to obey the lawful and reasonable orders of an employer or superior. The problem is, however, that nurses might not always agree morally with the lawful orders they have been given, and thus may sometimes find themselves in the uncomfortable position of having to perform acts which violate their reasoned moral judgments (Johnstone 1988, 1994).

There are many examples of nurses having been caught in both personal and professional dilemmas on account of legal demands to obey the lawful though morally controversial orders of doctors and nurse superiors. Several examples have already been given in this text, typically involving situations in which nurses have been ordered, against their will, to assist with morally controversial procedures such as abortion, euthanasia, electroconvulsive therapy (ECT) and organ transplantation. The difficulties nurses have encountered in such situations have been compounded by the fact that they have had little, if any, avenue for officially expressing their conscientious refusal without fear of losing their jobs or facing other threats.

Situations involving nurses' conscientious refusal to follow lawful but morally questionable orders invariably pose the age-old question of whether an individual can, all things considered, be decently expected to follow morally controversial or morally bad although legally valid laws — or, in this case, lawful orders.

As I have stated elsewhere (Johnstone 1988), the problem of legal–moral conflict is not new to philosophy. Questions of, for example, what is the proper relationship of morality to law, what is to count as a *good* legal system, or whether individuals ought to be compelled to obey immoral laws, are still matters of great philosophical controversy. Hart, an Oxford scholar and professor of jurisprudence, argues persuasively that existing law must not supplant morality 'as a final test of conduct and so escape criticism' (Hart 1957). He also argues that the demands of law must be submitted to the scrutiny and guidance of sound morality before they can be justly enforced (Hart 1961). Not surprisingly, these kinds of views have sparked enormous debates in both philosophy and law. It is beyond the scope of this text to discuss Hart's views and address the interesting questions concerning the philosophy of law that they raise. Nevertheless, it is assumed for argument's sake here that any law which fails the test of sound moral scrutiny should be either adjusted or rejected; it is also assumed that to punish autonomous moral agents for refusing to obey lawful but morally questionable orders is to commit a gross moral wrong.

A number of other important considerations are worthy of attention here. First, there is the persuasive view that forcing nurses to act against their reasoned or conscientious judgments is to not only ignore or diminish their moral autonomy, but also to violate the principles of critical morality itself — not least those of autonomy and reflectivity (Muyskens 1982b, p. 61). Perhaps even more troubling is the possibility that violating nurses' consciences would also unjustly violate their integrity as moral agents (Childress 1979).

Second, it is generally recognised that if people are forced constantly to violate their conscience their conscience will gradually weaken and lose its authority (Kant 1930 edn). This in turn makes it easier for individuals to avoid fulfilling their perceived moral duties and/or acting in accordance with autonomously chosen moral standards. As a result, there is likely to be a general breakdown in compliance with moral rules and principles, and a general erosion of individual moral responsibility and accountability. It takes little to imagine what would happen to the moral fabric of the community at large if all its members were forced, say, by order of the state, constantly to violate their reasoned moral judgments or consciences. No less consideration is due to what may ultimately happen to the moral fabric of the nursing profession if its individual members are constantly forced to abandon their reasoned moral judgments and consciences in favour of preserving the prescriptions and proscriptions of law and convention.

Related to this is a third consideration — that moral duty 'is mainly concerned with the avoidance of intolerable results' (Urmson 1958, p. 72). If fulfilling one's supposed duty does not avoid or prevent intolerable results, it seems reasonable to question whether in fact it was one's duty in the first place. As with the case of supererogatory acts (that is, acts above the call of duty, such as those performed by saints and heroes), care must be taken to distinguish those deeds which can be reasonably expected of 'ordinary' persons (or 'ordinary' nurses) from those which it would merely be nice of 'ordinary' persons (nurses) to perform, but which could never be reasonably *expected* of them (Urmson 1958, p. 68). On this point, Urmson (1958, p. 71) argues: '... a line must be drawn between what we can expect and demand of others and what we can merely hope for and receive with gratitude when we get it'.

Fourth, those who coerce others to act against their conscience erroneously presume that coercion vitiates moral responsibility. This, however, is not so. Just as more sophisticated claims of duty cannot be escaped or deceived, neither can claims of conscience. It is a mistake to hold that, if a person is forced to perform an act to which they are conscientiously opposed, they are less morally culpable for that act, and that they will feel less morally guilty for having performed it. What users of force fail to understand is that an instance of moral violation still stands, regardless of whether it has been caused by an act of coercion or an act of free will.

Fifth, nurses are not automata or robots, but thinking, reasoning, feeling, responsible human beings. Legal law recognises this by the very fact that it can and does hold nurses independently accountable for their actions (Johnstone 1994). Given this, it is a mistake to hold that nurses have an *unqualified* duty to obey the orders of a superior.

Lastly, it is ultimately more desirable than not to have a health care system comprised of conscientious nurses. Nurses comprise 70 per cent of the health care work force. The prospect of 70 per cent of health care providers being morally unconscientious is an overwhelmingly bleak one. In a culture which values objectivity and abstract detachment, the need is to cultivate moral motivation, not destroy it. Since most of us cannot be saints, but can be conscientious, we need to preserve and cultivate conscientiousness (Nowell-Smith 1954, p. 259; Garnett 1965, p. 91). Only by doing this can we be assured of achieving and maintaining some sort of moral order in health care domains. As Seeskin (1978) argues, '... we have no guarantee that our deliberations will be perfect or our moral sensibilities adequate' (p. 299); it is for this reason, among others, that conscience and moral conscientiousness should be given a place among the moral virtues. We might be condemned as fanatics if we hold conscience to be infallible, but if we do not at least acknowledge its ultimateness in the scheme of moral reasoning, we might be guilty of moral negligence and moral irresponsibility (Seeskin 1978; Kordig 1976).

The consequences of such views have interesting implications for policy makers attempting to respond to the conscientious objection problem. These views seem to suggest that, even if nurses' consciences are mistaken, on balance there are moral benefits to be gained by permitting their conscientious objections — not least, the benefits of fostering moral sensitivity and moral responsibility in the workplace. These views also suggest that, if nurses are not permitted conscientiously to object, then health care contexts, not to mention the community at large, will be morally worse off by virtue of being more at risk of suffering moral harms on account of receiving care that is not informed or guided by conscientious ethical beliefs and standards.

It might be objected here that permitting conscientious objection is not conducive to the efficient running of hospitals and other health services. There is, however, little support for this kind of claim. In the case of military service, for example, it has been found that objectors are rarely amenable to threats and usually make unsatisfactory soldiers if coerced, and that in fact there are generally not enough objectors to frustrate the community's purpose (Benn and Peters 1959, p. 193). I would suggest that something similar is probably true of objectors in nursing. As some of the examples in this text have shown, nurses have preferred to resign and risk dismissal than perform acts which they find morally offensive. Further to this, those nurses who have been coerced have not wholly complied with given orders. (For example, I know of nurses who have resuscitated patients in cases of controversial NFR orders, and not resuscitated patients in the case of controversial CPR orders. A more common disobedience, however, involves night nurses who secretly feed severely disabled newborns on whom a medical order has been given to withhold nourishing fluids with the purpose of hastening death.) It is also unlikely that there are enough objecting nurses to obstruct the efficient running of the hospital system. Lastly, it is likely that conscientious objectors would gain considerable community support if the extent of their personal and professional suffering was made public. I would argue, then, that it would be mutually beneficial to the state, the community and the nursing profession for formal procedures recognising conscientious objection to be adopted. If this is done, professional nurses can be spared the unnecessary and morally costly dilemma of whether to obey morally controversial but lawful orders; employers, in turn, can optimistically look forward to achieving a morally tolerable and harmonious clinical reality for both their employees and the communities they are serving.

Where lawful orders entail a demand to perform morally controversial procedures, there is considerable scope for arguing that a nurse has a firm moral basis upon which to conscientiously object. Issues such as abortion, organ transplants, electroconvulsive therapy, the enforced and involuntary treatment of psychiatric patients and euthanasia, are all morally controversial, and, as yet, no morally clear-cut grounds exist for resolving them. Until these issues can be resolved satisfactorily, it would be morally barbaric to insist that nurses must, when ordered, assist with abortion, organ transplantation, electroconvulsive therapy and euthanasia work — or any other work which is morally controversial. In other words, where a so-called 'standard' or 'reasonable' medical or nursing procedure is morally questionable, nurses cannot decently be forced to perform or participate in that procedure. Further, it is worth noting once again that what we have in a situation of extreme conscientious objection is radical moral disagreement — something which, as discussed in chapter 6, is unlikely to be resolved. The most amenable solution seems to be to permit conscientious objection.

CONSCIENTIOUS OBJECTION AND THE PROBLEM OF CONFLICT IN PERSONAL VALUES BETWEEN NURSE AND PATIENT

The International Council of Nurses' (1973) *Code for nurses* states that 'the nurse's primary responsibility is to those who require nursing care'. It further states that: '... the nurse, in providing care, promotes an environment in which the values, customs and spiritual beliefs of the individual are respected' (International Council of Nurses 1973). Sometimes, however, a nurse may find it difficult to respect a person's values, customs and spiritual beliefs, and for this reason may decline to be involved in caring for that person. Consider the following cases.

Case 1
A registered nurse working in a general medical ward was assigned a male patient who was known to be an orthodox Muslim. Upon

learning of the man's religion, the nurse refused to care for him, stating that she could not accept the attitudes of Muslim males towards women, and that if she cared for him she would be as good as condoning his views.

Case 2

A registered nurse working in an infectious diseases unit was assigned a male patient in the end stages of AIDS. Upon learning that the patient was a homosexual, the nurse refused to accept the assignment. He argued that as a Christian he could not condone homosexuality, and therefore it would be against his religious beliefs to care for the patient.

Case 3

A registered nurse working in a country hospital was asked to admit and care for a patient injured in a fight. When she recognised the patient as a member of a family who had been engaged in a feud with her own family for years, she declined to care for him. She stated as her reason that, were she to care for the man, she would be violating the loyalties she owed to her own family.

There is little doubt that all three registered nurses in the cases just given have sincere motivations behind their refusals to care for the patients in question. What is not so clear, however, is whether these motivations have a *moral* basis. For instance, their refusals to care for these patients seem to be based more on, for example, non-moral personal dislike, prejudice, fear, disdain or mere disapproval than on sincere moral motivation and the desire to achieve morally desirable ends. Second, it is not clear whether, by refusing to care for these patients, the nurses will preserve their moral integrity. In fact, it may be quite the reverse, since they have allowed personal interests to override the significant moral interests of their patients. Lastly, the professional demand to care for the patients in question is not *itself* morally controversial — at least, not in the same way that, say, the demand to care for and stabilise a 'brain dead' patient for organ donation is. While it may be imprudent to compel the nurses in these cases to care for the patients assigned to them, it is not immediately apparent that it would be immoral to do so. It might be concluded then that their refusals can, at least from a moral perspective, be justly over-ridden. Nevertheless, there may still exist pragmatic grounds for permitting their refusals. If they cannot be relied upon to give adequate care, for example, it might be better to allow their refusal. If their prejudices and personal feelings are of such a nature as to seriously cloud their prudential judgments and indeed their ability to *care* and engage in an effective therapeutic relationship, it may be that they should not be allocated the patients in question. This, however, may be more a practical consideration rather than a fully fledged moral one — although, granted, one which will probably have a significant moral dimension, namely, the patient's well-being.

CONSCIENTIOUS OBJECTION, THE FEAR OF CONTAGION, AND HOMOPHOBIA

The question of if, and when, and under what circumstances nurses may refuse to care for certain patients has become a particularly important and challenging one over recent years, largely because of the worldwide HIV/AIDS epidemic.

Questions are already being asked, both in Australia and overseas, about whether nurses can rightly refuse to care for HIV/AIDS patients (including infected newborns). Overseas research studies and opinion polls even suggest that some nurses would rather abandon their practices and nursing careers than place themselves at risk by caring for HIV/AIDS patients (Beard et al. 1988; Lester and Beard 1988; Huerta and Oddi, 1992). In one United States opinion poll, published in *Nursing 88*, it was revealed that 73 per cent of nurses surveyed were concerned about their own safety, and 47 per cent believed they had a right to refuse to care for HIV/AIDS patients; interestingly, an overwhelming majority (93 per cent) stated that they had never refused to care for an HIV/AIDS patient, despite their fears (Brennan et al. 1988). The poll also revealed that a staggering 80 per cent of nurses surveyed stated that their own families were concerned about their (the nurses') safety when caring for HIV/AIDS patients.

Other studies have found that nurses caring for HIV/AIDS patients have actually been shunned by family, friends and neighbours, and even by other health care workers, who apparently feared association 'with one who provides direct care' (Huerta and Oddi 1992, p. 221; *Nursing Times*, 29 October 1986, p. 10) — demonstrating further the complexity of the refusal to care issue, and the difficulties associated with answering the question: to what extent should nurses be expected to sacrifice their own important interests for the sake of those for whom they care?

Significantly, two of the most commonly cited reasons for refusing to care for HIV/AIDS patients are fear of contagion, and disapproval of patients' lifestyles (especially those involving either homosexuality or intravenous drug use) (Huerta and Oddi 1992, p. 223). A poignant example of how fear of contagion and disapproval of a patient's lifestyle can affect the ability of nurses to care and, in turn, the patient's overall well-being, is given below:

A client was diagnosed as having AIDS upon his admission to hospital. During his inpatient stay, nurses often cracked open the door and called in to him to learn of his condition, but would not enter the room. The hospital staff would not bathe him, and he was not allowed to shower. Bloody linens were not removed from the room. His emergency bedside signal [call bell] was left unanswered for as long as eight hours. A pamphlet was left at his bedside that described homosexuality as a sinful practice.

(Staff of the National Health Law Program 1991, p. 260)

Although this is an American case, the prejudicial attitudes it demonstrates are not restricted to the national borders of the United States. As recently as 1989 the respected Freemasons Hospital in Melbourne caused a public outcry when it imposed a ban on treating all people who had AIDS or who carried the HIV virus (Miller 1989). The decision to impose the ban was made by the hospital's medical advisory board, and was allegedly supported by both doctors and nurses working at the hospital, as well as by the Victorian Branch of the Australian Medical Association (AMA) (Athersmith 1989a; Price 1989). As a point of interest, it was later revealed that nurses had *not* in fact been consulted about the decision to effect the ban (Curtis 1989). The Freemasons' ban is believed to be the first case of its kind in Australia (Allender and Robinson 1989). The Victorian Government, meanwhile, has taken steps to outlaw hospital policies which effectively discriminate unjustly against HIV/AIDS patients.

The right of nurses to refuse to care for HIV/AIDS patients is a tough question, which may never find a wholly satisfactory answer. Nevertheless, a serious attempt must be made to address it.

It is doubtful whether HIV/AIDS (and/or other cases of infectious diseases — for example, hepatitis B and C) presents a situation in which conscientious objection claims would be valid. Certainly, claims in these sorts of cases do not seem to satisfy all the five criteria of genuine conscientious objection listed earlier. For example, it is not clear that claims in these cases are based on a distinctive moral motivation aimed at maintaining sound moral standards or achieving a desired moral end. Nor is it clear that claims in these cases are based on informed and critically reflective choice (many may, in fact, be based on misinformed, fearful and arbitrary self-interested choice). It is also not clear that the claims of conscientious objection in these cases are necessary as a 'last resort' in 'the defence of one's moral integrity'. For one thing, it has yet to be shown how, if at all, caring for someone who is HIV positive threatens the moral integrity or standards of a care giver (a point to be examined further shortly). Finally, it is far from clear that these cases involve a situation that is characteristically 'morally uncertain'. (It has yet to be shown convincingly that it is unethical to care for someone who is seriously ill with an infectious disease.) While the objector may recognise that others' conscientious claims are equally deserving in these cases, and thereby satisfy at least one of the five criteria listed, this is not enough to uphold a genuine claim of conscientious objection.

It should be noted, however, that, even though a claim of genuine conscientious objection might fail in cases of caring for people with potentially life-threatening infectious diseases, this does not necessarily mean that a given refusal to care by a nurse should not be permitted. Refusals to care for HIV/AIDS patients might, for example, sometimes be justified on pragmatic grounds — which, incidentally, as already pointed out, might also have morally significant dimensions. Consider the following.

There are, I believe, at least three conditions under which a refusal might arguably be permitted. The first of these is where an attending nurse would be placed at an unreasonable or an unacceptable risk of cross-infection — the point being, of course, that if cross-infection were to occur, the moral costs would be unacceptably high. It is worth noting here that in 1989 the number of health workers occupationally infected with the HIV/AIDS virus, most of whom were nurses (Pirrie 1989b), was 25 worldwide. Another case to be added to that figure was that of a New South Wales registered nurse who allegedly contracted HIV/AIDS after being pricked by an HIV/AIDS-infected needle during the course of her work (Sweet 1989). It was later reported that the nurse was still awaiting confirmation of an HIV/AIDS test for herself (Pirrie 1989b). The *Sunday Telegraph* (30 April 1989, p. 3), citing the incident, also reported that, of the 25 instances of occupational infection of health workers at that time, '[S]ixteen have resulted from needle stick injuries, seven from mucous membrane exposure and two from deep lacerations'. The report also quoted an American professor as confirming that the United States Centers for Disease Control were currently investigating fifty cases of HIV/AIDS infection in health care professionals 'where no risk factor had been identified' — implying that the virus had been contracted through occupation rather than lifestyle. A report in *The Age* later confirmed that in the United States it is estimated that health workers have one chance in two hundred of contracting the HIV/AIDS virus through needlestick injuries (Pirrie 1989b; see also Brown and Brown 1988). Meanwhile, a Victorian State Government survey revealed that 4 per cent of nurses suffered needlestick injuries over a six-month period in 1987 (Athersmith 1989b). For all this, it should not be forgotten that the likelihood of a nurse being cross-infected is considerably reduced by stringent adherence to approved infection control procedures. Also, research has found that the incidence of occupational infection of health care workers is low, and that the 'actual probability of contracting infection is extremely small' for these workers (Allen 1988).

A second condition under which a refusal might arguably be permitted is in instances where nurses are so distracted and so disturbed by their fear of contagion that they can no longer be relied upon to give safe and appropriate patient care. Thus, rather than facilitating the realisation of the moral benefits of nursing care, a terrified nurse might unwittingly thwart these. In such instances, if only for the patient's sake, it might be better not to assign the terrified nurse an HIV/AIDS patient. The patient's sense of well-being and self-worth in this case is hardly going to be maximised by being assigned a nurse who is too terrified to even enter the room, as happened in the case cited above. The issue of the nurse's well-being is also involved. While ideally nurses ought to try and overcome their fear of contagion, when they are genuinely unable to do so it is likely that little will be gained either by ridiculing the nurses' fears or censuring their refusal (for example, by threatening dismissal for non-compliance with a superior's order to care for an assigned HIV/AIDS patient). There is room to speculate here that the harms of coercion in the case of refusal to care for HIV/AIDS patients probably far outweigh the benefits: as already indicated, patients may find themselves receiving less than optimal nursing care, and nurses may end up suffering intolerable psychological distress.

A third and final condition under which nurses' refusal might, arguably, be permitted is in the case where a hospital does not have proper facilities to deal with infectious HIV/AIDS cases and associated cross-infection risks — a problem which is likely to increase as more infectious HIV/AIDS victims require hospitalisation. For example, not all hospitals have the resources necessary to institute full barrier nursing for significantly large numbers of patients — or, indeed, to offer the highly specialised care that these patients both need and are entitled to receive. These are all practical and very real considerations which have yet to be properly addressed. And until such time as these considerations are fully addressed, health workers probably do have reasonable grounds for concern about their safety in relation to the HIV/AIDS virus and the risk of cross-infection, as well as about their ability to provide the expert care that HIV/AIDS patients need during the end stage of their disease.

It is, I believe, questionable to assert, as some informally do, that nurses should nurse *all* patients as if they were infectious. Were nurses to follow this advice, and take it to its logical and absurd extreme, *every* patient would need to be barrier nursed to some degree. It is doubtful that the health care system could cope with this scenario, at least, not financially — a point which emphasises the need for a responsible and realistic approach to the HIV/AIDS crisis. The solutions are, I think, fairly obvious. Hospitals must look towards upgrading their facilities so as to be able to cope better with the HIV/AIDS epidemic. Health professionals need to be educationally prepared to better deal with the concerns raised by the HIV/AIDS epidemic, and not least their own fears and anxieties about the risks involved in caring for HIV/AIDS patients (see also Huerta and Oddi 1992; Gilmour 1992; McKenzie 1991; Almond 1990). Further to this, there is, I believe, a strong case for discretional routine testing of patients coming into hospitals and other related health care facilities. For unless nurses and other health workers *know* that a patient is HIV positive, they cannot take the precautions necessary to reduce and prevent the likelihood of cross-infection, nor can they rest assured that the likelihood of their being cross-infected is minimal. As Sipes (1988) comments:

> ... admission screening would not only allay fears of nurses and other health care professionals but also remind them to take appropriate precautions. For example, in one survey, nurses said they'd willingly care for an AIDS patient — if they knew the diagnosis. They felt this awareness would make them more vigilant about precautions.
>
> (Sipes 1988, p. 49)

Sipes' comments find further support from the poll conducted by Brennan et al. (1988, p. 63) which found that 70 per cent of nurses surveyed felt that an 'assurance of disclosure of known HIV/AIDS patients to staff' would be helpful to them in dealing with HIV/AIDS patients. Routine testing, then, need not be viewed as a draconian measure, but as a responsible one in terms of trying to contain the spread of the HIV virus. Further, there is a strong case for the discretional testing of health workers, in a bid to protect patients. Where risks of unjust discrimination are occurring, they can be anticipated and appropriately dealt with by implementing carefully formulated institutional policies and laws, and by preparing health professionals educationally to effectively uphold these policies and laws.

It needs to be acknowledged by all concerned that the problem of fear is by no means a trivial one. It is unrealistic to insist that nurses should not have fear, or that their fears are without basis. The reality is that nurses do have fear, as indicated by the *Nursing 88* opinion poll, and by a media report in *The Herald* (Giannoukos 1989). What is more, this fear is very real. Furthermore, even if it is conceded that the fear of contagion is without reasonable basis, the desire to protect oneself is not. The distinction between these two considerations is one warranting some attention in the refusal debate. As pointed out elsewhere in this text, morality does not generally require us to make large personal sacrifices on behalf of others. If some nurses believe the sacrifices they are being asked to make are too great, there may be grounds for permitting them to refuse to care for HIV/AIDS patients. Just what these grounds might be, however, remains very much a matter for moral and community debate.

The matter of fear is also hardly helped by an increasing distrust of the scientific medical community. Medical scientists do not always have a reputation for frankness and honesty, and some research activities have been known to be fraudulent and misleading, and to have yielded inaccurate and incorrect results (see, for example, Broad and Wade 1982). Further to this, as one medical commentator is reported as pointing out, many of the assurances given by the so-called 'AIDS experts' have later proved quite false. She is reported to have commented:

> They [the AIDS experts] said first of all that it [AIDS] was not transmitted by sex. Then it is. Then it's not transmitted by blood transfusions. Then it is. Then it's not 100 per cent fatal. Then it is. It's probably not transmitted by heterosexual sex. Now it is.
>
> (Pirrie 1989a, p. 2)

Given such considerations, there does seem to be room for suspicion that hospitals might 'not be getting the right messages about the real risks of AIDS', as Dr Bruce Shepherd of the AMA is reported to have pointed out (Price 1989), and that we have all been 'falsely reassured' about the AIDS virus (Morrell and Miller 1989). Rumours that full-blown AIDS patients have been admitted to general wards for full nursing care — without the attending nursing staff being told that these patients are infectious — have also hardly helped to allay nurses' fears about the risks of contagion. This fear is likely to increase as nurses come to terms with the fact that, of the world's known occupationally infected AIDS cases, most are nurses.

In the light of the points raised on this issue, I would argue that legislation alone will not resolve the dilemmas at hand, and may even exacerbate existing fears, anxieties and prejudices. A better solution might be found in education, negotiation, screening, increased funding for supporting lay carers, and improved infectious nursing facilities in general hospitals. The establishment of special HIV/AIDS treatment and caring units may also be a solution — although, it is acknowledged, one which is not without problems. As Huerta and Oddi (1992) point out, while the provision of separate units for the care of HIV/AIDS patients would enable the centralisation of resources and expertise, it might also inadvertently increase the risk of occupational infection by the disease, because nurses and others might be 'lulled into a false sense of security and fail to practice appropriate precautions' (p. 226). If this issue is not handled wisely, sensitively and competently, there is considerable room to suggest that we will not be able to cope with the intolerable suffering that this disease promises to cause. What, then, does this mean for the nursing profession? It means that nurses, like everyone else in the community, need to address the HIV/AIDS issue, and need to do so in a responsible, meaningful and carefully guided manner.

Another problem which needs to be addressed is that of homophobia (the 'irrational fear of homosexuality'), which, as Huerta and Oddi (1992, p. 223) argue, can further compound the fear of caring for HIV/AIDS patients. Significantly, attitudinal studies have found that some nurses feel uncomfortable with caring for male homosexuals and exhibit avoidance behaviour towards HIV/AIDS patients who belong to this group (Huerta and Oddi 1992, p. 223); nurses opposed to homosexuality also tend to believe that HIV/AIDS patients are 'responsible' for their disease, and, accordingly, these nurses 'blame the victim' (Viele et al. 1984). Equally significant are research findings which show that nurses who are homophobic manifest 'the greatest fear of HIV/AIDS and the least empathy for AIDS patients' (Huerta and Oddi 1992, p. 224).

While these studies are not conclusive, they nevertheless point to a need for nurses to examine their attitudes towards homosexuality and to explore ways in which prejudicial attitudes towards and fear of HIV/AIDS patients can be overcome. One study has found, for example, that nurses can be helped to gain a more positive attitude towards and less fear of homosexuality by participating in sexuality workshops where opportunities can be provided to explore and share feelings about the issue, and to engage in other learning activities (Young 1988).

One group of people who may not be amenable to this kind of education, however, are those who are fundamentally opposed to homosexuality on religious grounds. I have, for instance, heard some nurses who hold conservative religious beliefs express the view that they 'could not possibly care for a homosexual patient with HIV/AIDS, since to do so would be tantamount to condoning homosexuality, and thereby supporting a sinful practice'. (Similar arguments are used in the case of abortion; some nurses have expressed the view, for example, that caring for women who have had abortions is tantamount to condoning abortion.) The reasoning used here is, however, flawed. It is a fallacy to hold that caring for a particular class of patients is tantamount to condoning the lifestyles or life circumstances of those patients. If we were to accept this line of reasoning, we would be committed to accepting that, for example, caring for poor people is tantamount to condoning poverty, or that caring for unemployed people is

tantamount to condoning unemployment, or that caring for homeless people is tantamount to condoning homelessness. We would, I
think, reject the view that caring for these latter groups of people is
tantamount to condoning their respective lifestyles, or to providing
grounds upon which a morally defensible refusal to care for them
could be based. Since the acts of caring for HIV/AIDS patients are
demonstrably remote from the sexual acts to which some nurses
are opposed on religious grounds, and since caring for patients who
are homosexual does not entail performing acts proscribed by
religious doctrine, it is not clear that a refusal to care for patients
who are homosexual can be sustained. (Readers may also find
Fitzpatrick's [1988, pp. 128–34] discussion of the Catholic principles of cooperation/complicity helpful.)

It might be objected here, however, that, unlike homosexuality,
poverty, unemployment and homelessness are not 'sins' and therefore nurses opposed to sinful practices can care for people in these
groups without compromising their religious beliefs and moral
integrity. In fact, caring for these people might even be construed
as 'virtuous'. This, however, is not a satisfactory reply, since it fails
to show *why* caring for these groups of people is *not* tantamount to
condoning their lifestyles, which, significantly, can be shown to be
injurious to these groups of people's well-being and moral interests.
Let us explore this further.

Why, for instance, is caring for a homosexual patient regarded as
tantamount to condoning homosexuality, yet caring or an unemployed person *is* *not* regarded as tantamount to condoning
unemployment? If we take out the descriptive statements referring
to these groups whose respective lifestyles are in question, what
we end up with is something like this: *caring for members of group
X is tantamount to condoning their lifestyles, but caring for members
of group Y is not tantamount to condoning their lifestyles.* No reasons
are given why this is the case, however, demonstrating that the
thinking being used here is at best arbitrary and at worst fallacious. Even if it is conceded that what makes a morally significant difference in this case is the 'sinful' nature of homosexuality,
this will not help, since this seems to say that what makes caring
for a particular group of people tantamount to condoning their
lifestyles is the fact that what they do is 'sinful'. If nurses holding
conservative religious beliefs were to accept this, however, they
would be committed logically to accepting that caring for a whole
range of people would be tantamount to condoning their 'sinful'
lifestyles, and thus that there exists a whole range of people for
whom they should refuse to care. Nurses holding conservative
religious beliefs would, for instance, be obliged to refuse to care for
people who work on Sundays, bear false witness, steal, murder,
covet their neighbours' goods, fornicate, commit adultery, blas-
pheme, do not fear God, worship other gods, tell lies (including

telling children that Father Christmas is a real person and that tooth fairies bring money in the night), take contraception, have attempted suicide, and have performed a whole range of other acts deemed sins in the Bible or other religious texts. Clearly, if nurses were to accept the view that caring for people who commit sins is tantamount to condoning the sins in question, they would probably have to give up nursing altogether, since many people have committed the 'sinful' acts given above.

While the arguments presented here have had as their focus male homosexuals, they could, of course, be applied equally to the cases of other groups of people whose lifestyles some nurses regard as being problematic or sinful — for example, intravenous drug users and prostitutes.

CONSCIENTIOUS OBJECTION AND THE PROBLEM OF UNSAFE WORK CONDITIONS

A final type of situation to be considered here involves the common problem of nurses being expected to work in unsafe working conditions, most notably those caused by severe staff shortages. Typically, nurses might be ordered to work in an area with which they are unfamiliar and/or in which they are not educated to work, such as in an intensive care unit. They might also be expected to work at a staffing level which places patient safety and quality of care at risk. These two situations are inextricably linked. For example, if there was not a shortage of properly educated intensive care nurses, nurse administrators would not have to order an inexperienced nurse to go and 'help out' in the hospital's intensive care unit.

The problem of declining and unsafe working conditions is being increasingly responded to by nurses by all-out strike action, which, in many respects, might also qualify as a type of conscientious objection. Since this topic warrants in-depth attention, it is discussed separately later in this chapter.

Conscientious objection — issues and recommendations

For a conscientious objection policy to be effective and reliable, it must carry at least two minimal requirements (see Childress 1979). First, conscientious objectors must demonstrate that their claims are sincere. A given proof need not be religious in nature, nor necessarily absolute. As we have seen throughout this text, it is not always inconsistent for nurses (or for anyone) to have a 'moderate' position on the moral permissibility of certain procedures, such as abortion and organ transplants. Thus, it would not necessarily be inconsistent of nurses to, say, support abortion and to participate in most abortion procedures at their place of employment, yet nevertheless be opposed to a 'particular case' of abortion where the procedure in question fails to satisfy certain autonomously chosen moral standards. The same applies in the case of organ transplants. Conscientious objection policies, then, must recognise and make provision for the moderate's position, and accept that sometimes conscientious objectors might refuse to assist with a type of procedure they have previously assisted with, such as abortion.

A second minimal requirement is that employers must carry the burden of proof that no alternative is available when not permitting nurses to refuse on conscientious grounds to assist with a given procedure. Personally, I find it very difficult to accept that a claim of conscientious objection cannot be accommodated in cases where nurses have used rightful means in expressing a conscientious refusal — i.e. superiors have been given advance notice of an intention to refuse, reasons for refusal have been made explicit, replacement or other attending personnel have not been unduly compromised, other interests of comparable moral worth have not been sacrificed, and patients have not been stranded (Johnstone 1988, p. 153). Where an administrator does not accept a nurse's genuine conscientious objection claims, serious questions need to be asked about whether the administrator has sincerely tried to find viable alternatives which would make it possible for conscientiously objecting nurses to withdraw from situations they deem morally troubling or intolerable.

The key to settling the conscientious objection debate does not lie only in having enforceable mechanisms for protecting genuine conscientious objection claims, but also in having a demonstrable threshold beyond which nurses can base their claims. However, this threshold is one which can only be supplied by sound moral education (something which nursing education programs are only beginning to offer) and agreed moral standards within the profession.

Can superiors decently order nurses to perform tasks to which they are genuinely conscientiously opposed? The answer is 'no'. To compel nurses to act against their conscience is to risk weakening their moral conscientiousness and hence their ability to be moral. To deny moral conscientiousness in health care domains is also to risk the moral interests of those requiring health care. Furthermore, superiors simply do not have the moral authority to dictate to another which moral standards ought and ought not to be appealed to in a given situation.

There is much to support the view that a health care system comprised of morally conscientious and sensitive nurses would be much better than one without such nurses. This seems to support the conclusion that genuine conscientious objection is not only morally permissible, but may even, in the ultimate analysis, be morally required.

Strike action

In 1988, Dr Amelia Mangay-Maglacas, the chief nurse at the World Health Organization, urged nurses worldwide to engage in an unprecedented two-hour global strike. In defence of this initiative, Dr Mangay-Maglacas is reported to have argued that:

> ... a two hour global strike supported by all the world's nurses may be the only way to focus attention on the profession's problems.
>
> (*Nursing Times*, 6 April 1988, p. 5)

Rejecting the view that the nurses were mainly concerned with money, Dr Mangay-Maglacas responded that what nurses wanted was simply:

> ... the satisfaction of doing what they believe is right, developing and managing their own service and not being dictated to by others.
>
> (*Nursing Times*, 6 April 1988, p. 5)

In the past, strike action has been popularly viewed as the antithesis of professionalism, of caring, and even of professional responsibility (Kelly 1985, p. 187; Tschudin 1986, p. 15; Williams 1988, p. 6). One Melbourne writer would have us believe it is also the antithesis of 'feminine behaviour'! (see Women's Electoral Lobby 1987, p. 4). The underlying presumption of this view seems to be that *professionalism* is generally regarded as intrinsically 'other serving' (i.e. its end is the welfare of others, and to serve the public good), unlike *strike action*, which is generally considered to be 'self-serving' (i.e. its end is the welfare of self, sometimes even at the expense of the welfare of others). Nurses, both in Australia and overseas, have, I believe, been thoroughly persuaded by this view and have, at least until recent years, totally resisted any temptation to engage in the labours (or non-labours, as the case may be) of strike action.

The nursing profession's traditional (and universal) anti-strike position is nevertheless being gradually overturned as representative nursing associations and organisations around the world move to delete the 'no-strike' clauses from their rule books. However, such moves have not been without a sense of consternation, and have served to raise many serious questions about the professional integrity of nurses — both as individuals and as a group — in terms of their commitment to serving the public good in general, and the welfare of patients in particular.

This discussion attempts to address the questions of whether strike action by nurses is ever justified; and whether strike action by nurses entails a violation of both professional ethics and the interests of the community at large. In answering these questions I shall briefly outline some of the central professional and industrial issues which motivated the fifty-day-long Victorian nurses' strike of 1986; describe some of the extraordinary events which occurred during this strike; and critically examine some central philosophical and ethical arguments which might be raised both in criticism and in support of nurses' strikes in general.

Central issues of strike action

In Australia the 'no-strike' clause (section 31C) was deleted from the rules of the then Royal Australian Nursing Federation (RNAF), now the Australian Nursing Federation (ANF), after a national poll in 1984 found that 65 per cent of nurses were in favour of such a move (Gardner and McCoppin 1986, p. 31). As work conditions and standards of patient care continued to decline, and heavy and diverse workloads continued to increase, nurses around Victoria began to 'dig in their industrial toes' in a way they had never done before.

1984 saw work bans and short-duration strike action in support of a variety of long-standing issues ranging from 'non-nursing duties' to 'tertiary education for nurses'. Tired of the government's tardiness in settling these issues, and becoming increasingly suspicious of the government's overall intentions towards them, nurses decided once and for all to take their working futures firmly into their own hands. At a mass meeting on 11 October 1985 attended by over 5500 of Victoria's nurses, the decision to strike received overwhelming support. Settlement was reached by October 21 and the strike ended (Gardner and McCoppin 1986). Nevertheless, even a year later the issues at stake had still not been satisfactorily resolved. Propelled by the principle of 'last resort', the RANF (now the ANF) organised yet another mass meeting, this time for 30 October 1986, and it was here that the decision to strike 'indefinitely' was finally reached. Thus, less than three years after the removal of the 'no-strike' clause from the RANF's rules, an historic fifty-day-long nurses' strike took place (unprecedented in Victoria, and indeed in the Southern Hemisphere), affecting 70 per cent of Victoria's public and private hospitals.

While the central issues of the strike were long-standing, they were by no means extraordinary. I suspect they were thoroughly reminiscent of those for which nursing colleagues worldwide have fought in the past, and for which nurses everywhere are continuing to fight (see, for example, Williams 1988, pp. 6–7, 9–14; Bickley 1988, p. 6; *New Zealand Nursing Journal* 1988, p. 12). In brief, the issues at stake included:

1. career structure;
2. wage justice;
3. better nurse–patient ratios;
4. control over admissions and discharges;
5. role in decision making [the Australian Medical Association totally opposed this demand (Gardner and McCoppin 1986, p. 29)]; and
6. better supervision of student nurses (student nurses were often left in charge of wards during night shifts).

The consensus among nurses seemed to be that unless these issues were satisfactorily settled, the mass exodus of nurses from Victoria's hospitals would continue, as would the decline of patient care standards. It was estimated that as many as 56 per cent of registered nurses had already left active practice (Gardner and McCoppin 1986, p. 31). Given the issues at stake, nurses believed their cause to be just, in both professional and moral terms.

Events of the strike

As the strike progressed, nurses found themselves just as much victims of the strike as they stood to be its beneficiaries. The government threatened striking members with professional de-registration, dismissal, pay cuts, criminal charges for withdrawing labour (including charges of manslaughter in cases of patient deaths thought to be directly attributable to the strike), police intervention, and invoking the Essential Services Act (RANF 1986a; RANF 1987; Gardner and McCoppin 1986, p. 33). Meanwhile, previously recruited overseas nurses began arriving (Birnbauer 1986), and it was alleged that during the strike some student nurses were 'pushed out of hospital accommodation' in order to provide residence for these incoming recruits (RANF 1986c, p. 2).

As if the recruitment and arrival of the overseas nurses was not enough, the Government then added 'insult to injury' by publicly announcing a proposal to extend the range of duties carried out by the State's enrolled nurses (SENs) to include those otherwise carried out by registered nurses, such as drug administration, intravenous therapy maintenance, complex dressings, and the like. In effect, what the government was really saying was 'we can do without you' (the registered nurses). Significantly, this proposal was unanimously supported by the Australian Medical Association

(Davis 1986a; Cossar and Evans 1986). The RANF was quick to point out, however, that such an irresponsible move would place SENs in the legally indefensible position of practising outside the level of their skill and training, and thus negligently (RANF 1986e, p. 1; Davis and Menagh 1986b).

Tension between the government and the nurses mounted even further when it was publicly revealed that several hospitals were recruiting 'paid volunteers' to perform essential tasks for their inpatients (RANF 1987, p. 7). Angered by this blatant use of 'scab labour', the RANF agreed to the 'in-principle' support of a variety of non-nursing trade unions — including, among others, the Federated Engine Drivers' and Firemen's Association, the Electrical Trades Union, the Building Workers Industrial Union, and a number of 'blue collar' unions, to name a few (Davis and Menagh 1986a; Davis 1986b). Some nurses feared, however, that the involvement of non-nursing unions would undermine the already seriously tarnished professional image of nursing — a fear which was not unreasonable under the circumstances.

Picket lines, meanwhile, were beginning to have their effect, and hospital supplies were running seriously low. Intent on breaking both the strike and the nurses' morale, the government again threatened police intervention. Initially this angered the police, resulting in a public statement from Victoria's then Chief Commissioner of Police, Mr Miller, to the effect that 'no one had the right to use police as a threat' (Davis and Noble 1986). He went on to point out that the police had traditionally enjoyed an excellent rapport with the nursing profession 'and we propose to keep it that way' (Davis and Noble 1986). This admirable sentiment had evidently changed, however, when senior police took up positions to break the picket lines. Here the peacefulness of the nurses' protest ended.

In one incident, a nurse was removed by police by way of 'pressure being asserted on both carotid arteries in her neck — a technique that the SAS trains its "commandos" to use against enemy forces' (RANF 1987, p. 8). Thus what started as a just and noble cause was suddenly turned into something ugly and obscene. While many nurses received generous donations of food, money (donated to the RANF 'strike fund') and other items, just as many found themselves being evicted from their flats and subjected to physical, verbal and emotional abuse. Some were stood down by their employers (RANF 1986d, p. 2), while others suffered incredible ostracism by family, friends and colleagues. Grotesque cartoons appeared in the daily newspapers. One depicted a nurse with her entrails spilling out over the floor, following a surgical incision performed by a caricature figure of the minister of health dressed in surgeon's garb (see figure 13.1). Another blatantly sexist cartoon depicted the RANF Secretary, Irene Bolger, in bed with David

White, the Minister of Health, with each accusing the other of forcing them 'to do it' (see Figure 13.2).

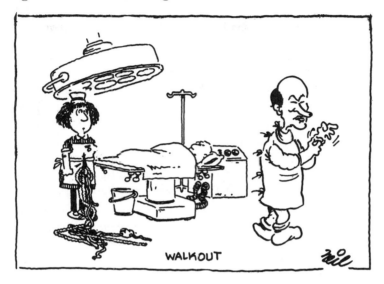

Figure 13.1 Cartoon published during the fifty-day nurses' strike in Victoria in 1986. (Cartoon by Neil, reproduced with permission from the Melbourne *Herald*, 6 November 1986, p. 6)

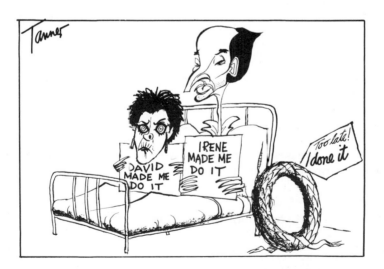

Figure 13.2 During the 1986 nurses' strike, Irene Bolger, Secretary of the Royal Australian Nursing Federation, and David White, Minister of Health, were caricatured in this cartoon by Tanner. (Reproduced with permission from *The Age*, 13 November 1986)

The media accused nurses of being 'unprofessional and ir-responsible', of abandoning or losing their professional ethics, and even of being inspired by Soviet trade unionism (Davis 1986c; Coster 1986). One particularly scathing editorial argued that nurses had engaged in 'industrial terrorism which, trampling on reason, ethics and compassion, turns the sick, the suffering and the scared into expendable hostages' (Forell 1986, p. 13).

Still other media reports piously asserted that there could be no justification for this kind of strike action by nurses, and repeatedly called upon them to end their strike (*The Herald* 1986; Cole-Adams 1986). As a point of interest, the 1988 spate of nurses' strikes in New Zealand met with similar abuses and accusations. In one reported incident, for example, the President of the Auckland Medical Association, Dr Stuart Ferguson, commented publicly 'that prostitutes were being more professional than striking nurses'. A number of prostitutes were quick to express their opinion in a letter to Dr Ferguson, a copy of which was sent to the *New Zealand Nursing Journal*. It reads:

> Thank you for your favourable comparison of the professionalism of prostitutes to that of nurses. We get very little positive comment in the media. We are aware, however, that throughout history nurses have strived to improve our working conditions.
>
> Nurses get one tenth of our hourly wage and often perform less pleasant duties. We therefore support them in their struggle for better working conditions.
>
> Signed: 14 'working girls of 'K' Road'.
>
> (*New Zealand Nursing Journal* 1988, p. 5)

Philosophical and ethical questions

Strike action by essential service workers such as nurses raises a number of interesting philosophical questions. Notable among these are:

1. Under what conditions, if any, might strike action by nurses be justified?

2. Does strike action by nurses necessarily entail a violation of (their) professional ethics?

3. Is strike action by nurses tantamount to an abdication of the profession's responsibility towards upholding the public good (i.e. the health and welfare interests of both immediate patients and the community at large)?

In attempting to answer these questions, let us examine a number of arguments which might be raised against the view that nurses do, in fact, have a just and morally defensible claim to engage in strike action.

Argument 1: *Patients have a right to receive health care in general, and nursing care in particular.* For nurses to withdraw their services as a mark of industrial dispute is seriously to interfere with patients' rights to receive the care they are otherwise entitled to receive. Since strike action by nurses entails violating other people's rights (in this instance, the patients'), it stands as morally objectionable (Rumbold 1986).

Argument 2: *Nurses have a fundamental moral and professional duty to provide safe care to their patients* (Benjamin and Curtis 1986, p. 156). Strike action undertaken by nurses necessarily entails a violation of the principle of safe nursing care. Unsafe nursing care is in itself a moral harm. Nurses who engage in strike action are, therefore, not only failing to fulfil their broader professional and moral obligations (and thus failing to prevent otherwise avoidable moral harm), but are also wittingly violating their professional ethics, and are guilty of actually *causing* moral harm.

Argument 3: *Nurses are morally bound to fulfil their otherwise immediate duties to provide (safe) nursing care.* The purposes of achieving some 'future good' (such as better future work conditions, patient care and the like) are not sufficient to override these more immediate duties, and thus strike action for these purposes can never be morally justified (Muyskens 1982b, pp. 174–5; 1982c).

Argument 4: *Strike action stands necessarily to cause otherwise avoidable (and in some instances irrevocable) harms* — such as patients suffering intolerable pain, deterioration in medical conditions, and even death. Where strike action does result in such harms, it stands as morally condemnable.

Argument 5: *The benefits (for example, improved patient care, better work conditions, salary justice) of strike action by nurses do not always outweigh the harms* (for example, loss of public trust, patient suffering, socioeconomic and political costs). Given this, nurses' strikes are morally unacceptable.

Argument 6: *Strike action by nurses necessarily entails holding patients 'hostage' for the purposes of advancing the nursing profession's interest* (Muyskens 1982b, p. 173). To use patients to further the nursing profession's interests is to treat patients as means to ends of others, or as 'objects', and not as ends in themselves or as entities with intrinsic moral worth. The failure to treat persons (patients) as ends in themselves is to seriously violate the moral principles of autonomy and respect for persons. Strike action which treats persons as means to ends (as objects) constitutes an intrinsic moral wrong.

Argument 7: *It is not the role — much less the duty — of nurses to seek improvements in seriously substandard health care systems.* Improving substandard health care systems is rightfully the domain of doctors, health care administrators and politicians, not nurses. By assuming such a role (or duty), nurses are usurping the moral responsibilities of others.

Argument 8: *Strike action might, in the final analysis, prove thoroughly self-defeating* (Baly 1984, p. 15). Nurses might, for example, find themselves being 'fairly' dismissed from their places of employment, charged with criminal negligence, and becoming the targets of bitter criticism from a mistrustful and unforgiving public. Such 'self-inflicted' harm or professional martyrdom constitutes a significant moral wrong.

Argument 9: *Strike action is not the best possible means of securing better patient care and work conditions for nurses* (Muyskens 1982a, p. 175). Other measures can be taken that might equally secure the benefits that strike action is intent on securing. Given this, strike action is in itself an avoidable harm which nurses are bound, for moral reasons, to reject.

Argument 10: *As professionals, nurses have a duty to serve the public interest and to uphold the 'service ideal'* (Newton 1981; Kelly 1985). To engage in strike action is to break the social contract that the nursing profession has with society, and the tacit promises inherent therein. To break one's contracts or promises (tacit or otherwise) is to commit a moral wrong (Freedman 1978).

Although the arguments raised against the notion of 'just' nurses' strikes are persuasive, they are not entirely unproblematic and are vulnerable to a number of possible counter-arguments. Consider the following.

1. Response to arguments 1 and 10. Since nurses are human beings, they too have fundamental moral interests deserving protection, such as to be respected as persons, to be treated fairly, and to be protected from harm in the workplace. To hold nurses to ransom just because they perform a certain type of work (Stephens 1986), or to deny nurses the right to strike on grounds of the special nature of their work, is to subject nurses to an act of blatant discrimination (i.e. unfair treatment on the basis of some distinguishing or differentiating characteristic that dominant others do not share or value). Where nurses' work conditions exploit them, and patient and/or employer expectations stand to cause them otherwise avoidable harms, employers, patients, and, indeed, society at large forfeit their rights to have the terms of the nurses' 'social contract' honoured, and thus to receive the services that nurses might otherwise be expected to give. Where nurses can demonstrate 'just cause', their right to strike is at least, prima facie, as weighty as the right to strike that others in the community enjoy (Rumbold 1986 pp. 145–6).

2. Response to arguments 2, 3, and 7. The ultimate end of nursing is the welfare of others (in this instance, patients). In upholding the welfare of others nurses must strive to prevent harm and promote good; this includes providing safe and ethically defensible nursing care, and alleviating patients' sufferings. In a seriously substandard health care system, nurses can no longer guarantee either the safety of their patients or the alleviation or prevention of patient suffering. Since nurses form a major component of health care systems, they are necessary contributors to the functionings (or dysfunctionings) of such systems. If nurses do nothing to correct a seriously substandard health care system (of which they are a part), they cannot escape culpability for that system's deficiencies and inadequacies; indeed, as Muyskens (1982a) argues, they sit as accomplices to them. It is morally naive to suppose that nurses do not have any real moral duties to correct the imbalance of moral harms and benefits in such instances. Given this, it is morally defensible to assert that, not only do nurses have a prima facie right to strike, but, in certain instances, they may even have a moral duty to do so. In the light of the morally compelling circumstances supplied by seriously substandard health care, not only would it be wrong to claim that strike action entails a violation of the principle of safe nursing care; it would also be wrong to assert that nurses do not have a duty to work towards some 'future good', particularly when this future good stands necessarily to include the realisation of the principle of safe and therapeutically effective nursing practice.

3. Response to arguments 4 and 5. Patients and the community do not always suffer on account of strike action undertaken by nurses. Indeed, during the Victorian nurses' strike, some claimed that nurse– patient ratios were better (safer) than they had been before the strike! Further to this, unlike other groups who take strike action, the nurses usually stop short of 'total walkouts' and work diligently to ensure that 'skeleton staff' are left to provide emergency and essential care. (As I overheard one nurse say one day, 'Nurses are the only ones I know who go on strike, but stay on duty!') Finally, such a view presumes that the suffering which supposedly occurs during an alleged strike action is greater than that which was already occurring before the strike action. Given the length of hospital waiting lists around the country and the declining quality of care in hospitals following the introduction of case-mix management, there is room to seriously question the validity of such a claim. There is also room to question here whether the harms of strike action do, in fact, outweigh the benefits, given the suffering caused by the dysfunctionings of a substandard health care system.

4. Response to argument 6. To expect nurses to perform demanding and responsible duties without fair reward, and to expect them to endure legally unsafe, physically and emotionally harsh, and even health-hazardous work conditions, is to exploit nurses and to treat them as *social and political slaves*. In short, it is to treat them as means to ends (objects), and not as ends in themselves (entities with intrinsic moral worth), which is, as already argued elsewhere, an intrinsic moral wrong. During just strike action it is not the nurses but the government and its hospital administrators who hold patients political 'hostages'.

5. Response to argument 8. To decline a morally obligatory act is to be morally negligent. To pay undue regard to one's own self-interests is to risk a very serious kind of moral error; it is to treat one's own interests as more deserving than the interests of others just because they are one's own interests, which is open to moral objection. Where a just nurses' strike stands to correct the otherwise avoidable and harmful inadequacies and deficiencies of a seriously substandard health care system, nurses are morally obliged to take such action — even though at some personal cost and inconvenience to self. Where nurses can act to prevent an otherwise avoidable harm from occurring without sacrificing anything of comparable moral importance, they are bound to perform that act (adapted from Singer 1979).

6. Response to argument 9. It is somewhat naively optimistic to suppose that those who are satisfied with a given status quo would be even remotely disposed to settle quickly a table of claims likely to incur significant financial costs. If there were other satisfactory measures for achieving a quick and functional settlement of claims, morality would, of course, compel people to use them. Where such measures are not readily accessible, the 'last resort' principle (i.e. the principle which sets 'moral deadlines') seems as weighty as any other in the face of potentially harmful odds.

Strike action by nurses can be justified in another way, and that is by appealing to certain criteria. Gonsalves (1985, p. 436), for example, argues that, in order for strike action to be just, it must satisfy at least four conditions: it must be for a just cause; it must have proper authorisation (i.e. be freely chosen by striking members, and backed by a democratically elected union body); it must be considered only as a last resort (i.e. after all other possible measures have failed); and, lastly, it must be carried out by rightful means (i.e. the property of others must be respected, protests must be conducted peacefully, and sabotage and violence must be avoided). He further argues that, even in cases where certain harms result, a given strike action can still be regarded as just, provided that:

- the strike action was necessary to bring about an equal distribution of harms and benefits (on this point Gonsalves contends, 'the more painful and widespread the evil, the greater must be the cause [or action] required to balance it');

- the strikers do not intend to bring about the evil or harmful consequences of their actions; and

- the strikers do not intentionally use the bad effects of their actions to bring about the good effects of their employer assenting to the demands made (here the bad effects must only 'accidentally put added pressure on the employer' to accede to the workers' demands).

There is not space here to discuss these criteria at length. It should be noted, however, that these criteria are not entirely unproblematic (particularly those which obviously derive from the doctrine of double effect; for more detailed examination of this doctrine, see chapter 10), and are vulnerable to a number of objections which might be raised against them. Nevertheless, Gonsalves' framework does, I believe, supply an instructive and useful starting point from which the nursing profession can begin to generate sound and morally defensible policies concerning strike action by its members.

Strike action — issues and recommendations

The arguments briefly considered in this discussion succeed, I think, in showing that, contrary to popular anti-strike views, just strikes are not wholly self-interested, and, indeed, can serve very effectively to promote and uphold the interests of others and/or the public good. While striking nurses may well be fighting to have their own interests justly protected, this is not the same as acting purely and simply out of self-interest; these two things are quite distinct and care must be taken to separate them.

In reply, then, to the three questions raised at the beginning of this discussion, there is room to answer, first, that strike action by nurses can be said to be morally justified when it stands, among other things, to prevent an otherwise avoidable harm from occurring or serves to correct a serious imbalance of harms over benefits. Second, given the nursing profession's broader moral responsibilities in terms of preventing harm and promoting good (i.e. alleviating suffering, conducting safe nursing care, upholding the welfare and interests of other human beings), strike action staged as a protest against a seriously substandard and harm-causing health care system does not entail a necessary violation of professional ethics; to the contrary, it upholds such a system of ethics. Third, where nurses succeed in achieving the moral ends of their action, it would be erroneous to hold that a just strike is tantamount to an abdication of the nursing profession's responsibility towards upholding the public good.

Whatever our personal experience or commitments, the decision to either support or refrain from strike action must always be made by way of rigorous and critical moral thinking and the application of sound moral standards. While nurses may well have the courage of their personal convictions, they must not lose sight of having also the courage of their caring. And neither must they lose sight of their duty as professionals to subscribe to a standard of morality 'more exacting' than that of the ordinary person in the street (Himsworth 1953). If nurses are to assert a supposed common right to strike, it must always and only be done on a sound moral basis and within the boundaries of sound moral considerations.

Institutional ethics committees

In March 1988, the Australian Health Ministers' Conference (AHMC) agreed to the establishment and membership of the National Bioethics Consultative Committee (NBCC). The NBCC was later charged with the responsibility of advising the health ministers on the social, ethical and legal issues arising from a full range of bioethical matters. As well as this, the Committee played an important role in offering guidance to the Commonwealth and State governments in the development of policy — particularly in the area of reproductive technology.

As a point of interest, one of the prime movers in getting the NBCC established and working was a registered general and psychiatric nurse, Marie-Louise Evans. Ms Evans was originally appointed Director of the Federal Government's Bioethics Unit. It was through this appointment that she acted as the NBCC's first executive director, and it was under her directorship that the Committee had its inaugural meeting in August 1988. In 1991, however, the Federal Government disbanded the NBCC, and its (the NBCC's) responsibility for advising the Government on bio-ethical issues was transferred to the National Health and Medical Research Council (NH & MRC) (*Bioethics News*, July 1991, p. 1).

At its 106th Session, in 1988, the NH & MRC approved and later publicly released a discussion paper, *Ethics of limiting life sustaining treatment*, signalling an expansion of its traditional and previously somewhat parochial role to include stimulating 'further discussion of important ethical issues within the community'. This paper raises the issue of patient care ethics committees and the kinds of roles they should play. The NH & MRC (1988) makes plain its recommendation:

> ... that patient care ethics committees in hospitals should be available to provide information, discussion of options, expert opinions and counsel for both patients and care-givers, but should never determine and direct what is to be done in any situation.
>
> (National Health and Medical Research Council 1988, p. 14)

Meanwhile, some Australian hospitals, residential care homes and other community-based health care agencies have already taken the initiative to establish ethics committees and others are rapidly following suit. The primary function of these ethics committees is to deal with the ethical issues arising from patient/client care, as opposed to the function of the more traditional institutional ethics committee, which has been primarily to approve, monitor, and/or disapprove *experimental human research projects* (see McNeill et al. 1990).

In most cases the workings of ethics committees remain concealed from the public eye; sometimes, however, their workings are made glaringly public, as occurred in the historical 1988 case of Mrs N, involving a 39-year-old woman suffering end stage motor neurone disease (Wilmoth and Pirrie 1988). Mrs N died after the St Vincent's Hospital medico-moral committee (alias institutional ethics committee) approved her conscious and rationally competent request to have the ventilator supporting her life removed (Cossar 1988). The case was reported as being 'the first time an Australian hospital has removed such a life-support system from a conscious patient to comply with the patient's wishes' (Pirrie 1988, p. 3). It was also probably the first time that an ethics committee had been actively involved in supporting such a request.

These relatively recent initiatives undoubtedly mark the beginning of a new conscientiousness in the Australian health care arena, and a recognition that *the system* (or, rather, those who comprise it) is ill prepared and inadequate to deal with the many moral complexities and controversies arising from orthodox medical practice and health care delivery. Whether institutional ethics committees will be the panacea for all the moral ills plaguing the health care system, however, remains to be seen. It is difficult to avoid asking the additional question: 'Will institutional ethics committees really help? Or will they emerge as little more than health care's "white elephants", as one writer warns that they might (Blake 1992)?'

Experience in the United States has shown that institutional ethics committees *can* help, and in a highly significant way. It has also shown, however, that the success of any given institutional ethics committee is conditional on a number of factors, notably its function, composition, authority/power, and accessibility. It is to examining these factors that this discussion now turns.

What is an institutional ethics committee?

In discussing the issue of institutional ethics committees, it is important first to be quite clear about what is being referred to. There is, for example, a common tendency for 'institutional ethics committee' to be used as a generic term for other health care institutional committees that are clinically oriented, such as critical care committees, organ transplant committees, research committees, optimal care committees, and prognosis committees (a tendency which, as a point of caution, can be misleading). As Brodeur (1984, p. 233) correctly points out: 'using the misnomer "ethics committee" to describe a committee whose function is different, muddles the medical decision making process'. It could be added here that it also 'muddles' the ethical issues at hand and creates the very real risk of ethical issues, once again, being translated into technical problems warranting clinical solutions.

Carol Levine defines a hospital ethics committee as:

> a group established by a hospital or health care institution formally charged with advising, consulting, discussing, or otherwise being involved in ethical decisions and policies that arise in clinical care . . . The committee may serve the entire hospital or a special unit, such as a neonatal intensive care nursery or a cardiac intensive care unit.
>
> (Levine 1984, p. 9)

While this is not the only definition of a hospital or institutional ethics committee, it is nevertheless an apt one, and it is thus the one which will tentatively be relied upon in this discussion. As a point of clarification, the notion of an 'institutional ethics committee' is to be distinguished from what I shall later refer to as a 'patient care ethics committee'.

Factors influencing the rise of institutional ethics committees

There are many factors which have contributed to the rise of institutional ethics committees. Special institutional ethics committees were formed in the United States as early as the 1920s to review sterilisation decisions, and in the 1950s to review abortion decisions (Levine 1984, p. 9). It was not until the mid-1970s, however, owing to the much publicised Karen Quinlan case (Muir 1978; Hughes 1978; Ross et al. 1986, pp. 5–8), that interest in institutional ethics committees began in earnest. This interest was primarily sparked by the New Jersey Supreme Court's decision in the Quinlan case, which made it clear:

> that the issue at stake was not definition of death, but rather the decision to stop treatment on one who has suffered serious neurological injury.
>
> (Veatch 1977, p. 22)

The next few years saw interest in institutional ethics committees heighten as physicians began to be charged with first degree murder for removing, at the request of the family or patients, life-supporting care and treatment (Cranford and Doudera 1984, p. 13). As doctors began increasingly to recognise their legal vulnerability (La Puma et al. 1988), and as nurses began to feel increasingly frustrated with having 'nowhere to go when confronted by ethical dilemmas' (Cranford and Doudera 1984, p. 15), so too the institutional ethics committee movement gained support, and eventually saw the establishment of working ethics committees in hospitals across the United States (see also Ross et al. 1986).

Factors influencing the rise of institutional ethics committees in Australia are similar to those which have influenced the American scene. With the increasing sophistication of medical technology has come increasing legal and public pressure to meet perceived legal and moral standards of care. The patients' rights movement is witnessing the rise of a public more willing and able to assert its rights to, in and against health care, together with the passage of major legislative reforms to protect these rights (Consumers' Health Forum of Australia 1990). And a more liberally educated health care work force is seeing the rise of a collective attitude demanding that moral/ethical considerations be given at least as much attention, if not more, as scientific considerations when making health care and medical treatment decisions. Inquiries into options for dying with dignity, patients' rights, medical malpractice, psychiatric care, the care of the aged and the disabled, and similar issues, have also created a greater awareness in both the professional and the lay communities of the need for developing reliable mechanisms for ensuring just decision making in health care contexts, and particularly in cases involving patient/client care.

Institutional ethics committees are a relatively new phenomenon in Australia. Some committees have been functioning for only a few years and, even then, only on an ad hoc basis, and have yet to receive mainstream support from the medical profession and hospital administrators. Doctors fear that the committees will erode their authority (Levine 1977, p. 26; McCormick 1984; Rudd 1992), and personal sources indicate that nurses are continuing to find that their presence on existing ethics committees is not wholly welcomed by dominant and conservative medical practitioners and hospital administrators. Academics, meanwhile, squabble about the merits and demerits of institutional ethics committees generally, and about what can and should be done to ensure that they achieve desired moral ends (Levine 1977 and 1984; Veatch 1977; Noble 1982; Randal 1983; McCormick 1984; Kuhse and Singer 1985; Kuhse 1988; Blake 1992).

Whatever the uncertainties and criticisms generated by the institutional ethics committee movement, the fact remains that Australia's State governments and hospitals are already committing themselves to supporting the establishment of working ethics committees and to taking the activities and findings of these committees seriously. Yet whether this commitment is well placed depends at least partially on what is expected of these committees, and how well they will in fact fulfil their given tasks. This raises the following questions.

1. What role or function should an institutional ethics committee have?

2. What authority and power should institutional ethics committees generally have?

3. Who should serve on institutional ethics committees?

4. Who should have access to them?

5. Do institutional ethics committees really work (i.e. what are their merits and demerits)?

6. Of what significance are institutional ethics committees to the nursing profession?

1. THE ROLE AND FUNCTION OF INSTITUTIONAL ETHICS COMMITTEES

There has been much debate on what the proper function or role of the institutional ethics committee should be (see, for example Levine 1977, 1984; Veatch 1977; Freedman 1981; Caplan 1982; anonymous 1983; Cranford and Doudera 1984; McCormick 1984;

Youngner et al. 1984; Blake 1992). Debate has centred on whether its function should be *decisional* (i.e. deciding morally hard cases); *prognostic* (i.e. establishing prognostic criteria and determining what a patient's actual prognosis is); *monitoring* (i.e. establishing quality assurance programs and evaluating health care practices); *advisory* (i.e. advising and supporting others on how and what to decide); *educational* (i.e. running workshops, seminars and conferences aimed at addressing ethical issues arising in clinical practice and preparing health providers to deal with these better); or a combination of all five.

Interestingly, the response in the philosophical literature has been almost unanimously supportive of the institutional ethics committee having a multi-purpose/multi-faceted role:

- *as a consultative/advisory/supportive mechanism* for assisting individuals (whether care givers or care receivers) to make their own moral decisions, and to help ensure that the decisions they make are reasonable and fair;

- *as an education and resource facility* aimed at preparing individuals and groups to better deal with moral problems and moral conflict in clinical practice (activities to be undertaken here include grand round discussions, seminars, workshops, and conferences, with a particular focus on ethical issues arising from clinical practice);

- *as a mechanism for policy formulation, development and review* (i.e. scrutinising past and existing policies for their moral adequacy and acceptability, and identifying areas where policy is lacking or where new policy is required, as in such areas as NFR procedures, the use and withdrawal of life-saving treatment, conscientious objection, and the like);

- *as a forum* where individuals can express their concerns and views without fear of ridicule or repercussions, and where moral disagreements among staff, patients and families can be aired and resolved;

- *as a reviewer of morally troubling (hard) cases*, offering advice and viewpoints to all those involved.

Whatever the role the institutional ethics committee in fact plays, it should never be viewed as being absolute or static in nature, and should always be subject to review as morality and experience demand.

2. THE AUTHORITY AND POWER OF INSTITUTIONAL ETHICS COMMITTEES

As with the question of function, there has also been considerable debate on the kind of power and authority that institutional ethics committees should have. Attention has mainly focused on whether the use of these committees and the demand to follow their findings should be voluntary/optional or compulsory/mandatory.

John Robertson (cited in Levine 1984, p. 11), of the University of Texas Law School, suggests that four possibilities are available to a committee:

1. *optional–optional* (it is optional for individuals to approach the ethics committee for consultation and advice, and optional to follow its recommendations);

2. *optional–mandatory* (it is optional for individuals to approach the ethics committee for consultation and advice, but if they do they must carry out its recommendations);

3. *mandatory–optional* (it is mandatory for individuals to approach the ethics committee for consultation and advice, but optional to follow its recommendations);

4. *mandatory–mandatory* (it is mandatory for individuals to approach the ethics committee for consultation and advice, and mandatory to follow its recommendations).

Levine (1984) points out that very few in the United States favour the *mandatory–mandatory* model, and that, in fact, many committees operate on the *optional–optional* model, although not altogether effectively. She also points out that there is mounting political pressure to make some cases the subject of mandatory review — particularly those involving severely disabled newborns, and the chronically and terminally ill from whom doctors wish to withhold life-supporting treatment.

Unfortunately, it is too early to tell at this stage which model Australian health care institutions and agencies will adopt. And it remains a matter of philosophical controversy just which model *should* be adopted. I suspect that the matter will largely be decided not by morality but by law, once questions are raised about the legal accountability of institutional ethics committees and whether and under what conditions they ought to refer 'hard cases' to the courts (see also Levine 1984; Freedman 1981; Ross et al. 1986, pp. 71–105). One possible solution might be to determine — through public debate, negotiation, and agreement — categories of cases which should rightly fall under each respective model. Either way, flexibility in this instance is of the essence in helping to reduce the risk of moral errors occurring.

At present, cases typically brought before institutional ethics committees involve moral dilemmas and moral controversies arising from treating the rationally incompetent, the critically ill and the hopelessly ill (i.e. those with poor prognoses), or in situations where health professionals (most notably treating doctors) are 'uncomfortable' with family demands (Brennan 1988, p. 803). These cases are commonly referred to by health professionals as 'hard cases' — that is, cases which are plagued by moral uncertainty and which are of a nature that defies easy resolution.

3. COMPOSITION OF INSTITUTIONAL ETHICS COMMITTEES

A third major issue to receive considerable attention in the bioethics literature is that pertaining to just who should rightly serve on the institutional ethics committee.

Many have worried that institutional ethics committees would become dominated by those representing the interests of the medical profession and hospital administrators — a fear not without some grounds. For example, a 1984 study in the United States found that 57 per cent of institutional ethics committee members were physicians (Levine 1984, p. 12).

There is general agreement in the philosophical literature that ethics committees should be *interdisciplinary* and should include lay persons independent of the institution. As a point of interest, Australia's National Bioethics Consultative Committee, referred to earlier, took stringent steps to ensure that no *one* professional, gender or age group dominated its membership. Membership was representative of expertise in the areas of science, medicine, health care (other than a doctor), economics, social science, ethics/philosophy, community/consumer interest, law, and moral theology. An effort was also made to ensure complete geographical representation. The committee was not culturally representative, however, and tended to be dominated by people of Anglo–Celtic white Australian backgrounds.

Institutional ethics committees in the United States typically include doctors, nurses, lawyers, social workers, hospital administrators, psychologists, members of the clergy, and at least one non-staff member (Levine 1984; Ross et al. 1986, pp. 37–42). Whether these people are the most appropriate to serve on the committees is a matter of some controversy. First, as Kuhse and Singer (1985) point out, the composition tends to give 'too much power to the institution' (p. 183). Thus, even if 'outsiders' are represented on the committee, there is still the risk of the committee deciding in favour of the hospital's or the institution's interests. Second, there is no guarantee that this kind of composition will in fact result in appropriate and effective moral decision making. While the people represented may well be technically expert, this in no way guarantees their expertise as moral decision makers. As Veatch (1972) has argued in relation to another matter, 'technical competency does not a value judgment expert make' (p. 536). Thus, rather than pooled moral knowledge and competence, such a committee may only yield pooled moral ignorance and incompetence. Third, such a composition may be self-defeating; for example, if all members have radically different views on the matters brought before the committee, they may be quite unable to offer constructive advice and guidance to the people seeking assistance. This is a problem which may be exceedingly difficult to resolve. Fourth, and last, it is not clear why some of these entities should be on an ethics committee at all. While the need for a lawyer can be appreciated (given that some ethical decisions could have serious legal ramifications), and while the need for clinical practitioners (such as doctors, nurses and social workers) can be appreciated (in so far as these people are in a unique position to contribute relevant factual information to the decision-making process), it is far from clear that the presence of a theologian or clergyman is needed. As Dr Swan, producer and presenter of ABC Radio's 'Health Report', is reported as saying:

> I would love to hear a good reason why a Jew should be subjected to an Anglican's view even though he may try to hide his dogma behind an objective gloss. Why should a Catholic be subject to a rabbi or a Hindu to the local priest.
>
> (Voumard 1988, p. 17)

Further to this, Kuhse and Singer (1985) point out that, while 'some experienced ethicists are also members of the clergy', it is not the case that 'all members of the clergy are knowledgeable about ethics' (p. 182). In the light of these and similar comments, it seems that there is no compelling reason for a member of the clergy to be included in the composition of an ethics committee.

Many of the difficulties identified here can be overcome by ensuring that those who are included in the committee's member-ship are morally sensitive and responsible (Freedman 1981), are respectful of the other committee members' views, have good com-munication skills, and have at least a working knowledge of bioethics (Levine 1984) and are able to think critically and use a 'problem-solving approach that is primarily reflective' (Ross et al. 1986, p. 37). Humility and a willingness and ability 'to work co-operatively with people who come from different levels within the hospital hierarchy' are also essential attributes (Ross et al. 1986, p. 38). Youngner et al. (1984) argue further that full cooperation between members is essential if 'resentment, political discord, and dysfunction' are to be avoided. However, even if all these things are attended to, there remains the uneasy feeling that the typical composition of institutional ethics committees might still not be *right*, particularly in terms of their role in advising, and possibly even deciding on behalf of a patient, what is to count as an ultimate 'good'.

A study in the mid-1980s of patient attitudes towards institutional ethics committees found, significantly, that, while 76 per cent of patients surveyed felt that institutional ethics committees 'could be useful', only 12 per cent felt that an ethics committee should 'make the final decision' (Youngner et al. 1984, p. 23). When asked what they thought the 'ideal purpose' of an institutional ethics committee should be, the overwhelming majority (76 per cent) stated that it should be only to 'provide consultation and advice' (Youngner et al. 1984, p. 27). Meanwhile 43 per cent indicated that the committee should become involved only in cases 'where there is disagreement and uncertainty'. As well, 76 per cent felt that 'all patients and family should be automatically informed about the committee's existence upon admission to the hospital'. Also of interest are the patients' views on who should serve on institutional ethics committees: 96 per cent chose physicians, with nurses ranking a close second at 74 per cent. Only 58 per cent thought clergymen should serve, and only 55 per cent thought social workers should serve (Youngner et al. 1984).

Some argue that, in cases of specific patient care dilemmas, perhaps what is called for is not a committee comprised of *hospital and health care agency* care givers, but rather one which is comprised of persons belonging to the *patient's own support group*. Levine (1977), for example, suggests that patients' interests might, in the end, be better served by a committee (a true patient care ethics committee) made up of the patient's own family, friends, clergyman, lawyers, and the like. This seems a most plausible possibility, as long as conditions are carefully defined, and one which should be seriously considered by policy makers and law reformers. Attending health professionals and hospital administrators need not feel threatened by this suggestion, since there need be nothing stopping them from declaring their concerns and interests and imparting their clinical knowledge and other relevant clinical facts to the patient committee. Indeed, there is room to suggest that the only role that attending health professionals and administrators should play is that of giving the relevant clinical information necessary for the patient committee to make an informed choice.

In some respects the new role of the public advocate is already giving legitimacy to the notion of patient representatives (usually family members or friends) assuming some or all of the burden of decision making in hard cases, rather than this task falling solely into the hands of doctors or the health care team or some other bureaucratic mechanism such as the court. In cases where there is no one to assume the burden of decision making, clearly the need exists for a facility, such as an interdisciplinary institutional ethics committee, to help to decide the most morally appropriate course of action to take.

4. ACCESS TO INSTITUTIONAL ETHICS COMMITTEES

The question of who should have access to institutional ethics committees has not been as widely addressed as the other more complex questions have been. Nevertheless, this in no way implies that the question of accessibility is any less important. Interestingly, again, the general view is fairly unanimous, with arguments tending to favour committees being accessible to virtually anyone (patients, staff, families) who requires assistance in working through a moral problem and making moral decisions. Since this is a relatively uncontroversial matter, I do not propose to say anything more about it here.

5. CAN INSTITUTIONAL ETHICS COMMITTEES HELP?

There is increasing evidence that institutional ethics committees and related consultation services are achieving very positive results. La Puma et al. (1988), for example, cite a one-year study involving physicians at a university teaching hospital who used the hospital's ethics consultation service between 1 July 1986 and 30 June 1987. Of those interviewed, 71 per cent of requesting physicians stated that the ethics consultation they had was 'very important' in patient management, 'in clarifying ethical issues, or in learning about medical ethics' (p. 809). Of those physicians who used the ethics consultation service, 96 per cent indicated that they intended 'to request an ethics consultation in the future' (La Puma et al. 1988, p. 809). Significantly, there is a paucity of research on the subject of whether nurses have access to and use ethics consultation services, and, if so, whether they have found them beneficial.

A number of other benefits have also been postulated in the bioethics literature. Brodeur (1984), for example, suggests that institutional ethics committees help to ensure good decision making, which in turn will help to limit the risk of legal liability. More importantly, from a moral perspective, the committees help to re-emphasise *patient care* as *the* central goal of health care practice. Cranford and Doudera (1984), like Brodeur, see institutional ethics committees as ensuring better and more systematic moral decision making. They also see the committees as helping to identify previously unrecognised moral issues on which there is no general consensus, thus paving the way for moral negotiation and the realisation of just moral outcomes. Caplan (1982), on the other hand, sees the benefit of allowing moral expertise to have a place in technical domains as, quite simply, that of improving moral understanding (see also Moreno 1991).

Institutional ethics committees are not without their problems, however. They are obviously unable to *guarantee* the quality and appropriateness of their moral analyses and decision making, and are at risk of merely replacing, rather than changing and improving, the traditional loci of decision making. They are also vulnerable to breeding what McCormick (1984, p. 154) calls 'inhouse protectionism' (i.e. where committee members 'operate protectively for the institution and its practitioners'), 'legal accommodationism' (i.e. where the committee becomes too narrowly focused on the law to the point that ethical considerations become diluted and even lost), and 'oversensitivity' (i.e. where committees become 'oversensitive to the felt need of consensus' to the point where they lose all the moral ingredients which otherwise distinguish them as ethically imperative). McCormick identifies the further concern that institutional ethics committees, by their very nature, may also provide the ultimate breeding ground for 'whistleblowers', particularly if the committee keeps minutes of its activities and findings or documents them in some other way. Just why this should be any more of a problem for institutional ethics committees than it is for any other kind of committee whose proceedings are confidential is not clear; it may even be, as one colleague has suggested, a *benefit*. Another problem is that institutional ethics committees can be rather cumbersome and clumsy — particularly in situations demanding 'a quick response, without prior notice, at any hour of the day or night' (Kuhse and Singer 1985, p. 183).

Such problems are not insurmountable, however, and with careful forethought and planning can be prevented and/or overcome. Australia is at a distinct advantage in that it can look to the experience in the United States and learn from the mistakes made there. (A particularly helpful resource on this matter is Ross et al's [1986] *Handbook for Institutional ethics committees.*) Australia also has the advantage of having the required expertise to draw upon in planning and establishing institutional ethics committees. All that is required now is the intellectual maturity to look to those who have the relevant expertise (and sensitivity) to guide initiatives in setting up ethics committees and evaluating their effectiveness. By doing this, the Australian health care system will move a step closer towards achieving a morally tolerable clinical reality for all concerned.

6. IMPLICATIONS FOR THE NURSING PROFESSION

The last question to be addressed here is: what are the implications of institutional ethics committees for members of the nursing profession?

Possible answers to this question will depend very much on the function, power, composition and accessibility of any given ethics committee. If committees take on a multi-purpose role, as outlined earlier, it is likely that the implications for nurses will be positive. Nurses will have somewhere to go to air their concerns and will gain the opportunity of resolving moral disagreement formally. They will also gain the opportunity of developing a deeper awareness and understanding of moral issues arising from clinical practice and developing their moral problem-solving skills. And they will have the unique opportunity of gaining insights into and understanding of the kinds of moral problems and personal difficulties that other members of the health care team also experience, which will pave the way for more harmonious and interdependent working relationships. If ethics committees adopt only a narrow mono-dimensional role, however, the implication for nurses might not be so positive; indeed, the position of nurses will probably be just as frustrating as it was before any thought was given to the establishment of institutional ethics committees in the first place.

A committee's power and authority perhaps stand to have the most serious implications of all for the nursing profession — particularly in cases involving mandatory review and mandatory compliance. Where mandatory decisions stand to impinge on and infringe standards of nursing care (for example, in cases involving the withholding of food and fluids), the nursing profession will be faced with a serious problem. The only viable option in such cases might be conscientious objection. If, however, the committee is charged with the responsibility for determining genuine claims of conscientious objection, the viability of this option may be considerably reduced. What this warns, I think, is that careful attention needs to be given not only to the authority and power of an institutional ethics committee, but also to the possible moral costs of its having mandatory authority and power.

Related to this concern is the question of composition. While it is generally accepted in the philosophical literature that nurses should be represented on ethics committees, in practice there is little sympathy for the view (at least, from non-nurses). Nurses are having to 'fight' and play the usual 'games' to gain representation on these committees — something which is quite intolerable and unacceptable. The point — as is made evident throughout this text — is that nurses are just as vulnerable to moral problems and controversies as are doctors and others. As well as this, nurses have very real moral as well as legal responsibilities towards those who require nursing care. It is then right and proper that a 'grass roots' clinical nursing perspective be represented on ethics committees. To exclude a substantive clinical nursing perspective would be to allow the committee to have less integrity than it perhaps should have if it is to function appropriately and effectively as a mechanism for guiding and assisting the resolution of moral conflict in health domains.

The degree of accessibility also has the potential to affect nurse practitioners. If accessibility means that the committee is literally open to all who need it, nurse practitioners need not fear suffering any undue burdens or disadvantages. If access is restricted, however, this would pose a different situation altogether. In the unlikely event of access being restricted, nurses might well suffer disproportionate burdens and disadvantages through not having the opportunity to experience the kinds of benefits that a multi-purpose ethics committee could offer.

If nurses are finding that they are not achieving fair representation on established ethics committees, or are being denied access commensurate with their needs, one solution is for nurses to establish their own working ethics committees. Indeed, many nurses have already established — or are in the process of establishing — their own nursing ethics committees. There are sound justifications for doing this. As I have discussed elsewhere (Johnstone 1992, p. 4.31), unlike the broader institutional or hospital ethics committees, which have as their focus more general concerns relating to patient care and institutional activities, nursing ethics committees focus specifically on the moral concerns and experiences of *nurses*, and on the kinds of moral problems that nurses encounter when planning and delivering nursing care to patients. One of the major advantages of establishing nursing ethics committees is that these can provide nurses with a unique opportunity to identify and examine bioethical issues from a *nursing* point of view, and not from the point of view of those whose dominant interests tend to dictate which ethical issues will be addressed by a broader institutional ethics committee, and how, when, and by whom. This means that nurses can have the 'space', for want of a better word, to identify what *they* consider to be important ethical issues, and to determine how, when and by whom they consider these issues should be addressed. Another major advantage of nursing ethics committees is that these can provide an opportunity for nurses to identify what their (educational, support, policy reform and other) needs are and how these needs can best be met. With broader-based institutional ethics committees, these kinds of opportunities to nurses might not always be available.

Nursing ethics committees are not without disadvantages, however. Indeed, they can fall prey to exactly the same kinds of problems that more general institutional ethics committees can experience. For example, a nursing ethics committee may be lacking in institutional authority, may be lacking in direction, may have a membership which serves the interests more of the institution than of nurses and patients, may be dominated by a particular faction of nurses (for example, nursing administrators), may lack the expertise necessary for dealing with the kinds of ethical problems nurses face in their day-to-day practice, may be plagued by radical moral disagreement among committee members, may be unable or powerless to implement its decisions, may be reluctant to 'rock the boat', and so on. Despite these and like problems, however, the establishment of nursing ethics committees is a welcome and long overdue initiative in Australia. What is also needed, though, is a nursing ethics committee network through which nurses can share their knowledge and experiences; keep each other informed of the activities and achievements of their respective committees; and contribute generally to the achievement of moral practices in the health care institutions and facilities in which they work.

Institutional ethics committees — issues and recommendations

As indicated at the beginning of this discussion, it remains to be seen whether institutional ethics committees will provide the panacea so desperately needed for all the moral ills plaguing health care domains. It is likely that they will not — at least, not on their own — and that they will need to function collaboratively with other mechanisms such as true patient-care ethics committees, smaller-unit ethics committees and ethical consultation services, public advocates, patient representatives, cultural and language interpreters, and even the courts, in order to achieve their goals. This is not to say that institutional ethics committees do not have an important role to play; it merely means that they do not have an ultimate role to play. In the final analysis, the success of any given institutional ethics committee will always depend on the moral commitment, sensitivity and moral competence of those who comprise it, run it and evaluate its activities and outcomes. It will also depend on whether the patient and patient care really are the central goals of the committee, or whether there are other goals such as those of self-interest, profit, and academic or professional prestige resting at the core of its endeavours.

An earlier version of the discussion on strike action was presented as a paper entitled 'Professional responsibility and the dilemma of strike action' at the New Zealand Nurses' Association International Conference, Challenges–options–choices, *held Rotorua, 5 August 1987, in conjunction with the International Council of Nurses' Representatives meeting, Auckland. The paper has been revised for publication in this text.*

An earlier version of the discussion of conscientious objection was presented as a paper entitled 'Conscientious objection and professional obligation — a contradiction in terms?' at the Nursing Law and Ethics, 2nd Victorian State Conference. Dealing with dilemmas, *Monash University, 5 May 1989 (organised by the School of Nursing, Phillip Institute of Technology). The paper has been revised for publication in this text.*

The discussion on institutional ethics committees was presented as a paper entitled 'The role of an institutional ethics committee' at the 14th Australian and New Zealand Scientific Meeting on Intensive Care, Conrad International Hotel, Gold Coast, Queensland 3–6 December 1989.

References

For the reader's convenience, references are arranged under the subject headings 'Conscientious objection', 'Strike action' and 'Institutional ethics committees'.

Conscientious objection

Allen, J. R. (1988). Health care workers and the risk of HIV/AIDS transmission. In *Hastings Center Report, Special Supplement — AIDS. The responsibilities of health professionals*, April/May, pp. 1–5.

Allender, J. and Robinson, P. (1989). Hospital AIDS ban to be outlawed. *The Australian*, 8 March, p. 1.

Almond, B. (ed.) (1990). *AIDS — a moral issue: the ethical, legal and social aspects*. Macmillan, Houndmills, Basingstoke, Hampshire.

Athersmith, F. (1989a). Hospital's ban on AIDS to be made illegal. *The Age*, 8 March, p. 3.

Athersmith, F. (1989b). Four per cent of nurses hurt by needles, survey finds. *The Age*, 5 May, p. 3.

Beard, B., Lester, L., Ivy, S. and Prince, N. (1988). Obstetrical nurses' attitudes about AIDS: an international study. *4th International Conference on AIDS. Book 1: Final program. Abstracts, Monday June 13, Tuesday June 14.* Stockholm International Fairs, Stockholm, Sweden, p. 505 (no 9116).

Beardshaw, V. (1982). A question of conscience. *Nursing Times* 78 (9), pp. 349–51.

Beauchamp, T. L. and Childress, J. F. (1989). *Principles of biomedical ethics*, 3rd edn. Oxford University Press, New York.

Benn, S. I. and Peters, R. S. (1959). *Social principles and the democratic state*. George Allen & Unwin, London.

Brennan, L. and the editors of *Nursing 88* (1988). The battle against AIDS: a report from the nursing front. *Nursing 88* 18 (4), April, pp. 60–4.

Broad, C. D. (1940). Conscience and conscientious action. First published in *Philosophy*, volume 15; reprinted in J. Feinberg, *Moral concepts*, Oxford University Press, Oxford, 1969, pp. 74–9.

Broad, W. and Wade, N. (1982). *Betrayers of the truth*. Oxford University Press, Oxford.

Brown, B. L. and Brown, J. W. (1988). The third international conference on AIDS: risks of AIDS in health workers. *Nursing Management* 19 (3), pp. 33–5.

Childress, J. F. (1979). Appeals to conscience. *Ethics* 89, pp. 315–35.

Crabbe, G. (1988). The lonely dilemma. *Nursing Times* 84 (9), p. 18.

Curtis, M. (1989). Nurse AIDS anger. *The Sun*, 10 March, p. 3.

Fitzpatrick, F. J. (1988). *Ethics in nursing practice: basic principles and their application.* The Linacre Centre, London.

Fletcher, J. (1966). *Situation ethics.* SCM Press, Bloomsbury Street, London.

Garnett, A. C. (1965). Conscience and conscientiousness. First published in *Rice University Studies,* volume 51; reprinted in K. Kolenda (ed.), *Insight and vision,* Trinity University Press, 1966, pp. 71–83; subsequently reprinted in J. Feinberg, *Moral concepts,* Oxford University Press, Oxford, 1969, pp. 80–92.

Giannoukos, T. (1989). Nurse AIDS fear over needle jabs. *The Herald,* 5 May, p. 3.

Gilmour, J. (1992). *Michael: a mother's battle for the rights of her child.* Little Hills Press, Sydney.

Gonsalves, M. A. (1985). *Right and reason.* Times Mirror/Mosby College Publishing, St Louis.

Hart, H. L. A. (1957). Positivism and the separation of law and morals. *Harvard Law Review* 71, pp. 593–629.

Hart, H. L. A. (1961). *The concept of law.* Oxford University Press, Oxford.

Hicks, C. (1982). Why I am opposing the doctors. *Nursing Times* 76 (36), pp. 1579–80.

Huerta, S. R. and Oddi, L. F. (1992). Refusal to care for patients with human immunodeficiency virus/acquired immunodeficiency syndrome: issues and responses. *Journal of Professional Nursing* 8 (4), pp. 221–30.

Hume, D. (1888 edn). A *treatise of human nature.* Oxford University Press, London.

International Council of Nurses (1973). *Code for nurses.* International Council of Nurses, Geneva, Switzerland.

Johnstone, M.-J. (1988). Law, professional ethics and the problem of conflict with personal values. *International Journal of Nursing Studies* 25 (2), pp. 147–57.

Johnstone, M.-J. (1994). *Nursing and the injustices of the law.* W. B. Saunders/Baillière Tindall, Sydney.

Kant, I. (1930 edn). *Lectures on ethics* (translated by L. Infield and J. MacMurray). Methuen, London. See in particular 'Conscience', pp. 129–35.

Kordig, C. R. (1976). Pseudo-appeals to conscience. *Journal of Value Inquiry* 10, pp. 7–17.

Lester, L. and Beard, B. (1988). Student nurses' fear of AIDS. *4th International Conference on AIDS. Book 1: Final program. Abstracts, Monday June 13, Tuesday June 14.* Stockholm International Fairs, Stockholm, Sweden, p. 504 (no 9113).

Lewy, G. (1970). Superior orders, nuclear warfare, and the dictates of conscience. In R. A. Wasserstrom, *War and morality,* Wadsworth, Belmont, California, pp. 115–34.

Machan, T. (1983). Individualism and the problem of political authority. *The Monist* 66 (4), October, pp. 500–16.

McKenzie, N. F. (ed.) (1991). *The AIDS reader: social, political, ethical issues.* Meridian, New York.

Mill, J. S. (1962 edn). Utilitarianism (reprinted from 1861 edn). In M. Warnock (ed.), *Utilitarianism,* Fontana Library/Collins, London, pp. 251–87.

Miller, C. (1989). Outrage as hospital bans AIDS. *The Herald* (Melbourne), 7 March, p. 1.

Morrell, S. and Miller, C. (1989). Doctors call AIDS summit. *The Herald* (Melbourne), 8 March, p. 1.

Muyskens, J. L. (1982). *Moral problems in nursing: a philosophical investigation.* Rowman & Littlefield, Totowa, New Jersey.

Nowell-Smith, P. H. (1954). *Ethics.* Penguin Books, Harmondsworth, Middlesex.

Nursing Mirror (1984). ECT nurse loses appeal. 158 (24), 20 June, p. 2.

Nursing Times (1982). Secret Wexham report slams Walsh. 78 (38), 22 September, p. 1573.

Nursing Times (1982). MP calls for conscience clause in Bill. 78 (42), 20 October, p. 1738.

Nursing Times (1983). Third nurse sacked over ECT issue. 79 (14), 6 April, p. 17.

Nursing Times (1983). Sacked ECT student presses for new hearing. 79 (32), 10 August, p. 18.

Nursing Times (1986). Health staff avoid nurses tending AIDS patients. 82 (44), 29 October, p. 10.

Nursing Times (1986). Nurse loses appeal over refusing to give ECT. 82 (52), 31 December, p. 7.

Parsons, L. (1982). Why ECT is an ethical issue. *Nursing Times* 78 (9), 3 March, p. 352.

Pirrie, M. (1989a). Maverick tackles doctors in AIDS war. *The Age*, 29 April, p. 2.

Pirrie, M. (1989b). Woman health worker catches AIDS virus from patient. *The Age*, 1 May, p. 1.

Price, T. (1989). New fears on AIDS: hospital ban may spread. *The Sun*, 8 March, p. 3.

Rawls, J. (1971). *A theory of justice*. Oxford University Press, Oxford.

Seeskin, K. R. (1978). Genuine appeals to conscience. *Journal of Value Inquiry* 12, pp. 296–300.

Sipes, C. (1988). Should hospital patients be screened for AIDS? *Nursing 88* 18 (2), February, p. 49.

Staff of the National Health Law Program (1991). Health benefits: how the system is responding to AIDS. In N. F. McKenzie (ed.), *The AIDS reader: social, political, ethical issues*, pp. 247–72.

Sunday Telegraph (1989). Nurse catches AIDS from needle at work. 30 April, p. 3.

Sweet, M. (1989). Australian nurse gets AIDS from infected needle. *Sunday Observer*, 30 April, p. 1.

Timms, N. (1983). *Social work values: an enquiry*. Routledge & Kegan Paul, London. (See in particular chapter 3, 'Conscience in social work: towards the practice of moral judgment', pp. 33–44.)

Urmson, J. O. (1958). Saints and heroes. First published in A. I. Melden (ed.), *Essays in moral philosophy*, University of Washington Press, pp. 198–216; reprinted in J. Feinberg, *Moral concepts*, Oxford University Press, Oxford, 1969, pp. 60–73.

Viele, C., Dodd. M. and Morrison, C. (1984). Caring for acquired immune deficiency syndrome patients. *Oncology Nursing Forum* 11, pp. 56–60.

Vousden, M. (1985). Swallow your pride, or lose your job? *Nursing Mirror* 160 (1), 2 January, p. 23.

Young, E. W. (1988). Nurses' attitudes toward homosexuality: analysis of change in AIDS workshops. *Journal of Continuing Education in Nursing* 19 (1), pp. 9–12.

Strike action

Baly, M. (1984). *Professional responsibility*, 2nd edn. H. M. & M. Nursing Publications, Division of John Wiley & Sons, Chichester, UK.

Benjamin, M. and Curtis, J. (1986). *Ethics in nursing*, 2nd edn. Oxford University Press, New York.

Bickley, J. (1988). Why NZNA supports direct action. *New Zealand Nursing Journal* 81 (3), March, p. 6.

Birnbauer, B. (1986). Government wants to hire 500 UK nurses to ease waiting lists. *The Age*, 30 January, p. 3.

Cole-Adams, P. (1986). As public support fades, the nurses reach a turning point. *The Age*, 12 December, p. 1.

Cossar, L. and Evans, J. (1986). Nurses: wider role closer for 'aides'. *The Herald*, 12 December, p. 1.

Coster, P. (1986). After 39 days in a crisis the doctors battle for patients — the nurses to keep their patience. *The Herald*, 8 December, p. 1.

Davis, M. (1986a). Use nursing aides, AMA urges. *The Age*, 11 December, p. 10.

Davis, M. (1986b). Unions plan strike to support nurses. *The Age*, 26 November, p. 5.

Davis, M. (1986c). Casualty nurses to walk out today. *The Age*, 8 December, p. 1.

Davis, M. and Menagh, C. (1986a). Bans threat as unions back nurses' strike. *The Age*, 19 November, p. 1.

Davis, M. and Menagh, C. (1986b). Nurses angered by aides plan. *The Age*, 13 December, p. 1.

Davis M. and Noble, T. (1986). Threats to nurses upset police. *The Age*, 5 November, p. l.

Freedman, B. (1978). A meta-ethics for professional morality. *Ethics* 89, pp. 1–19.

Forrell, C. (1986). Concerned nurses should walk out on their leadership. *The Age*, 10 December, p. 13.

Gardner, H. and McCoppin, B. (1986). Vocation, career or both? Politicization of Australian nurses, Victoria 1984–1986. *Australian Journal of Advanced Nursing* 4 (1), September–November, pp. 25–35.

Gonsalves, M. A. (1985). *Right and reason: ethics in theory and practice*, 8th edn. Times Mirror/Mosby College, St Louis.

Himsworth, Sir Harold (1953). Change and permanence in education for medicine. *The Lancet* 6790, 17 October, pp. 789–91.

Kelly, L. (1985). *Dimensions of professional nursing*, 5th edn. Macmillan, New York.

Muyskens, J. L. (1982a). Collective responsibility and the nursing profession. In V. Barry (ed.), *Moral aspects of health care*, Wadsworth, Belmont, California, pp. 120–7.

Muyskens, J. L. (1982b). *Moral problems in nursing: a philosophical investigation*. Rowman & Littlefield, Totowa, New Jersey.

Muyskens, J. L. (1982c). Nurses' collective responsibility and the strike weapon. *Journal of Medicine and Philosophy* 7 (1), February, pp. 101–12.

Newton, L. (1981). Lawgiving for professional life: reflections on the place of the professional code. *Business and Professional Ethics Journal* 1 (1), Fall, pp. 41–53.

New Zealand Nursing Journal (1988). Prostitutes support nurses. 81 (4), April, p. 5.

Nursing Times (1988). Nurses urged to strike worldwide. 84 (14), 6 April, p. 5.

Royal Australian Nursing Federation (RANF) (Vic.) (1986a). *Newsflash*. 10 November, Melbourne.

Royal Australian Nursing Federation (RANF) (Vic.) (1986b). *Nurses Action*. September, RANF, Melbourne.

Royal Australian Nursing Federation (RANF) (Vic.) (1986c). *Nurses Action*. October, RANF, Melbourne.

Royal Australian Nursing Federation (RANF) (Vic.) (1986d). *Nurses Action*. November, RANF, Melbourne.

Royal Australian Nursing Federation (RANF) (Vic.) (1986e). *Nurses Action*. December, RANF, Melbourne.

Royal Australian Nursing Federation (RANF) (Vic.) (1987). *Nurses Action.*
February, RANF, Melbourne.
Rumbold, G. (1986). *Ethics in nursing practice.* Baillière Tindall, London.
Singer, P. (1979). Famine, affluence, and morality. In R. A. Wasserstrom (ed.),
Today's moral problems, 2nd edn, Macmillan, New York, pp. 561–72.
Stephens, P. (1986). Should essential workers lose their right to strike?
The Age, 12 December p. 13.
The Herald (1986). The achievement of Irene Bolger. Editorial comment,
2 December, p. 6.
Tschudin, V. (1986). Ethics in nursing: the caring relationship. Heinemann
(Nursing), London.
Williams, G. (1988). Industrial Report. *New Zealand Nursing Journal* 81 (3),
pp. 6–14.
Women's Electoral Lobby (1987). Comment reported in *Victorian Diary
Newsletter* (February), Melbourne.

Institutional ethics committees

anonymous (1983). AMA judicial chairman sees emergence of hospital ethics
panels as an inevitability. *Federation of American Hospitals Review* 16,
November/December, pp. 30–2.
Bioethics News (1991). National Bioethics Consultative Committee disbanded.
10 (4), July, p. 1.
Blake, D. C. (1992). The hospital ethics committee: health care's moral
conscience or white elephant? *Hastings Center Report* 22 (1), pp. 6–11.
Brennan, T. A. (1988). Ethics committees and decisions to limit care. *Journal
of the American Medical Association* 260 (6), 12 August, pp. 803–7.
Brodeur, Rev. D. (1984). Towards a clear definition of ethics committees.
Linacre Quarterly 51 (3), August, pp. 233–47.
Caplan, A. L. (1982). Mechanics on duty: the limitations of a technical
definition of moral expertise for work in applied ethics. *Canadian Journal of
Philosophy,* supplementary vol. 8, pp. 1–17.
Consumers' Health Forum of Australia (1990). *Legal recognition and protection
of the rights of health consumers.* Consumers' Health Forum of Australia,
Curtin, ACT.
Cossar, L. (1988). Hospital helps woman to die. *The Herald,* 22 March, p. 1.
Cranford, R. E. and Doudera, J. D. (1984). The emergence of institutional
ethics committees. *Law, Medicine and Health Care* 12 (1), February,
pp. 13–20.
Freedman, B. (1981). One philosopher's experience on an ethics committee.
Hastings Center Report 11 (2), April, pp. 20–2.
Hughes, Judge C. J. (1978) In the matter of Karen Quinlan. In T. L.
Beauchamp and S. Perlin (eds), *Ethical issues in death and dying.*
Prentice Hall, Englewood Cliffs, New Jersey, pp. 290–8.
Johnstone, M.-J. (1992). *Ethics and Nursing, Module 601E: a distance
education package for registered nurses.* Royal College of Nursing, Australia,
Melbourne.
Kuhse, H. (ed.) (1988). Ethics Committees. *Bioethics News* 7 (4), July, special
supplement.
Kuhse, H. and Singer, P. (1985). *Should the baby live?* Oxford University Press,
Oxford.
La Puma, J., Stocking, C. B., Silverstein, M. D., DiMartini, A. and Siegler, M.
(1988). An ethics consultation service in a teaching hospital. *Journal of the
American Medical Association* 260 (6), 12 August, pp. 808–11.
Levine, C. (1977). Institutional ethics committees: a guarded prognosis.
Hastings Center Report 7 (3), June, pp. 25–8.

Levine, C. (1984). Questions and (some very tentative) answers about institutional ethics committees. *Hastings Center Report* 14 (3), June, pp. 9–12.

McCormick, R. A. (1984). Ethics committees: promise or peril? *Law, Medicine and Health Care* 12 (4), September, pp. 150–5.

McNeill, P. M., Berglund, C. A. and Webster, I. W. (1990). Reviewing the reviewers: a survey of institutional ethics committees in Australia. *Medical Journal of Australia* 152 (March), pp. 289–96.

Moreno, J. D. (1991). Ethics consultation as moral engagement. *Bioethics News* 10 (2), January, *Ethics committees: a special supplement*, pp. 3–13.

Muir, Judge R. (1978). Opinion in the matter of Karen Quinlan. In T. L. Beauchamp and S. Perlin (eds), *Ethical issues in death and dying*. Prentice Hall, Englewood Cliffs, New Jersey, pp. 285–90.

National Health and Medical Research Council (1988). *Discussion paper on the ethics of limiting life sustaining treatment*. NH & MRC, Woden, ACT.

Noble, C. N. (1982). Ethics and experts. *Hastings Center Report* 12 (3), June, pp. 7–9.

Pirrie, M. (1988). Woman's request to stop respirator had legal basis: hospital. *The Age*, 23 March, p. 3.

Randal, J. (1983). Are ethics committees alive and well? *Hastings Center Report* 13 (6), December, pp. 10–12.

Ross, J., Wilson, Bayley C., Michel, V. and Pugh, D. (1986). *Handbook for hospital ethics committees: practical suggestions for ethics committee members to plan, develop, and evaluate their roles and responsibilities*. Americal Hospital Publishing, Chicago.

Rudd, S. (1992). Ethics committees — a forum for nurses? *Australian Medicine* 4 (12), July 6, p. 15.

Veatch, R. (1972). Medical ethics: professional or universal? *Harvard Theological Review* 65, pp. 531–9.

Veatch, R. (1977). Institutional ethics committees: is there a role? *Hastings Center Report* 7 (3), June, pp. 22–5.

Voumard, S. (1988). Ethics committees out of kilter with public opinion, says doctor. *The Age*, 18 May, p. 17.

Wilmoth, P. and Pirrie, M. (1988). Whose life is it anyway? *The Age* (Saturday Extra), 23 April.

Youngner, S., Coulton, C., Juknialis, B. W. and Jackson, D. L. (1984). Patients' attitudes toward institutional ethics committees. *Law, Medicine and Health Care* 12 (1), February, pp. 21–5.

Chapter

14

Where to from here?

IN THE PREFACE OF THIS TEXT IT WAS argued that the outcome of the bioethics debate will depend not only on its content, but also on who leads it, who contributes to it, whose interests are at stake, and how wisely it is conducted. It was contended that, unless nurses have a working knowledge of bioethics and actively respond to the ethical issues arising from nursing practice, they will continue to find themselves in the intolerable position of having to comply with questionable standards of behaviour imposed on them by others, and will thereby be further constrained in their attempts to deliver morally responsible and accountable nursing care.

The examples given in this text have shown that the bioethics debate has been less than impartial because it has been over-whelmingly dominated by the views and values of society's controlling — mostly male — elite, including doctors, philosophers, judges, politicians, and media editors. They have also shown that nurses have had to and are continuing to bear intolerable moral, legal, professional and personal burdens on account of these dominant views and values shaping the content and conclusions of ongoing bioethical debates — particularly those concerning the issues of abortion, euthanasia, organ transplantation, and patients' rights. Equally significantly, these examples have shown that bioethics has been transformed — undesirably in my view — into a political issue capable of having electoral repercussions. The danger of this is, of course, that the development of social policies on ethical issues might be unduly influenced by public opinion, which, as we have seen, is not always a reliable moral guide.

The moral, legal, professional and political consequences of failing to contribute a substantive nursing perspective to current and future bioethical debates are already proving disastrous for both nurses and patients. This emphasises the point that nurses cannot afford to be either complacent about or ignorant of bio-ethical issues and their potential to affect — sometimes positively, sometimes negatively — standards of nursing care. Merely being aware about the impact of bioethics on nursing standards, however, is not enough; much, much more is required of the nursing profession and the individuals who comprise it. In this final chapter, a number of recommendations will be outlined and suggestions made on how the nursing profession can better prepare its members to function as ethical professionals and, further, how it might better prepare itself to contribute substantially to the bioethics debate. The recommendations and suggestions given will be considered under the respective areas of education, research, lobbying, and policy and law reform. It should be noted that these headings are not intended to represent any particular order or priority. All are of equal value and importance, and are mutually interdependent and reliant on one another. For example, without education, there cannot be an informed awareness of the issues at hand and the ability to conduct research on these; without education and research, there cannot be effective lobbying; without effective lobbying, there cannot be meaningful policy and law reform; without constructive and meaningful policy and law reform, there cannot be change; and so the circle turns.

Education

Crucial to the ability of nurses to practise as ethical professionals is a substantive ethics education aimed at preparing them to uphold the demands of a sound professional ethic and to deal effectively with moral problems in the workplace. Without appropriate moral education, nurses will not be able to function effectively as moral practitioners nor contribute effectively to resolving moral problems in the contexts in which they work. As I hope this text has shown, without at least a working knowledge of bioethics (its theories, terms, concepts, principles, and the practical application of these), nurses are at risk of making serious moral mistakes in the course of planning and delivering nursing care. At least three questions arise here, notably:

1. What should be taught in nursing ethics courses?
2. How should it be taught?
3. Who should teach it?

1.   What should be taught?

In identifying the content of moral education for nurses, it is important to recognise that many of the ethical problems faced by nurses are quite distinct from those faced by doctors (Pence 1983, p. 373; Hilliard 1990). It would, then, be quite misleading to suggest that the moral education of nurses should be based on 'lessons learned from examining physician-related dilemmas', or to suggest that the lessons learned from medico–moral problems (as opposed to nursing–moral problems) can always be meaningfully applied in nursing contexts. This is not to say that nurses and doctors do not share similar moral problems or that they cannot learn from each other's experiences — quite the reverse: it means, simply, that moral education must be *relevant to* and fully *cognizant of* the kinds of moral problems that arise from *nursing practice* and thus from what *nurses are actually experiencing* or are likely to experience at some stage during their professional nursing careers.

One particular concern which nursing ethics courses need to take into account involves the special problems arising from power conflicts (Beauchamp and Childress 1983, Preface). As Yarling and McElmurry (1986) point out, the authority and power that superiors and institutions have over a nurse can seriously restrict a nurse's ability to act as an autonomous moral agent. A second important concern which nursing ethics courses need to address is that of developing appropriate moral attitudes as an essential ingredient of ethical nursing care (Kitson 1987). Unfortunately, not all of us are born with an appropriate moral attitude; as moral psychology and cultural anthropology would probably tell us, this is as much a product of conditioning and life experience as it is of inherent disposition. What this instructs is that moral education should aim not only at developing nurses' moral reasoning and decision-making skills, but also at developing their moral sensibilities and their personal sense of moral responsibility.

A third consideration is that there needs to be a major change in thinking about ethics — its nature, content and ultimate ends. Among other things, it is important to understand that ethics — and, more specifically, bioethics — is not just about how to apply moral principles or how to solve the 'big' moral questions in health care, such as those which are commonly associated with exotic issues such as abortion, euthanasia, organ transplantation and reproductive technology. Ethics is also fundamentally about how to *be* moral, and about how to encourage a more reflective, sensitive, aware, knowledgeable empathetic, compassionate, kind, caring, just, wise and humane way of being, deciding and acting in health care contexts (see also Solomon et al. 1991). It is also about recognising human vulnerability and being committed, at a very personal level, to responding in appropriate ways to remedy this vulnerability, to overturn the conditions contributing to it, and to prevent the avoidable suffering that can and does occur as a result of it being exploited, overlooked or ignored.

What, then, should nurses be taught in nursing ethics courses? As with any subject, it is important that attention be given to both theory and practice. The theory component, however, ought to be kept at a level substantial enough to provide a basis for sound moral decision making, but not so theory-based as to overwhelm students and cause them to lose sight of the practical issues needing to be addressed, or even to lose interest in the topic altogether.

It is important to remember that the aim of ethics courses for nurses is not to transform them into nurse-ethicists (this requires a specialist education program of its own), but merely to give them a working knowledge of ethics which can be used and relied upon to help resolve moral problems arising from nursing practice and to guide ethical conduct generally. I would suggest that the level of theory given in this text is more than sufficient for the purposes of nursing ethics courses. In the case of undergraduates, the material may need to be reduced, depending on the learning abilities and needs of the group.

It is important that the practical issues discussed in nursing ethics courses be relevant to the nurse practitioner's area of practice and experience, otherwise nursing ethics education will not be seen to be meaningful. The content of this text reflects issues which have been consistently raised by the thousands of nurses I have spoken to at various seminars, workshops and conferences around Australia, New Zealand and Singapore, and to whom those reading this text owe a debt of gratitude. The issues chosen here, however, are by no means an exhaustive selection, and I acknowledge that nurses specialising in given areas are likely to have an interest in a number of other bioethical issues besides those covered here. Midwives, and maternal and child health nurses, for example, would be likely to have an interest in the ethical issues arising from, for example, in vitro fertilisation, surrogacy, contraception, adoption, genetic engineering and therapeutic genetic manipulation, women's health, children's rights, child abuse, mandatory reporting, counselling, and research investigating these issues. On the other hand, nurses specialising in psychiatric nursing would probably be more interested in the ethical issues arising from, for example, culpable and exculpable 'unreason' (madness); the uses and misuses of psychosurgery, electroconvulsive therapy, psychotropic drugs and behaviour modification programs; suicide; involuntary treatment; and the political misuse of psychiatry. Those practising as theatre nurses would want to explore more fully such issues as sterilisation and abortion, organ transplantation, allocation of scarce resources and malpractice. Nursing administrators might benefit from a course examining ethical issues arising from, for example, staff appointments (including selection criteria), promotion (including promotional criteria) and dismissal; peer review and staff appraisal mechanisms; professional reference writing; racism and sexism in the workplace; budget allocation; complaints procedures; and similar issues.

A golden rule in any given nursing ethics course is that it must be flexible enough to allow *need* (including community need) to determine content, but firm enough to ensure that those undertaking the course emerge with the moral skills necessary to function as ethical practitioners. Such an approach, however, clearly requires that the lecturer taking such a course be highly skilled and knowledgeable about the subject matter under discussion. On this point, it is questionable practice to allocate the task of teaching ethics to someone who is 'interested' in the topic but has no appropriate qualifications to teach it — a point to which I shall return shortly.

2. How should ethics be taught?

The question of how ethics should be taught (and, indeed, *whether* it can be taught!) is a matter of some controversy (see, for example, Carse 1991; McCullough and Jonsen 1991; Solomon et al. 1991; Waithe and Ozar 1990; Goodpaster 1982; Mahowald and Mahowald 1982; Arcskar 1977; Cochrane et al. 1979). In addressing this question it would be wise to consider the example set by the great Greek philosopher and teacher, Socrates. Socrates' method of philosophical reasoning encouraged dialogue, discussion and critical thinking among his students. As discussed in chapter 6 of this text, Socrates' aim was not to rebut but 'to show people how to think for themselves'. Given the well tested Socratic method of teaching (a method which, incidentally, has been used by the Harvard law and business schools since the 1930s), there is room to suggest that the first golden rule in the *how* of teaching ethics to nurses is: encourage open dialogue and discussion, stimulated by carefully planned questions aimed at showing the students/nurses how to think for themselves. This, in turn, needs to be backed up by strategies aimed at instilling in students/nurses a sense of confidence in their own thoughts. One way of achieving this is to take care not to 'rebut' their views, and to show them that what they have to say is just as valid as what anybody else has to say — an approach which I have found to be enormously successful with both undergraduate and postgraduate nursing students.

On a more practical level, and drawing on the experience of teaching ethics to students in undergraduate and postgraduate nursing ethics courses, I have found short (12–15-minute) and full-length videos depicting both real-life and hypothetical case scenarios, newspaper clippings, television and media reports, and real-life anecdotal case studies from the students themselves, extremely appropriate and useful in helping students to learn to recognise moral problems in the workplace, as well as to analyse these, identify possible solutions, and plan an effective course of action for dealing with them. This has also served to stimulate their interest in the topics under discussion — for the simple reason, I believe, that the cases presented are all realistic. Such teaching strategies and methods have proved successful in assisting nurses to gain the skills they require to be more effective moral decision makers, moral mediators and moral negotiators in patient-care contexts.

One question which I am commonly asked is: should ethics be taught to nurses as a discrete subject or as an integrated subject? There is, I believe, a strong case for teaching ethics as a discrete subject, for reasons which I hope this text has made self-evident. For one thing, teaching ethics as a discrete subject allows full attention to be given to the intricacies of ethical reasoning and to coming to terms with the implications of bioethical issues for nursing practice. Further to this, as already mentioned, ethics is after all a *distinct* discipline of its own — something which many nurses have yet to appreciate fully. At a seminar I was conducting recently, for example, a registered nurse commented to me: 'It's such a pity you can't *do* ethics.' When I asked what she meant by this comment, she replied: 'Well, you can't go to a university and just study it, can you . . .? It took quite some minutes for me to clarify that ethics can most certainly be studied, and that courses are available through the philosophy departments of most universities. This experience was both enlightening and concerning, in several ways: first, it made me realise that some nurses do not have a very good understanding of the nature of ethics as a discipline, and, second, there still seems to be a prevailing view among some nurses that ethics is merely a matter of personal opinion, and thus not something warranting serious attention, either in nursing education programs or in other professional nursing domains.

Teaching ethics as an *integrated* subject also carries certain benefits. One advantage is that it allows students to become familiar with the relevance and application of ethics across the spectrum of nursing practice. One major disadvantage of this approach, however, is that many nurse educators/lecturers are simply not appropriately qualified to teach ethics in their respective lecturing areas. This can have the unfortunate consequence of students being misled in their moral thinking, sometimes with disastrous consequences. Another major difficulty is that it does not allow students to gain a firm basis upon which they can build their moral knowledge.

My own view is that there are advantages in teaching ethics to nurses *both* as a discrete *and* as an integrated subject — provided the students have had some practical experience beforehand to enable them to relate to the subject matter being taught and to contribute to the discussions being advanced. I have found that undergraduate students who have had at least eighteen months' experience are better able to deal with ethics lectures than those who are novices to an undergraduate nursing program.

Like other areas of nursing education, it is important that moral education be an ongoing process. It would be concerning if graduates left a course with the impression that when they have completed a given nursing ethics subject they know all there is to know on the matter. The ongoing moral education of nurses can be facilitated in many ways. These include the now familiar activities of ethics workshops, seminars and conferences — all of which also provide an important and unique opportunity for sharing knowledge, ideas and experiences. Another valuable mode of ethical education is through conducting ethical rounds in the clinical area, a practice which is becoming increasingly popular in hospitals in the United States.

3.   Who should teach ethics?

In some respects, the question of 'who should teach ethics?' is a trivial one, and some might wonder why I have raised it at all. The answer to this is very simple: the nursing profession is faced with the problem of not having many nurses who are appropriately qualified (by which I mean dually qualified in both nursing *and* philosophy/ethics) to teach bioethics to nurses. One unfortunate consequence of this has been that nursing students have received only a very limited moral education, or a misguided moral education, or, in cases where no lecturer was available, no moral education at all.

Some nursing education programs have overcome the problem of 'who should teach' by having moral philosophers from other departments on campus to teach the ethics component of the nursing curriculum. While there are advantages in having moral philosophers involved in teaching nurses (see, for example, Beauchamp 1982; Singer 1982), there are also disadvantages. For instance, moral philosophers (like most people in the community) tend to have a very poor understanding of the nature of nursing practice and of the special kinds of moral problems that nurse practitioners all too frequently encounter when giving nursing care.

I would further suggest that philosophers who do not have a good understanding of the kinds of moral issues and problems nurses face will find it difficult to make their material meaningful and relevant to nursing students. This might, in turn, have the unfortunate consequence of the students simply 'switching off' — as did happen to one moral philosopher teaching ethics in the first-year program of an undergraduate nursing course.

Another disadvantage is that philosophers may attempt to educate nursing students in the classical rationalistic tradition at the expense of other moral viewpoints — such as those considered in chapters 4 and 5 of this text. As I have already discussed the problem of the incompatibilities between Western moral philosophy, feminist moral theory, transcultural ethics and holistic nursing philosophy in this text, I shall not say anything more on it here.

Research

There is an appalling lack of nursing research in both Australia and New Zealand on ethical issues arising from nursing practice. This has made it very difficult for nurses to speak authoritatively on the many moral problems they face in health care contexts. Just why this neglect has occurred is a matter for speculation. It may be because few nurses are knowledgeable enough about the bioethics movement generally, and about nursing ethics in particular, to undertake research in this area. Another reason is that nursing research groups have yet to recognise ethics as a distinct and separate area of inquiry, and thus one warranting its own research agenda. Jameton and Fowler (1989), however, suggest that the neglect of scholarly philosophical/ethics research in nursing can also be linked to the popular though mistaken view that scholarly research is not 'proper' research — unlike empirical research, which is seen to conform fully with traditional definitions of 'research'. Fortunately, this view is beginning to change.

At present, nursing research interests are typically divided into three main categories, namely, administration, clinical practice, and education. While it is appreciated that ethical issues arise in all three of these areas of nursing, this is not enough to justify denying ethics a research category of its own. Until the nursing profession starts to give ethics prominence on its own agenda, there is room to speculate that there is little chance of it being given prominence on the agendas of others — much less those controlling the bioethics debate, and, of course, the resulting law and policy reforms. The direction the nursing profession would be well advised to take on this matter is, I think, self-evident. This text has identified some of the issues which warrant investigation, and which would benefit from further formal research, including non-empirical scholarly research, empirical research, or a mixture of both these approaches (see Jameton and Fowler 1989).

Lobbying

The nursing profession has not been very successful in getting its voice heard and in getting the public to understand what nursing ethics is about. We have seen examples in this text of how the nursing perspective on bioethical issues has been conspicuously absent from history, the media, interdisciplinary conferences, and other influential domains of public activity. There can be little doubt that it is time for the nursing profession to develop a well organised action lobby, just as other professional groups have done, to remedy this situation. There is nothing unprofessional or dishonourable about engaging in lobbying activities, and there is no reason for suggesting that the nursing profession should not 'pick up the gauntlet', so to speak. Furthermore, as the National Women's Consultative Council (1988) points out:

> Action can be fun. Even when you know that it's mainly symbolic it's still more gratifying to act collectively than to fume privately. Action means getting together with other people to talk things over, finding out that other people have the same concerns that you have, and then taking those concerns to the people in power and publicly demanding that they do something about it.
>
> (National Women's Consultative Council 1988, p. 4)

As there are already several publications available on how to lobby, including, in particular, the National Women's Consultative Council's *Women into Action* (1988), I do not propose to say anything more about it here. What does warrant mention, however, is that the nursing profession would be well advised to be much better organised than it presently is if it is to make an impact. Among other things, the nursing profession would benefit from having a core group of informed, active, articulate and committed people who can scrutinise and respond to policy-making initiatives, political debate, and media activities (i.e. conduct a media watch). This group could be formally charged with the responsibilities of ensuring that a substantive nursing perspective is sought and fully represented in policy and law reforms. It could also play a fundamental role in coordinating media releases aimed at publicly declaring the nursing profession's position on matters which stand to significantly affect both its own and the public's interests. Unless the nursing profession assumes a much higher public and political profile than it has until now, it may, in the final analysis, find that it is in no position to fulfil its broader moral as well as professional responsibilities towards the community at large.

Policy and law reform

Another area which has been sorely neglected by the nursing profession is that of policy and law reform — an area which I consider to be a primary target for action lobbying by nurses.

However we look at it, the fact is that nurses have suffered intolerable burdens on account of inadequate or inappropriate legal laws and institutional policies (see in particular Johnstone 1994, *Nursing and the injustices of the law*). In the light of the examples given in this text and elsewhere (see, for example, Johnstone 1994), I would suggest that the nursing profession has a significant moral interest in researching the inadequacies and deficiencies of existing legal laws, institutional policies and similar areas, and in actively lobbying for those inadequate and deficient laws and policies to be reformed — or, in cases where laws or policies are intolerable to accountable and responsible nursing practice, even abandoned altogether. The nursing profession would also benefit from identifying areas where policy guidelines are seriously lacking — such as those pertaining to conscientious objection, Not for Resuscitation orders, informed consent, and the withholding of food and fluids. Until policy and law reforms are achieved in these and similar areas, nurses will never be free to practise nursing as they have been taught to practise it, as nursing research suggests it should be practised, and as the public is entitled to have it practised; nor will they be free to be moral — that is, free to practise as morally accountable and responsible professionals (Yarling and McElmurry 1986).

Conclusion

I want to conclude this text by paying tribute to two very special nurses. These nurses have been chosen not because of any great startling deeds they have performed, but because of their enormous integrity as professional care givers, and because they have set a powerful example for other nurses to follow.

The first of these nurses is unknown. She is, however, a real person, and is recorded as once having made an important difference to a patient's well-being and survival. The patient in this instance was none other than the internationally reputed medical sociologist, Ann Oakley. Upon being greatly moved by the action and care of her 'invisible nurse', Oakley (1986) devoted a full chapter to the importance of nurses in her celebrated book, *Telling the truth about Jerusalem* (1986). Oakley had been admitted to hospital for treatment of a tumour on her tongue. She writes:

> I remember silently crying in front of the consultant the day the tumour was diagnosed. All he said was, 'What are you crying about? The treatment won't affect your appearance.' My appearance was not what I was worried about.

> (Oakley 1986, p. 182)

It was after this that, for the first time, despite her fifteen-year career as a medical sociologist studying health services, Oakley became aware of, and began to respect, the contributions nurses make to health care. Like so many others, Oakley had simply taken the presence of nurses 'for granted'.

Oakley's awareness changed when one day, lying in bed with a radioactive implant stitched to her tongue, she realised that her disease might be fatal — an insight which caused her to become acutely distressed. A young nurse entering the room at that moment to collect a lunch tray saw that Oakley was upset and, instead of continuing the task of removing the tray, immediately sat down to comfort and to talk to her. Oakley discussed her fears and worries — most of which derived from a lack of information about the nature of her tumour and likely prognosis. Upon learning of this, the young nurse went immediately to read Oakley's medical history and came back and informed her that, in her 'limited medical opinion' she 'would probably be all right' (Oakley 1986, p. 182).

Discussing the nurse's actions that day, Oakley writes:

> ... she stayed with me for nearly an hour, which she should not have done. I was radioactive and no one was meant to spend any longer than 10 minutes at a time with me. She was also, presumably, not supposed to tell me what was in my case-notes, so she was breaking at least two sets of rules. I never saw this nurse again after I left hospital, but I would like her to know that she was important to my survival.
>
> (Oakley 1986, p. 182)

The personal and professional apology offered by Ann Oakley to the 'invisible nurses' of this world is long overdue. It is difficult to comprehend how a researcher can spend *fifteen years* observing health care contexts and not notice nurses. In fairness to Oakley, she at least has had the integrity to 'admit to a certain blindness with respect to the contributions nurses make to health care' (p. 181), and to offer a public apology — an action which is by no means insignificant.

The truly morally praiseworthy person in this case, however, is not Oakley, but the 'invisible nurse' who broke 'at least two sets of rules' in order to enhance the well-being of a stranger in the grip of unnecessary and avoidable suffering. The moral outcomes of this nurse's simple actions show that one does not always have to be heroic to be moral, but merely *aware of* and *sensitive to* the vulnerability of human beings, and sufficiently committed to patient well-being to take the actions that may be necessary in order to prevent patients from suffering unnecessarily.

The second nurse to whom tribute is owed is widely known, despite some rather extraordinary attempts by the Australian medical profession to have her achievements denied formal recognition. The nurse being referred to here is Elizabeth Kenny, a controversial figure who gained notoriety for her marvellous care and rehabilitation of polio victims during the 1930s (Willis 1979). Predictably, Kenny's methods of care and treatment were not favourably received by members of the Australian medical profession, who clearly felt threatened by what they considered an invasion of their own territory.

Kenny's work, however, had enormous public support, and her methods were widely acclaimed both in the United States and the United Kingdom (Willis 1979, p. 34). Thus, despite fierce opposition from the Australian medical profession, and despite the negative and frankly biased findings of a number of public inquiries (all of which, incidentally, were carried out entirely by doctors) into her methods, various State governments around Australia went ahead and established Kenny clinics.

Gradually the most successful of Kenny's methods were taken over and incorporated into orthodox medical treatments, thus lessening the differences between her own success rates and those of the doctors. Significantly, as Willis (1979, p. 34) points out, the medical profession took Kenny's methods 'without any acknowledgment being given to [her]'.

Like the 'invisible nurse' discussed above, Elizabeth Kenny deserves ultimate moral praise. She defied the rules of convention, and in doing so promoted the health and well-being (moral ends) of thousands of polio sufferers around the world. The moral outcomes of this nurse's somewhat complex actions show, again, that nurses do not necessarily have to be heroic to be moral; sometimes it is enough just to be committed, shrewd and determined. The Kenny experience also shows the importance of nurses having public support (something which Florence Nightingale recognised long ago).

Where to from here? The answer is: to *doing*. To *doing* whatever needs to be done to make health care contexts morally tolerable — whether in a patient's own home, in the community or in an isolated unit of some major university teaching hospital. To *doing* whatever needs to be done to protect people, and to prevent them from suffering unnecessary moral harms. And to *doing* whatever needs to be done to achieve peaceable solutions to the radical moral disagreements which may arise among patients, patients' families, friends, lay carers and health professionals.

Nurses may not be able to change the world. They can, however, make a difference to the way a person experiences it. Whether this experience is hostile or friendly, traumatic or peaceable, painful or pleasurable, depends, in the end, not on science, or even on reason, but on an appropriate moral attitude and on the virtues of human care, compassion, empathy, kindness, friendship, generosity, altruism and love.

References

Aroskar, M. A. (1977). Ethics in the nursing curriculum. *Nursing Outlook* 25 (4), April, pp. 260–4.

Beauchamp, T. L. (1982). What philosophers can offer. *Hastings Center Report* 12 (3), June, pp. 13–14.

Beauchamp, T. L. and Childress, J. F. (1983). *Principles of biomedical ethics*, 2nd edn. Oxford University Press, New York.

Carse, A. L. (1991). The 'voice of care': implication for bioethical education. *Journal of Medicine and Philosophy* 16 (1), pp. 5–28.

Cochrane, D. B., Hamm, C. M. and Kazepides, A. C. (1979). *The domain of moral education*. Paulist Press, New York.

Goodpaster, K. E. (1982). Is teaching ethics 'making' or 'doing'? *Hastings Center Report* 12 (1), February, pp. 37–9.

Hilliard, M. T. (1990). Nursing, ethics, and professional roles. *Hastings Center Report* 20 (1), p. 2.

Jameton, A. and Fowler, M. D. M. (1989). Ethical inquiry and the concept of research. *Advances in Nursing Science* 11 (3), pp. 11–24.

Johnstone, M.-J. (1994). *Nursing and the unjustices of the law*. W. B. Saunders/Baillière Tindall, Sydney.

Kitson, A. L. (1987). A comparative analysis of lay-caring and professional (nursing) caring relationships. *International Journal of Nursing Studies* 24 (2), pp. 155–65.

Mahowald, M. B. and Mahowald, A. P. (1982). Should ethics be taught in a science course? *Hastings Center Report* 12 (4), August, p. 18.

McCullough, L. B. and Jensen, A. R. (1991). Bioethics education: diversity and critique. *Journal of Medicine and Philosophy* 16 (1), pp. 1–4.

National Women's Consultative Council (1988). *Women into action*. CPN Publications, Canberra.

Oakley, A. (1986). *Telling the truth about Jerusalem*. Basil Blackwell, Oxford.

Pence, T. (1983). Nursing ethics. *Teaching Philosophy* 6 (4), October, pp. 373–80.

Singer, P. (1982). How do we decide? *Hastings Center Report* 12 (3), June, pp. 9–11.

Solomon, M., Jennings B , Guilfoy, V., Jackson, R., O'Donnell, L., Wolf, S., Nolan, K., Koch-Weser, D. and Donnelley, S. (1991). Toward an expanded vision of clinical ethics education: from the individual to the institution. *Kennedy Institute of Ethics Journal* 1 (3), pp. 225–45.

Waithe, M. E. and Ozar, D. T. (1990). The ethics of teaching ethics. *Hastings Center Report* 20 (4), pp. 17–21.

Willis, E. (1979). Sister Elizabeth Kenny and the evolution of the occupational division of labour in health care. *Australian and New Zealand Journal of Sociology* 15 (3), November, pp. 30–8.

Yarling, R. R. and McElmurry, B. J. (1986). The moral foundation of nursing. *Advances in Nursing Science* 8 (2), pp. 63–73.

APPENDIX I

CODE FOR NURSES
Ethical concepts applied to nursing, 1973*

International Council of Nurses

The fundamental responsibility of the nurse is fourfold: to promote health, to prevent illness, to restore health and to alleviate suffering.

The need for nursing is universal. Inherent in nursing is respect for life, dignity and rights of man. It is unrestricted by considerations of nationality, race, creed, colour, age, sex, politics or social status.

Nurses render health services to the individual, the family and the community and coordinate their services with those of related groups.

Nurses and people

The nurse's primary responsibility is to those people who require nursing care.

The nurse, in providing care, promotes an environment in which the values, customs and spiritual beliefs of the individual are respected.

The nurse holds in confidence personal information and uses judgement in sharing this information.

Nurses and practice

The nurse carries personal responsibility for nursing practice and for maintaining competence by continual learning.

The nurse maintains the highest standards of nursing care possible within the reality of a specific situation.

The nurse uses judgement in relation to individual competence when accepting and delegating responsibilities.

The nurse when acting in a professional capacity should at all times maintain standards of personal conduct which reflect credit upon the profession.

Nurses and society

The nurse shares with other citizens the responsibility for initiating and supporting action to meet the health and social needs of the public.

Nurses and co-workers

The nurse sustains a cooperative relationship with co-workers in nursing and other fields.

---

* This code was adopted by the ICN Council of National Representatives, Mexico City, in May 1973 Reprinted by permission of the International Council of Nurses, Geneva.

The nurse takes appropriate action to safeguard the individual when his care is endangered by a co-worker or any other person.

Nurses and the profession

The nurse plays the major role in determining and implementing desirable standards of nursing practice and nursing education.

The nurse is active in developing a core of professional knowledge.

The nurse, acting through the professional organization, participates in establishing and maintaining equitable social and economic working conditions in nursing.

APPENDIX II

CONSUMER HEALTH RIGHTS*

The Consumers' Health Forum of Australia promotes the following set of principles, rights and responsibilities to enhance the health rights of consumers individually and collectively within Australia.

Principles

A. We are entitled to a healthy and safe environment in which to live and work. That is:

- our basic needs are met;
- the physical environment enhances our quality of life;
- we are protected from health hazards.

B. We are entitled to adequate, accurate information and education enabling us to make informed decisions which promote health and prevent ill health and disability.

C. We are entitled to participate in the development, monitoring and implementation of social and economic policies and programs.

D. We are entitled to equal access to health services which:

- promote health;
- prevent and alleviate ill health and disability; and
- provide health care.

E. We are entitled to determine whether or not to seek assistance from health workers.

Rights

The Consumers' Health Forum of Australia supports the rights outlined below for all consumers. These rights are not all currently enforceable by law in Australia. The Forum recognises that, in exceptional circumstances, individuals may be unable to exercise their rights. In some cases a person independent of the care giver and institution may be required to act on an individual's behalf.

---

* Reprinted by permission of the Consumers' Health Forum of Australia Inc., Curtin, ACT.

1. I have a right to appropriate, quality health care, when I need it.
2. I have the right to determine what happens to me, including:
   - to choose to leave my condition untreated;
   - to give my explicit consent before any procedure can be carried out;
   - to withdraw my consent to a procedure;
   - to refuse to allow a procedure to be carried out;
   - to refuse health care from a particular health worker (including medical practitioners, allied health professionals and alternative health practitioners);
   - to refuse health care from students;
   - to refuse to participate in research and experiments.
3. I have the the right to an adequate explanation, in terms and language I can understand, of
   - the nature of my ill health and the likelihood of my return to good health;
   - the details of any proposed procedures and therapies (e.g. consultations, tests, examinations, treatment), as well as possible alternatives, including:
   — expected outcome,
   — adverse and after effects,
   — chances of success,
   — risks,
   — costs and availability,
   — whether the procedure is experimental or to be used in research;
   - the results of any procedures which have been carried out and the implication of those results;
   - the possible consequences of not taking the advice of the health worker;
   - the name, position, qualifications and experience of health workers who are carrying out the procedures.
4. I have the right to receive health care in privacy and to be treated with respect and dignity.
5. I have the right to decide who will be present when I receive health care.
   - I can require the presence of other people, including a friend, family member, advocate, interpreter, etc.
   - I can refuse the presence of:
   — health workers not directly involved in my care, — students,
   — researchers, and
   — others, including family members.
6. I have the right to seek information and advice from other sources.

7. I have the right to seek treatment from other health workers of my choice.

8. I have the right to have all identifying personal information kept confidential. Thus no identifying information about me, my condition or treatment will be made available to anyone else without my consent.

9. I have the right of access, and to seek amendment or additions, to all information relating to my health care and condition, either personally or through another person I nominate.

10. I have the right to comment on, or complain about, my health care.

11. I have the right to receive compensation for injuries or illness caused, or aggravated by, health care or health care advice provided by a health care worker.

12. I have the right to refuse admission to, and to leave, a health care facility, regardless of my physical condition or against medical advice, and regardless of whether I have paid the bill.

Responsibilities

Exercising responsibilities in the health system can be as important as exercising rights.

However, there are many areas of life in which people find it difficult to exert control. In many instances consumers find it difficult to make an informed choice.

Nevertheless, it is in our best interests to assume as much responsibility for our health as possible.

After all, it is *our* health at stake!

In order to promote partnership between the consumer and health workers, the Consumers' Health Forum of Australia recommends that consumers:

- provide information that enables the health care worker to provide adequate advice and care;

- actively seek health care information;

- treat seriously any agreement to action chosen in partnership with a health worker;

- acknowledge responsibility for the consequences of their decision to accept or reject advice;

- recognise that choices concerning their lifestyle affect their health;

- advise the appropriate authority of any complaint they may have concerning their health care so that corrective action can be taken.

APPENDIX III

CODE OF ETHICS FOR NURSES IN AUSTRALIA

Introduction

Nursing practice is undertaken in a variety of settings. Any particular setting will be affected to some degree by factors which are not within a nurse's control or influence. These include resource constraints, institutional policies, management decisions, and the practice of other health care providers. Nurses also recognise the potential for conflict between one person's needs and those of another, or of a group or community. Such factors may affect the degree to which nurses are able to fulfil their moral obligations and/or the number and type of ethical dilemmas they may face.

The Code contains six broad value statements. Nurses may use these statements as a guide in reflecting on the degree to which their practice demonstrates the stated value. As a means of assisting in interpretation of the six expressed values, a number of explanatory statements are provided. These are not intended to cover all the aspects a nurse should consider, but can be used as an aid in further exploration and consideration of ethical concerns in nursing practice.

A Code of Ethics is not intended to provide direction for the resolution of specific ethical dilemmas, nor can this document adequately address the definitions and exploration of terms and concepts which are part of the study of ethics. Nurses are encouraged to undertake discussion and educational opportunities in order to clarify for themselves issues related to the fulfilment of their moral obligations.

Nurses are independent moral agents and sometimes may have a personal moral stance which conflicts with participation in certain procedures. Nurses are morally entitled to refuse to participate in procedures which would violate personal moral beliefs (conscientious objection). However, nurses should not refuse involvement if there is any possibility of danger to the life or welfare of any person. Nurses accepting employment positions where they foresee they may be called on to be involved in situations at variance with their beliefs, have a responsibility to acquaint their employer or prospective employer with this fact. Employers and colleagues have a responsibility to ensure that such nurses are not discriminated against in their workplace.

The Code of Ethics will be enhanced by the Code of Conduct presently being developed by the nurse registering authorities. While the Code of Ethics focuses on the morals and ideals of the profession, the Code of Conduct identifies the minimum requirements for practice in the profession and focuses on the clarification of professional misconduct and unprofessional conduct. These two Codes, together with Australian nursing's published practice standards, provide a working framework for nursing practice.

Both the Code of Ethics and the Code of Conduct need to be responsive to the needs and changes within the profession and, in time, these Codes will need to change in relation to changes in nursing and in society. This Code of Ethics will be reviewed within five years, or earlier if necessary.

Preamble

Nurses support and enable individuals, families and groups to maintain, restore or improve their health status, or to be cared for and comforted when deterioration of health has become irreversible. A traditional ideal of nursing is the concern for the care and nurture of human beings regardless of race, religion, status, age, gender, diagnosis or any other ground.

Nursing care is based on the development of a helping relationship and the implementation and evaluation of therapeutic processes. Therapeutic processes include health promotion and education, counselling, nursing interventions and empowerment of individuals, families or groups to exercise maximum choice in relation to their health care. Nurses provide care and support before and during birth and throughout life, and alleviate pain and suffering during the dying process.

The Code of Ethics has been developed for nursing in the Australian context and is relevant to all nurses working in Australia. The Code of Ethics outlines nursing's intentions in practice and is supported by policies and position statements from organisations representing nurses and nursing. The Code of Ethics is complementary to the International Council of Nurses (ICN) Code for Nurses (1973).

Thus, the purpose of this Code of Ethics is to:

- identify the fundamental moral commitments of the profession.

- provide nurses with a basis for professional and self reflection and a guide to ethical practice; and,

- indicate to the community the values which nurses hold.

Code of Ethics

Value statement 1

Nurses respect persons' individual needs, values and culture in the provision of nursing care.

Explanatory statements

1. Nursing care for any individual or group should not be compromised because of ethnicity, gender, spiritual values, disability, age, economic, social or health status, or any other ground.

2. Respect for a person's needs includes recognition of the individual's place in a family and community. Nurses should, therefore, facilitate the participation of significant others in the care of the individual if, and as, the person and the significant others wish.

3. Respect for individual needs, beliefs and values includes culturally sensitive care, and the provision of as much comfort, dignity, privacy and alleviation of pain and anxiety as possible.

Value statement 2

Nurses respect the rights of persons to make informed choices in relation to their care.

Explanatory statements

1. Individuals are entitled to make decisions related to their own welfare, based on accurate information given by health care providers. If persons are not present or able to speak for themselves, nurses have a role in ensuring that someone is present to accurately represent the person's perspective.

2. Nurses have a responsibility to inform people about the nursing care that is available to them, and people have free choice to accept or reject such care. Nurses respect the decisions made by each person.

3. Illness and/or other factors may compromise a person's capacity for self-determination. Where able, nurses need to provide such persons with the opportunities for choice to enable them to maintain some degree of self-direction and self-determination.

Value statement 3

Nurses promote and uphold provision of quality nursing care for all people.

Explanatory statements

1. Quality nursing care includes competent care provided by appropriately qualified individuals.

2. Promotion of quality nursing care includes valuing continuing education as a means of maintaining and increasing knowledge and skills. Continuing education refers to all formal and informal opportunities for education.

3. Standards of care are one measure of quality. Nurses implement procedures to evaluate nursing practice in order to raise standards of care, and to ensure that such standards are ethically defensible.

4. Research is necessary to the development of the profession of nursing. Research should be conducted in a manner that is ethically defensible.

Value statement 4

Nurses hold in confidence any information obtained in a professional capacity, and use professional judgement in sharing such information.

Explanatory statements

1. The nurse respects persons' rights to determine who will be provided with their personal information and in what detail. Exceptions may be necessary in circumstances where the life of the person or of other persons may be placed in danger if information is not disclosed.

2. When personal information is required for teaching, research or quality assurance procedures, care must be taken to protect the person's anonymity and privacy. Consent must always be obtained.

3. Nurses protect persons in their care against inadvertent breaches of privacy by confining their verbal communications to appropriate personnel and settings, and to professional purposes.

4. Nurses have a moral obligation to adhere to practices which limit access to personal records (whether written or computerised) to appropriate personnel.

Value statement 5
Nurses respect the accountability and responsibility inherent in their roles.

Explanatory statements
1. As morally independent agents, nurses have moral obligations in the provision of nursing care.

2. Nurses participate with other health care providers in the provision of comprehensive health care, recognising the perspective and expertise of each team member.

3. Nurses may have personal values which may cause them to experience moral distress in relation to participating in certain procedures. Nurses have a moral right to refuse to participate in procedures which would violate their reasoned moral conscience (that is, they are entitled to conscientious objection).

Value statement 6
Nurses value the promotion of an ecological, social and economic environment which supports and sustains health and well being.

Explanatory statements
1. Nursing includes involvement in the detection of ill effects of the environment on the health of persons, the ill effects of human activities on the natural environment, and assisting communities in their actions on environmental health problems aimed at minimising these effects.

2. Nurses value participation in the development, implementation and monitoring of policies and procedures which promote safe and efficient use of resources.

3. Nurses acknowledge that the social environment in which persons reside has an impact on their health, and in collaboration with other health professionals and consumers, initiate and support action to meet the health and social needs of the public.

Bibliography
American Nurses' Association. 1985. *Code for Nurses*. American Nurses' Association, Kansas City.
Australian Nursing Federation. 1992. *Draft policy on conscientious objection*. Australian Nursing Federation, Melbourne.

Bandman, E. & Bandman, B. 1985. *Nursing Ethics Through the Life Span.* Prentice Hall, New York.

Beauchamp, T. & Childress, J. (1989). *Principles of Biomedical Ethics.* Oxford University Press, New York.

Canadian Nurses Association. 1989. *Code of Ethics for Nursing.* Canadian Nurses Association, Ottawa.

Consumers' Health Forum of Australia. 1989. *Consumer Health Rights.* Consumers' Health Forum of Australia, Canberra.

Husted, G. & Husted, J. 1981. *Ethical Decision Making in Nursing.* Mosby, St. Louis.

International Council of Nurses. 1973. *Code for Nurses: Ethical Concepts Applied to Nursing.* ICN, Geneva.

Johnstone, M. J. 1989. *Bioethics: A Nursing Perspective.* W. B. Saunders, Sydney.

The New Zealand Nurses' Association. 1988. *Code of Ethics.* The New Zealand Nurses' Association, Wellington.

Woodruff, A. 1991. Discussion paper: Code of Ethics and Code of Conduct. ANRAC Competencies Steering Committee, Adelaide.

Feedback from the Code of Ethics Think Tank. 1992.

July 1993

APPENDIX IV

PATIENTS' BILL OF RIGHTS*

Australian Nursing Federation (Western Australian Branch) Position Paper

The ANF (WA Branch) believes that patients/clients, as the consumers of health care, are responsible for making decisions about their own health care.

This Patients' Bill of Rights is presented as a guide for nurses to enable them to assist patients/clients whether in the hospital or community setting, to be aware of their rights and responsibilities.

1. The legal rights of patients/clients in any health care setting are:

1.1 Right to a clear, understandable explanation in lay persons' terms of their condition, problems or disease.

1.2 Right to a clear, understandable explanation of all proposed procedures and possible alternatives. The explanation should include the nature of the condition; the proposed treatment; other alternative forms of treatment; the nature of the risks involved in the different types of treatment; and the chances of success or failure of the different types of treatment.

1.3 Right to seek 'alternative health care' and to receive such care from any person competent to provide it. 'Alternative health care' includes acupuncture, chiropractice, herbalism, homeopathy, hypnotherapy, naturopathy, osteopathy and the like.

1.4 Right to obtain a professional opinion of anyone of their choice at any stage of the health care programme. (Subject to the patients/clients or insurer paying for same.) Patients/clients also have the right to know the identity, professional status and qualifications of those providing health services.

1.5 Right to refuse any specific treatment, drug, examination or other health care procedure.

1.6 Right to change their mind and refuse treatment to which they have previously agreed.

1.7 Right to decline admission to hospital or any other health care facility.

* Reprinted by permission of the Australian Nursing Federation (WA), formerly the Royal Australian Nursing Federation (WA).

1.8   Right to leave the health care facility regardless of their physical con-
       dition or financial status (exceptions to the right to discharge may
       occur if an infectious disease has been diagnosed or if the patient
       has been certified as mentally ill).

1.9   Right to be informed of any research and/or experimental proce-
       dures which may involve them and be given the option to agree or
       refuse to participate.

1.10   Right to have their case history kept confidential, except when they
       consent to have such information divulged or where it is required by
       law to be divulged.

1.11   Right to seek compensation for injuries or illness resulting from
       health care.

1.12   Right to refuse examination, treatment or observation by, or in the
       presence of, students.

1.13   Right to specify in writing any treatments that they would not wish
       to have carried out should they lose consciousness or the ability to
       communicate.

1.14   Right to be consulted before decisions are made to transfer them to
       any other health facility.

The above rights are entitlements of all legally competent health care
consumers (that is, sane persons over the age of eighteen). In the case of
children or wards of the State, parents or guardians may exercise any of
the above rights on behalf of their children or wards, provided that in
exercising these rights the best interests of the patients are paramount.

**2.   The ANF (WA Branch) also believes that patients/clients should be
entitled to:**

2.1   A high standard of health care, regardless of social status, age, sex,
       race, religion, political beliefs or source of payments.

2.2   Prompt and appropriate treatment, according to health needs,
       provided in a humane manner with considerate and respectful care.

2.3   Receive information on the contents of their health record. (Legally
       patients/clients can appoint an agent, such as a solicitor, to obtain
       this information should such an action be required.)

2.4   Right of access to people outside the health care facility (parents
       should be able to stay with their children and nominated support
       persons should be able to stay with terminally ill patients twenty-four
       hours a day. In the case of midwifery patients, they should be able to
       have their partner or nominated support person with them through-
       out labour, delivery and the immediate post-partum period).

2.5   Be informed, by means of an information booklet or other method, of
       the layout of the facilities available in the health care agency.

2.6   The services of a qualified interpreter should they be required.

2.7   Nominate an advocate or representative to join the patient/client and
       their health therapist in making decisions.

2.8 Expect adequate instruction in self-care and for an appropriate lifestyle before being discharged from hospital; and that relatives or friends who will be caring for them receive such instruction and that arrangements be made for necessary support services.

3. The ANF (WA Branch) also believes that patients/clients have certain responsibilities. If a person is in need of health care they should, in their own interests:

3.1 Seek information as to their rights and see that their rights are satisfactorily applied.

3.2 Ensure that they have understood the purpose of all tests, treatments or other procedures, the reason for them and possible alternatives before agreeing to them.

3.3 Take responsibility for postponing, terminating or continuing part or all of the proposed health care programme, including operations. They should insist upon explanations until they feel suitably informed and should consult with all relevant persons before reaching a decision.

3.4 Know their own and their family's health history.

3.5 Keep appointments or inform those concerned of their intention not to do so.

3.6 Comply with treatment or inform the therapist of their intention not to do so.

3.7 Accept the consequences of their own informed decision.

3.8 Inform their health practitioner if they are currently in consultation with or under treatment from another practitioner in connection with the same complaint.

Acknowledgments

Medical Consumer Association of NSW: *Patients' rights*
American Hospitals Association: *A Patient's Bill of Rights*
Health Care Consumers Association of the ACT: *Patients' Bill of Rights and Responsibilities*
Health Care Consumers Association of WA: *Patients' Rights and Responsibilities*
ANF (Vic. Branch): *Patients' Bill of Rights*

The ANF (WA Branch) advises that the legal rights as set out in Section 1 may vary according to the particular circumstances that the patient or health professional find themselves in.

February 1984

APPENDIX V

PATIENTS' BILL OF RIGHTS*

Australian Nursing Federation (Victorian Branch) Position Paper

Australian Nursing Federation (Victorian Branch) believes that nurses must have a clear understanding of the entitlement of all patients to certain 'rights' concerning the delivery of health care, both in the hospital setting and in the community. The following statement has been formulated as a guide to nurses.

Statement

Consumers of health care are becoming increasingly aware that they have a right and responsibility to take an active part in decision making regarding a healthy lifestyle, and when necessary to enlist the intervention of health professionals to make an informed choice regarding the nature of treatment and care.

Australian Nursing Federation (Victorian Branch) believes all nurses should respect the following 'rights' of patients no matter what the personal beliefs of the nurse may be.

1. The right to health care

- right to the highest standards of health care, regardless of social status, age, sex, race, religion or political belief; this care to be prompt and appropriate;
- right to nominate a medical practitioner of their own choice.

2. The right to be informed

- right to be informed about the health care system and facilities available for their specific requirements;
- right to know the identity and professional status and qualifications of those providing health services;
- right to be able to request that their medical practitioner obtain a report regarding their care in any health agency and to ensure that they have access to this information;
- right to obtain a second opinion from professional persons of their choice at any stage of the health care programme;

---

* Reprinted by permission of the Australian Nursing Federation (Vic.), formerly the Royal Australian Nursing Federation (Vic.).

- right to be acquainted, whether by means of an 'information booklet' or other method, with the layout of the facilities available in the hospital or health care agency for their personal assistance, safety and comfort;
- right to be informed that students are present in any group wishing to interview or examine the patient;
- right to ask for assistance from appropriate personnel if not satisfied with care and to make any suggestions which it is felt may improve this care;
- right to expect adequate instructions in self-care and for an appropriate lifestyle before being discharged from hospital; that relatives and friends who will be caring for them receive such instructions and that arrangements are made for necessary support services;
- right to receive itemised details of the total, final account for services rendered.

3. The right to consent to treatment

- right to participate in the decision regarding any treatment programme after:
  a. a clear, concise explanation in understandable terms, with the use of a qualified interpreter if necessary, of all proposed procedures, health problems, disease processes, diagnostic tests and prognosis;
  b. being informed of anything that is of an experimental nature, or for the purposes of research, in the proposed treatment;
  c. being informed of any known risks and of any possible alternative avenues of treatment;
  d. knowing who will be concerned in their treatment;
  e. being informed of any financial costs.

4. The right to refuse treatment

- right to refuse any specific treatment, drug, examination or health procedure;
- right to refuse to participate in any research and/or experimental procedures;
- right to refuse to be attended by a particular member of the health team;
- right to refuse to be interviewed or examined by medical or paramedical students;
- right to reverse permission previously given regarding any treatments, to be informed of the likely consequences of such a refusal and to accept the responsibility for this action;
- right to seek alternative health care, but to have the possible risks of such a decision clearly explained in a factual, non-judgmental manner;
- right to leave the health care facility regardless of their physical condition or financial status, accepting that they can be requested to

sign a release stating that they are leaving against the medical judgment of the doctor or hospital. Persons under compulsory treatment do not have the right to leave the health agency. This includes:

— serving prisoners of the state;
— the criminally insane;
— those in quarantine;
— those with certain specific infectious diseases.

5. The right to confidentiality

- right to have their medical history kept confidential, except where the individual consents to have any information divulged or where it is required to be divulged by law.

6. The right to access of persons of their own choice

- right to access of people outside the health care facility; to assistance in seeing a minister of religion, counsellor or solicitor; also to request that specified persons not be permitted to visit;

- right of patients, e.g., children, terminally ill, to have a relative or close friend to remain with them during hospitalization and take part in their care when appropriate;

- right of midwifery patients to have their partner or nominated support person with them throughout labour, delivery and the immediate post-partum period, subject to certain medical restrictions and dependent on facilities available and the rights of other patients;

- right to nominate a friend, advocate or representative to join with the patient and health professional in making decisions and to determine who should be informed of their condition.

7. The right to compensation

- right to compensation for injuries or illness incurred in hospital care facilities or aggravated by the health professional.

8. The right to maintenance of dignity

- right to be treated in a humane manner, with considerate and respectful care in an atmosphere of privacy;

- right not to be subjected to any procedure or treatment without an adequate explanation of what is involved;

- right to die with dignity.

The recognition of patients' rights implies the acceptance of responsibility on the part of the health care consumer for:

- following a life-style appropriate to the maintenance of health and carrying out self-help programmes which demonstrate assumption of their accountability for their own health status;

- seeking information about their rights;

- divulging any information known to them about their own or their family's medical history, which may have relevance to their own health care;

- keeping appointments and complying with treatment, or alternatively informing the health professional of their intention not to do so;

- accepting the consequences of their own informed decision;

- ensuring that they and their visitors at all times act in such a manner that others are not disturbed or inconvenienced;

- respecting the privacy of others and keeping in confidence any information they gain about them;

- notifying the appropriate authority of any complaints so that any necessary corrective action may be taken.

October 1984

APPENDIX VI

ASSURING QUALITY CARE FOR THOSE WHO ARE DYING*

Australian Nursing Federation

Preamble

Nurses place high value on the worth, dignity, and autonomy of human beings, and on the maintenance of integrity in caring for them throughout the life cycle. These values and responsibilities are reflected in the Code for Nurses issued by the International Council of Nurses of which ANF is a member, and in the ANF Standards for Nursing Practice adopted in April 1983. Nurses are accountable for exercise of judgement in accepting and delegating responsibility, and for demonstrating practice that conforms with these values and standards.

Clinical nursing practice, with its attendant responsibilities, has become increasingly complex as rapid advances have been made in technology and science, including pharmacology. Societal changes have resulted in citizens being more concerned with issues of freedom of choice. They are seeking greater involvement in decision making about their care, and voicing a strong belief that care should be guided by the wishes of the patient and significant others.

In the practice setting, nurses frequently encounter ethical dilemmas which arise from a conflict of values, standards, and expectations, and from inappropriate or unprofessional behaviour by health care providers. Limitations of material resources, and lack of time and appropriate education to care for those with health problems threaten the integrity of the nurse. Research shows that conflict engendered by failure to identify and openly discuss these ethical issues impacts negatively on patient care and contributes to stress, burnout, and drop-out among nurses.

Nursing, medical and hospital administrators have the responsibility for establishing an environment in which quality care can be provided in accordance with patient choices; in which interdisciplinary problems can be discussed and solutions posed and tested; and in which staff can develop professionally. It is imperative that ways be found for health care providers to deal professionally with the dilemmas which face them. A prime example of a situation fraught with dilemmas is care of the dying.

---

* Reprinted by permission of the Australian Nursing Federation (formerly the Royal Australian Nursing Federation). Acknowledgment is made of the contributions from State branches, and in particular of those from the Oncology Nurses Special Interest Group of the Victorian Branch.

The present health care system is oriented to curing disease. In this situation the dying person can become an enigma. Cure is no longer possible and treatment must be directed towards comfort, alleviation of symptoms, and psychological support. It is often difficult to disregard the modern tools of invasive procedures and sophisticated drugs in the interests of patient comfort.

The Australian Nursing Federation calls upon boards of management and health care administrators to acknowledge the complex issues of care of those who are dying, to generate policies and to develop guidelines that take account of the multicultural nature of Australian society and facilitate the professional process of care.

These policies and guidelines should minimise the conflicts generated by the dilemmas outlined above and make provision for:

- a range of services including home care;
- the establishment of multidisciplinary teams to provide comprehensive care;
- the patient, family or significant others to make informed decisions and choices regarding the care and its setting;
- mechanisms to achieve and maintain quality of care;
- sufficient staff with specialised knowledge and skills to permit a professional standard of care;
- work release for staff to attend specific development programs designed to equip them with the knowledge and skills to provide an effective service for the dying;
- forums to assist staff to resolve personal and professional dilemmas arising from care of the dying.

Dying is one of life's most difficult experiences. A person should have the right to die with dignity and at peace. Dying at home should be the right of all who request it. Multidisciplinary care of the dying person in our culturally and socially diverse community requires imagination, education, maturity, and emotional support.

In the multidisciplinary team, the nurse has a principal role acting as comforter and advocate, and carrying out independent, interdependent and dependent nursing functions. In fulfilling this role, the nurse can be put in a situation of conflict when treatment is not primarily geared to the patient's comfort or in accordance with the patient's wishes. In order to provide a desirable standard of care for a dying person in an appropriate environment, it is crucial that professional conflict is resolved and good communication fostered among all concerned.

Care of the dying can pose many dilemmas and threaten the integrity of the nurse, particularly when:

- the nurse is not privy to the information which has been given to the patient, his/her family or significant others, or where information is withheld from the patient and/or family;
- the wishes of the patient are disregarded;

- there is no clear direction regarding resuscitation measures for particular patients — for example, those with advanced carcinoma, severely malformed infants, irreversible illness and trauma such as head injury etc;

- the plan of care is not formulated by a multidisciplinary team in consultation with the patient, family and significant other, and when care is provided on a 'stop' 'go' basis;

- infrequent review of the patient's condition prevents realistic management;

- life is maintained in situations that provide no hope of recovery and the rationale for treatment is unclear;

- the wishes of the patient and/or the family or significant other are disregarded;

- the personal and professional values are in conflict.

APPENDIX VII

CODE OF ETHICS*

New Zealand Nurses' Association

Preamble

Nursing is defined as a specialised expression of caring concerned primarily with enhancing the abilities of individuals and groups to achieve their health potential within the realities of their situation.

Nursing is an integral part of the society out of which it has grown and with which it continues to evolve. It is a profession concerned with health; it exists in response to the health needs of society, the client is the central focus of nursing.

The contribution of nursing is one of professional caring for human beings in varying states of health. This caring enhances the capacity to cope with real or potential threats to well being.

(Social Policy NZNA 1985)

Introduction

By the act of becoming a nurse the individual is seen to embrace the expressed ethical beliefs of the professional body. While the nurse does make individual moral choices, the professional body of nursing represents to society a standard of ethical practice to which a nurse subscribes.

The professional ethic comprises the principles of conduct as accepted by a specific profession. This code of ethics sets out a system of principles of conduct as expressed in values and behaviours which express standards and limitations for nurses practising in New Zealand.

The code identifies the basic moral commitments of nursing and serves as a source for education and reflection. It also provides a basis for self evaluation and for peer review. For those outside nursing the code may serve to establish expectations regarding the ethical conduct of nurses.

This *Code of Ethics* is a modification of the International Council of Nurses' *Code of Ethics* (1973). The format of the Canadian Nurses' Association *Code of Ethics for Nursing* provides the basis for the Code.

---

* Reprinted by permission, from the New Zealand Nurses' Association, *Code of Ethics* (April 1988), prepared by the Professional Services Committee of the New Zealand Nurses' Association.

Definition of terms

Ethical problems fall into two distinct categories: ethical violations and ethical dilemmas. An ethical violation involves the neglect of a moral obligation, e.g. a nurse who neglects to provide competent care to a client because of the race of the client. This document provides illustrations with respect to the avoidance of ethical violations.

An ethical dilemma on the other hand arises when ethical reasons both for and against a course of action are present, i.e. when either action will result in equally undesirable consequences e.g. resuscitation of a young person who is chronically and seriously disabled. This code cannot serve to provide clear direction with respect to ethical dilemmas. There is room within the profession of nursing for conscientious disagreement among nurses. The resolution of a dilemma often depends upon the specific circumstances of the case in question. For each nurse, resolution depends upon the relative weight given to the opposing principles, a matter about which reasonable people may disagree. There is no particular resolution which defines good nursing practice.

The code constitutes an attempt to provide guidance for those nurses who face ethical dilemmas. For example, a client who refuses some form of appropriate health care may not be coerced into consent by the nurse. Neither may a nurse deceive the client about the nature of the care to be provided. [See value 2, p. 538.]

The following statements are designed to assist with the interpretation of this document.

— **Values** express broad ideals of nursing. They establish the correct directions for nursing. In the absence of a conflict of ethics, the fact that a particular action promotes a value of nursing may be decisive in some specific instances. Nursing behaviour can always be appraised in terms of values: how closely did it approach the value, how widely did it deviate from it? Because they are so broad, values may not give specific guidance in difficult instances.

— **Behaviours** consistent with the values are included as examples to aid interpretation.

— **Limitations** are provided to suggest exceptional circumstances in which a value cannot receive its usual expression. It is also important to emphasise that even when the expression of a value must be limited, it nonetheless carries moral weight. For example, a nurse who is compelled to testify in a court of law regarding confidential matters is still subject to the values and standards of confidentiality. [See value 5, limitation, p. 539.]

The satisfaction of some ethical responsibilities requires action to be taken by the nursing profession as a whole. The fourth section of the Code contains values and behaviours concerned with those collective responsibilities of nurses and are particularly addressed to professional associations. Ethical reflection must be an ongoing affair, and its facilitation is a continuing responsibility of the New Zealand Nurses' Association.

CODE OF ETHICS

The body of the Code is divided into sections that correspond to the sources of nursing obligations.

Values relating to:	Ethical values
I CLIENTS	1. Respect for clients' individual needs and values.
	2. Respect for clients' right of choice.
	3. Respect for the right of clients to control their own care.
	4. The advocacy of clients' interests.
	5. Respect for the confidentiality of client related information.
	6. Respect for the dignity of clients.
	7. Competency in the care of clients.
II HEALTH TEAM	8. Cooperation between health professionals.
III SOCIAL CONTEXT	9. Advocacy of the ethics of nursing.
	10. Public and consumer trust in nurses and nursing.
	11. Respect for the worth of nurses.
IV THE PROFESSIONAL ASSOCIATION	12. Collective responsibility for ethical nursing conduct.

SECTION I: CLIENTS

Value	Examples of behaviour
1. Respect for clients' individual needs and values.	1.1 The nurse's care of clients is not compromised by factors such as clients' age, race, ethnicity, sexual orientation, social and health status.
	1.2 The nurse acknowledges the expectations and normal life patterns of clients, and designs individualised programmes of nursing care to accommodate the needs of clients.
	1.3 The nurse assists clients to express their needs and values related to health care.

2. Respect for clients' right of choice	2.1 The consent of competent clients is an essential precondition to the provision of health care.
	2.2 The nurse obtains informed consent for nursing care and facilitates informed consent for other care.
	2.3 The nurse does not employ force, coercion or manipulative tactics in obtaining consent.
	2.4 When illness or other factors compromise clients' capacity for self direction, the nurse provides them or their agent with opportunities for choices within their capabilities.
	2.5 Any information given to clients is presented in a truthful, understanding and sensitive manner.
	2.6 The nurse responds freely to clients' requests for information and explanation when in possession of the knowledge required.
	2.7 When clients require information beyond the authority of the nurse to provide, the nurse takes steps to ensure that clients receive that information.
3. Respect for the right of clients to control their own care.	3.1 The nurse informs clients about the nursing care options available to them.
	3.2 The nurse assists clients to be active participants in their care to the maximum extent that circumstances permit.
	3.3 With clients' consent the nurse facilitates the participation of significant others in their care.
4. Advocacy of clients' interest.	4.1 The nurse ensures clients' perspectives are accurately represented.
	4.2 When speaking professionally to public issues or in court, the nurse provides factual and relevant information.

5. Respect for the confidentiality of client related information.

    5.1   Clients are informed when care requires that other members of the health team have access to relevant information.

    5.2   The nurse respects clients' rights to determine who, apart from the health care team, will be told of their condition and in what detail.

    5.3   When discussions of clients' care may be required for teaching, research or quality assurance the nurse takes special care to protect the clients' anonymity. Whenever possible clients should be informed of these requirements at the onset of care.

    5.4   The nurse institutes and maintains practices which protect clients' confidentiality, e.g. by limiting access to records.

LIMITATION

When compelled to testify in a court of law the nurse must reveal only that confidential information which is pertinent to the case in hand, and such information must be given only within the appropriate context.

6. Respect for the dignity of clients.

    6.1   Nursing care is carried out with consideration for the personal modesty of clients.

    6.2   When discussing clients' care in their presence the nurse actively involves the clients.

    6.3   In assisting clients who are dependent the nurse takes measures to provide as much comfort, dignity and freedom from anxiety and pain as possible.

7. Competency in the care of clients

    7.1   The nurse engages in continuing education and in the upgrading of skills relevant to the practice setting.

7.2 The nurse ensures that accurate performance appraisal is carried out regularly and feedback provided to employees and students.

7.3 In seeking or accepting employment the nurse accurately states areas of competence and limitations.

7.4 The nurse manager ensures that the competencies of personnel are used efficiently.

7.5 The nurse required in emergency situations to work outside areas of present competence provides the best care that circumstances, experience and education permit.

7.6 When competent care is threatened due to inadequate resources or for some other reason the nurse manager acts to minimise the present danger and to prevent future harm.

LIMITATION

A nurse is not ethically obliged to provide care when compliance would violate personal moral beliefs held. When the request falls within recognised forms of health care the client should be referred to a more appropriate health care practitioner. Nurses who have or are likely to encounter such situations are morally obliged to seek to arrange conditions of employment so that the care of the client is not jeopardized.

SECTION II: HEALTH TEAM

Value

8. Cooperation between health professionals

Examples of behaviour

8.1 The nurse recognises the strengths and the limitations of each team member.

8.2 The nurse participates with other health professionals in the assessment, planning, implementation and evaluation of comprehensive programmes of care for clients.

8.3 The nurse accepts a responsibility to work with others (through professional associations) to secure quality care for clients.

8.4 The nurse who suspects incompetence or unethical conduct takes appropriate measures to ensure the welfare of present and future clients.

i. The nurse ascertains the facts of the situation before deciding on the appropriate course of action.

ii. The nurse uses organisational mechanisms for reporting incidents or risks of incompetent or unethical care.

iii. The nurse will not participate in any effort to deceive or mislead the client.

LIMITATION

When a situation can be resolved (without prejudice to present or future clients) by direct discussion with the colleague who has acted incompetently or unethically, the nurse follows that course of action.

SECTION III: SOCIAL CONTEXT

Value	**Examples of behaviour**
9. Advocacy of the ethics of nursing.	9.1 The nurse serving on committees concerned with health care or research actively promotes nursing's professional ethic. 9.2 When involved in civic activities the nurse furthers the objectives of nursing as well as fulfilling the duties of a citizen.
10. Public and consumer trust in nurses and nursing.	10.1 The nurse does not knowingly accept employment in situations where the values of the Code cannot be upheld. 10.2 The nurse does not promote health products in a misleading way.

11. Respect for the worth of nurses.	11.1 The nurse is provided with adequate health and safety measures in any situation which could result in a health risk for the nurse.
	11.2 The nurse has conditions of service which reflect the worth of nurses.
	11.3 The nurse recognises the right of other nurses to express their commitment in different but equally appropriate ways.
	11.4 The professional association ensures policies and actions reflect the best interests of nurses.

LIMITATION

In situations of industrial unrest the nurse recognises professional responsibility toward present as well as future clients in determining the nature of industrial action.

The nurse maintains emergency services during any industrial action.

SECTION IV: THE PROFESSIONAL ASSOCIATION

Value	**Examples of behaviour**
12. Promotion of ethical nursing conduct	12.1 Communication between all nursing representative bodies is maintained to ensure an overall code of ethical nursing practice.
	12.2 The association represents nursing interests and perspectives before non nursing bodies, including legislative bodies, employers, the professional organisations of other health disciplines and the public media.
	12.3 The association encourages its members to consider the ethics of nursing on a regular and continuing basis and provides assistance to those concerned with its implementation.

12.4 The association promotes education of the ethical aspects of nursing and actively supports or develops structures designed toward this end.

12.5 The association actively supports the nurse who, in fulfilling ethical oblications, is placed in conflict with the employer.

References

Code of Ethics for Nursing. Canadian Nurses' Association February 1985.
Code of Ethics. Internatonal Council of Nurses 1973.
Nursing — A Social Policy Statement. New Zealand Nurses' Association 1985.

APPENDIX VIII

CODE OF PROFESSIONAL CONDUCT

United Kingdom Central Council for Nursing, Midwifery and Health Visiting* (June 1992)

Each registered nurse, midwife and health visitor shall act, at all times, in such a manner as to:

- safeguard and promote the interests of individual patients and clients;
- serve the interests of society;
- justify public trust and confidence and
- uphold and enhance the good standing and reputation of the professions.

As a registered nurse, midwife or health visitor, you are personally accountable for your practice and, in the exercise of your professional accountability, must:

1. act always in such a manner as to promote and safeguard the interests and well-being of patients and clients;
2. ensure that no action or omission on your part, or within your sphere of responsibility, is detrimental to the interests, condition or safety of patients and clients;
3. maintain and improve your professional knowledge and competence;
4. acknowledge any limitations in your knowledge and competence and decline any duties or responsibilities unless able to perform them in a safe and skilled manner;
5. work in an open and co-operative manner with patients, clients and their families, foster their independence and recognise and respect their involvement in the planning and delivery of care;
6. work in a collaborative and co-operative manner with health care professionals and others involved in providing care, and recognise and respect their particular contributions within the care team;
7. recognise and respect the uniqueness and dignity of each patient and client, and respond to their need for care, irrespective of their ethnic

---

* Reproduced with permission of the United Kingdom Central Council for Nursing, Midwifery and Health Visiting.

origin, religious beliefs, personal attributes, the nature of their health problems or any other factor;

8. report to an appropriate person or authority, at the earliest possible time, any conscientious objection which may be relevant to your professional practice;

9. avoid any abuse of your privileged relationship with patients and clients and of the privileged access allowed to their person, property, residence or workplace;

10. protect all confidential information concerning patients and clients obtained in the course of professional practice and make disclosures only with consent, where required by the order of a court or where you can justify disclosure in the wider public interest;

11. report to an appropriate person or authority, having regard to the physical, psychological and social effects on patients and clients, any circumstances in the environment of care which could jeopardise standards of practice;

12. report to an appropriate person or authority any circumstances in which safe and appropriate care for patients and clients cannot be provided;

13. report to an appropriate person or authority where it appears that the health or safety of colleagues is at risk, as such circumstances may compromise standards of practice and care;

14. assist professional colleagues, in the context of your own knowledge, experience and sphere of responsibility, to develop their professional competence, and assist others in the care team, including informal carers, to contribute safely and to a degree appropriate to their roles;

15. refuse any gift, favour or hospitality from patients or clients currently in your care which might be interpreted as seeking to exert influence to obtain preferential consideration and

16. ensure that your registration status is not used in the promotion of commercial products or services, declare any financial or other interests in relevant organisations providing such goods or services and ensure that your professional judgement is not influenced by any commercial considerations.

Notice to all Registered Nurses, Midwives and Health Visitors

This code of Professional Conduct for the Nurse, Midwife and Health Visitor is issued to all registered nurses, midwives and health visitors by the United Kingdom Central Council for Nursing, Midwifery and Health Visiting. The Council is the regulatory body responsible for the standards of these professions and it requires members of the professions to practice and conduct themselves within the standards and framework provided by the Code.

The Council's Code is kept under review and any recommendations for change and improvement would be welcomed and should be addressed to the:

Registrar and Chief Executive
United Kingdom Central Council for Nursing, Midwifery and Health Visiting
23 Portland Place
London
W1N 3AF

APPENDIX IX

AMERICAN NURSES' ASSOCIATION CODE FOR NURSES*

Preamble

A code of ethics makes explicit the primary goals and values of the profession. When individuals become nurses, they make a moral commitment to uphold the values and special moral obligations expressed in their code. The Code for Nurses is based on a belief about the nature of individuals, nursing, health, and society. Nursing encompasses the protection, promotion, and restoration of health; the prevention of illness; and the alleviation of suffering in the care of clients; including individuals, families, groups and communities. In the context of these functions, nursing is defined as the diagnosis and treatment of human responses to actual or potential health problems.

Since clients themselves are the primary decision makers in matters concerning their own health, treatment, and well-being, the goal of nursing actions is to support and enhance the client's responsibility and self-determination to the greatest extent possible. In this context, health is not necessarily an end in itself, but rather a means to a life that is meaningful from the client's perspective.

When making clinical judgments, nurses base their decisions on consideration of consequences and of universal moral principles, both of which prescribe and justify nursing actions. The most fundamental of these principles is respect for persons. Other principles stemming from this basic principle are autonomy (self-determination), beneficence (doing good), nonmaleficence (avoiding harm), veracity (truth-telling), confidentiality (respecting privileged information), fidelity (keeping promises), and justice (treating people fairly).

In brief, then, the statements of the code and their interpretation provide guidance for conduct and relationships in carrying out nursing responsibilities consistent with the ethical obligations of the profession and with high quality in nursing care.

Introduction

A code of ethics indicates a profession's acceptance of the responsibility and trust with which it has been invested by society. Under the terms of the implicit contract between society and the nursing profession, society grants the profession considerable autonomy and authority to function in the conduct of its affairs. The development of a code of ethics is an essential activity of a profession and provides one means for the exercise of professional self-regulation.

---

* Reproduced with the permission of the American Nurses' Association, © 1976, 1985. *The Code for Nurses with Interpretive Statements* is published by the American Nurses' Association.

Upon entering the profession, each nurse inherits a measure of both the responsibility and the trust that have accrued to nursing over the years, as well as the corresponding obligation to adhere to the profession's code of conduct and relationships for ethical practice. The *Code for Nurses with Interpretive Statements* is thus more a collective expression of nursing conscience and philosophy than a set of external rules imposed upon an individual practitioner of nursing. Personal and professional integrity can be assured only if an individual is committed to the profession's code of conduct.

A code of ethical conduct offers general principles to guide and evaluate nursing actions. It does not assure the virtues required for professional practice within the character of each nurse. In particular situations, the justification of behavior as ethical must satisfy not only the individual nurse acting as a moral agent but also the standards for professional peer review.

The Code for Nurses was adopted by the American Nurses' Association in 1950 and has been revised periodically. It serves to inform both the nurse and society of the profession's expectations and requirements in ethical matters. The code and the interpretive statements together provide a framework within which nurses can make ethical decisions and discharge their responsibilities to the public, to other members of the health team, and to the profession.

Although a particular situation by its nature may determine the use of specific moral principles, the basic philosophical values, directives, and suggestions provided here are widely applicable to situations encountered in clinical practice. The Code for Nurses is not open to negotiation in employment settings, nor is it permissible for individuals or groups of nurses to adapt or change the language of this code.

The requirements of the code may often exceed those of the law. Violations of the law may subject the nurse to civil or criminal liability. The state nurses' associations, in fulfilling the profession's duty to society, may discipline their members for violations of the code. Loss of the respect and confidence of society and of one's colleagues is a serious sanction resulting from violation of the code. In addition, every nurse has a personal obligation to uphold and adhere to the code and to ensure that nursing colleagues do likewise.

Guidance and assistance in applying the code to local situations may be obtained from the American Nurses' Association and the constituent state nurses' associations.

Code for nurses

1. The nurse provides services with respect for human dignity and the uniqueness of the client unrestricted by considerations of social or economic status, personal attributes, or the nature of health problems.

2. The nurse safeguards the client's right to privacy by judiciously protecting information of a confidential nature.

3. The nurse acts to safeguard the client and the public when health care and safety are affected by the incompetent, unethical, or illegal practice of any person.

4. The nurse assumes responsibility and accountability for individual nursing judgments and actions.

5. The nurse maintains competence in nursing.

6. The nurse exercises informed judgment and uses individual competence and qualifications as criteria in seeking consultation, accepting responsibilities, and delegating nursing activities to others.

7. The nurse participates in activities that contribute to the ongoing development of the profession's body of knowledge.

8. The nurse participates in the profession's efforts to implement and improve standards of nursing.

9. The nurse participates in the profession's efforts to establish and maintain conditions of employment conducive to high quality nursing care.

10. The nurse participates in the profession's effort to protect the public from misinformation and misrepresentation and to maintain the integrity of nursing

11. The nurse collaborates with members of the health professions and other citizens in promoting community and national efforts to meet the health needs of the public.

APPENDIX X

CODE OF ETHICS FOR NURSING*

Canadian Nurses Association

Preface

In 1955, the Canadian Nurses Association adopted its first Code of Ethics, based on a code developed by the International Council of Nurses (ICN). This code (with minor changes) continued to guide members in their ethical decision-making well into the 1970s.

Over the years, however, a growing need was expressed for an ethical code tailored to nursing in Canada. At the CNA's 1978 Annual Meeting, the development of a new national code was made a priority, and in 1979, Sister Simone Roach was appointed as project director. In February 1980, the Board approved *CNA Code of Ethics: an ethical basis for nursing in Canada.* But shortly afterwards, many members began to voice concern over certain aspects of the new Code — Section Three in particular — which appeared to violate the nurse's right to equitable working conditions. It was also felt that the code should be written in a form that could be used in everyday practice.

As a result, in February 1981, the Board decided that a completely new code would need to be written, using the 1980 document as background. Two months later, an ad hoc committee was established, consisting of nursing leaders, a consultant ethicist/writer, and a CNA staff resource person.

Throughout the drafting and revision process, the committee sought input from nurses all across Canada — to ensure the new Code would be truly national in scope. In February 1984, a draft Code was published in the CNA journals, and members were encouraged to provide feedback. Their comments, plus consultations with member associations, led to several changes that clarified and improved the Code. This process of 'sifting and sorting' through ideas — so crucial to the development of our profession — could have been extended even further. However, the Committee felt that this document represented the 'state of the art' for the profession, and that it was time to give the Code a chance to 'live'.

To avoid confusing this Code with others, it should be emphasised that ethical codes can be understood at three levels — provincial, national, and international — each expressing different values. In several provinces, the registering/licensing bodies have adopted codes of ethics or guidelines that set standards specifically for nurses working in those jurisdictions. The

---

* Adopted in 1985. Reprinted here with permission of the Canadian Nurses Association. This Code is currently under review.

national guidelines, on the other hand, express the values shared by nurses across Canada, while the ICN Code reflects those values shared by nurses all over the world.

The work of arriving at a national code, acceptable to the majority of the membership, has been a long and arduous task. On behalf of the Board of Directors, I would like to thank Stephany Grasset, Jocelyn Hezekiah, Judith Lougheed, Jeanette Pick, and Anne Thorne for their dedicated work on the Ad Hoc Committee. Dr. Benjamin Freedman also provided valuable consulting services, and Marianne Lamb acted as the CNA staff resource.

The Code is now a living document — and one that we can live with for some time to come. Provision has been made for the Code to be reviewed at least every five years to keep it responsive to changing needs and values, both within our profession and within society. Change is inevitable; however, certain truths will always remain for us to identify and respond to in our work with the human condition. This Code, it is hoped, will provide an ethical framework to guide us in this process.

Lorine Besel
President

Preamble

Nursing practice can be defined generally as a 'dynamic, caring, helping relationship in which the nurse assists the client to achieve and maintain optimal health'.[1] Nurse educators, administrators and researchers, although not necessarily assisting the client directly, have too as their ultimate goal, the maintenance and improvement of nursing practice. 'Nurses direct their energies toward the promotion, maintenance and restoration of health, the prevention of illness, the alleviation of suffering and the ensuring of a peaceful death when life can no longer be sustained'.[2]

The nurse, by entering and maintaining a commitment to the profession, is committed to its professional ethics. As persons and as citizens, nurses continue to be bound by the moral and legal norms shared by all other participants in society. In addition, nurses assume a professional commitment to the health and the well-being of clients. Nursing as such encompasses moral activities.

The adoption of this Code represents a conscious undertaking on the part of the Canadian Nurses Association and its members to be responsible for upholding the following statements (values, standards, and limitations). This Code expresses and seeks to clarify those ethical principles that are definitive of ethical nursing activity. For those entering the profession, this Code identifies the basic moral commitments of nursing and may serve as a source for education and reflection. For those within the profession, the Code also serves as a basis for self-evaluation and for peer review. For those outside the profession, this Code may serve to establish expectations regarding the ethical conduct of nurses.

Ethical Problems and Dilemmas

Ethical *problems* fall into two distinct categories:

(a) Ethical *violations* involve the neglect of moral obligation; for example, a nurse who neglects to provide competent care to a client because of personal inconvenience has ethically failed the client.

(b) Ethical *dilemmas*, however, arise when ethical reasons both for and against a particular course of action are present. For example, a nurse whose client is likely to refuse some appropriate form of health care presents the nurse with an ethical dilemma. In this case, substantial moral reasons may be offered on behalf of several opposed options.

This Code provides clear direction with respect to the avoidance of ethical violations. When a course of action is mandated by the Code, and there exists no opposing ethical principle, ethical conduct requires that course of action.

This Code cannot serve the same function for all ethical dilemmas. There is room within the profession of nursing for conscientious disagreement among nurses. The resolution of a dilemma often depends upon the special factual circumstances of the case in question. Resolution may also depend upon the relative weight of the opposing principles, a matter about which reasonable people may disagree.

For dilemmas, no particular resolution may be definitive of good nursing practice. However, the Code constitutes an attempt to provide *guidance* for those nurses who face ethical dilemmas. A proper consideration of the Code may rule out some suggested resolutions of the ethical dilemmas. For example, a nurse whose client is likely to refuse some form of appropriate health care, as was noted, presents the nurse with an ethical dilemma. Even so, it would be wrong for the nurse to engineer consent by deceiving the client about the nature of the care to be provided. (For example, see Value II, Standard 4).

Elements of the Code

This Code contains different elements designed to help the nurse in its interpretation. The values and standards are presented by topic and not in order of importance. There is variation in the normative (the nurse *should* or *ought* to or is *obliged* to) terminology used in the Code. These terms have been used interchangeably and no difference in moral force of the statements is intended. A number of distinctions between ethics and morals may be found in the literature. Since no distinction has been uniformly adopted by writers on ethics, these terms are used interchangeably in this Code as well.

- *Values* express broad ideals of nursing. They establish the correct directions for nursing. In the absence of a conflict of ethics, the fact that a particular action promotes a *value* of nursing may be decisive in some specific instances. Nursing behavior can always be appraised in terms of values: how closely did it approach the value, how widely did it deviate from it. Because they are so broad however, values may not give specific guidance in difficult instances.

- *Standards* are moral obligations that have their basis in nursing values. Standards provide more specific direction for conduct than do values, however; they spell out what a value requires under particular circumstances.

- *Limitations* describe exceptional circumstances in which a value or standard cannot receive its usual application. Limitations have been included separately to emphasize that, in the ordinary run of events, the values and standards will be decisive.

It is also important to emphasize that even when a value or standard must be limited, it nonetheless carries moral weight. For example, a nurse who is compelled to testify in a court of law regarding confidential matters is still subject to the values and standards of confidentiality. While the requirement to testify is a justified limitation upon confidentiality, in other respects confidentiality must be observed. The nurse must only reveal that confidential information which is pertinent to the case at hand and such revelation must take place within the appropriate context. The general obligation to preserve the client's confidences remains despite particular limiting circumstances.

Rights and Obligations

Clients possess *rights*, both legal and moral. In general, the statements in this Code are cast in the form of the moral obligations of nurses rather than in terms of the rights of clients. Those legal and moral rights exist with or without professional acceptance. The obligations of nurses *exceed* that which would be required by the legal rights of clients and this Code tries to reflect that fact. (For example, see Value II, Standard 3.) In many instances, it is beyond the power of nurses to *secure* the right of a client. A client's right to be treated in a dignified fashion must be reflected in the nurse's own behavior towards the client and in attempts to influence the actions of other members of the health care team. The task of this Code is to state clearly the moral obligations that are incumbent upon nurses.

Nurses too possess legal and moral rights, as persons and as nurses. It is beyond the scope of this Code to address the personal rights of nurses. To the extent that conditions of employment are essential to the establishment of ethical nursing, however, this Code must deal with that issue.

The satisfaction of some ethical responsibilities requires action taken by the nursing profession as a whole. The fourth section of the Code contains values and standards concerned with those collective responsibilities of nursing and are particularly addressed to professional associations. Ethical reflection must be an ongoing affair, and its facilitation is a continuing responsibility of the Canadian Nurses Association.

The body of the Code is divided into sections that correspond to the sources of nursing obligations:

- *Clients*
- *Health Team*
- *The Social Context of Nursing*
- *Responsibilities of the Profession*

Clients

I.   A nurse is obliged to treat clients with respect for their individual needs and values.

Standards

1.   Factors such as the client's race, religion, ethnic origin, social status, sex, age or health status may not be permitted to compromise the nurse's commitment to that client's care.

2. The expectations and normal life patterns of clients are acknowledged. Individualized programs of nursing care are designed to accommodate the psychological, social, cultural and spiritual needs of clients, as well as their biological needs.

3. The nurse does more than respond to the requests of clients, by accepting an affirmative obligation to aid clients in their expression of needs and values within the context of health care.

4. Recognizing the client's membership in a family and a community, the nurse, with the client's consent, attempts to facilitate the participation of significant others in the care of the client.

II. Based upon respect for clients and regard for their right to control their own care, nursing care should reflect respect for the right of choice held by clients.

Standards

1. The competent client's consent is an essential precondition to the provision of health care. Nurses bear the primary responsibility to inform clients about the nursing care that is available to them.

2. Consent may be signified in many different ways. Verbal permission or knowledgeable cooperation are the usual forms in which clients consent to nursing care. In each case, however, a valid consent represents the free choice of the competent client to undergo that care which is to be provided.

3. Consent properly understood is the process by which a client becomes an active participant in care. All clients should be aided in becoming active participants in their care to the maximum extent that circumstances permit. Professional ethics may require of the nurse actions that exceed the legal requirements of consent. For example, although a child may be legally incompetent to consent, nurses should nevertheless attempt to inform and involve the child in treatment.

4. Force, coercion and manipulative tactics must not be employed in the obtaining of consent.

5. Illness or other factors may compromise the client's capacity for self-direction. Nurses have a continuing obligation to value autonomy in such clients, for example, by creatively providing them with opportunities for choices, within their capabilities, thereby aiding them to maintain or regain some degree of autonomy.

6. Whenever information is provided to a client, this must be done in a truthful, understandable and sensitive way. It must proceed with an awareness of the individual client's needs, interests and values.

7. Nurses should respond freely to their client's requests for information and explanation when in possession of the knowledge required to respond accurately. When the questions of the client require information beyond that of the nurse, the client should be informed of that fact and referred to a more appropriate health care practitioner for a response.

III. The nurse is obliged to hold confidential all information regarding a client learned in the health care setting.

Standards

1. The rights of persons to control the amount of personal information that will be revealed applies with special force in the health care setting. It is, broadly speaking, up to clients to determine who shall be told of their condition, and in what detail.

2. In describing professional confidentiality to a client, its boundaries should be revealed:

    (a) Competent care requires that other members of a team of health personnel have access to or be provided with the relevant details of a client's condition.

    (b) In addition, discussions of the client's care may be required for the purpose of teaching, research or quality assurance. In this case, special care must be taken to protect the client's anonymity.

    Whenever possible, the client should be informed of these necessities at the onset of care.

3. An affirmative duty exists to institute and maintain practices that protect client confidentiality, for example, by limiting access to records.

Limitations

The nurse is not morally obligated to maintain confidentiality when the failure to disclose information will place the client or third parties in danger. Generally, legal requirements to disclose are morally justified by these same criteria. In facing such a situation, the first concern of the nurse must be the safety of the client or third party.

Even when the nurse is confronted with the necessity to disclose, confidentiality should be preserved to the maximum possible extent. Both the amount of information disclosed and the number of people to whom disclosure is made should be restricted to the minimum necessary to prevent the feared harm.

IV. The nurse has an obligation to be guided by consideration for the dignity of clients.

Standards

1. Nursing care should be carried out with consideration for the personal modesty of clients.

2. A nurse's conduct at all times should acknowledge the client as a person. For example, discussion of care in the presence of the client should actively involve or include that client.

3. As ways of dealing with death and the dying process change, nursing is challenged to find new ways to preserve human values, autonomy and dignity. In assisting the dying client, measures must be taken to afford as much comfort, dignity and freedom from anxiety and pain as possible. Special consideration is given to the need of the client's family to cope with their loss.

V.   The nurse is obligated to provide competent care to clients

Standards

1. Nurses should engage in continuing education and in the upgrading of skills relevant to the practice setting.

2. In seeking or accepting employment, nurses should accurately state their areas of competence as well as limitations.

3. Nurses who are assigned to work outside of an area of present competence should seek to do that which, under the circumstances, is in the best interests of their clients. Supervisors or others should be informed of the situation at the earliest possible moment so that protective measures can be instituted. As a temporary measure, the safety and welfare of clients may be better served by the best efforts of the nurse under the circumstances than by no nursing care at all.

4. When called upon outside of an employment setting to provide emergency care, nurses fulfill their obligations by providing the best care that circumstances, experience and education permit.

Limitations

A nurse is not ethically obliged to provide requested care when compliance would involve a violation of her or his moral beliefs. When that request falls within recognized forms of health care, however, the client should be referred to a more appropriate health care practitioner. Nurses who have or are likely to encounter such situations are morally obligated to seek to arrange conditions of employment so that the care of clients is not jeopardized.

VI.   The nurse is obliged to represent the ethics of nursing before colleagues and others.

Standards

1. Nurses serving on committees concerned with health care or research should see their role as including the vigorous representation of nursing's professional ethics.

2. Many public issues include health as a major component. Involvement in civic activities may afford the nurse the opportunity to further the objectives of nursing as well as to fulfill the duties of a citizen.

VII.   The nurse is obligated to advocate the client's interest.

Standards

1. Advocating the interests of the client includes assistance in achieving access to quality health care. For example, by providing information to clients privately or publicly, the nurse enables them to satisfy their rights to health care.

2. When speaking to public issues or in court as a nurse, the public is owed the same duties of accurate and relevant information as are clients within the employment setting.

VIII. In all professional settings, including education, research and administration, the nurse retains a commitment to the welfare of clients. The nurse bears an obligation to act in such a fashion as will maintain trust in nurses and nursing.

Standards

1. Nurses accepting professional employment must ascertain that conditions will permit provision of care consistent with the values and standards of the Code. Prospective employers should be informed of the provisions of the Code so that realistic and ethical expectations may be established at the beginning of the nurse–employer relationship.

2. Accurate performance appraisal is required by a concern for present and future clients and is essential to the growth of nurses. Nurse administrators and educators are morally obligated to provide timely and accurate feedback to nurses, and their supervisors, student nurses and their teachers.

3. Administrators bear special ethical responsibilities that follow from a concern for present and future clients. The nurse administrator seeks to ensure that the competencies of personnel are used efficiently. Working within available resources, the administrator seeks to ensure the welfare of clients. When competent care is threatened due to inadequate resources or for some other reason, the administrator acts to minimize the present danger and to prevent future harm.

4. An essential element of nursing education is the student–client encounter. This encounter must be conducted in accordance with ethical nursing practices, with special attention to the dignity of the client. The nurse educator is obligated to ensure that nursing students are acquainted with and comply with the provisions of the Code.

5. Research is necessary to the development of the profession of nursing. Nurses should be acquainted with advances in research, so that established results may be incorporated into practice. The individual nurse's competencies and circumstances may also be used to engage in, or to assist and encourage research designed to enhance the health and welfare of clients.

The conduct of research must conform to ethical nursing practice. The self-direction of clients takes on added importance in this context. Further direction is provided in the Canadian Nurses Association publication entitled, *Ethical Guidelines for Nursing Research Involving Human Subjects.*

Health Team

IX. Client care should represent a cooperative effort, drawing upon the expertise of nursing and other health professions. Acknowledging personal or professional limitations, the nurse recognizes the perspective and expertise of colleagues from other disciplines.

Standards

1. The nurse participates in the assessment, planning, implementation and evaluation of comprehensive programs of care for clients. The

scope of a nurse's responsibility should be based upon education and experience, as well as legal considerations of licensure or registration.

2. The nurse accepts a reponsibility to work with others through professional nurses' associations to secure quality care for clients.

X.   The nurse, as a member of the health care team, is obliged to take steps to ensure that the client receives competent and ethical care.

Standards

1. The first consideration of the nurse who suspects imcompetence or unethical conduct should be the welfare of present clients or potential harm to future clients. Subject to that principle, the following should be considered:

   a) The nurse is obliged to ascertain the facts of the situation in deciding upon the appropriate course of action.

   b) Institutional mechanisms for reporting incidents or risks of incompetent or unethical care should be followed.

   c) It is unethical for a nurse to participate in efforts to deceive or mislead clients regarding the cause of their injury.

   d) Relationships in the health care team should not be disrupted unnecessarily. If a situation can be resolved without peril to present or future clients by direct discussion with the colleague suspected of providing incompetent or unethical care, that should be done.

2. The nurse who attempts to protect clients threatened by incompetent or unethical conduct may be placed in a difficult position. Colleagues and professional associations are morally obliged to support nurses who fulfill their ethical obligations under the Code.

3. Guidance concerning those activities that may be delegated by nurses to assistants and other health care workers is found in legislation and policy statements. When functions are delegated, the nurse should be satisfied regarding the competence of those who will be fulfilling these functions. The nurse has a duty to provide continuing supervision in such a case.

The Social Context of Nursing

XI.   Conditions of employment should contribute to client care and to the professional satisfaction of nurses. Nurses are obliged to work towards securing and maintaining conditions of employment that satisfy these connected goals.

Standards

1. In the final analysis, the improvement of conditions of nursing employment is often to the advantage of clients. Over the short term however, there is a danger that action directed toward this goal will work to the detriment of clients. Nurses bear an ethical responsibility to present as well as future clients and so the following principles should be noted:

a) The safety of clients should be the first concern in planning and implementing any job action.

b) Individuals and groups of nurses participating in job actions share this ethical commitment to the safety of clients. However, their responsibilities may lead them to express this commitment in different, but equally appropriate ways.

c) Clients whose safety requires ongoing or emergency nursing care are entitled to have those needs satisfied throughout the duration of any job action. Members of the public are entitled to know of the steps that have been taken to ensure the safety of clients.

d) Individuals and groups of nurses participating in job actions have a duty of coordination and communication to take steps reasonably designed to ensure the safety of clients.

Responsibility of the Profession

XII. Professional nurses' organizations recognize a responsibility to clarify, secure and sustain ethical nursing conduct. The fulfillment of these tasks requires that professional organizations remain responsive to the rights, needs and legitimate interests of clients and nurses.

Standards

1. Sustained communication and cooperation between the Canadian Nurses Association, provincial associations and other organizations of nurses, is an essential step towards securing ethical nursing conduct.

2. Professional nurses' associations must at all times accept responsibility for assuring quality care for clients.

3. Professional nurses' associations have a role in representing nursing interests and perspectives before non-nursing bodies, including legislatures, employers, the professional organizations of other health disciplines and the public media of communication.

4. Professional nurses' associations should provide and encourage organizational structures that facilitate ethical nursing conduct.

   a) Changing circumstances may call for reconsideration and adaption of this Code. Supplementation of the code may be necessary in order to address special situations. Professional associations should consider the ethics of nursing on a regular and continuing basis and be prepared to provide assistance to those concerned with its implementation.

   b) Education in the ethical aspects of nursing should be available to nurses throughout their careers. Nurses' associations should actively support or develop structures designed towards this end.

Notes

1. Canadian Nurses Association, *A Definition of Nursing Practice, Standards for Nursing Practice*, Ottawa, Canadian Nurses Association, 1980, p. vi.

2. Ibid, p. v.

Index

This index was prepared by Glenda Browne, a registered member of the
Australian Society of Indexers.

A

Aboriginals, AIDS tests, 203
abortion, 290-320
  clinics vandalised, 313
  conscientious objection, 12, 291-
    93, 316
  fathers' legal action, 309-10
  fetuses as hospital property, 17,
    51-52
  late v. early, 292, 296, 301
  law, 291-92, 294
  moral disagreement, 174
  nurses, 81-82, 294-99, 315-16
  opinion polls, 53, 305
Abraham myth, 122
absolute rights defined, 79
access to health care, 215-20
accident victims, organ retrieval,
    424-25
accountability in hierarchies, 54-56
act-deontology, 82
act-utilitarianism, 89
active euthanasia, 324, 332-33
  law v. ethics, 41
  medical opinion, 53
  v. passive euthanasia, 174, 344-45
admission screening for AIDS, 463
adoption option, 303
adversary method of evaluation,
    118-19
advocacy, 270-87
Aesara of Lucania, 105
age, and NFR orders, 405-6
Age, The, 5-8
  abortion polls, 53, 305
AIDS
  false predictions, 464
  occupational infection, 461-62

  testing, 203, 463
AIDS patients
  confidentiality, 253, 256
  hospitals, 218-19, 458-67
  lay care, 218-19
alternative health care, 219-20
altruism, 128
  abortion, 309
  euthanasia, 335-36, 338-39
Alzheimer's disease, 321
AMA
  on AIDS, 203, 460
  on complaints, 261-63
  on euthanasia, 326, 340
  on informed consent, 223
  members as witnesses, 231
  on NFR orders, 165
  on nurses' strike, 471
American Nurses' Association (ANA)
    code, 11-12, 46
amoralism, 169-70
amputation, cultural differences,
    219-20
anaesthetics consent form, 228
anaesthetised patients experimented
    on, 15-17
analgesia, 351-52, see also narcotic
    analgesia
ancient Greece, 39, 362-64
ancient Rome, 362-64
anencephalic infants as organ
    donors, 438
animal rights activists, 428, 437
animals as organ donors, 427-28,
    436-37
anti-rejection drugs, 425, 427, 438
anxiety from abortion work, 295
appropriate health care, 219-22

Aquinas, St Thomas, 109, 301, 367–68
Arete of Cyrene, 105
Aristotle, 108–9
  on suicide, 363
Arthur, Dr Leonard, 350–52
artificial hearts, 376–77, 436–37
assisted suicide, 321, *see also* euthanasia
atheists
  moral development, 111
  in religious hospitals, 66
attempted suicide, 359, 370–72, 386–87
attitudes, 69–70, 172–73, 180, 503
  homosexuality and AIDS, 458–67
  towards nurses, 1–2, 230–31, 510–11
Auckland Medical Association, 474
Australia
  abortion, 305, 313–14
  ethics committees, 483–94
  organ transplantation, 422–23, 425–27
Australian Nurses Journal, 291
Australian Nursing Federation
  on care for the dying, 329
  on patients' rights, 210–11
  strike action, 470–74
  Victorian Human Tissue Bill, 437
authority and power
  ethics committees, 486–87
  health care institutions, 19
  rationality, 110–11
autocides, 359
autonomy, 91–92, 99, 147
  advocacy, 277–78, 280–81, 285
  confidentiality, 253–54
  conscientious objection, 452–55
  cultural differences, 146–51
  euthanasia, 334, 336–37
  informed consent, 224, 232
  justice theories, 98
  NFR orders, 171, 405
  overridden if incompetent, 243–44, 246–49
  suicide, 379–85
Aztec blood sacrifices, 427

B

babies *see* disabled newborns; newborns
baboon's heart transplants, 436–37
Baby Fae, 436
Bailey, Dr Harry (Chelmsford), 160–62
Bailey, Dr (heart transplant), 436
Barnard, Dr Christiaan, 427
barrier nursing, 462

'beating heart' organ donation, 428, 438
Belgian abortion law, 312
beneficence, 93–95, 98
  and euthanasia, 331
Bentham, Jeremy, 86–87
Bible, *see also* Christian beliefs
  on abortion, 300
  on suicide, 365–66
bioethics, 3–29, *see also* nursing bioethics
  conferences, 9–10
  defined, 37–39
blood transfusions for Jehovah's Witnesses, 67, 94–95, 231
Blum, Lawrence, 127
Bocchi, Dorotea, 106
bone marrow transplantation, 309
Bonham, Professor Dennis, 15, 19
Bonhoeffer, Dietrich, 82
Bormann defence, 55
Bosnia, rape victims' abortions, 303, 314–15
brain-death criteria, 429–31
  and human relationships, 438
  organ harvesting, 174–75, 426, 428
  problems of diagnosis, 433, 435
  v. death, 426
Brazil, organ trading, 423–24
breast cancer, 50, 216–17
Britain
  nurses on euthanasia, 324
  transplant program, 425–26
Brown Sisters (Nazi), 22, 195
burdensome illnesses, 335–36, 338–39
burial after suicide, 368–70

C

cadavers *see* corpses
Canadian abortion law, 291–92, 311
cancer
  breast, 50, 216–17
  information on diagnosis, 147–51, 177–79, 181, 183–91
  nursing care, 510–11
  patients' concerns, 393
  quality of life, 392
  second opinions, 50
  significant others, 182, 194, 196
cardiac emergency, 48–49, *see also* NFR orders
cardiopulmonary resuscitation *see* NFR orders
care, 132–33, *see also* nursing care
  and context, 122–24
  morality, 113–14, 123, 132, 195–96, 198
  right to quality, 220–22

support for, 218–19
v. rationality, 126
carer's pension, 218–19
categorical imperative, 26, 68
Catholicism
  abortion, 301, 314–15
  euthanasia, 341
  narcotic pain relief, 347
  principles of
    cooperation/complicity, 466
  suicide, 367, 369
Central America, organ trading,
  423–24
Centre for Human Bioethics
  conferences, 6, 9–10
Cervical Cancer Inquiry (NZ), 12–19,
  208, 273
Char, Walter, 294–99
Charaka's set of standards, 25
Chelmsford Private Hospital, 160–62,
  208
  confidentiality, 255
child health nurses, bioethical
  issues, 504
children
  Nazi research, 20–21
  sedatives, 351–52
  suicide, 360
choice see autonomy;
  decision–making
Christian beliefs, see also
  Catholicism; clergy
  abortion, 300–301
  conscientious objection, 458
  homosexuality, 465–67
  suicide, 362, 365–72, 379
Christian deaconesses and
  matrons, 26
Christian Science, 67
claims rights, 80
Clark, Barney, 376–77
clergy on ethics committees, 488–89
client, defined, 212, see also patient
clinical-moral Gestalt shift, 165–66
Clinton, Pres. Bill on abortion, 313
codes of conduct, 1, 84
  Encyclopedia of Bioethics, 28
  ICN, 25, 457
  legal status, 47
codes of ethics, 25–27
  ANA, 11–12, 46
  legal status, 46–47
  patient advocacy, 281
  v. ethics, 45–48, 281
collective action, 446, see also
  lobbying; strike action
Collison, Dr, 17–18
coma depasse, 429
common-sense ethics, 40

comparative justice, 98
competence see rational competence
complaints procedures, 208, 225,
  261–63
conferences on nursing bioethics,
  9–10
confidentiality, 251–57
  AIDS and syphilis, 115–16, 203
  interpreters, 240
  and patient care, 387
conflict of duty, 120–21, 177–79
conflict of interests, 179–80
conflict of rights, 80–81
conscience, 449–52, 454–56, 468
conscientious objection, 11–12,
  447–69
  abortion, 291–93, 316
  mandatory ethics committees, 492
  moderate position, 467–68
  moral disagreement, 451
  narcotic analgesia, 347, 349
  NFR orders, 399–400, 417, 420
  nursing position statements, 448
  organ transplantation, 437–38
  personal conflict, 457–59
  superiors' orders, 453–57
  theological ethics, 67
  unsafe work conditions, 467
consequences, 83–85
consequentialist ethics see
  teleological ethics
consumerist rights, 283, see also
  patients' rights
contagion risk, 459–67
context see decontextualisation
contractarianism, 74–76
Copeland, Dr Jack, 436–37
cornea transplantation, 428, 437
Corporal Works of Mercy, 26
corpses
  organ harvesting, 174–75, 434, 438
  suicide, 368–69, 371
cost-effectiveness of medical
  technology, 216–17
CPR see NFR orders
cross-infection risk, 461–63
cultural differences, see also
  transcultural ethics
  advocacy, 273, 279
  autonomy, 92
  care, 219
  informed consent, 235
Curtin, Leah, 275–77

D

Danville case, 352–53
death, see also corpses
  definitions, 429–31, 438
  from narcotic analgesia, 345–50

human relationships, 438–39
painless induction, 330–32
deception *see* lying
decision-making, 240–41, *see also*
    informed consent; rational
    competence
advocacy, 276, 281–82
ethics committees, 483–84, 490–91
model for, 183–91
patient representatives, 489–90
patients, 92, 229–30
potential conflict, 44–45
surrogate, 244–45, 249–50
Declaration on euthanasia, 341
decontextualisation, 121–22, 125,
    131, 147–51
deep sleep therapy, 160–62
definitions, 36–37
deontological theory, 64–83
    v. teleological, 90
Department of Public Prosecutions
    and euthanasia, 324
dependency, 37, 133, 338, 396
    on physicians, 1
depression
    abortion work, 295
    suicide, 381–82, 384, 387
developing countries, moral
    development, 111
diagnosis
    cost of machinery, 216–17
    errors, 339–40, 433, 435
    information given, 147–51, 177–79,
        181, 183–91
dignity *see* dying with dignity
disabled fetuses, 315, 438
disabled newborns, 347
    anencephalic organ donors, 438
    ethics committees, 486
    euthanasia, 8–9, 325, 344, 350–53,
        456
    key terms in article, 6
    Nazi killing and research, 20
discrimination, 340–341, *see also*
    employers
dismissal *see* employers
distributive justice, 97–98
    access to health care, 215
Do Not Resuscitate *see* NFR orders
doctor–nurse relationship, 110, 189
doctor–patient relationship and
    nurses, 167–68, 238
doctors, 18–19, 44–45, 293–94, *see*
    also medical treatment
    abortions, 292, 297
    ethics committees, 484, 487–90
    euthanasia, 321, 324–28, 342–43,
        349–50
    informed consent, 222–30

injury to patients, 206
NFR orders, 413–14
nursing bioethics, 3–5
patients' rights, 208–10, 263, 284
suicide, 371
doctrine of double effect, 347–48
strike action, 479
Dogma of the Immaculate
    Conception, 301
Down's syndrome patients
    hysterectomy, 49–50, 165–66
    infant euthanasia, 350–52
drug errors, moral response, 197–98
drug overdoses *see* narcotic
    analgesia
Dutch nurses and euthanasia,
    323–24
duty, 65, 68–69, 72, 80–82, 84–86
    conflict, 120–21, 177–79
    conscientious objection, 451–52
    euthanasia, 334, 336–37
    rights, 34–35, 80
    strike action, 475–78
duty to die, 335–36, 338–39
duty to warn, 252
dying with dignity, 257–61, 328–29,
    334–35, 337, 340, 401
Dying with dignity: interim guidelines,
    328–29

E

economics *see* resource allocation
editorial bias, 6, 23
education *see* moral education;
    nursing bioethics, education
Elizabeth of Bohemia, 106
embryo as a human being, 301
emergencies, consent waived, 239
emotion (philosophical concept), 113,
    116, 127–28, 194–95, 450
emotions
    abortion work, 296
    nurse–patient relationship, 194–95
    professional behaviour, 295
    suicide, 381–82, 384
emotivism, 69–71
    and conscience, 450
employers and conscientious
    objection, 11–12, 21, 292–93,
        399–400, 448, 453–57, 468
Encyclopedia of bioethics, 23–28
enforcement, non–moral, 189–90
Engelhardt, H. Tristram, 60
equality
    health care access, 215–19
    justice theories, 97–98, 215
    women, 106, 120
ethical egoism, 84, 86–87
ethical elitism, 84

ethical parochialism, 84
ethical universalism, 84
ethics, 34–60, 158, 506, *see also*
    bioethics; codes of ethics; feminist
    moral theory; moral philosophy;
    nursing bioethics; transcultural
    ethics
ethics committees, 480–94
ethics consultation services, 490
ethnocentrism *see* transcultural
    ethics
etiquette, 48–50
European Community and
    abortion, 312
European Court of Human
    Rights, 312
euthanasia, 37, 321–58, *see also* life-
    support removal; NFR orders
    biblical, 366
    brain-death criteria, 429
    defined, 330–32
    disabled newborns, 8–9, 325, 344,
        350–53, 456
    Go Slow codes, 409
    law, 8–9, 42–43, 321, 323–29, 334,
        352
    letting die v. killing, 174, 342–49
    Nazi Germany, 19
    'nursing care only', 349–53, 413–14
    rational competence, 203, 299,
        341–42
    surveys, 7–9, 324
    v. suicide, 321, 377–78
Evans, Marie–Louise, 480
existential advocacy, 277–80
experiential approach to moral
    problems, 191–96
experimental medicine
    artificial heart, 376–77
    ethics committees, 481
    organ transplantation, 436–37
    unethical, 12–19
expert medical witnesses, 229–31
expert nurse witnesses, 353
eyes for transplantation, 428, 437

F
families
    ethics committees, 485, 487
    euthanasia, 193, 325, 327, 353
    NFR orders, 401–2, 405–6, 408
    organ harvesting, 422–26, 432–36
    Pythagorean philosophy, 105
    role, 115, 119–21, 279, 286, 387
    transcultural ethics, 147–50,
        177–79
Family Cultural Advocacy
    Communication Model, 279
Family Planning Association, 314

fathers and abortion, 309–11
fear of AIDS contagion, 462–65
feelings *see* emotions
Feinberg, Joel, 77–78
feminist moral theory, 65, 103–34,
    180–82
fetuses
    blessing, 51–52, 295
    organ donors, 309, 438
    personhood and rights, 174, 301–2,
        304–9, 315
fluids *see* withholding of food and
    fluids
folk healers, 38–39
food *see* withholding of food and
    fluids
Free v. Holy Cross Hospital, 168
freedom, 120
Freemasons Hospital
    (Melbourne), 460
friends, 119–20, 127
    advocacy, 286
funding for lay carers, 218–19

G
Gadow, Sally, 277–80
gas chambers, nurses' role, 21
Gauthier, David, 59–60
gender differences, *see also* women
    books and meetings, 10, 23–24
    moral thinking, 108–14, 122,
        124–30
Germany
    abortion law, 312
    human organ trading, 424
Gestalt clinical-moral shift, 165–66
Gilligan, Carol, 111–14
'Go Slow' codes, 408–9, 411
God *see* religious beliefs
golden rule (Christian), 68
greatest happiness principle, 87–88
Greek patients, 147–50, 219–20, 231
    cleaners as interpreters, 240
    information about diagnosis,
        150–51, 177–79
    informed consent, 225–26
Green, Dr Herbert, 13–15, 19
gut response, 182
    and NFR orders, 405
    v. ethics, 56–57

H
Hare, Richard, 59
harm, 180–81
harmonia, 104–5, 133
Harvard criteria for brain death, 429
Hawaiian abortion laws, 294
health, 38

Health Call (Vic.), 225, 261, 263
health care, 213–22
  complaints, 208, 225, 261–63
  moral conscientiousness, 468–69
  providers, 38
  substandard, 476–78, 480
Health Care Complaints Bill
  (NSW), 262
Health Department, NSW, 293–94,
  328, 403
Health Department Victoria
  donor cards, 432–34
  NFR orders, 403
Health Issues Centre, 225, 261, 263
health professionals
  with AIDS, 461–63
  NFR orders, 404
  patient trust, 253
  scientific, 38–39
health services commissioner,
  261–62
*Health Services (Conciliation and
  Review) Act* 1987 (Vic.), 208,
  261–63
heart transplants, 427, 436–37
  artificial, 376–77, 436–37
hedonistic utilitarianism, 86–88
hepatitis patients
  conscientious objection, 460
  heart transplant, 437
Herbert, Clarence, 343–44
hierarchical authority, 54–56
High Court of Australia, 223
HIV infection *see* AIDS
Hobbes, Thomas, 57
holistic health care philosophy
  brain-death criteria, 439
  lay carers, 219
  resources and rights, 214
  scientific professionals, 220
Holland, euthanasia, 323–25
homicide v. euthanasia, 324,
  330–31, 350–53
homophobia, 459–67
homosexual patients, 458–67
homosexuals, carers' pensions, 218
Honduras, organ trading, 423
hopelessness and suicide, 381–82,
  384–87
hospital administrators on ethics
  committees, 487, 489
hospital ethics committees *see* ethics
  committees
hospitals
  AIDS patients, 218–19, 458–67
  efficiency and objectors, 456–57
  etiquette v. ethics, 48–50
  NFR orders, 402–3, 406
  patients' rights, 15–16, 209, 250

  wastage in, 216
human advocacy, 275–77
human beings defined, 174, 304–6,
  see also fetuses
human experiment *see* experimental
  medicine
human life *see* quality of life
human relationships, 123, 145
  and brain-death criteria, 430–31,
  438
  transcultural ethics, 144–45, 151
human rights, 77, 278, *see also*
  patients' rights
  and patients, 211–12, 276, 283
human sacrifices, 427
humane disposition, 58–59
Hume, David, 57, 70
hunger suppression and euthanasia,
  347, 350–52, 456
hurt (concept), 180–82
Hyde Amendment, 313
hysterectomy, Down's syndrome girl,
  49–50

I

iatrogenic illness, 217, 270
ICN *Code for Nurses,* 25, 457
  confidentiality, 251–52
  legal standing, 46–47
ICN Ethics of Nursing Committee, 25
ICN position statement on the rights
  and duties of nurses, 34–35
Illinois Department of Children and
  Family Services, 353
imperialist model of morality, 143–44
*In re alleged unfair dismissal of
  Ms K. Howden by the City of
  Whittlesea,* 47
inalienable rights, 79
independence *see* autonomy;
  dependency
India, early formal standards, 25
individualistic sense of justice, 105
individuals, *see also* self–interest
  action by, 446
  and groups, 134
  as moral agents, 115, 119
industrialised societies, morality,
  144–45
infants *see* disabled newborns;
  newborns
infectious diseases and care, 459–67
information, *see also* lying
  about nursing procedures, 250
  about risks, 223
  cancer diagnosis, 147–51, 177–79,
  181, 183–91
  culturally appropriate, 147–51
  informed consent, 232–41, 250–51

overseas abortions, 312
patient advocacy, 280, 282
patient autonomy, 92
reasonable doctor standard, 229
informed consent, 222–51, see also
   decision-making; rational
   competence
abuses, 12–19, 160–62, 203, 208,
   224–27, 273
dying with dignity, 260
forms, 160, 206–7, 228
life-support removal, 349
NFR orders, 401, 411
organ harvesting, 424–26, 428,
   431–36
spine operation, 226–27
v. advocacy, 283
Inquiry into options for dying with
   dignity, 401–3
institutional policies, 167–69, see
   also ethics committees
informed consent, 250
NFR orders, 406
suicide, 387–88
intensive care units, 216
NFR orders, 398–401, 407–8, 411
intentionality
   euthanasia, 342–43
   Go Slow codes, 409
   murder charge, 350
   narcotic analgesia risk, 345–49
   suicide, 374–76
interdependency see dependency
interests
   conflict of, 179–80
   and rights, 77–78, 80
   self-interest, 173, 478–79
internal moral disagreement, 172–74
International Code of Medical Ethics,
   251–52
International Council of Nurses see
   ICN
interpreters, 225–26, 239–40, see
   also non-English speaking
intuitionism, 71–74, 96
   and conscience, 450
'invisible nurse', 510–11
involuntary euthanasia, 332–33, 349
involuntary hospitalisation of suicide
   attempters, 372–73
Irish abortion law, 312
Italian patients, 150–51
IUD practice insertion, 15–16

J

Jehovah's Witnesses, blood
   transfusions, 67, 94–95, 231
Jewish beliefs
   accidental abortion, 301

suicide, 365, 379
Jocasta, suicide, 362
justice, 75–76, 95–99, 123
   confidentiality, 253–54
   euthanasia, 335, 338
   stage in moral development,
      111–14

K

Kant, Immanuel, 57–58, 125
   categorical imperative, 26, 68
   on dignity, 258–59
   rationalism, 68–69, 77
   women's morality, 110
Kenny, Elizabeth, 512
Kervorkian, Dr Jack, 321
kidney transplantation, 424, 427–28,
   432–33
King Baudouin on abortion, 312
King Solomon and the mother, 122
Kohlberg, Lawrence, 111–14
Kohlberg-Gilligan debate, 111–14
Kohnke, Mary, 280–83
Kolf, Willem, 376
Kyneton (Vic.) youth suicides, 359

L

language see moral language
Larundel Hospital patient
   suicides, 387
late abortions, 292, 296, 301
law, 2–3, 41–47, see also specific
   actions (e.g. abortion, law)
   confidentiality, 251, 256
   ethics committees, 491
   lobbying for reform, 510
   moral conflict, 46–47, 167–69,
      453–57
   patients, 209, 281
   v. position statements, 210
Law Reform Commissions on
   consent, 208
lawyers on ethics committees, 488
lay carers, 38–39
   of AIDS sufferers, 218–19
leukemia patient court case, 325–26
liberty, 120
life see quality of life; right to life
Life (organisation) and
   euthanasia, 350
life-support removal, 342–44, see
   also euthanasia
   and brain-death criteria, 429–31
   by nurses or doctors, 327
   ethics committees, 481, 483, 486
lifestyles and refusal to care, 458–60,
   465–67
liver transplant unit (Qld), 425

lobbying, 250, 508–9
  medical, 208, 263, 325, 371
  needed on patients' rights, 263–64
love ethic, Wittgenstein, 128
lying, *see also* truth telling sanctions
  confidentiality, 254
  pain avoidance, 173
  patients' autonomy, 92
  rules and principles, 99
  transcultural, 150–51

M

MacIntyre, Alasdair, 126–27
Mackie, John, 58–59
majority views *see* public opinion
male moral thinking
  new directions, 124–30
  v. female thinking, 108–14
maleficence *see* non–maleficence
mammography, 216–17
management, nurses excluded, 221
mandatory decisions by ethics
    committees, 486, 492
Mangay-Maglacas, Dr Amelia, 469
Maori tradition, premature fetus,
    51–52, 295
mastectomy, 50, 217
maternal and fetal rights, 305–11
maternal nurses, bioethical
    issues, 504
McDermott, John, 294–99
McEwan, John, 203–4, 222
media
  abortion, 290
  Cervical Cancer Inquiry, 13
  lobbying, 509
  nursing bioethics, 2, 5–9
  organ donation, 290, 421–22
  Victorian nurses' strike, 472–74
  voluntary euthanasia, 290
medical defence unions, 230–31
medical ethics, 38, 490
medical profession *see* doctors
medical research *see* experimental
    medicine
medical technology
  cost–effectiveness, 216–17
  dying with dignity, 334–35
  patients' interests, 270–72
  reproductive, 480
medical treatment, *see also* doctors
  v. health care, 213–14, 217
Medical Treatment Act 1988 (Vic.),
    207, 328, 411
medicalisation of suicide, 371–73
medicide, 321
medicine, 43, 131
mental illness, *see also* psychiatric
    treatment

  competency and choice, 243–48
  confidentiality breaches, 256
  suicide, 385
mercy killing *see* euthanasia
midwives
  abortions in UK, 292
  bioethical issues, 504
Mill, John Stuart, 87, 115
  on women, 106–7, 120
Monash University Centre for
    Human Bioethics, 6, 9–10
moral action, 189–91, 195–96, 446
moral blindness, 163–66
moral complacency, 170–71
moral decision-making model,
    183–91
moral dilemmas, 158, 176–82
moral disagreement, 172–76, 451
  ethics committees, 485
  moral pluralism, 152–53
moral education, 111, 189–90, 192,
    288, *see also* nursing bioethics,
    education
moral emotion *see* emotion
moral fanaticism, 171–72
moral indifference, 166–69
moral language, 35–57, 82, 133
  amoralists, 170
  transcultural discourse, 143, 154
moral law, 41
moral negotiation, 189–90
moral obligations, 85–87
moral philosophy, 39–40, 64–100,
    116, *see also* ethics
moral pluralism, 142, 152–54
moral principles, 59, 90–99, 133
moral problems, 157–200
  experiential approach, 191–96
  systematic approach, 182–91
moral thinking, 107–14, 124–30,
    133–34
moral unpreparedness, 159–63
moral-legal conflict, 167–69, 453–57
morality, 127, 144–45, *see also* duty;
    ethics; rules; virtues
  overriding, 68–69
  stages of development, 111–14
  v. ethics definition, 34, 37
morphine *see* narcotic analgesia
mothers' rights, 308–9
motor neurone disease patient, 481
multicultural ethics *see*
    transcultural ethics
murder v. euthanasia, 324, 330–31,
    350–53
Muslim beliefs, abortion, 300

N

narcotic analgesia, 169, 327, 345–52
  death from, 55, 345–50
  morphine, 55, 182, 345–46
  under-administered, 347
National Bioethics Consultative
    Committee, 480–81 487
National Health & Medical Research
    Council *see* NH&MRC
National Kidney Foundation
    (U.S.), 423
National Women's Consultative
    Council, 509
National Women's Hospital
    (Auckland), 12–18, 160, 208
Natural Death Act 1983 (S.A.), 328
natural rights theory, 76–77
Nazi Germany, 172
  Brown Sisters (nurses), 22, 195
  ethics, 19–23, 298, 452
  law v. ethics, 41–42
  obedience not an excuse, 55, 447
  school suicide, 365
needlestick injuries, 461
negligence
  euthanasia, 350–51
  NFR orders, 411–12
negotiated patient goals, 92
Netherlands, euthanasia, 323–25
neurological death *see* brain-death
    criteria
New South Wales Complaints Unit,
    262–63
New South Wales Health
    Department, 293–94, 328, 403
New Zealand Nurses' Association, 18
New Zealand Nurses Journal, 291
New Zealand nurses' strikes, 474
newborns, *see also* disabled
    newborns
  AIDS, 459
  heart transplant, 436
  vaginal swabs, 14–15
newspapers *see* media
NFR orders, 7, 10, 165, 397–421
  conscientious objection, 417, 420,
    456
  decision–making, 207–8, 404–7,
    416–17, 420
  documentation, 399, 407–8,
    410–14, 416
  informed consent, 240 401,
    418–19
  legal liability, 409, 411
  nurses, 327, 397–98, 417
  residential care homes, 170–71,
    417
NH&MRC, 481
  NFR guidelines, 403
  organ transplantation code, 434

Nightingale, Florence, 25–27
Nile, Rev Fred, 313–14
No Code see NFR orders
nocebo phenomenon, 148–50
non-comparative justice, 98–99
non-English speaking patients,
    consent, 207, 225–26, 235,
    239–40
non-maleficence, 92–93, 180–82
  confidentiality, 253–54
  moral dilemmas, 176–77
  transcultural questions, 152
non-voluntary euthanasia, 332–33,
    349
Not For Resuscitation *see* NFR
    orders
nourishment *see* withholding of food
    and fluids
NSW Health Department, 293–94,
    328, 403
nurse–patient relationship, 3–4, 168
  advocacy, 270–84, 286
  moral sensibilities, 194–95
nurses, 510–13, *see also*
    conscientious objection;
    obedience
  attitudes towards, 1–2, 230–31,
    510-11
  decisions, 44–45
  and doctors, 25, 110, 167–68,
    189, 238
  on ethics committees, 484, 488–89,
    492–94
  moral action, 98, 161–62, 446–95
  moral development assessed, 112
  patients' rights, 48–50, 210–11
  role, 19, 110, 221, 297, 351
  working conditions, 98, 467,
    469–74
Nurses Society of New Zealand, 16
nursing administrators, 504–5
nursing bioethics, 1–30, 130–32,
    145, 501–13, *see also* care
  defined, 38
  education, 24, 112, 196–98, 502–8
  research, 508
nursing care, 43, 132–33, *see also*
    care
  abortions, 290–92, 297–98, 315–16
  AIDS patients refused, 458–67
  cancer patients, 510–11
  culturally appropriate, 140, 154
  dying patients, 260–61, 328–29
  euthanasia, 299, 321–24, 327, 329,
    353–55
  informed consent, 237–38, 249–51
  narcotic administration, 348–49
  NFR orders, 397–98, 403, 407–8,
    414–15, 417

nursing strikes, 475, 477–78
organ transplantation, 437–39
standards, 351
'nursing care only' orders, 349–54,
410, 413–14
nursing codes *see* codes of conduct;
codes of ethics
nursing ethics committees, 493–94,
see also ethics committees
nursing homes *see* residential care
homes
nursing journals and ethical
issues, 291

O

Oakley, Ann, 238, 510–11
obedience to a superior, 110
conscientious objection, 453–57
duties v. obligations, 86
Florence Nightingale, 27
not an excuse, 55, 447
power conflicts, 503
v. ethics, 54–56
obligations (moral), 85–87
occupational AIDS infection, 461–62,
464–65
Office of the Health Services
Commissioner, 261–62
Ombudsman (Vic.), 210, 263
operating theatre *see* theatre nurses
operation consent form, 228
opinion polls *see* surveys
organ transplantation, 421–39, *see
also* brain-death criteria
animals, 427–28, 436–37
anti-rejection drugs, 425, 427, 438
families, 423, 432–36
fetal donors, 309, 438
informed consent, 423, 425–26,
428, 431–36
law, 428–31
moral issues, 36, 77, 115, 174–75,
437–38
nurses, 437–49
opting-out laws, 422, 428, 430
recipients, 425, 428, 434–35
stabilisation and removal, 432–33,
435–36
oxygen humidifiers, 216

P

pain, *see also* analgesia; suffering
quality of life, 394–96
suicide, 384
parents
abortion rights, 308–10
and euthanasia, 325, 353
partial codes, 409

passive euthanasia *see* euthanasia
paternal rights and abortion, 309–11
patient care *see* nursing care
patient care ethics committees, 481,
489–90
patients, 212, *see also* autonomy;
informed consent
advocacy, 270–84, 286
injury by doctors, 206
lifestyles and care, 458–60, 465–67
representatives, 208, 489
safety and staffing levels, 467
patients' rights, 15–16, 203–64, 278,
287–88
books on, 208–9
defined, 211–12
doctors, 208–10, 263, 284
ethics committees, 481, 483,
489–90
human rights, 276, 283
NFR orders, 403–8, 411–12,
414, 420
nurses, 48–50, 210–11
treatment refusal, 328
v. patient care, 387
perception examples, 163–64
Perictone I, 105
personal values conflict, 457–59
personhood, 36, 306–7, *see also*
fetuses
physicians *see* doctors
Plato
on euthanasia, 330
Republic on family, 120
on suicide, 363
task of morality, 57
police
euthanasia ignored, 324
intervention during strike, 472
policies, 52, 509–10
conscientious objection, 456–57
ethics committees, 485
polio treatment, 512
politics and abortion, 313–14
polls *see* surveys
Pope on abortion, 314–15, s*ee also*
Catholicism
Portia, suicide, 363
Portugal, organ retrieval, 424–25
power *see* authority and power
prejudice against homosexuals,
459–67
preference utilitarianism, 88
preferences *see* decision-making
pregnancy quality and abortion,
303–4, 308
prima facie duties, 85
prima facie judgments, 72
prima facie moral rules, 100

prima facie rights, 79
principles, moral, 59, 90–99, 133
privacy and confidentiality, 254
pro-life movement see right to life
procedural principle of justice, 75–76
professionalism, see also codes of
    conduct
  social contract view, 75
  strike action, 469
professionals see health
    professionals
promise keeping and
    confidentiality, 253
prostitutes compared to striking
    nurses, 474
psychiatric nurses, bioethical
    issues, 504
psychiatric treatment
  competence to choose, 243–48
  conscientious objection, 448
  suicide attempters, 371–72
psychiatrists
  duty to warn, 252–53
  nurses and abortion work, 294–99
public opinion, see also surveys
  euthanasia, 324
  Kenny polio clinics, 512
  v. ethics, 53–54
Pythagorean philosophers, 104–5,
    133
  justice and caring, 123
  on suicide, 363

Q
quadriplegia
  euthanasia, 203–4, 340
  risk and informed consent, 226–27,
    229–30, 238
quality of life, 37, 391–97
  abortion rights, 309
  NFR orders, 404, 406
  organ harvesting, 175
Queen Victoria Hospital, 325
Quinlan, Karen, 483

R
radical moral disagreement, 174–76
  conscientious objection, 457
rape, 303, 311–15
rational competence, 241–49
  euthanasia, 203, 299, 341–42
rationalism, 68–69
  and brain-death criteria, 430
rationality, 41, 117–19, 125–26, see
    also moral thinking
  conscience, 449–50
  and emotivism, 71
  and intuition, 73–74

medicine, 131
  moral maturity, 113
  rights, 77
  utilitarianism, 87
Rawls, John, 60
  justice theory, 96–97, 111–14
reason defined, 132, see also
    rationality
reasonable doctor standard model of
    consent, 222–23, 228–30
reasonable patient standard model of
    consent, 222, 228–31
relationships see human
    relationships
religious beliefs, see also Christian;
    Jehovah's Witnesses; Jewish;
    Muslim
  discrimination, 293, 457–58
  nursing practice, 67
  suicide, 362, 379
religious ethics, 66–67, 76–77
relinquishing mothers, 303
removal of life-support see life-
    support removal
reproductive technology policy, 480
research, see also experimental
    medicine
  moral development, 111–14
  Nazi, 20–21
  nursing bioethics, 508
residential care homes
  combination locks, 244
  conflict of interests example,
    179–80
  large narcotic doses, 346
  NFR orders, 402–3, 405–6,
    413, 417
resource allocation, 213–16, 218
  distributive justice, 98
  nurses' role, 221
respirators see life-support removal
resuscitation, see also NFR orders
  and suicide, 325–26, 382
Resuscitation by the nurse, 412
right to die, 323, 325, 334, see also
    euthanasia; NFR orders
right to health care, 213–22
right to life, 79
  fetal, 302, 305–11
  organisations, 313, 324, 340–41,
    350
  women's, 302, 308
right to privacy, 79
right to strike, 477, 480
right and wrong see conscience
rights, 76–82, see also patients'
    rights
  and duty, 34–35, 80
rights claims, 80–81

rights view of ethics, 86
Role of the nurse, 6, 10
Ross, Stephen, 59
Rousseau, Jean-Jacques, 109–10
Royal Australian Nursing Federation,
470–74, *see also* Australian
Nursing Federation
Royal College of Nursing (Aust.), 210
Royal Dutch Medical Association,
324–25
rule-deontology, 82–83
rule-utilitarianism, 89
rules, 59, 99–100

S

sacrifices, human, 427
sanctions, 43
sanctity of life
abortion, 301
analgesia risk, 346–47
euthanasia, 339
moral dilemmas, 176–77
NFR orders, 405
organ harvesting, 174–75
scientific health professionals, 38–39
screening for AIDS, 463
second medical opinions
etiquette, 48–50
moral v. legal law, 210
secrecy *see* confidentiality; lying
security officer removed grieving
friend, 182, 194, 196
sedatives, 327
children, 351–52
self-concept, 307, 392
self-defence and abortion, 302
self-determination *see* autonomy
self-interest, 86–88, 173
strike action, 478–79
SENs *see* state enrolled nurses
sense of right and wrong *see*
conscience
sentience and rights, 78, 302, 308
sentiments *see* emotions
sex-selected abortions, 315
sexuality workshops, 465
Siamese twins euthanasia case,
352–53
significant others *see* families;
friends
sin *see* religious beliefs
situation ethics, 82
situations *see* decontextualisation
skeleton staff and strike action, 477
social abortions, 292
social contract theory, 74–76
Social Development Committee,
401–3
Social Security Act, 218

social workers, 488–89
Socrates, suicide, 363
Socratic dialogue, 67, 118, 505
Somera, Lorenza, 56, 96
spina bifida infant, euthanasia, 325
spinal surgery consent, 226–27,
229–30, 238, 241
St Augustine, 367–68
St Thomas Aquinas, 109, 301,
367–68
St Vincent's Hospital, 326, 481
staffing levels, 467, 477
stages of moral development, 111–14
standards of conduct, 90–91
transcultural, 145–46
Starzl, Dr Thomas, 437
state enrolled nurses, 471–72
sterilisation
informed consent, 225
moral objection, 293
Nazi, 21
Stevenson, Charles, 70–71
stickers on NFR orders, 410, 412–14
Stoic philosophy on suicide, 363
strike action, 469–80
distributive justice, 98
New Zealand, 474
working conditions, 467
stroke patients, euthanasia, 162,
344, 346
student nurse supervision, 471
Subjection of women, 106–7
suffering, *see also* pain
euthanasia, 331, 333–35, 337–38
suicide, 383–84
unwanted NFR orders, 406
suicide, 359–88, *see also* euthanasia
autonomy, 379–85
competency, 243, 246
defined, 373–79
economic considerations, 363–64,
373
intervention, 325–26, 380–85
Kervorkian's machine, 321
law, 370–73
property rights, 364, 369, 371
socio-cultural attitudes, 361–73
statistics, 359–60, 367, 369–70,
374
taboos, 363–64, 372, 377
v. euthanasia, 322–23
Suicide Act 1961 (England), 371
supererogatory acts, 455
superior's orders *see* obedience to a
superior
Supreme Court on euthanasia,
325–26
supreme principle of morality,
57–58, *see also* categorical

imperative
surrogate decision making, 244–45,
  249–50
surrogate uterus, 308–9
surveys, *see also* public opinion
  abortion, 305
  AIDS nursing, 459
  euthanasia, 333
  NFR orders, 415
  organ transplantation, 423
  risks, 54
  Victorian nurses, 324
suttee, 363–64
swabs from newborns, 14–15
Swan, Dr Norman, 488
symptom distress, 392–93
systematic ethics, 40, 182–91

T

taboos, suicide, 363–64, 372, 377
*Tarasoff v. Regents of the University
  of California*, 252–53
Task force on patients' rights
  (SA), 208
Taylor, Harriet, 106
technology *see* medical technology
teleological ethics, 64, 83–90
  lying, 254
telephone complaints service, 225,
  261, 263
Telling the truth about Jerusalem,
  510–11
terminally ill patients, *see also*
  euthanasia: NFR orders
  euthanasia, 325–26, 328
  value of life, 338
Theano I, 104–5
theatre nurses
  and consent abuses, 16–17
  moral issues, 225, 504
theologians on ethics committees,
  488–89
theological ethics, 66–67, 76–77
third-world countries moral
  development, 111
tissue donation *see* organ
  transplantation
Tolstoyan ethic, 129
trade unions and nurses' strike, 472
transcultural ethics, 37, 55, 139–55,
  178–79, *see also* Greek patients;
  Italian patients; phrases
  beginning with cultural
transcultural nursing, 140, 154
'Trihard, Sally', 96
trust, 248, 253
truth-telling sanctions, 43, *see also*
  lying
Tuma v. Board of Nursing of the State

of Idaho, 167–68, 238
Turkey, organ trading, 424

U

Unborn Child Protection Bill, 313–14
understanding
  informed consent, 233, 235–36,
    238, 241
  nursing procedures, 250
  rational competency, 243
United Kingdom, abortion, 292–93,
  309–10
United Nations Declaration of
  Human Rights, 214
United Nations War Crimes
  Commission, 447
United States
  abortion, 292, 310, 313
  ethics committees, 483
universal moral principles, 40, 68,
  75, 87, 112
utilitarianism, 84, 86–89

V

vaginal examination without
  consent, 14–17
value–neutral reasoning, 117–19,
  121, *see also* decontextualisation
Vatican, *see also* Catholicism
  Declaration on euthanasia, 341
  on narcotics, 347
ventilators *see* life–support removal
victimisation and informed
  consent, 241
Victorian AIDS Council carers, 219
Victorian Central Health Interpreters
  Service, 239–40
Victorian government
  on AIDS discrimination, 460
  nurses' strike, 471–73
  ombudsman, 210, 263
  Social Development Committee,
    401–3
Victorian Human Tissue Bill, 437
Victorian nurses
  euthanasia survey, 324
  strike, 470–74
Victorian Nursing Council, 412
virtues, 105, 127
voluntary euthanasia, 321, 332–33

W

wages and strike action, 471
Waikato Hospital (NZ), 55
Walker, Fred, 404–6
war atrocities, 59
*Warthen v. Toms River Community
  Memorial Hospital*, 11–12, 46, 168

wastage in hospitals, 216
Webster, Alasdair, 314
Western moral philosophy, 64–100
Westmead Hospital mammography
    study, 216–17
whistleblowers, 491
widows, suicide, 363–64
will to live, 148–50
Williams, Bernard, 125–26
withholding of treatment *see* life-
    support removal; NFR orders;
    'nursing care only' orders
withholding of food and fluids, 327,
    331, 343–45, 353
  disabled newborns, 350–53, 456
Wittgenstein, Ludwig, 117, 128–30
Wollstonecraft, Mary, 106

women
  excluded from medicine, 131
  feminist moral theory, 65, 103–34,
      180–82
  philosophers on, 106–7, 120
  thinking style, 108–14
Women into Action, 509
working conditions, 98, 467, 469–74
World Health Organization, 469

Y

youth suicide, 359–60

Z

Zeno, suicide, 363

TO THE OWNER OF THIS BOOK

We are interested in your reaction to *Bioethics: A nursing perspective*, 2nd Edition, by Megan-Jane Johnstone.

1. What was your reason for using this book?

_____ university course   _____ continuing education course
_____ college course   _____ personal interest
_____ TAFE course   _____ other (specify)

2. In which school are you enrolled?_____

3. Approximately how much of the book did you use?

_____1/4 _____ 1/2 _____3/4 _____ all

4. What is the best aspect of the book?

5. Have you any suggestions for improvement?

6. Would more illustrations/diagrams help?

7. Is there any topic that should be added?

Fold here

- -

(Tape shut)

No postage stamp req
if posted in Aus

| |

REPLY PAID 5
Managing Editor, College Division
Harcourt Brace & Company, Australia
Locked Bag 16
MARRICKVILLE, NSW 2204